Library of Congress Cataloging-in-Publication Data

Heart disease and rehabilitation / Michael L. Pollock, Donald H.
    Schmidt, editors. -- 3rd ed.
            p.   cm.
        Includes bibliographical references and index.
        ISBN 0-87322-588-0
        1. Heart--Diseases.   2. Heart--Diseases--Patients--Rehabilitation.
    I. Pollock, Michael L.   II. Schmidt, Donald H.
        [DNLM: 1. Heart Diseases--rehabilitation.   WG 200 H4365 1995]
    RC681.H363   1995
    616.1'2--dc20
    DNLM/DLC
    for Library of Congress   94-12879
                                                                            CIP

ISBN: 0-87322-588-0

This book is a revised edition of *Heart Disease and Rehabilitation* (2nd Edition) published in 1986 by John Wiley & Sons, Inc.

Developmental Editor: Judy Patterson Wright, PhD
Assistant Editors: Jacqueline Blakley, Julie Lancaster, John Wentworth, and Hank Woolsey
Copyeditors: Jay Thomas and Dawn Barker
Proofreaders: Dawn Barker and Myla Smith
Indexer: Margie Towery
Typesetters: Sandra Meier, Julie Overholt, and Yvonne Winsor
Text Designer: Keith Blomberg
Layout Artists: Denise Lowry and Sandra Meier
Cover Designer: Jack Davis
Cover Photograph: Provided by Rami A. Gal, MD
Cover Description: A two-dimensional transthoracic exercise echocardiogram, four-chamber view
Mac Artists: Thomas E. Janowski and Kathy Fuoss
Printer: Braun-Brumfield

Printed in the United States of America

10   9   8   7   6   5   4   3   2   1

Human Kinetics
P.O. Box 5076, Champaign, IL 61825-5076
1-800-747-4457

Canada: Human Kinetics, Box 24040,
Windsor, ON N8Y 4Y9
1-800-465-7301 (in Canada only)

Europe: Human Kinetics, P.O. Box IW14, Leeds LS16 6TR, England
(44) 532 781708

Australia: Human Kinetics, Unit 5, 32 Raglan Avenue,
Edwardstown 5039, South Australia
(08) 371 3755

New Zealand: Human Kinetics, P.O. Box 105-231, Auckland 1
(09) 309 2259

This book is dedicated to Mr. and Mrs. Norman Soref, Mr. and Mrs. Bernard Soref, Mrs. Milton Soref, Mr. Robert Miller, and those who desired to remain anonymous for their creative generosity in both time and worldly goods to the Cardiovascular Disease Program and Cardiac Rehabilitation Program of Sinai Samaritan Medical Center, Milwaukee, Wisconsin. With great pleasure we acknowledge our indebtedness to them and to the American College of Sports Medicine, American Heart Association, and the American Association of Cardiovascular and Pulmonary Rehabilitation for their leadership and pioneering spirit in preventive and rehabilitative medicine. Special acknowledgments go to Herman K. Hellerstein, MD, professor emeritus, Case Western Reserve University School of Medicine, and to Thomas K. Cureton, Jr., PhD, professor emeritus, University of Illinois, for their dedication to and research in the fields of Adult Fitness and Cardiac Rehabilitation. Their pioneering spirit and inspiration will always be felt.

Contents

Preface

It has been interesting and exciting to have witnessed much of the development of the subspecialties of primary prevention and cardiac rehabilitative medicine over the past 35 years. It is always difficult to identify who was first or how a field of study or discipline was started. In the modern era the studies of Levine and Lown in 1951 concerning the importance of getting patients out of bed (arm chair exercise) and, in 1957, Hellerstein and Fords' article in the *Journal of the American Medical Association* on cardiac rehabilitation had major impacts on making physicians and allied health professionals aware of the importance of cardiac rehabilitation.

In 1972 the American Heart Associations' committee on Exercise (now called Exercise and Cardiac Rehabilitation) published its first guidelines on exercise testing and training of apparently healthy persons, and in 1975 for patients with heart disease and those at high risk. Their latest *Exercise Standards* were published in 1990 and updated in 1994. At its first Aspen conference in 1971, the American College of Sports Medicine began the development of its "Guidelines for Graded Exercise Testing and Exercise Prescription" (first edition, 1975) and certification conference for program directors in cardiac rehabilitation (1975). The establishment of a formal curriculum for developing professionals in the field of cardiac rehabilitation began in the 1960s at the University of Wisconsin, Madison, under direction of Bruno Balke, MD, and at San Diego State University by Fred Kasch, PhD, and Jack Boyer, MD. Further developments in curriculum were made by Phillip Wilson, EdD (University of Wisconsin, La Crosse), and by Paul Ribisl, PhD, and Henry Miller, Jr., MD (Wake Forest University).

In 1972, the Airlie conference postgraduate course "Physiology and Psychology of Exercise Testing and Training of Coronary Disease Patients and Coronary-Prone Subjects: Principles, Techniques, Applications and Effects" set the stage for more organized and multidisciplinary rehabilitation programs. Proceedings from the conference were published by Naughton, Hellerstein, and Mohler in 1973, and they summarized much of the research data available on cardiac rehabilitation at that time. Five years later, in an attempt to further update the field of cardiac rehabilitation, Michael Pollock, PhD, then at Mount Sinai Medical Center (MSMC) in Milwaukee, and Donald Schmidt, MD, Chief of the Cardiovascular Disease section of MSMC, organized a conference called "Heart Disease and Rehabilitation: State of the Art." The proceedings of this conference were published in 1979 as the first edition of *Heart Disease and Rehabilitation*. From the roots of this meeting a plan was formed to produce a specialty journal in cardiac rehabilitation. In 1981, the *Journal of Cardiac Rehabilitation* was first published, with Michael Pollock, PhD, and Victor Froelicher, MD, as its co-editors (the journal has since changed its name to the *Journal of Cardiopulmonary Rehabilitation*). The *Journal* is in its 14th year of publication with Barry Franklin, PhD, the current editor.

The field of cardiac rehabilitation showed a major development when the Association of Cardiovascular and Pulmonary Rehabilitation was formed in 1986. The development of an association has been a catalyst for the formation of many state organizations and the forum for the presentation and sharing of ideas and knowledge of cardiac rehabilitation.

In 1979, when the first edition of *Heart Disease and Rehabilitation* was published, the field of cardiac rehabilitation was in its infancy. The first edition was written by experts who helped develop cardiac rehabilitation and formed the first programs to practice it. The second edition, published in 1986, included a major updating and revision of chapters of the first edition. It included the latest information on clinical assessment of CHD, assessment of risk factors associated with the development of CHD, and the effect of risk factor modification on both primary and secondary prevention. It also included the latest information on exercise testing and prescription and the management of patients through their stages of recovery.

This third edition includes work by 37 new authors, all contributing in their area of expertise. Information, topics, and areas have been condensed and reorganized; instead of 38 chapters, there are now 30, 28 of which have been completely rewritten. All of these efforts in this latest edition have been done with the aim of accomplishing one thing: to provide a compact and comprehensive state-of-the-art volume that is the quintessential text for all current and future practitioners in the field of cardiac rehabilitation.

The currency of this volume is reflected by both the agreement and disagreement among the contributing authors. Indeed, the reader will discover a number of controversies. The effect that exercise has on morbidity, mortality, and risk; the virtues of medical versus surgical management of the coronary patient; the manner in which exercise should be prescribed, monitored, and supervised; and the procedures by which graded exercise testing should be performed and evaluated are only a few of these controversial issues. Because of its extensiveness, this book may well raise more questions than it answers, thus whetting our appetite for future inquiry and research. To this point, suggestions as to how the field of cardiac rehabilitation will be practiced in the future "managed care" environment is discussed.

The future looks bright for the field of cardiac rehabilitation. Our thanks go to the professional organizations and many health-care professionals who have devoted their time and energies to treating patients and developing the field of cardiac rehabilitation. To this end, it is our hope that this volume truly represents the "state of the art."

Acknowledgments

The editors wish to acknowledge and thank Linda Martin and Robert Henderson for their secretarial and organizational support in the preparation of the manuscript materials for this third edition. A special appreciation goes to Lorna Grade for her editorial assistance. Further appreciation goes to Judy Patterson Wright, PhD, our developmental editor at Human Kinetics for her advice and technical assistance in the preparation of this text.

Michael L. Pollock, PhD
Donald H. Schmidt, MD

PART I

Epidemiology of Heart Disease

and reduced vital capacity in women are also important risk factors for coronary disease and cardiac failure. Elevated fibrinogen continues to contribute to coronary disease and stroke in persons of advanced age. ECG evidence of LVH and nonspecific repolarization abnormalities often indicate a compromised coronary circulation in elderly persons and are associated with an increased risk of coronary events, stroke, and cardiac failure.

There is also evidence that recurrent cardiovascular events are influenced by the same cardiovascular risk factors that predispose people to initial events (25). The risk of cardiovascular events following an MI is greater in persons of advanced age. Clinical trials suggest that risk is increased in relation to elevated cholesterol and is reduced by controlling lipid levels. Control of hypertension can reduce instances of stroke and cardiac failure following an MI. Quitting smoking can reduce fatal reinfarction and sudden death and can slow progression of peripheral arterial disease. Weight reduction can improve all risk factors and increase exercise tolerance. Exercise can improve lipid levels and work capacity and may possibly improve survival rates (see chapter 11).

Although proof of the efficacy of modifying risk factors in older persons is limited, available information, as well as recent general declines in coronary and stroke mortality in the United States, justifies optimism. Although more evidence of the efficacy of modifying risk factors in the elderly is sorely needed, it seems likely that the benefits of preventive measures in middle-aged persons can be extrapolated to the elderly.

Risk Factors in Myocardial Infarction Patients

Age-adjusted analysis of 459 MI survivors in the Framingham cohort showed the risk of reinfarction to be positively associated with BP and serum cholesterol (25). Coronary mortality was strongly associated with blood sugar, SBP, serum cholesterol, HR, and diabetes. In multivariate analysis, SBP, serum cholesterol, and diabetes remained independently predictive. Relative weight was inversely associated with reinfarction.

Following an MI, women usually appear to be at higher risk of reinfarction and death than men. However, when adjustment is made for the effects of the higher level of risk factors, women with MIs have only half the risk of death from CVD that men have. The higher baseline risk factors in women

sustaining MIs tends to obscure the survival advantage of women over men even following an MI.

Familial Predisposition

An innate susceptibility to CVD was noted in the Framingham cohort when there was a family history of premature CVD. Framingham Study subjects who had a brother afflicted with CVD had more than double the risk of developing CVD; this excess risk was not attributable to shared risk factors (26). CVD does cluster in families, but there has been uncertainty as to whether a positive family history is an independent risk factor. A family history of death due to CVD occurring in parents of the Framingham cohort was associated with an independent increased risk of CVD of 30%. The effect of a positive family history was stronger for someone who had a family member with an early CVD event than a later outcome (27). This effect of a parental history of CVD death on risk was not entirely mediated by shared risk factors. A history of early CVD occurring in either parent carried the same risk before the age of 60. For parental CVD occurring after age 60 years, maternal CVD death was a stronger predictor of CVD in offspring.

Multivariate Risk Profiles

CHD can now be predicted with reasonable accuracy from little more than ordinary office procedures and simple laboratory tests. Trials have been undertaken to examine the prospects for primary prevention by correcting such risk factors as BP and blood lipids in CHD candidates. Whereas cholesterol-lowering trials in subjects with elevated cholesterol have proved efficacious, antihypertension trials have been disappointing, probably because of failure to improve the multivariate risk profile, including blood lipids, BP, and LVH (18).

Categorical assessments of risk according to the number of risk factors arbitrarily defined can identify high-risk persons, but they tend to overlook other persons at high risk because of multiple marginal abnormalities. This is the segment of the population that experiences most of the coronary events, and it is important not to neglect them. To facilitate office and public-health cardiovascular risk assessments, multivariate risk factor formulations have been developed in the form of handbooks, personal-computer software, and small electronic calculators.

A Framingham Stroke Risk Profile has been produced from data on more than 500 strokes that occurred in persons who were followed for more than 34 years. The components of the profile include cardiac disease, atrial fibrillation, SBP, LVH, age, diabetic status, and cigarette smoking (Figure 1.9) (28). The risk formulation assigns a number to each component weighted by the strength of its contribution to stroke incidence. The sum score of these weighted risk factors yields an estimate of the conditional probability of a stroke. By demonstrating risks and possible benefits the multivariate profile should help physicians prevent strokes in their elderly hypertensive or cardiac patients and might motivate patients to comply with recommended preventive measures.

A similar multivariate profile is now available for coronary risk assessment as well (29). The score from this formulation enables physicians to assess the need for preventive management without overlooking high-risk persons with multiple marginal risk factor abnormalities (Figure 1.10).

Secular Trends

Declining cardiovascular mortality in the United States over the past three decades is well documented, but the reasons for the decline are speculative. The Framingham Study analyzed cohort data to examine changes in risk factors in relation to cardiovascular mortality over three decades (30). Ten-year incidence of CVD and death were examined in men aged 50-59 years at baseline in 1950, 1960, and 1970 to assess secular trends in the incidence of CVD relative to predisposing risk factors and to medical care.

The 10-year cumulative cardiovascular mortality rate in the 1970 cohort was found to be 43% lower than that in the 1950 cohort, and 37% less than that in the 1960 cohort. Among the men who were free from CVD at baseline, the 10-year cumulative incidence of CVD declined approximately 19%, whereas the 10-year cardiovascular death rate declined 60%.

Significant improvements in risk factors for CVD between 1950 and 1970 in men free from CVD were found: these factors included lower serum cholesterol and SBP and reduced cigarette smoking. Improvement in cardiovascular risk factors in the 1970 cohort over values seen in previous decades for this cohort appear to have made an important contribution to the 60% decline in mortality noted. However, a decline in the incidence of CVD and improved medical care may also have contributed significantly to the observed decline in mortality (30).

Preventive Implications

The epidemiologic data demonstrating the hazards of elevated BP and blood lipids prompted trials to examine the benefits of treating mild levels of hypertension and hypercholesterolemia. These trials and the availability of a variety of pharmaceuticals, which, by different modes of action, can effectively lower BP, raise HDL cholesterol, and reduce LDL cholesterol without inducing dangerous side effects, stimulated promulgation of national guidelines for early detection and control of blood lipids and blood pressure. Trials to test the efficacy of lowering cholesterol by drugs and diet have convincingly shown benefits for CHD, angiographically evaluated lesions, and xanthomata regression. The trials of antihypertensive treatment have been consistently successful in preventing strokes but have been disappointing in preventing CHD (18), except for a study that evaluated isolated systolic hypertension (31). For patients with CHD it appears that longer treatment with agents that do not adversely affect other features of the coronary risk profile are preferable.

Although exercise, weight control, smoking abatement, and control of hyperglycemia appear to be rational features of a comprehensive risk reduction program, controlled trial evidence to show their benefits is lacking. Nonetheless, these actions can be recommended because they are likely to be effective and are worthwhile for other reasons. Also, preventive management is likely to be optimal only if it is multifactorial. Preventive strategies should include public-health measures that will improve the ecology by shifting the distribution of risk factors to more favorable levels, education that will enable people to preserve their own health, and preventive medicine for high-risk candidates who require drugs. It is important to note, however, that implementation of such hygienic measures as diet modification, exercise, smoking abatement, and weight reduction require well-developed skills in behavior modification on the part of the patient and health care provider.

1. Find points for each risk factor:

Men

Age		SBP		HYP RX	DB	CVD	Cigs	AF	LVH
54-56	0	95-105	0	No 0	No 0	No 0	No 0	No 0	No 0
57-59	1	106-116	1	Yes 2	Yes 2	Yes 3	Yes 3	Yes 4	Yes 6
60-62	2	117-126	2						
63-65	3	127-137	3						
66-68	4	138-148	4						
69-71	5	149-159	5						
72-74	6	160-170	6						
75-77	7	171-181	7						
78-80	8	182-191	8						
81-83	9	192-202	9						
84-86	10	203-213	10						

Women

Age		SBP		HYP RX	DB	CVD	Cigs	AF	LVH
54-56	0	95-104	0	No 0	No 0	No 0	No 0	No 0	No 0
57-59	1	105-114	1	If Yes, see below	Yes 3	Yes 2	Yes 3	Yes 6	Yes 4
60-62	2	115-124	2						
63-65	3	125-134	3						
66-68	4	135-144	4						
69-71	5	145-154	5						
72-74	6	155-164	6						
75-77	7	165-174	7						
78-80	8	175-184	8						
81-83	9	185-194	9						
84-86	10	196-204	10						

If currently under antihypertensive therapy, add the following points depending on systolic level

SBP	95-104	105-114	115-124	125-134	135-144	145-154
Points	6	5	5	4	3	3

SBP	155-164	165-174	175-184	185-194	195-204
Points	2	1	1	0	0

2. Add up points for all risk factors:

Age ___ + SBP ___ + HYP RX ___ + Diabetes ___ + Cigs ___ + CVD ___ + AF ___ + LVH ___ = Point total ___

3. Look up 10-year risk corresponding to point total:

Men

Points	Risk	Points	Risk	Points	Risk
1	2.6%	11	11.2%	21	41.7%
2	3.0%	12	12.9%	22	46.6%
3	3.5%	13	14.8%	23	51.8%
4	4.0%	14	17.0%	24	57.3%
5	4.7%	15	19.5%	25	62.8%
6	5.4%	16	22.4%	26	68.4%
7	6.3%	17	25.5%	27	73.8%
8	7.3%	18	29.0%	28	79.0%
9	8.4%	19	32.9%	29	83.7%
10	9.7%	20	37.1%	30	87.9%

Women

Points	Risk	Points	Risk	Points	Risk
1	1.1%	11	7.6%	21	43.4%
2	1.3%	12	9.2%	22	50.0%
3	1.6%	13	11.1%	23	57.0%
4	2.0%	14	13.3%	24	64.2%
5	2.4%	15	16.0%	25	71.4%
6	2.9%	16	19.1%	26	78.2%
7	3.5%	17	22.8%	27	84.4%
8	4.3%	18	27.0%		
9	5.2%	19	31.9%		
10	6.3%	20	37.3%		

4. Compare to average 10-year risk:

Age	Men's risk	Women's risk
55-59	5.9%	3.0%
60-64	7.8%	4.7%
65-69	11.0%	7.2%
70-74	13.7%	10.9%
75-79	18.0%	15.5%
80-84	22.3%	23.9%

Key to risk factors:

SBP = Systolic blood pressure; HYP RX = Under antihypertensive therapy?; Diabetes = History of diabetes?; Cigs = Smokes cigarettes?; CVD = History of cardiovascular disease (myocardial infarction, angina pectoris, coronary insufficiency, intermittent claudication, or congestive heart failure)?; AF = History of atrial fibrillation?; LVH = Left ventricular hypertrophy on electrocardiograph?

Figure 1.9 Stroke risk factor prediction chart. Framingham Study.

From Wolf, P.A., D'Agostino, R.B, Belanger, A.J., & Kannel, W.B. Probability of Stroke: A Risk Profile From the Framingham Study. *Stroke,* **22**:312-318, 1991. Figure © American Heart Association. *Risk Factor Prediction Kit,* 1990. Reprinted by permission.

1. Find points for each risk factor:

Age (women)		Age (men)		HDL cholesterol		Total cholesterol		SBP		Other factors
30	-12	30	-2	25-26	7	139-151	-3	98-104	-2	Smoker:
31	-11	31	-1	27-29	6	152-166	-2	105-112	-1	Yes = 4
32	-9	32-33	0	30-32	5	167-182	-1	113-120	0	No = 0
33	-8	34	1	33-35	4	183-199	0	121-129	1	
34	-6	35-36	2	36-38	3	200-219	1	130-139	2	Diabetes:
35	-5	37-38	3	39-42	2	220-239	2	140-149	3	Yes (male) = 3
36	-4	39	4	43-46	1	240-262	3	150-160	4	Yes (female) = 6
37	-3	40-41	5	47-50	0	263-288	4	161-172	5	No = 0
38	-2	42-43	6	51-55	-1	289-315	5	173-185	6	
39	-1	44-45	7	56-60	-2	316-330	6			LVH:
40	0	46-47	8	61-66	-3					Yes = 9
41	1	48-49	9	67-73	-4					No = 0
42-43	2	50-51	10	74-80	-5					
44	3	52-54	11	81-87	-6					
45-46	4	55-58	12	88-96	-7					
47-48	5	57-59	13							
49-50	6	60-61	14							
51-52	7	62-64	15							
53-55	8	65-67	16							
58-60	9	68-70	17							
61-67	10	71-73	18							
68-74	11	74	19							

2. Add up points for all risk factors:

____ + ____ + ____ + ____ + ____ + ____ + ____ = ____
Age   HDL cholesterol   Total cholesterol   SBP   Smoker   Diabetes   LVH   Point total

3. Look up risks corresponding to point total:

Points	5-year	10-year	Points	5-year	10-year	Points	5-year	10-year
≤1	<1%	<2%	12	3%	7%	23	12%	23%
2	1%	2%	13	3%	8%	24	13%	25%
3	1%	2%	14	4%	9%	25	14%	27%
4	1%	2%	15	5%	10%	26	16%	29%
5	1%	3%	16	5%	12%	27	17%	31%
6	1%	3%	17	6%	13%	28	19%	33%
7	1%	4%	18	7%	14%	29	20%	36%
8	2%	4%	19	8%	16%	30	22%	38%
9	2%	5%	20	8%	18%	31	24%	40%
10	2%	6%	21	9%	19%	32	25%	42%
11	3%	6%	22	11%	21%			

4. Compare to average 10-year risk:

Age	Women's risk	Men's risk
30-34	<1%	3%
35-39	<1%	5%
40-44	2%	6%
45-49	5%	10%
50-54	8%	14%
55-59	12%	16%
60-64	13%	21%
65-69	9%	30%
70-74	12%	24%

Key to risk factors:

HDL cholesterol = High-density lipoprotein cholesterol level; Total cholesterol = Total cholesterol level; SBP = Systolic blood pressure; Smoker = Smokes cigarettes?; Diabetes = History of diabetes?; LVH = Left ventricular hypertrophy on electrocardiograph?

Figure 1.10 Coronary artery disease risk factor prediction chart. Framingham Study. From Anderson, K., Wilson, P., Odell, P., & Kannel, W.B. An Updated Coronary Risk Profile. *Circulation*, 83:356-362, 1991. Figure © American Heart Association. *Risk Factor Prediction Kit*, 1990. Reprinted by permission.

Summary

Four decades of prospective epidemiologic investigation at the Framingham Study have documented the importance of major risk factors that predispose to atherosclerotic cardiovascular disease. The major contributors identified include atherogenic personal attributes and living habits that promote atherosclerosis. The relation of serum cholesterol to coronary heart disease derives from the LDL component, and there is also a protective HDL fraction that is inversely related to CHD risk. At any serum total cholesterol, the rate of atherogenesis varies depending on the total/HDL cholesterol ratio, which reflects the two-way traffic of cholesterol entering and leaving the arterial intima. Hypertension, impaired glucose tolerance, and fibrinogen are other atherogenic traits that independently affect risk of atherosclerotic cardiovascular events.

Lifestyles that predispose to accelerated atherogenesis are typified by a too-rich diet, sedentary habits, unrestrained weight gain, and cigarette smoking. Alcohol or coffee consumption is acceptable in moderation. Acquired abdominal obesity worsens the entire cardiovascular risk profile promoting dyslipidemia, hypertension, left ventricular hypertrophy, insulin resistance, and glucose intolerance.

Preclinical compromise of the circulation can be conveniently detected by static and exercise ECG examination. A strong family history of cardiovascular disease occurring at an early age identifies susceptibles. Occurrence of menopause promptly escalates risk of cardiovascular disease in women.

Optimal cardiovascular risk assessment requires a quantitative synthesis of multiple risk factors into a composite estimate. This provides the conditional probability of an event and includes those at high risk because of multiple marginally elevated risk factors that are often overlooked.

Preventive management should also be multifactorial. Although efficacy of interventions against all relevant risk factors is unproven, such measures are rational and worthy of prevention-minded physicians.

References

1. Kannel, W.B. Some lessons in cardiovascular epidemiology from Framingham. Am. J. Cardiol. 37:289-292; 1976.

2. Kannel, W.B. Contribution of the Framingham heart study to preventive cardiology. Bishop lecture. J. Am. Coll. Cardiol. 15:206-211; 1990.

3. Epstein, F.H. Predicting, explaining, and preventing coronary heart disease. An epidemiological view. Modern Concepts of Cardiovascular Disease. 48:7-12; 1979.

4. Report of intersociety commission for heart disease resources. Optional resources for primary prevention of atherosclerotic diseases. Circulation. 70:157A-205A; 1984.

5. Cupples, L.A.; D'Agostino, R.B.; Kiely, T. Some risk factors related to the annual incidence of cardiovascular disease and death. Framingham study. 30-year follow-up. NIH Publication No. 87-2703, pp. 1-462. Washington, DC: U.S. Department of Commerce, National Technical Information Service; 1987.

6. Kannel, W.B. New perspectives in cardiovascular risk factors. Am. Heart J. 114:213-219; 1987.

7. Kannel, W.B.; McGee, D.L.; Castelli, W.P. Latest perspective on cigarette smoking and cardiovascular disease: The Framingham study. J. Cardiac Rehab. 4:267-277; 1984.

8. Kannel, W.B.; Wolf, P.A.; Castelli, W.P.; D'Agostino, R.B. Fibrinogen and risk of cardiovascular disease. The Framingham study. JAMA. 258:1183-1186; 1987.

9. Harris, T.; Cook, E.F.; Kannel, W.B.; Goldman, L. Proportional hazards analysis of risk factors for coronary heart disease in individuals aged 65 or older. The Framingham heart study. J. Am. Geriatr. Soc. 36:1023-1028; 1988.

10. Higgins, M.; Kannel, W.B.; Garrison, R.; Pinsky, J.; Stokes, J., III. Hazards of obesity. The Framingham experience. Acta Med. Scand. [Suppl.]. 723:23-36; 1987.

11. Kannel, W.B.; Wilson, P.W.F.; Blair, S.N. Epidemiologic assessment of the role of physical activity and fitness in development of cardiovascular disease. Am. Heart J. 109:876-885; 1985.

12. Kannel, W.B.; Dawber, J.R.; McGee, D.L. Perspectives in systolic hypertension: The Framingham study. Circulation. 61:1179-1182; 1980.

13. Kannel, W.B. Hypertension: Relationship with other risk factors. Drugs. [Suppl.]. 1:1-11; 1986.

14. Wilking, S.; Van, B.; Belanger, A.; Kannel, W.B.; D'Agostino, R.B.; Sfiel, K. Determinants of isolated systolic hypertension. JAMA. 260:3451-3455; 1988.

15. Kannel, W.B. High density lipoproteins: Epidemiologic profile and risks of coronary artery disease. Am. J. Cardiol. 52:93-123; 1983.

16. Kannel, W.B. Lipids, diabetes and coronary heart disease: Insights from the Framingham study. Am. Heart J. 110:1100-1107; 1985.

17. The expert panel: Report of the national cholesterol education program expert panel on detection, evaluation and treatment of high blood cholesterol in adults. Arch. Intern. Med. 148:36-39; 1988.

18. MacMahon, S.W.; Cutler, J.D.; Furberg, C.D.; Payne, G.H. The effects of drug treatment of hypertension

on morbidity and mortality from cardiovascular disease: A review of randomized trials. Prog. Cardiovasc. Dis. [Suppl.]. 29:99-118; 1986.

19. Reaven, G.M. Banting lecture 1988. Role of insulin resistance in human disease. Diabetes. 37:1595-1607; 1988.

20. Kannel, W.B.; McGee, D.L. Diabetes and glucose intolerance as risk factors for cardiovascular disease. The Framingham study. Diabetes Care. 2:110-126; 1979.

21. Kannel, W.B.; Sytkowski, P.A. Atherosclerosis risk factors. Pharmacol. Ther. 32:207-235; 1987.

22. Eaker, E.D.; Haynes, S.B.; Feinleib, M. Spouse behavior and coronary heart disease in men: Prospective results from the Framingham heart study. II. Modification of risk in type A husbands according to the social and psychological status of their wives. Am. J. Epidemiol. 118:23-41; 1983.

23. Ernst, E.; Hammerschmidt, M.D.; Bagge, U.; Matrai, A.; Dormandy, J.A. Leukocytes and the risk of ischemic diseases. JAMA. 257:2318-2324; 1987.

24. Kannel, W.B.; Dannenberg, A.L.; Levy, D. Population implications of electrocardiographic left ventricular hypertrophy. Am. J. Cardiol. 60:851-931; 1987.

25. Wong, N.D.; Cupples, L.A.; Ostfeld, A.M.; Levy, D.; Kannel, W.B. Risk factors for long-term coronary prognosis after initial myocardial infarction: The Framingham study. Am. J. Epidemiol. 130:469-480; 1989.

26. Snowden, E.B.; McNamara, P.M.; Garrison, R.J.; Feinleib, M.; Kannel, W.B.; Epstein, F.H. Predicting coronary heart disease in siblings—a multivariate assessment. The Framingham study. Am. J. Epidemiol. 115:217-222; 1982.

27. Schildkraut, J.M.; Myers, R.H.; Cupples, L.A.; Kiely, D.; Kannel, W.B. Coronary risk associated with age and sex or parental heart disease in the Framingham heart study. Am. J. Cardiol. 64:555-559; 1989.

28. Wolf, P.A.; D'Agostino, R.B.; Belanger, A.J.; Kannel, W.B. Probability of stroke: A risk profile from the Framingham study. Stroke. 22:312-317; 1991.

29. Anderson, K.M.; Wilson, P.W.F.; Odell, P.M.; Kannel, W.B. An updated coronary risk profile. A statement for health professionals. Circulation. 83:356-362; 1991.

30. Sytkowski, P.A.; Kannel, W.B.; D'Agostino, R.B. Changes in risk factors and the decline in mortality from cardiovascular disease. The Framingham heart study. N. Engl. J. Med. 322:1635-1641; 1990.

31. SHEP Cooperative Study Group. Prevention of stroke by antihypertensive drug treatment in older persons with isolated systolic hypertension. Final results of systolic hypertension in the elderly program (SHEP). JAMA. 265:3255-3264; 1991.

PART II

The Heart Disease Patient: Pathophysiology, Diagnosis, and Treatment

Chapter 2

Morphological Findings in the Coronary Arteries of Patients With Myocardial Ischemia and Its Myocardial Consequences

William Clifford Roberts

Atherosclerotic coronary artery disease (CAD) is the most common cause of death in the Western world. In the United States, one person dies every minute because of CAD, and about 6 million people have symptomatic myocardial ischemia due to CAD. About 250,000 coronary artery bypass grafting (CABG) and 300,000 coronary angioplasty procedures were performed in 1990 in the United States. The cause of atherosclerosis is now clear: the evidence is overwhelming that atherosclerosis is a cholesterol problem. The higher the blood total cholesterol level (specifically low-density lipoproteins [LDLs]) the greater the chance of developing symptomatic CAD and of having a fatal CAD and the greater the extent of atherosclerotic plaques. Furthermore, lowering the blood total cholesterol level decreases the chances of having symptomatic or fatal CAD and increases the chance that some atherosclerotic plaques will actually regress. Although pathologists have examined the coronary arteries by visual inspection at necropsy for over a century, only in recent years has the extent of the atherosclerotic process in patients with symptomatic or fatal CAD become appreciated. This chapter first reviews the status of the major epicardial coronary arteries in various subsets of patients with fatal atherosclerotic CAD. It then describes the effects of angioplasty on these arteries, some observations in patients having thrombolytic therapy, CABG, and various complications of myocardial ischemia.

Number of Major Epicardial Coronary Arteries Severely Narrowed in Various "Coronary Events"

The most common method for describing the severity of CAD in patients with clinical evidence of myocardial ischemia is by the number of major epicardial coronary arteries that are narrowed by more than 50% in luminal diameter, as determined by angiography. Thus, patients are divided into groups of single-vessel, double-vessel, triple-vessel, and left main CAD. Because a 50% diameter reduction is essentially equivalent to a cross-sectional area narrowing of 75%, this latter value is the cutoff point for significant luminal narrowing at necropsy. Physiologically, there is no obstruction to arterial blood flow until the lumen is narrowed by more than 75% in cross-sectional area.

Table 2.1 summarizes the number of major (right, left main, left anterior descending, and left circumflex) epicardial coronary arteries narrowed by more than 75% in cross-sectional area by atherosclerotic plaque alone in a study of 129 patients with fatal CAD (1). All 516 of their major coronary arteries were examined at necroscopy and of them 345 (67%) showed significant narrowing. In contrast, of 40 control subjects, who were mainly victims of acute leukemia and who had no clinical evidence of myocardial ischemia during life, all 160 major epicardial coronary arteries were examined and of them 60 (37%) showed significant narrowing. Among the 129 patients with fatal CAD, only 11 (8%) had a single coronary artery significantly narrowed (controls = 23%); 37 (29%) had two arteries so narrowed (controls = 13%); 64 (50%) had three arteries so narrowed (controls = 5%), and 17 (13%) had all four major arteries significantly narrowed (controls = 0). Thus, of the 4 major coronary arteries in the CAD patients an average of 2.7 were significantly narrowed compared to 0.7 among the controls.

The average number of major coronary arteries severely narrowed by atherosclerotic plaque

Table 2.1   Number of Major (Right, Left Main, Left Anterior Descending, and Left Circumflex) Coronary Arteries Narrowed > 75% in Cross-Sectional Area by Atherosclerotic Plaque in Fatal Coronary Artery Disease

| Coronary event | Patients (n) | Mean age (yrs) | Number of four arteries/Pt > 75% ↓ in CSA by plaque | | | | |
			4	3	2	1	Mean
Sudden coronary death	31	47	3	20	6	2	2.8
Acute myocardial infarction	27	59	3	14	10	0	2.7
Healed myocardial infarction							
Asymtomatic	18	66	0	7	7	4	2.2
Chronic CHF without aneurysm	9	63	0	3	5	1	2.2
Left ventricular aneurysm	22	61	1	12	6	3	2.5
Angina pectoris/unstable	22	48	10	8	3	1	3.2
Total (%)	129	56	17 (13)	64 (50)	37 (29)	11 (8)	2.7
Controls (%)	40	52	0 (0)	5 (5)	12 (13)	21 (23)	0.7

CHF = congestive heart failure; CSA = cross-sectional area.
Reprinted from Roberts, W.C. *Am. J. Cardiol.* (see reference 1). Used by permission.

among the various subsets of CAD patients was relatively similar except for the unstable angina patients (Table 2.1). Among the 31 patients who experienced sudden coronary death (2), all of whom died outside the hospital, an average of 2.8 of the 4 major arteries were severely narrowed. This number was virtually identical to that of the 27 patients with transmural acute myocardial infarction (MI) (3), all of whom died in a coronary care unit. Only 2 of the 31 sudden death victims and none of the 27 acute MI victims had single-vessel disease.

The group with healed MI was divided into three subgroups. One consisted of patients who had had an acute MI that had healed and thereafter had no clinical evidence of myocardial ischemia. These patients died from a noncardiac cause, usually cancer (4). Nevertheless, the average number of major coronary arteries severely narrowed at necropsy was 2.2 of 4. The second subgroup consisted of patients who had chronic congestive heart failure (CHF) after healing of an acute MI but in the absence of a left ventricular aneurysm (5). The average number of major coronary arteries severely narrowed in this group was also 2.2. The third subgroup of healed MI patients had a true left ventricular aneurysm (6); the average number of major coronary arteries severely narrowed was 2.5.

The final subgroup consisted of 22 patients with unstable angina pectoris; all of them underwent CABG within 7 days of death (7). Preoperatively, all had normal left ventricular function and none

had a clinically apparent acute MI or CHF. The average number of major coronary arteries severely narrowed was 3.2 of 4, and 10 of the 22 patients had severe narrowing of the left main coronary artery as well as of the other three major coronary arteries. (Another study [8] has shown that severe narrowing of the left main coronary artery usually indicates that the other three major arteries are also severely narrowed.) The unstable angina group thus had the largest average number of major coronary arteries severely narrowed of any of the subgroups; nevertheless, this group of patients had excellent left ventricular function.

A Quantitative Approach to Atherosclerotic Coronary Artery Disease

Although the single-, double-, triple-, and quadruple-vessel designations for evaluating the severity of CAD has been useful clinically, this is considered a qualitative analysis that usually does not discern differences in degrees of coronary narrowing in the various subsets of patients. To obtain a better appreciation of the extent of the atherosclerotic process in patients with fatal CAD, we examined every 5-mm long segment of each of the four major coronary arteries (1). In adults, the average length of the right coronary artery is 10 cm; the left main artery, 1 cm; the left anterior descending artery, 10 cm; and the left circumflex artery, 6 cm.

Thus, an average of 27 cm of major epicardial coronary arteries were available for examination in each adult, or fifty-four 5-mm segments. This approach allows us to ask how many of the 5-mm segments are narrowed 76% to 100% (i.e., how many are significantly narrowed), but also 51% to 75%, 26% to 50%, and 0% to 25% in cross-sectional area. This approach may be considered a quantitative one.

The patients described in Table 2.1, in which the qualitative approach was used, were also examined at necropsy by the quantitative method; the findings are summarized in Table 2.2. A total of 6,461 5-mm segments were sectioned and later examined histologically. The findings in the 129 patients with fatal CAD were compared with those in 1,849 5-mm segments from the 40 control subjects. In each CAD subgroup, the 5-mm segments from each of the four major coronary arteries were pooled so that the amount of narrowing in an individual patient was not discernible. The proportion of 5-mm segments narrowed by 76% to 100% was 35% for the CAD patients and 3% for the control subjects; the proportion narrowed by 51% to 75% was 36% for the CAD patients and 22% for the control subjects. Thus, 71% of the 5-mm segments in the CAD patients and 25% in the control subjects were narrowed more than 50% in cross-sectional area. In contrast, only 29% of the 5-mm segments in the CAD patients were narrowed less than 50% and only 8% less than 25%; 75% of the 5-mm segments in the control subjects were narrowed less

than 50% and 31% less than 25%. Thus, in the CAD patients, 92% of the 6,461 5-mm segments were narrowed more than 25% in cross-sectional area by atherosclerotic plaque. Accordingly, the coronary atherosclerotic process is diffuse in patients with fatal CAD.

Among the various subsets of CAD patients, those with sudden coronary death (2) and acute MI (3) had similar proportions of 5-mm segments narrowed 76% to 100% in cross-sectional area by plaque (36% and 34%, respectively); patients with healed MI (4-6) had the least severe narrowing (31% of segments narrowed more than 75%), and the patients with unstable angina pectoris (7) had the most severe narrowing (48% of segments narrowed more than 75%).

Distribution of Severe Narrowing in the Three Longest Epicardial Coronary Arteries in Fatal Coronary Artery Disease

In all of the aforementioned quantitative coronary arteries studies, the amount of luminal narrowing of cross-sectional area by atherosclerotic plaque in the right, left anterior descending, and left circumflex coronary arteries was similar when the 5-mm segments in each of the three longest coronary arteries was pooled together from a number of patients.

Table 2.2   Amounts of Cross-Sectional Area Narrowing of Each 5-mm Segment of the Four Major (Right, Left Main, Left Anterior Descending, and Left Circumflex) Epicardial Coronary Arteries by Atherosclerotic Plaques in Subjects With Fatal Coronary Artery Disease

Subgroup	Patients (n)	Mean age (yrs)	Number 5-mm segments	Percent segments narrowed 0-25%	26-50%	51-75%	76-100%	Mean score	Mean % narrowing/ 5-mm segments
Sudden coronary death	31	47	1,564	7	23	34	36	2.98	67
Acute myocardial infarction	27	59	1,403	5	23	38	34	3.01	68
Healed myocardial infarction									
Asymptomatic	18	66	924	11	23	35	31⎱	2.87	64
Chronic CHF without aneurysm	9	63	529	11	23	37	29 ⎬31%	2.78	61
LV aneurysm	22	61	992	4	21	42	33⎰	3.03	68
Angina pectoris	22	48	1,049	11	12	29	48	3.12	70
Total	129	56	6,461	8	21	36	35	2.98	67
Controls	40	52	1,849	31	44	22	3	1.97	32

CHF = congestive heart failure; LV = left ventricular.
Reprinted from Roberts, W.C. *Am. J. Cardiol.* (see reference 1). Used by permission.

In a single patient, however, the proportion of 5-mm long coronary artery segments severely narrowed in one major epicardial coronary artery may be greater or less than that of another major coronary artery. However, when the segments from one coronary artery (right, for example) were pooled together from several patients with fatal CAD and compared with pooled 5-mm segments from another coronary artery (left anterior descending, for example) from several patients with fatal CAD, the proportion of segments narrowed in each of the four categories of cross-sectional area narrowing in each artery were similar. Thus, the quantity of atherosclerotic plaque is similar for similar lengths of the right, left anterior descending, and left circumflex coronary arteries, and because the amount of atherosclerotic plaque is similar, the amount of resulting luminal narrowing also is similar. The cholesterol thesis would likely not be tenable if the amount of atherosclerotic plaque were highly different in the different major epicardial coronary arteries, given that the same serum cholesterol level presumably is present in each major coronary artery.

Clinical Usefulness of the Quantitative Approach to Assessing Coronary Artery Disease

The information derived at necropsy quantitating the severity and extent of atherosclerosis in the four major epicardial coronary arteries in patients with fatal CAD is potentially useful to live patients in two areas: (1) interpreting degrees of coronary narrowing by angiography during life and (2) deciding how many of the major coronary arteries need a conduit at the time of CABG.

Without coronary angiography neither CABG nor angioplasty could be done. The only way during life to obtain information on the status of the coronary arteries is by angiography, a procedure that revolutionized diagnosis of CAD, just as CABG revolutionized CAD therapy. But angiography—as good as it is—has certain deficiencies. Angiography is a luminogram that fluoroscopically visualizes the coronary arteries. Narrowed segments are compared with less narrowed segments that are assumed to be normal. The angiogram does not delineate the internal elastic membrane of the artery, so the true size of the artery's lumen remains uncertain (Figures 2.1 and 2.2).

The aforementioned quantitative studies demonstrated in patients with fatal CAD that 92% of the 5-mm long segments of the four major epicardial coronary arteries were narrowed by more than 25% in cross-sectional area by atherosclerotic plaque. Thus, only 8% of the 5-mm segments even approached normal, and virtually none was normal. Thus, in fatal CAD at least, and probably also in live patients with symptomatic myocardial ischemia, it is infrequent that a segment of a coronary artery determined angiographically as severely narrowed can be compared with a segment of coronary artery that is actually normal. In other words, in patients with symptomatic myocardial ischemia, the coronary angiogram measures degrees of narrowing by comparing severely narrowed segments to segments which are simply less narrowed and probably not normal (Figure 2.1). Accordingly, coronary angiograms in patients with symptomatic myocardial ischemia usually underestimate the degrees of luminal narrowing (10,11).

The unit of measuring degrees of narrowing by angiography is different from the unit of measurement at necropsy. In the anatomical quantitative studies presented herein, the unit was *cross-sectional–area* narrowing. The unit of angiography is *diameter* narrowing. As noted, a 75% narrowing in cross-sectional area is equivalent to a 50% reduction in diameter; therefore, a reduction in diameter of 50% or more during life has generally been considered the cut-off point between clinically significant and clinically insignificant coronary narrowing.

The second potential usefulness of the information derived from the quantitative CAD studies at necropsy is the appreciation that the atherosclerotic process in patients with symptomatic myocardial ischemia is usually diffuse and severe and that therefore more rather than fewer aortocoronary conduits should provide a higher frequency of relief or improvement in symptoms of myocardial ischemia, an improvement in results of exercise testing, and a prolongation of life. From a study at necropsy of 102 patients dying either early (≤ 60 days) or late (2.5-108 months; mean = 35) after CABG, Waller and Roberts (12) found that the bypassed and nonbypassed native coronary arteries had similar degrees of severe luminal narrowing by atherosclerotic plaque. Specifically, in 213 (94%) of the 226 bypassed native arteries and in 73 (91%) of 80 nonbypassed native arteries, the lumens were narrowed more than 75% in cross-sectional area by atherosclerotic plaque. The reason the native arteries were not bypassed was not that they were too small or severely narrowed distally, but because by angiogram the lumens were

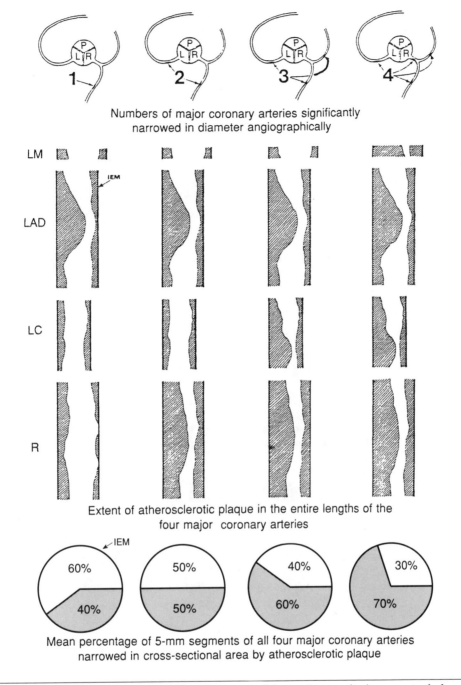

Numbers of major coronary arteries significantly
narrowed in diameter angiographically

Extent of atherosclerotic plaque in the entire lengths of the
four major coronary arteries

Mean percentage of 5-mm segments of all four major coronary arteries
narrowed in cross-sectional area by atherosclerotic plaque

Figure 2.1   Number of coronary arteries significantly narrowed by angiogram (*top*), amount of plaque in the entire lengths of the four major or epicardial coronary arteries (*middle*), and cross-sectional view (*bottom*) of the average amount of plaque in each 5-mm segment of the entire length of the arteries according to the numbers of major arteries significantly narrowed by angiogram. (LAD = left anterior descending; LC = left circumflex; LM = left main; R = right.)

Reprinted with permission from Roberts, W.C. Coronary "Lesion," Coronary "Disease," "Single-Vessel Disease," "Two-Vessel Disease": Word and Phrase Misnomers Providing False Impressions of the Extent of Coronary Atherosclerosis in Symptomatic Myocardial Ischemia. *Am. J. Cardiol.* **66**:121-123, 1990.

judged not to be sufficiently narrowed to warrant the insertion of a conduit. Thus, if two of the major coronary arteries are severely narrowed by angiogram and the third major artery is "insignificantly" narrowed and if CABG is to be done, the need for insertion of a conduit in all three major coronary arteries could be reasonably argued. There is, of course, potential danger to inserting a conduit in

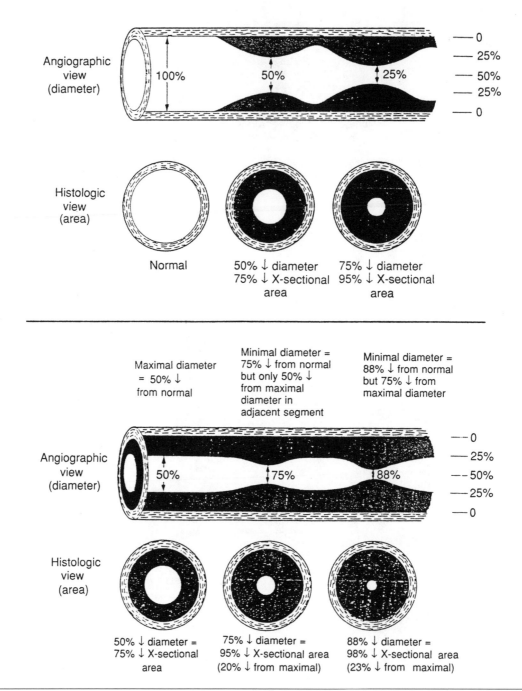

Figure 2.2 Differences in units used for designating degrees of narrowing by angiography (diameter reduction) and for histological examination (cross-sectional area narrowing) of coronary arteries. In general, a 50% diameter reduction (by angiography) is equivalent to a 75% cross-sectional area narrowing. The upper panel shows a segment of a coronary artery that is entirely normal. This situation rarely exists in persons with symtomatic myocardial ischemia. The usual situation in this condition is depicted in the lower panel, which indicates that the severist narrowing is compared to an adjacent area, which by angiography may be considered to be normal but in actuality is simply less narrowed.

Reprinted with permission from Arnett et al. Coronary Artery Narrowing in Coronary Heart Disease. *Ann. Intern. Med.* **91**:350-356, 1979.

an artery insignificantly narrowed; nevertheless, it may be more advantageous to err on the side of too many conduits than too few. At necropsy, triple-vessel disease is far more frequent than double-vessel disease, and even when only two of the three major arteries at necropsy are narrowed more than 75% in cross-sectional area, the third one is usually narrowed 51%-75% (12,13). Thus, an appreciation of the diffuse nature of coronary atherosclerosis in fatal CAD and probably also in symptomatic myocardial ischemia encourages the tilt towards more rather than fewer conduits being placed during CABG.

Significance of Coronary Arterial Thrombus in Transmural Acute Myocardial Infarction

Thrombi in the coronary arteries of necropsy patients with transmural acute MI have been observed in numerous studies (14-16). Herrick (17) found thrombi in 4 patients with fatal acute MI, and for many decades thrombi were believed to precipitate acute MI (which is why the term *coronary thrombosis* was used for years to describe the event that physicians now call acute MI). To evaluate the significance of coronary thrombi in acute MI, Brosius and Roberts (18) examined in detail the coronary arteries containing thrombi in 54 autopsied patients who had died from transmural acute MI. Of 235 patients with fatal acute MI, 99 had histologic sections available from every 5-mm segment of each of the four major coronary arteries. Movat-stained histological sections, approximately 55 per patient, were reviewed, and a thrombus was found in one of the four major coronary arteries in 54 of the 99 patients (55%). In the coronary artery containing the thrombus, the maximal degree of cross-sectional area narrowed by atherosclerotic plaque was determined at the site of the thrombus, in the 2-cm portion of artery proximal to the thrombus, and in the 2-cm segment of coronary artery below the distal site of attachment of the thrombus. The length of the thrombus was determined by the number of 5-mm long segments of coronary artery that contained thrombus.

A coronary arterial thrombus was defined as a collection of fibrin (with or without engulfed erythrocytes) or platelets or both within the residual lumen with attachment of the fibrin and platelets to the luminal surface of the artery. Among the 54 patients with fatal acute MI, the luminal surface was always the surface of an underlying atherosclerotic plaque. The thrombus was always attached to the intimal surface in its distal portion, but in a few patients it was not attached in its most proximal portion. The thrombus was considered occlusive when it totally occupied the residual lumen of the artery, that is, the portion not occupied by atherosclerotic plaque. The thrombus was considered nonocclusive when it filled the residual lumen incompletely.

All patients had an acute MI that involved the entire inner half of the left ventricular wall and a portion or all of the outer half of the left ventricular wall. Twenty patients also had one or more transmural scars. The 54 patients ranged in age from 38 to 92 years (mean = 62 years); 41 were men and 13 were women.

The thrombi were occlusive in 47 patients (87%) and nonocclusive in 7 (13%). The coronary arterial systems containing thrombi were the left anterior descending artery in 22 patients (41%), the right coronary artery in 19 (35%), and the left circumflex artery in 13 (24%). The coronary thrombi ranged from 0.5 to 10 cm in length (mean = 1.6 cm).

The maximal luminal narrowing caused by atherosclerotic plaques alone at the site of the thrombus varied from 33% to 98% (mean = 81%); the maximal coronary luminal narrowing caused by the thrombus alone varied from 2% to 67% (mean = 19%) in the 47 patients with occlusive thrombi and from 2% to 24% (mean = 7%) in the 7 patients with nonocclusive thrombi. The maximal luminal narrowing caused by atherosclerotic plaques in the 2-cm segment of coronary artery proximal to the thrombus ranged from 26% to 98% (mean = 75%) and in the 2-cm segment distal to the distal site of attachment of the thrombus, from 43% to 98% (mean = 76%). No significant differences were noted in the amount of maximal luminal narrowing at, proximal to, or distal to the thrombus between the 47 patients with occlusive thrombi and the 7 with nonocclusive thrombi. Likewise, no significant differences were observed in the amount of maximal luminal narrowing at, proximal to, or distal to the coronary thrombus in the three major coronary arteries.

In 52 (96%) of the 54 coronary arteries with thrombi, the lumens of the arteries at, proximal to, or distal to the thrombi were already narrowed 76% to 100% in cross-sectional area by atherosclerotic plaques: in 27 of 42 arteries (64%) examined proximal to the thrombus (in 12 arteries the thrombi began at, or nearly at, the origin of the coronary artery from the aorta or left main coronary artery), in 35 (66%) of 53 arteries examined distal to the distal site of attachment of the thrombus, and in 41 (76%) of the 54 coronary arteries (or patients) at the site of attachment of the thrombus. Furthermore, in 26 (48%) of the 54 coronary arteries, the lumens of the arteries at, proximal to, or distal to the thrombi were narrowed 91% to 98%

in cross-sectional area by atherosclerotic plaques. In 16 (30%) of 54 coronary arteries with thrombi, the site of most severe narrowing by atherosclerotic plaque in the portion of artery examined was within the 2-cm segment proximal to the thrombus. The site of most severe narrowing in the coronary arteries was not significantly different between patients with occlusive and nonocclusive thrombi.

At the site of attachment of thrombi, the underlying atherosclerotic plaques contained extravasated erythrocytes in 21 (39%) of the 54 patients. In none of the 21, however, did the hemorrhage into the pultaceous debris of the plaque appear to compromise the lumen.

The Brosius and Roberts study (18) raises questions about the importance of coronary thrombi in patients with fatal transmural acute MI. The major finding at autopsy is that, among patients with fatal acute MI, thrombi are found in major coronary arteries that already are severely narrowed by old atherosclerotic plaques at, immediately proximal to, and immediately distal to the site of thrombosis. The lumen of the coronary artery containing the thrombus was already narrowed an average of 79% (range = 26% to 98%) in cross-sectional area by atherosclerotic plaque alone at and within the 2-cm segments proximal to and distal to the thrombus; that is, an "average" coronary artery with a thrombus was severely narrowed ($\geq$ 75% in cross-sectional area) at three sites: at, proximal to, and distal to the thrombus.

The average coronary arterial narrowing at the site of thrombus, however, actually underestimates the severity of the narrowing in the vicinity of the thrombus. The site of most severe narrowing was within the 2 cm proximal to the thrombus in 16 of 54 (30%) coronary arteries, at the site of thrombus in 25 (46%) subjects, and within the 2-cm segment distal to the thrombus in 13 (24%) subjects. At the site of most severe narrowing, 96% of the coronary arteries were narrowed 76% to 98% in cross-sectional area by atherosclerotic plaque, and half were narrowed 91% to 98%. In contrast, the proportion of coronary lumen narrowed by thrombus alone averaged 19% of the original cross-sectional area of the artery (range = 2% to 67%) in the 47 patients with occlusive thrombi and 7% (range = 2% to 24%) in the 7 patients with nonocclusive thrombi. Thus, if thrombi were the only luminal material, the amount of thrombus within the coronary artery, with a few exceptions, probably would not by itself diminish or slow blood flow. Moreover, the frequent need for CABG or angioplasty after successful thrombolysis is readily

understandable. A corollary is that among necropsy patients with fatal acute MI, the coronary thrombus, when present, is always superimposed on an atherosclerotic plaque. The exception is coronary embolism, when a clot may be present without underlying atherosclerotic plaque (19).

The length of coronary thrombi in necropsy patients with fatal acute MI is usually short. Among the 54 patients studied by Brosius and Roberts (18), the average coronary thrombus was 1.6 cm long (range = 0.5 to 10 cm), and the occlusive thrombi were longer than the nonocclusive thrombi (1.8 versus 0.7 cm). Also, occlusive thrombi in the right coronary arteries tended to be longer than those in the left anterior and circumflex coronary arteries (2.4 versus 1.4 and 1.1, respectively). Because the right and left anterior descending coronary arteries in adults are more than 10 cm long and the left circumflex artery is usually about 6 cm long, the actual length of a coronary artery occupied by thrombus is small, and in no patient was the entire length of a coronary artery occupied by a thrombus. In the right coronary artery, there was a weak, but significant, positive correlation between the length of an occlusive thrombus and the duration of survival of a patient between the time of acute MI and death. This relation suggests that thrombi may lengthen or "grow" with time.

Cardiac Morphological Findings in Acute Myocardial Infarction Treated With Thrombolytic Therapy

Until thrombolytic and revascularization therapies for acute MI were introduced, virtually all acute MIs observed at necropsy were nonhemorrhagic. Treatment with thrombolytic agents has been shown to restore the patency of occluded coronary arteries, but this has been associated with an apparently marked, although heretofore undetermined, increase in the frequency of hemorrhagic infarcts. It has been suggested that myocardial hemorrhage after coronary reperfusion is confined to zones of the myocardium that were already necrotic and that the hemorrhage is probably a consequence of severe microvascular injury and not its cause. Gertz et al. (20) studied at necropsy the hearts of 52 patients who had received recombinant tissue plasminogen activator (rt-PA) during acute MI and compared clinical and cardiac morphological findings in patients with hemorrhagic infarcts with those with nonhemorrhagic infarcts. The acute MIs were hemorrhagic by gross inspection (with histological confirmation) in 23, nonhemorrhagic in 20, and not grossly visible in 2; in 7, there was no acute necrosis by either gross or histological examination of multiple sections of the myocardium. In 4 of these 7 patients without acute MIs, the interval from chest pain to death was less than 10 hours, which is often too early to detect the presence of necrosis by histologic examination.

No significant differences were found between patients with hemorrhagic and nonhemorrhagic MIs with respect to mean age, heart weight, interval from chest pain to rt-PA infusion, interval from chest pain to peak creatinine kinase, interval from chest pain to death, location of the myocardial necrosis, frequency of left ventricular dilatation, frequency of myocardial rupture (left ventricular free wall or ventricular septum), or frequency of cardiogenic shock, fatal arrhythmias, or fatal bleeding. Furthermore, the frequencies of thrombi and plaque rupture in coronary arteries and the sizes of the infarct were similar in patients with hemorrhagic and nonhemorrhagic MIs. Thus, although the frequency of hemorrhagic infarction increases after thrombolytic therapy, the hemorrhage does not appear to extend the MI or to increase the frequency of complications of the MI.

In a separate study, Gertz et al. (21) compared cardiac findings at necropsy in 23 patients who had received thrombolytic therapy (i.e., rt-PA) during acute MI with those in 38 patients with acute MI who had not received thrombolytic therapy. Although each group of patients had similar baseline characteristics, the patients receiving rt-PA had a greater frequency of platelet-rich (fibrin-poor) thrombi in the infarct-related coronary arteries, more nonocclusive than occlusive thrombi, and a lower frequency of myocardial rupture.

Composition of Atherosclerotic Plaques in Fatal Coronary Artery Disease

Kragel et al. (22,23) studied at necropsy atherosclerotic plaque composition in the four major coronary arteries in 15 patients who died from the consequences of acute MI, in 12 patients with sudden coronary death without associated MI, and in 10 patients with isolated unstable angina pectoris with pain at rest. Among the three subsets of patients, there were no differences in plaque composition among any of the four major coronary arteries. Within all three groups the major component

of plaque was a combination of dense acellular and cellular fibrous tissue with much smaller portions of plaque composed of pultaceous debris, calcium, foam cells with and without inflammatory cells, and foam cells alone (Figure 2.3). Within all three groups, plaque morphology varied as a function of cross-sectional–area narrowing of the segments. The amount of dense, relatively acellular fibrous tissue, calcified tissue, and pultaceous debris (amorphous debris containing cholesterol clefts, presumably rich in extracellular lipid) increased linearly with increasing degrees of cross-sectional–area narrowing of the segments. Multiluminal channels were most frequently observed in the subgroup with unstable angina pectoris. The studies by Kragel et al. (22,23) are the first to quantitatively analyze the composition of coronary arterial plaques in various subsets of CAD patients.

Effects of Percutaneous Transluminal Coronary Angioplasty on Atherosclerotic Plaques and Relation of Plaque Composition and Arterial Size to Outcome

To delineate their relation to outcome of percutaneous transluminal coronary angioplasty (PTCA), Potkin and Roberts (24) determined the atherosclerotic plaque composition and coronary artery size in 82 5-mm long segments at 28 PTCA sites in 26 patients undergoing PTCA. The 26 patients were subdivided into three groups according to the degree of angiographic patency at the end of the PTCA procedure and to the duration of survival after PTCA (≤ 30 or > 30 days): early success (13 patients, 16 PTCA sites, and 49 5-mm segments), early failure (4 patients, 4 PTCA sites, and 16 5-mm segments), and late success (9 patients, 8 PTCA sites, and 17 5-mm segments). The mean proportion of plaque composed of fibrous tissue among the three groups, respectively, was 80% ± 18%, 71% ± 23%, and 82% ± 16%; the mean proportion of plaque composed of lipid was 17% ± 16%, 21% ± 24%, and 16% ± 15%; and mean proportion of plaque composed of calcium was 3% ± 4%, 8% ± 10%, and 2% ± 3%. The mean coronary arterial internal diameter was 3.3 ± 0.6, 3.9 ± 1.2, and 3.2 ± 0.7 mm, respectively. A plaque tear was present in one or more histologic sections in 25 of the 26 patients; the 1 patient without a tear had the longest interval (nearly 3 years) between PTCA and death. A plaque tear extending from the intima into the media with dissection was observed only

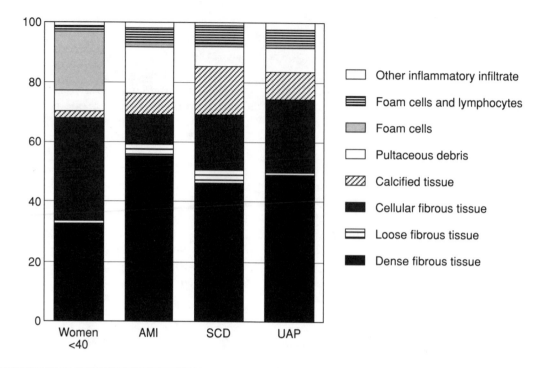

Figure 2.3   Atherosclerotic plaque composition (mean percent) in histologic sections of 5-mm sections of the four major epicardial coronary arteries narrowed greater than 75% in cross-sectional area. The patients included 8 women aged 31-39 years (mean = 34) with fatal coronary artery disease and 35 patients over 40 years of age (mean = 59) with fatal acute myocardial infarction (AMI), sudden coronary death (SCD), and unstable angina pectoris (UAP). The dominant component of the atherosclerotic plaques in all groups was fibrous tissue.
Reprinted with permission from Dollar, A.L., Kragel, A.H., Fernicola, D.J., Waclawiw, M.A., and Roberts, W.C. Composition of Atherosclerotic Plaques in Coronary Arteries in Women < 40 Years of Age With Fatal Coronary Artery Disease and Implications for Plaque Reversibility. *Am. J. Cardiol.* **67**:1223-1227, 1991.

in the early- and late-success groups. A hemorrhage into the plaque was present in 16 (80%) of 20 PTCA sites in the early-success and early-failure groups and in 3 (37%) of 8 sites in the late-success group. Occlusive thrombus and plaque debris in residual lumens were insignificantly different among the three groups. Plaques that had > 25% lipid content had an increased frequency of hemorrhage into the plaque, occlusive thrombus and plaque debris in residual lumens. These findings suggest that coronary arterial size and plaque composition are strong determinants of PTCA outcome. The ideal coronary arterial atherosclerotic narrowing for both technically and clinically successful PTCA appears to be a small (< 3.3 mm in internal diameter) artery in which the plaque contains relatively little calcium and lipid.

Morphological Findings in Saphenous Veins Used as Coronary Arterial Bypass Conduits

Saphenous veins, when used as aortocoronary conduits, undergo changes in their intimal, medial,

and adventitial layers. The predominant late intimal change is a proliferation of fibrous tissue, a finding observed within 2 months after CABG. Other late changes include lipid deposits, thrombi, and, rarely, aneurysm formation. Most published studies describing changes in saphenous veins used as bypass conduits have involved few necropsy patients, involved only operatively excised specimens, or involved cases with relatively short intervals from coronary bypass to death or reoperation. Kalan and Roberts (13) studied at necropsy the hearts and grafts of 53 patients who lived longer than 1 year after coronary bypass. They examined 123 saphenous vein grafts and 1,865 5-mm segments of the grafts in the 53 patients, some of whom died of consequences of myocardial ischemia and some of whom died of noncardiac conditions.

The 53 patients died 13 to 53 months (mean = 58) after a single aortocoronary bypass operation. Of the 53 patients, 32 (60%) died of a cardiac cause; of their 72 saphenous vein aortocoronary conduits, 36 (49%) were narrowed at some point more than 75% in cross-sectional area by atherosclerotic plaque. The remaining 21 patients (40%) died of a noncardiac cause; of their 50 saphenous vein conduits, 10 (20%) were narrowed at some point more than 75% in cross-sectional area by plaque. Thus, the noncardiac mode of death in a large proportion of the patients suggests that the bypass operation prolonged life to a degree sufficient for another condition to develop. The 123 saphenous vein conduits were divided into 5-mm segments, and a histological section was prepared from each. Of the 1,104 5-mm segments in the 32 patients who died as a consequence of myocardial ischemia, 291 (26%) were narrowed more than 75% in cross-sectional area by plaque; in contrast, of the 761 5-mm segments of veins in the 21 patients with a noncardiac mode of death, 86 (11%) were narrowed more than 75% by plaque. Of the total, 1,865 5-mm segments of vein, only 395 (21%) were narrowed 25% or less in cross-sectional area by plaque. Thus, in patients dying late after coronary bypass, the atherosclerotic process continues in all segments of the saphenous veins used as aortocoronary conduits. Therapy after the operation must be directed toward prevention or progression of the atherosclerosis in the "new" coronary "arteries."

In the study by Kalan and Roberts (13), the amount of luminal narrowing in the saphenous veins used as aortocoronary conduits was significantly greater in those patients who died of cardiac causes compared with those who died of noncardiac causes. Additionally, the proportion of vein conduits and the proportion of 5-mm segments of the vein conduits that were totally or at least 95% occluded in cross-sectional area were significantly greater in patients who died of cardiac causes compared with those who died of noncardiac causes.

Surprisingly, the interval from CABG to death did not correlate with either the proportion of vein conduits or the proportion of 5-mm segments of vein conduit narrowed more than 75% in cross-sectional area by plaque. The percentage of severely narrowed venous conduits was similar in the 18 conduits (7 patients) that were in place from 13 to 24 months and in the 9 conduits (5 patients) in place for longer than 10 years. Moreover, the proportion of severely narrowed 5-mm segments of saphenous vein conduit was similar in the 35 patients surviving up to 5 years compared with the 18 patients surviving more than 5 years.

Why some saphenous vein conduits became severely narrowed or occluded and others did not may be related more to the status of the native coronary artery containing the graft than to the graft itself. Of the 123 native coronary arteries containing a saphenous vein conduit, 49 (40%) of the arteries distal to the anastomotic site were narrowed more than 75% in cross-sectional area by plaque, and the anastomosed saphenous vein was severely narrowed in 33 (67%) of them. In contrast, of the 74 native coronary arteries narrowed less than 75% distal to the anastomotic site, the attached saphenous vein was severely narrowed in only 14 (19%). Thus, the amount of narrowing in the native coronary artery distal to the anastomotic site plays a major determining role in the fate of the attached saphenous vein.

The composition of the plaques in the saphenous venous conduits was similar to that in the native coronary arteries. Fibrous tissue or fibromuscular tissue was the dominant component of the plaques in the saphenous vein conduits just as it is the dominant component of plaques in the native coronary arteries of patients with fatal CAD who did not undergo CABG. Lipid was present in plaques in saphenous veins in much smaller amounts than was fibrous tissue. Intracellular lipid was found in a saphenous vein as early as 14 months after CABG, and it did not increase in either frequency or amount as the interval from surgery to death increased. Extracellular lipid was first seen at 26 months after CABG, and it did not appear to increase thereafter as the interval from surgery increased. Hemorrhage into plaque, which occurred almost entirely into extracellular lipid deposits (containing cholesterol clefts within pultaceous debris), was first seen at 32 months after CABG. Intraluminal thrombus was found in saphenous veins in 14 patients (26%) and was first observed at 32 months. Thrombus was always superimposed on underlying lipid plaque. Calcific deposits were found in saphenous vein conduits in 11 patients (21%); they were first noted at 34 months after CABG, and calcific deposits did increase in frequency with time.

The frequency of the various modes of death among the patients dying late after CABG is different from that of patients with symptomatic myocardial ischemia who did not have CABG. Of the 53 CABG patients studied, only 32 (60%) died of cardiac causes. Among patients with symptomatic myocardial ischemia who do not have CABG, approximately 95% die of cardiac causes. The fact that 40% of the CABG cases studied died of noncardiac causes supports the view that the CABG operation in many patients prolongs life long enough in many for various fatal noncardiac conditions to develop. Of the 53 CABG patients studied by Kalan and Roberts (13), 10 (19%) died of cancer, a proportion far higher than patients with symptomatic myocardial ischemia not having CABG.

The Kalan and Roberts study reemphasizes that CABG is useful but that it does not deter progression of the underlying atherosclerotic process. In a slight way the CABG operation might even cause acceleration of the atherosclerotic process, in that in about 25% of persons having the surgery, serum total cholesterol and body weight increase substantially during the first year after operation. Because lowering the serum (or plasma) total cholesterol level causes some portion of atherosclerotic plaques to regress and the chances of a subsequent fatal or nonfatal atherosclerotic event to decrease, a strong case can be advanced for combined simultaneous initiation of both low-fat, low-cholesterol diet therapy and lipid-lowering drug therapy as soon as is reasonably feasible after CABG (25).

Morphological Features of Complications of Transmural Acute Myocardial Infarction

Cardiogenic Shock

Cardiogenic shock is the leading cause of death in patients hospitalized for acute MI. Since the advent of coronary care units (CCUs), the frequency of cardiogenic shock in patients with fatal acute MI has at least doubled (40% to about 80%). Necropsy studies have shown important differences in the hearts of patients with acute MI and cardiogenic shock compared with that of patients with acute MI who have died of other complications, such as arrhythmias and emboli. The major differences are the amount of myocardium damaged and the frequency of coronary arterial thrombi. The location of myocardial necrosis bears no relation to the occurrence of cardiogenic shock. Shock occurs with approximately equal frequency in patients with anterior wall MI and in those with posterior wall MI. The size of the MI, in contrast, correlates with the occurrence of shock. Shock is more frequent in patients having large rather than small acute MIs, and myocardial scars are more frequent in patients with cardiogenic shock than in those without. Thus, the total amount of damaged myocardium appears to be more important than the size of the acute MI in determining the occurrence of cardiogenic shock.

To determine the extent of myocardial necrosis and fibrosis, Page et al. (26) studied 20 patients with fatal acute MI and cardiogenic shock and 14 others with fatal acute MI without shock. Of the 20 with acute MI and shock, 19 had lost 40% to 70% of the left ventricular myocardium, and 1 had lost 35%; 13 had combined recent and old MIs and 7 had recent MIs only. Of the 14 patients with acute MI without shock, 12 had lost 30% or less of the left ventricular myocardium, 1 had lost 35%, and 1, 40%; 6 had combined recent and old infarcts, and 8 had recent MIs only. The patients with cardiogenic shock, in contrast to those with MI without shock, had microscopic foci of necrotic myocardial cells at the edges of the infarcts and at other sites in both the left and right ventricles. Similarly, widespread microscopic foci of necrosis were also observed in the hearts of the 20 patients dying of shock not due to acute MI. Thus, cardiogenic shock in acute MI is associated with extensive left ventricular myocardial damage due to recent or to both recent and healed MIs, and additional widespread acute myocardial damage appears to occur secondary to the shock.

A second important feature of cardiogenic shock in acute MI is its association with a high frequency of recent coronary thrombosis. Of 37 patients with fatal acute MI studied by Walston et al. (27), 24 (65%) had cardiogenic shock. No differences between the two groups of patients were observed in extent of coronary atherosclerosis, which was extensive and severe in all but two patients. The frequency of coronary arterial thrombi in the two groups differed greatly: thrombi were found in 17 (71%) of 24 patients with, and in only 2 (15%) of 13 patients without, cardiogenic shock. Of the 37 patients, 19 had coronary arterial thrombi and 17 (90%) had cardiogenic shock; of the 18 patients without thrombi, 7 (39%) had shock. Of the 20 patients with cardiogenic shock, 5 had coronary occlusions from hemorrhage into old atherosclerotic plaques, whereas occlusion due to this mechanism occurred in only 1 of the 13 patients without shock. Thus, 22 (88%) of the 24 patients with cardiogenic shock had coronary occlusions due to thrombus or intramural hemorrhage, whereas only 3 of 13 patients without shock had an acute occlusion. Kurland et al. (28) also studied the association of acute coronary occlusion and cardiogenic shock in fatal acute MI. Of 46 patients with cardiogenic shock, 31 (67%) had acute coronary occlusions; of 81 patients without shock, 39 (48%) had acute coronary occlusions. In the study by Page et al. (26), a high frequency (90%, or 18 of 20 patients) of coronary thrombosis occurred in patients with cardiogenic shock and fatal MI, but a high frequency

(78%, or 11 of 14 patients) was also found in their patients with fatal MI without shock.

In other studies of fatal acute MI, the frequency of coronary arterial thrombosis has varied from 21% to 100% (15). Several factors probably contributed to this variation: (1) the inclusion of cases of subendocardial MI and sudden death ("acute cardiovascular collapse in the absence of myocardial necrosis") with cases of transmural necrosis, (2) the varying frequency of cardiogenic shock in the different studies, and (3) the differing techniques used in studying the coronary vascular tree.

On the basis of the thrombolytic-infusion studies during acute MI, it would appear that the clinical frequency of coronary thrombosis during the infarction is higher than might be discerned from the necropsy studies. Coronary thrombus is diagnosed clinically by injection of contrast material into a coronary artery, finding the lumen to be totally occluded, and, after infusing a thrombolytic agent and injecting contrast material again, finding that the lumen is patent. This sequence clearly suggests that a thrombus was present and that it was dissolved by thrombolysis. Diagnosing thrombus by contrast material, however, is a presumption, and the coronary lumen has become patent during infarction in several patients when saline, rather than a thrombolytic agent, was infused into the occluded coronary artery. Exactly what a 2- or 3-hour-old thrombus looks like is unclear. At this stage, it probably consists mainly or entirely of platelets, and it may or may not be adherent to the intimal lining of the artery. The lack of fibrin and the possible lack of adherence of the thrombus to the intimal lining clearly make the early thrombus quite distinct from the later thrombus. Possibly these early thrombi are missed at necropsy or they dissolve after death.

Papillary Muscle Dysfunction

Recognizing the importance of the left ventricular papillary muscles to closure of the mitral orifice during ventricular systole represented a significant 1960s advance in cardiology (29). Hypoxemia, necrosis, and fibrosis of the left ventricular papillary muscles may be associated with varying degrees of mitral regurgitation. Although coronary atherosclerosis is the most common cause of papillary muscle disease, scarred or necrotic papillary muscles have been observed in a number of conditions in which the coronary arteries were normal. Despite increased awareness of disorders of the papillary muscles, a number of discrepancies indicate that knowledge about these structures is in-

complete. For example, some patients without precordial murmurs during life have been observed at necropsy to have severe necrosis and/or fibrosis of one or both left ventricular papillary muscles. Severe mitral regurgitation during or after acute myocardial infarction has been found at necropsy to be associated with normal papillary muscles, normal mitral leaflets and chordae tendineae, and normal-sized mitral annuli.

Rupture of the Left Ventricular Free Wall and Ventricular Septum

In the period before the introduction of CCUs, the reported frequency of cardiac rupture (of the left ventricular free wall or ventricular septum) among necropsy cases of fatal acute MI varied from 4% to 24% (mean = 8%) (30). Since the introduction of CCUs, the reported frequency has varied from 16% to 21% (mean = 17%). Reddy and Roberts (30) described the frequency of rupture of the left ventricular free wall or ventricular septum in 648 necropsy patients studied by them from 1968 to 1988. Of 648 such patients, 204 (31%) had rupture of the left ventricular free wall or ventricular septum. Rupture occurred in 171 (40%) of 431 patients without healed MI (who did not have grossly visible left ventricular scars) and in 29 (13%) of 217 patients with a healed MI. Thus, the frequency of rupture of the left ventricular free wall or ventricular septum during acute MI appears to have increased substantially since the widespread use of CCUs. Also, the frequency of rupture was nearly three times greater in those in whom rupture occurred during the first acute MI compared to those with a previous MI that had healed.

The reason the frequency of cardiac rupture during acute MI appears to have increased since the widespread use of CCUs is unclear. The most plausible explanation is that the frequency of fatal arrhythmias during acute MI has significantly decreased; if the frequency of one cause of death, namely, arrhythmias, has decreased, another cause of death must increase, and that other cause appears to be cardiac rupture. A much less likely explanation is the increased use of nonsteroidal anti-inflammatory drugs during the past 2 decades. Anecdotal evidence has been presented by one center that patients with acute MI receiving nonsteroidal anti-inflammatory agents for "pericarditis" had a higher frequency of cardiac rupture than did patients who did not receive these drugs during acute MI. Corticosteroid therapy might also increase the frequency of cardiac rupture because these drugs delay the healing process.

It also has been suggested that thrombolytic therapy might increase the frequency of rupture of the left ventricular free wall or ventricular septum during acute MI and that this increase accounts for the higher mortality during the first 24 hours after onset of acute MI compared with patients not treated with thrombolytic agents. Among the 648 necropsy patients studied by Reddy and Roberts (30), 56 (9%) had received either streptokinase or rt-PA during the first few hours after onset of MI: 18 (32%) had rupture of the left ventricular free wall or ventricular septum, a proportion similar to that in the patients who had not received thrombolytic therapy (31%).

Rupture of the Left Ventricular Free Wall

Mann and Roberts (31) compared clinical and necropsy findings in 138 patients (69 men, 69 women) with rupture of the left ventricular free wall during acute MI with those 50 patients who died during their first acute MI without rupture. The frequency of systemic hypertension (55% versus 52%), angina pectoris (13% versus 22%), and congestive heart failure (CHF) (0% versus 0%) before the fatal acute MI was similar for both rupture and nonrupture groups. Mean heart weights for men (479 versus 526 g) and women (399 versus 432 g) with and without rupture were also similar. A left ventricular scar that was present before the MI that ruptured was present in 18 patients (13%); previous necropsy studies of fatal acute MI without rupture indicated that 50% have left ventricular scars. The rupture group had a significantly more frequent lateral wall location of the MI (12% versus 2%). The number of major coronary arteries narrowed more than 75% in cross-sectional area at some point was significantly lower in the rupture group (39% versus 58%). The proportion of the arteries totally occluded more than 95% in cross-sectional area also was significantly less in the rupture group (12% versus 26%). Analysis of each 5-mm long segment of these arteries in each group disclosed that the rupture group had significantly less narrowing than the nonrupture group. Of the 3,287 5-mm segments of artery examined in the rupture group (66 patients), 512 (15%) were narrowed more than 75% in cross-sectional area; in contrast, of the 1,848 5-mm segments in the nonrupture group (38 patients), 508 (28%) were narrowed to this degree. Thus, rupture of the left ventricular free wall is primarily a complication of a patient's first acute

MI and is associated with considerably less amounts of coronary narrowing than fatal acute MI without rupture.

Rupture of the Ventricular Septum

Mann and Roberts (32) studied at necropsy 38 unoperated patients (24 men and 14 women) with an acquired ventricular septal defect during acute MI (rupture group) and compared their clinical and necropsy findings with those in 50 patients who died during their first acute MI without rupture (nonrupture group). The frequency of systemic hypertension (54% versus 52%), angina pectoris (28% versus 22%), and CHF (5% versus 0%) before the fatal acute MI was similar for both rupture and nonrupture groups. Mean heart weights for men (498 versus 526 g) and women (397 versus 432 g) with and without septal rupture also were insignificantly different. Whereas previous studies of fatal acute MI cases have shown that 50% of patients with fatal acute MI without rupture have left ventricular scars, only four (10%) of the rupture cases had a left ventricular scar before the MI that ruptured. The rupture group had a significantly more frequent posterior location of the MI (74% versus 40%) and therefore a higher frequency of associated right ventricular MI (50% versus 18%). The number of major coronary arteries narrowed at some point more than 75% in cross-sectional area from atherosclerotic plaque was the same in both groups. The proportion of arteries totally occluded more than 95% in cross-sectional area was significantly less in the rupture group compared with the nonrupture group (9% versus 26%). Analysis of each 5-mm segment of these arteries in each group disclosed that the rupture group had significantly less narrowing than the nonrupture group. Of the 825 5-mm segments of artery examined in the rupture group (18 patients), only 101 (13%) were narrowed more than 75% in cross-sectional area. In contrast, of the 1,848 5-mm segments in the nonrupture group (38 patients), 508 (28%) were narrowed to this degree. Thus, rupture of the ventricular septum is primarily a complication of the first acute MI. It is associated with less severe coronary arterial narrowing than is observed in fatal acute MI without rupture, and it is a more frequent complication of posterior (inferior) than anterior wall acute MI.

Mann and Roberts (33) also described cardiac morphological findings in 16 necropsy patients having operative closure of an acquired ventricular septal defect during acute MI. Of the 16 patients,

6 were women (mean age = 60 ± 7 years) and 10 were men (mean age = 60 ± 11 years). The acute MI associated with the ventricular septal defect was the first coronary event in 13 patients (81%). At least 6 patients had a history of systemic hypertension. Conduction disturbances were diagnosed by electrocardiogram (ECG) in 5 patients (31%). The median interval from the onset of the acute MI to death was 11 days, and from the onset of the acute MI to operative closure of the ventricular septal defect, 4 days. Eight patients died in the operating room or within 2 hours of operation. CABG was performed simultaneously with the ventricular septal defect closure in 7 patients. Death was attributed to unsuccessful ventricular septal defect closure in 5 patients, to an inadequate left ventricular cavity after resection of necrotic myocardium in 5 patients, and to inadequate viable left ventricular myocardium in 4 patients. Heart weights were increased in 14 patients (88%). The acute MI associated with the ventricular septal defect was anterior in 9 patients and posterior (inferior) in 7. Healed MIs were present in 3 patients. All 16 patients had severe narrowing of one or more of the major coronary arteries.

On rare occasions, both the ventricular septum and the left ventricular free wall may rupture (double rupture) during acute MI. Such was the case in 7 necropsy patients described by Mann and Roberts (34).

True Left Ventricular Aneurysm

Some left ventricular wall motion abnormality—hypokinesia, akinesia, or dyskinesia—occurs at the time of transmural acute MI. After healing of the MI, a few patients are left with focal convex left ventricular protrusions, some during ventricular systole only (functional aneurysm) and some during both ventricular systole and diastole (anatomic aneurysm) (35). Cabin and Roberts (36) analyzed clinical and necropsy findings in 28 patients with true anatomic aneurysms at sites of healed left ventricular MI. Twenty-four of the 28 patients were men, a greater sex difference than in other subsets of CAD patients. Also, in contrast to other subsets of CAD patients, chronic congestive cardiac failure was frequent (22 patients); angina pectoris was infrequent (4 patients) and when present was of a mild degree; recurrence of acute MI (2 patients), sudden death (2 patients), and clinical events compatible with systemic emboli (one patient) were infrequent; survival for longer than 5 years after

healing of the MI was limited (in 3 of 21 patients with clinically diagnosed MI); and survival for longer than 12 months after aneurysmectomy was lacking (none of 7 patients). Additionally, most patients (23 of 28) had large hearts (> 400 g [mean = 523 g]), 26 had dilated nonaneurysmal portions of the left ventricle, and all but 1 had large (> 30% of left ventricular wall) MIs.

Thus, from studies of necropsy patients with true anatomic left ventricular aneurysms and healed MIs, the following conclusions appear justified:

- The MIs are large.
- The cardiac weights are increased, and non-scarred left ventricular walls hypertrophied.
- The nonaneurysmal portions of the left ventricular cavities are dilated.
- The major epicardial coronary arteries are severely narrowed.
- Chronic CHF is frequent and is the most common cause of death.
- Angina pectoris is infrequent, as is recurrence of acute MI.
- Clinical events compatible with systemic emboli are infrequent despite frequent intra-aneurysmal thrombus.
- The long-term prognosis is poor.
- Sudden death is infrequent.
- The clinical diagnosis of the left ventricular aneurysm without left ventricular angiography or echocardiography is infrequent, despite the high (up to 20%) occurrence in cases with MI at autopsy examination.

Atherosclerotic Coronary Artery Disease, Healed Myocardial Infarction Without Aneurysm, and Chronic Congestive Heart Failure

Ross and Roberts (37) described clinical and necropsy findings in 81 patients (aged 29 to 91 years [mean = 62 years]; 77 [95%] men) with severe CHF of more than 3 months in duration, left ventricular transmural scar, and cross-sectional–area narrowing of more than 75% by atherosclerotic plaque of one of the major coronary arteries. The duration of symptoms from initial onset of acute MI (59 patients), CHF (18 patients), or angina pectoris (2 patients) to death ranged from 0.5 to 18 years (mean = 7.1 years); the duration for 2 patients was unknown. Angina pectoris occurred at some time, however, in 31 patients (38%). The mode of death was CHF in 48 patients (59%), sudden (arrhythmia) in 16 (20%), acute MI in 11 (14%), and emboli in 6 (7%). The heart weight ranged from 410 to 800 g (mean = 585 g). Left or right ventricular thrombi or both occurred in 37 patients (46%), only 4 (10%) of whom had systemic emboli; of the 44 patients without intracardiac thrombi, none had any form of emboli. The severity of coronary narrowing was variable. In 24 patients (30%), only one artery was narrowed more than 75% in cross-sectional area; in 22 patients (27%), two arteries were so narrowed; in 32 patients (39%), three arteries; and in three patients (4%), four arteries. The size of the left ventricular scar also varied. Of the 81 patients, 58 (72%) had large scars (involving more than 40% of the left ventricular wall); 10 (12%) had moderate-sized scars (6% to 40% of the wall); and 13 (16%) had small scars (≤ 5% of the wall). The size of the left ventricular scar correlated with a history of habitual alcoholism: of the 16 habitual alcoholics, 6 (38%) had small and 8 (50%) had large left ventricular scars; of the 65 non-alcoholics, 7 (11%) had small and 50 (77%) had large left ventricular scars. Chronic CHF in the 68 patients with either moderate- or large-sized left ventricular scars is readily attributed to the left ventricular damage. In the 13 patients with small left ventricular scars, however, chronic CHF more reasonably may be attributed to another factor, such as alcoholism, despite coronary artery narrowing similar in severity to that seen in the patients with large left ventricular scars.

Atherosclerotic Coronary Artery Disease, Chronic Congestive Heart Failure, Without Myocardial Infarction

Ross and Roberts (38) described clinical and necropsy findings in 18 patients (aged 38 to 73 years [mean = 58 years]; 16 [89%] men) studied at necropsy who had had chronic CHF of more than 3 months in duration, greater than 75% cross-sectional area narrowing of one or more of the major coronary arteries, and no left ventricular fibrosis or necrosis. The duration of symptoms from onset of CHF to death ranged from 0.3 to 13 years (mean 5.7 years). Angina pectoris occurred in two patients (11%). The cause of death was CHF in 12 (67%), sudden death (arrhythmia) in 5 (28%), and emboli in 1 (5%). Heart weight ranged from 410 to 890 g (mean = 632 g). Of 72 major coronary

arteries in the 18 patients, 30 (42%) were narrowed 76% to 100% in cross-sectional area (1.7 per patient). Left and right ventricular thrombi were found in 9 patients (50%); of these, 1 had a systemic embolus; of the 9 patients without intraventricular thrombi, none had systemic emboli. Because grossly visible myocardial lesions were absent, the severe chronic CHF in the 18 patients cannot reasonably be attributed to CAD. It is most reasonable to believe that this group of patients had idiopathic dilated cardiomyopathy and that the CAD was coincidental.

Right Ventricular Infarction

Acute MI secondary to coronary arterial narrowing virtually always involves the left ventricular free wall and often also the ventricular septum. Involvement of the right ventricular free wall secondary to coronary luminal narrowing has, until recently, rarely been diagnosed clinically, and few morphologic studies have focused on its frequency or extent. Infarctions were previously found in the right ventricle of 14% of autopsied patients with MI (39). Isner and Roberts (40) examined the frequency of right ventricular infarction in patients with associated transmural left ventricular infarction and determined its extent and relation to the accompanying location of the infarct of the left ventricular wall.

A total of 236 necropsy patients with transmural acute MI of the left ventricular wall were studied. The patients were divided into two groups: those with transmural myocardial necrosis (acute MI) and those with transmural myocardial fibrosis (healed MI). When both fibrosis and necrosis were grossly visible in the same heart (34 patients), which was more extensive determined the patient's category. The hearts then were further subdivided by location of the left ventricular infarction into two additional groups: anterior wall and posterior wall.

Of the 236 patients, 116 had acute and 120 had healed left ventricular MI. The MI involved the anterior wall in 97 patients and the posterior wall in the other 139. Of the 97 patients with anterior left ventricular infarction (acute in 56 [40%] and healed in 83 [60%]), 33 (24%) had associated right ventricular infarction. Of the total 236 patients, 133 had transmural infarction of the ventricular septum, 68 had anterior left ventricular infarction, and 65 had posterior left ventricular infarction. All 33 patients with a right ventricular infarction were also in the group of 65 patients with a posterior left ventricular infarction, associated with transmural infarction of the ventricular septum. Of the 74 patients with posterior left ventricular infarction without associated transmural infarction of the ventricular septum, none had right ventricular infarction. Among the patients with isolated anterior wall left ventricular infarcts, irrespective of whether the ventricular septum was involved, none had associated right ventricular infarcts. The right ventricular wall was hypertrophied (> 5 mm thick) in only 1 of the 33 patients, whereas right ventricular dilatation was present in 12. Right ventricular thrombus occurred in 3 patients. The infarct of the right ventricle was limited to its posterior wall (Type I or II) in 36 patients and to both posterior and anterolateral right ventricular free walls (Types III and IV) in the other 7.

Comparison of the 33 patients who had posterior left ventricular wall infarction with associated right ventricular wall infarction with the 106 patients who had posterior wall left ventricular wall infarction but without associated right ventricular wall infarction disclosed no significant differences in the patients' age, sex, length of survival after onset of symptoms of myocardial ischemia, or the presence of right ventricular hypertrophy or thrombosis. Right ventricular dilatation, however, was significantly more frequent among the group with posterior left ventricular infarction with associated right ventricular wall infarction.

The major coronary arteries were examined in detail in 87 (63%) of the 139 patients with left ventricular posterior wall infarcts. Twenty-eight of them had associated right ventricular infarcts and 59 did not. No significant differences among the patients with posterior left ventricular infarcts were observed in the percentage of cross-sectional–area luminal narrowing greater than 75% due to old atherosclerotic plaques in each of the major coronary arteries between patients with versus without right ventricular infarcts. The degree of narrowing of the right coronary artery was similar in the patients with and without right ventricular infarcts. The proportion of patients in whom the right coronary artery was narrowed 76% to 100% in cross-sectional area by old atherosclerotic plaque was significantly greater than those in whom the left anterior descending coronary artery was narrowed to this degree, irrespective of whether or not the infarction involved the right ventricular wall.

Among patients with a fatal MI secondary to severe coronary arterial luminal narrowing, right ventricular infarction occurred only when the left ventricular infarct involved its posterior wall. Of the 139 patients with posterior left ventricular infarcts, 33 (24%) had associated right ventricular infarcts. Even among the patients with posteriorly located left ventricular infarcts, however, transmural infarction of the ventricular septum was a prerequisite for development of right ventricular infarction. Of the 139 patients with posterior left ventricular infarcts, 74 did not have transmural infarction of the ventricular septum and none had associated right ventricular infarction. Of the 65 with transmural infarction of the ventricular septum, 33 (50%) had associated right ventricular infarction. Thus, right ventricular infarction was a complication exclusively of transmural posterior left ventricular infarction.

Right ventricular hypertrophy was not an important predisposing factor for the development of right ventricular MI but rather was more frequent among the patients without associated right ventricular MI. Right ventricular hypertrophy was observed at necropsy in only 1 (3%) of the 33 patients with right ventricular MI and in 12 (6%) of the 203 patients with left ventricular MI unassociated with right ventricular MI. Furthermore, none had necropsy evidence of cor pulmonale. Although extensive right ventricular scarring has been described in various entities associated with right ventricular hypertrophy (including chronic pulmonary emboli and hypertrophic cardiomyopathy in the absence of significant coronary arterial luminal narrowing), Isner and Roberts excluded such cases unless they were associated with left ventricular scarring and significant coronary arterial luminal narrowing. Right ventricular dilatation was the single anatomic feature distinguishing the patients with right ventricular MI from those without it. Among the 139 patients with posterior wall left ventricular MIs, the right ventricular cavities were dilated in 21 (36%) of the 33 patients with and in 10 (9%) of 106 patients without associated right ventricular MIs. Right ventricular dilatation occurred in only 16 (16%) of the 97 patients with anterior wall left ventricular MI, a significantly lower proportion than in the patients with right ventricular MI.

Right ventricular mural thrombus is another necropsy finding reported to be more frequent among patients with associated right ventricular wall MI than in patients with isolated left ventricular wall MI. In the 237 patients with left ventricular wall MI, however, right ventricular thrombi occurred with similar frequency in those with and in those without associated infarction of the right ventricular wall.

Among the patients with posterior wall left ventricular MIs, the proportion with 76% to 100% cross-sectional–area luminal narrowing of the right coronary artery was similar (about 90%) in the patients with compared with those without right ventricular infarcts. All patients with right ventricular MI had severe luminal narrowing of the dominant coronary artery; that is, either the right or the left circumflex that was responsible for perfusing the posterior ventricular wall.

Diagnosis during life of a right ventricular MI in patients with left ventricular MI secondary to severe coronary arterial luminal narrowing is, at best, difficult. If the left ventricular MI is isolated to the anterior wall, the chance of an associated right ventricular MI is minimal. Thus, a posterior location of the left ventricular MI is a prerequisite for right ventricular MI. Nearly one-quarter of patients with a posterior wall MI of the left ventricle had an associated right ventricular MI. If, however, the ventricular septum is transmurally infarcted, the frequency of associated right ventricular MI doubles (becomes 50%). One finding suggestive of right ventricular MI is right ventricular dilatation, an occurrence nearly three times more frequent in patients with right ventricular MI than in those without. Right ventricular hypertrophy is rare in patients with right ventricular MI secondary to coronary narrowing and is, therefore, not helpful from a diagnostic standpoint.

Before the introduction of newer noninvasive techniques, especially myocardial imaging, clinical validation of right ventricular MI was limited to cardiac catheterization. The finding of elevated right atrial (or right ventricular end-diastolic) pressure has been suggested as the characteristic hemodynamic profile of right ventricular MI. Three of the 4 patients studied by Isner and Roberts with necropsy-confirmed right ventricular MI had hemodynamic profiles that were not suggestive of associated right ventricular MI. The hemodynamic profile previously considered characteristic of right ventricular MI is less diagnostically sensitive than previously believed, and right ventricular MI may still occur in the presence of normal or near-normal intracardiac pressures. Conversely, in the absence of pericardial or valvular heart disease, the hemodynamic abnormalities described for right ventricular MI appear to be relatively specific.

Cumulative clinical experience with right ventricular MI complicating left ventricular MI has clearly established the existence of a specific hemodynamic syndrome of right ventricular dysfunction, characterized by underfilling of the left ventricle as a result of impaired right ventricular contractility. In patients with this syndrome right ventricular dilatation is the sole compensatory mechanism by which right ventricular contractility may be augmented. Under such circumstances, volume administration may be critical to maintain an optimal right ventricular filling pressure. Indeed, supplemental fluid administration in patients with elevated right-sided pressures and a normal or near-normal left ventricular filling pressure (i.e., patients with right ventricular MI) has produced marked hemodynamic improvement. Thus, it is important to recognize clues to the often occult syndrome of right ventricular dysfunction or right ventricular MI. Evidence of an inferior wall MI combined with the evidence of right ventricular dilatation should make one particularly suspicious of the presence of right ventricular MI.

Modes of Death in Fatal Atherosclerotic Coronary Artery Disease

Roberts et al. (41) described the mode of death; frequency of a healed or an acute MI, or both; number of major coronary arteries severely narrowed by atherosclerotic plaque; and heart weight at necropsy in 889 patients 30 years of age or older with fatal atherosclerotic CAD. No patient had undergone CABG or PTCA. The 889 patients were classified into four major groups, with each major group classified into two subgroups: (1) acute MI without (306 patients) or with (119 patients) a healed MI, (2) sudden out-of-hospital death without (121 patients) or with (118 patients) a healed MI, (3) chronic CHF with a healed MI and without (137 patients) or with (33 patients) a left ventricular aneurysm, and (4) sudden in-hospital death without (20 patients) or with (35 patients) unstable angina pectoris.

The mean age of the 687 men (77%) was 60 ± 11 years and of the 202 women (23%), 68 ± 13 years. Although men included 77% of all patients, they made up approximately 90% of the out-of-hospital (nonangina) sudden death group. The frequency of systemic hypertension and angina pectoris was similar in each of the four major groups. The frequency of diabetes mellitus was least in the sudden out-of-hospital death group and similar in the other three groups.

The mean heart weight and the percent of patients with a heart of increased weight were highest in the chronic CHF group; values were lower and similar in the other three groups. All patients in the chronic CHF group (by definition) had a healed left ventricular MI, which was similar in frequency in the other three groups. The proportion of patients in whom three or four of the 4 major coronary arteries were severely narrowed was highest in the unstable angina subgroup and similar in all other major groups.

Of the 437 patients (49%) with one or more grossly visible left ventricular scars, the fatal coronary event in 119 (27%) was an acute MI; in 118 patients (27%) it was sudden out-of-hospital (or nearly so) cardiac arrest; in 170 patients (39%) it was chronic, intractable CHF; and in 30 patients (7%) it was sudden in-hospital death with or without preceding unstable angina pectoris. Of the 452 patients (51%) without a grossly visible left ventricular scar, the fatal coronary event in 306 (68%) was an acute MI; in 121 patients (27%) it was sudden out-of-hospital cardiac arrest; and in 25 patients (5%) it was sudden in-hospital cardiac arrest with or without preceding unstable angina pectoris. Thus, the patients without a previous acute MI were more likely (nearly 70%) to die from an acute MI, and the fatal events in the patients with a previous acute MI were more or less equally divided among the subgroups with fatal acute MI, sudden out-of-hospital cardiac arrest, and chronic CHF.

One of the tragedies of CAD is the relative youth of its victims. The average age at death was roughly 10 years less than the average life expectancy for men and women in the United States (42).

Although many reports have described findings at necropsy in patients with CAD, it is difficult and often meaningless to compare the present data with those reported in earlier decades. These comparisons are probably not useful for several reasons (one exception will be described later).

- Older reports contain outdated cardiac terms that were never defined or imprecisely defined.
- Older reports contain different inclusion and exclusion criteria.
- Older reports report relatively few cases.
- Older reports have data collected by numerous physicians with little expertise in cardiovascular disease versus data collected by a single or relatively few individuals who specialize in cardiovascular disease.
- The treatment of patients usually differs from one time period to another, and the different treatments may alter frequency in the various modes of death and necropsy cardiac findings.

The Rochester, Minnesota Study

A superb study of the modes of death from CAD and of cardiac findings at necropsy in its victims was reported by Spiekerman et al. (43). Their study analyzed deaths of residents in a single community (Rochester, Minnesota) during a 5-year period, 1947 to 1952. During that period, 1,026 persons (50% women, 50% men) aged 20 years or older died, and necropsy was performed in 691 (67%). Of the 1,026 patients, 563 (55%) died in the hospital and autopsy was done in 377 (67%), and 463 (45%) died outside the hospital and necropsy was done in 314 (68%). Of the 691 patients aged 20 years or over studied at necropsy, 221 (32%) had died from CAD (40% of the men and 22% of the women). Of the patients aged 30 to 64 years, 54% had died from CAD, and in the age group 65 years or older, 38% had died from CAD. In this study, the modes of death in the 221 patients with fatal CAD were as follows: "acute coronary failure" (sudden death), 94 patients (43%); acute MI, 87 patients (39%); CHF, 32 patients (14%); and "thromboembolism," 8 patients (4%). A healed MI was seen at necropsy in 115 (52%) of the 221 patients, a proportion virtually identical to that of the study by Roberts et al. (41).

Association Between Heart Weight and Coronary Artery Disease

Cardiomegaly (heart weight > 400 g in men and > 350 g in women) occurred in 80% of the 889 patients studied by Roberts et al. (41). The average heart weight in the men was 505 g and in the women, 427 g. Of the 170 patients with CHF, 162 (95%) had a heart of increased weight; in contrast, of the 239 patients who died suddenly outside the hospital, 178 (74%) had a heart of increased weight. Of all 889 patients, only 20% had a heart of normal weight.

References

1. Roberts, W.C. Qualitative and quantitative comparison amounts of narrowing by atherosclerotic plaques in the major epicardial coronary arteries at necropsy in sudden coronary death, transmural acute myocardial infarction, transmural healed myocardial infarction and unstable angina pectoris. Am. J. Cardiol. 64:324-328; 1989.
2. Roberts, W.C.; Jones, A.A. Quantitation of coronary arterial narrowing at necropsy in sudden coronary

death. Analysis of 31 patients and comparison with 25 control subjects. Am. J. Cardiol. 44:39-45; 1979.

3. Roberts, W.C.; Jones, A.A. Quantification of coronary arterial narrowing at necropsy in acute transmural myocardial infarction. Analysis and comparison of findings in 27 patients and 22 controls. Circulation. 61:786-790; 1980.

4. Virmani, R.; Roberts, W.C. Non-fatal healed transmural myocardial infarction and fatal noncardiac disease. Qualification and quantification of coronary arterial narrowing and of left ventricular scarring in 18 necropsy patients. Br. Heart J. 45:434-441; 1981.

5. Virmani, R.; Roberts, W.C. Quantification of coronary arterial narrowing and of left ventricular myocardial scarring in healed myocardial infarction with chronic eventually fatal congestive cardiac failure. Am. J. Med. 68:831-838; 1980.

6. Cabin, H.S.; Roberts, W.C. True left ventricular aneurysm and healed myocardial infarction. Clinical and necropsy observations including quantification of degree of coronary arterial narrowing. Am. J. Cardiol. 46:754-763; 1980.

7. Roberts, W.C.; Virmani, R. Quantification of coronary arterial narrowing in clinically isolated unstable angina pectoris. An analysis of 22 necropsy patients. Am. J. Med. 67:792-799; 1979.

8. Bulkley, B.M.; Roberts, W.C. Atherosclerotic narrowing of the left main coronary artery. A necropsy analysis of 152 patients with fatal coronary heart disease and varying degrees of left main narrowing. Circulation. 53:823-828; 1976.

9. Isner, J.M.; Wu, M.; Virmani, R.; Jones, A.A.; Roberts, W.C. Comparison of degrees of coronary arterial luminal narrowing determined by visual inspection of histologic sections under magnification among three independent observers and comparison to that obtained by video planimetry. An analysis of 559 five-mm segments of 61 coronary arteries from eleven patients. Lab. Invest. 42:566-570; 1980.

10. Arnett, E.N.; Isner, J.M.; Redwood, D.R.; Kent, K.M.; Baker, W.P.; Ackerstein, M.; Roberts, W.C. Coronary artery narrowing in coronary heart disease: Comparison of cineangiographic and necropsy findings. Ann. Intern. Med. 91:350-356; 1979.

11. Isner, J.M.; Kishel, J.; Kent, K.M.; Ronan, J.A., Jr.; Ross, A.M.; Roberts, W.C. Accuracy of angiographic determination of left main coronary arterial narrowing. Angiographic-histologic correlative analysis in 28 patients. Circulation. 63:1056-1064; 1981.

12. Waller, B.F.; Roberts, W.C. Amount of narrowing by atherosclerotic plaque in 44 nonbypassed and 52 bypassed major epicardial coronary arteries in 32 necropsy patients who died within 1 month of aortocoronary bypass grafting. Am. J. Cardiol. 46:956-962; 1980.

13. Kalan, J.M.; Roberts, W.C. Morphologic findings in saphenous veins used as coronary arterial bypass conduits for longer than 1 year: Necropsy analysis of 53 patients, 123 saphenous veins, and 1865 five-mm segments of veins. Am. Heart J. 119:1164-1184; 1990.

14. Wartman, W.B.; Hellerstein, H.K. The incidence of heart disease in 2000 consecutive autopsies. Ann. Intern. Med. 28:41; 1948.

15. Roberts, W.C.; Buja, L.M. The frequency and significance of coronary arterial thrombi and other observations in fatal acute myocardial infarction. A study of 107 necropsy patients. Am. J. Med. 52:425-443; 1972.

16. Kragel, A.H.; Gertz, S.D.; Roberts, W.C. Morphologic comparison of frequency and types of acute lesions in the major epicardial coronary arteries in unstable angina pectoris, sudden coronary death, and acute myocardial infarction. J. Am. Coll. Cardiol. 18:801-808; 1991.

17. Herrick, J.B. Thrombosis of the coronary arteries. JAMA. 72:387; 1919.

18. Brosius, F.C., III; Roberts, W.C. Significance of coronary arterial thrombus in transmural acute myocardial infarction. A study of 54 necropsy patients. Circulation. 63:810-816; 1981.

19. Roberts, W.C. Coronary embolism. A review of causes, consequences, and diagnostic considerations. Cardiovasc. Med. 3:699-710; 1978.

20. Gertz, S.D.; Kalan, J.M.; Kragel, A.H.; Roberts, W.C.; Braunwald, E.; The TIMI Investigators. Cardiac morphologic findings in patients with acute myocardial infarction treated with recombinant tissue plasminogen activator. Am. J. Cardiol. 65:953-961; 1990.

21. Gertz, S.D.; Kragel, A.H.; Kalan, J.M.; Braunwald, E.; Roberts, W.C.; The TIMI Investigators. Comparison of coronary and myocardial morphologic findings in patients with and without thrombolytic therapy during fatal first acute myocardial infarction. Am. J. Cardiol. 66:904-909; 1990.

22. Kragel, A.H.; Reddy, S.G.; Wittes, J.T.; Roberts, W.C. Morphometric analysis of the composition of atherosclerotic plaques in the four major epicardial coronary arteries in acute myocardial infarction and in sudden coronary death. Circulation. 80:1747-1756; 1989.

23. Kragel, A.H.: Reddy, S.G.; Wittes, J.T.; Roberts, W.C. Morphometric analysis of the composition of coronary arterial plaques in isolated unstable angina pectoris with pain at rest. Am. J. Cardiol. 66:562-567; 1990.

24. Potkin, B.N.; Roberts, W.C. Location of an acute myocardial infarct in patients with a healed myocardial infarct: Analysis of 129 patients studied at necropsy. Am. J. Cardiol. 62:1017-1023; 1988.

25. Roberts, W.C. Lipid-lowering therapy after an atherosclerotic event. Am. J. Cardiol. 65:16F-18F; 1990.

26. Page, D.L.; Caufield, J.B.; Kastor, J.A.; DeSanctis, R.W.; Sanders, C.A. Myocardial changes associated with cardiogenic shock. N. Engl. J. Med. 285:133; 1971.

27. Walston, A.; Hackel, D.B.; Estes, H.E. Acute coronary occlusion and the "power failure" syndrome. Am. Heart J. 79:613; 1970.

28. Kurland, G.S.; Weingarten, C.; Pitt, B. The relation between the location of coronary occlusions and the occurrence of shock in acute myocardial infarction. Circulation. 31:646; 1965.

29. Roberts, W.C.; Cohen, L. Left ventricular papillary muscles. Description of the normal and a survey of conditions causing them to be abnormal. Circulation. 46:138-154; 1972.

30. Reddy, S.G.; Roberts, W.C. Frequency of rupture of the left ventricular free wall or ventricular septum among necropsy cases of fatal acute myocardial infarction since introduction of coronary care units. Am. J. Cardiol. 63:906-911; 1989.

31. Mann, J.M.; Roberts, W.C. Rupture of the left ventricular free wall during acute myocardial infarction: Analysis of 138 necropsy patients and comparison with 50 necropsy patients with acute myocardial infarction without rupture. Am. J. Cardiol. 62:847-859; 1988.

32. Mann, J.M.; Roberts, W.C. Acquired ventricular septal defect during acute myocardial infarction: Analysis of 38 unoperated necropsy patients and comparison with 50 unoperated necropsy patients without rupture. Am. J. Cardiol. 62:8-19; 1988.

33. Mann, J.M.; Roberts, W.C. Cardiac morphologic observations after operative closure of acquired ventricular septal defect during acute myocardial infarction: Analysis of 16 necropsy patients. Am. J. Cardiol. 60:981-987; 1987.

34. Mann, J.M.; Roberts, W.C. Fatal rupture of both left ventricular free wall and ventricular septum (double rupture) during acute myocardial infarction: Analysis of seven patients studied at necropsy. Am. J. Cardiol. 60:722-724; 1987.

35. Cabin, H.S.; Roberts, W.C. Left ventricular aneurysm, intraaneurysmal throbus and systemic embolus in coronary heart disease. Chest. 77:586-590; 1980.

36. Cabin, H.S.; Roberts, W.C. True left ventricular aneurysm and healed myocardial infarction. Clinical and necropsy observations including quantification of degrees of coronary arterial narrowing. Am. J. Cardiol. 46:754-763; 1980.

37. Ross, E.M.; Roberts, W.C. Severe atherosclerotic coronary artery disease, healed myocardial infarction and chronic congestive heart failure: Analysis of 81 patients studied at necropsy. Am. J. Cardiol. 57:44-50; 1986.

38. Ross, E.M.; Roberts, W.C. Severe atherosclerotic coronary arterial narrowing and chronic congestive heart failure without myocardial infarction: Analysis of 18 patients studied at necropsy. Am. J. Cardiol. 57:51-56; 1986.

39. Wartman, W.B.; Hellerstein, H.K. The incidence of heart disease in 2000 consecutive autopsies. Ann. Intern. Med. 28:41; 1948.

40. Isner, J.M.; Roberts, W.C. Right ventricular infarction complicating left ventricular infarction secondary to coronary heart disease. Frequency, location, associated findings and significance from analysis of 236 necropsy patients with acute or healed myocardial infarction. Am. J. Cardiol. 42:885-894; 1978.

41. Roberts, W.C.; Potkin, B.N.; Solus, D.E.; Reddy, S.G. Mode of death, frequency of healed and acute myocardial infarction, number of major epicardial coronary arteries severely narrowed by atherosclerotic plaque, and heart weight in fatal atherosclerotic coronary artery disease: Analysis of 889 patients studied at necropsy. Am. J. Cardiol. 15:196-203; 1990.

42. Roberts, W.C.; Kragel, A.H.; Potkin, B.N. Ages at death and sex distribution in age decade in fatal coronary artery disease. Am. J. Cardiol. 66:1379-1381; 1990.

43. Spiekerman, R.E.; Brandenburg, J.T.; Anchor, R.W.P.; Edwards, J.E. The spectrum of coronary heart disease in a community of 30,000. A clinicopathologic study. Circulation. 25:57-65; 1962.

Chapter 3

Biobehavioral Aspects of Coronary Artery Disease: Considerations for Prognosis and Treatment

Rachel E. Burnett
James A. Blumenthal

The roles of behavioral, psychological, and social factors have become increasingly recognized in the etiology, course, and treatment of coronary artery disease (CAD). We review here evidence for the importance of these factors to prognosis and treatment in patients with CAD. We consider first the prognostic value of traditional medical variables and then review biobehavioral variables as predictors of health outcomes. Finally, we address the therapeutic value of psychological and behavioral interventions, including exercise, modification of Type A behavior, and stress management.

Medical Predictors of Prognosis After Myocardial Infarction

Health professionals use a variety of medical procedures for determining prognosis in the post–myocardial infarction (MI) patient; each contributes different information with various degrees of prognostic value. The most accurate prognosis is one that considers all predictive variables, although certain measures carry more weight than others.

Although this chapter focuses on the post-MI patient, this section reviews those physiological factors relevant to the prognosis of CAD patients in general. Although CAD is used here as a broad term, there are significant differences in the severity, extent, and location of lesions in the coronary arteries, as well as in the amount of damage to the myocardium. This information also should be considered in making prognostic estimates.

Prognostic Variables From Clinical Assessment

In terms of the predictive information elicited from clinical assessment, six prognostic variables have emerged as significant in at least two of seven major studies (Coronary Artery Surgery Study, Cleveland Clinic Registry, Duke University Database, European Coronary Surgery Study, Life Insurance studies, Seattle Heart Watch Registry, and Veterans Administration Cooperative Trial) (1). These variables are age, gender, cardiac risk factors, pain and ischemic symptoms, myocardial damage, and peripheral vascular disease (PVD).

In these studies, increased age was associated with a worsened prognosis in patients with established CAD. Castello et al. (2) suggest, however, that although age is an independent prognostic factor for late mortality when any degree of heart failure is present, elderly patients cannot be considered a homogeneous group of high risk patients. Among elderly CAD patients, there are high- and low-risk subgroups based on clinical variables present at the time of the MI, such as gender; the presence of diabetes mellitus, elevated cholesterol, or high blood pressure; more than two risk factors; a history of angina; and a history of a previous MI.

Gender appeared only marginally important in establishing a prognosis in the seven major studies listed. Separate data from Dittrich et al. (3) indicate that gender had no independent predictive value when variables that included age, congestive heart failure (CHF) in the hospital, history of CHF, prior MI, and diabetes were considered.

Traditional cardiac risk factors, such as smoking, hypercholesterolemia, hypertension, and diabetes, are considered to be more important in the development of CAD than in the prognosis of patients with established disease (1). However, in a follow-up of the Framingham Study, Wong et al. (4) found that the standard risk factors, particularly elevated systolic blood pressure (BP), elevated serum cholesterol, and diabetes, remained important predictors of long-term prognosis in post-MI patients.

Another prognostic variable studied in initial clinical assessment is angina. Chronic symptoms of angina suggest the presence of established CAD and a worsened prognosis. This finding is supported by Yeung et al. (5) in a study in which post-MI patients with symptomatic ischemia had a worse prognosis than patients without symptoms. Fioretti et al. (6), however, concluded that exercise-induced angina does not identify patients with a worsened prognosis at 4 years post-MI. However, there are numerous problems with relying on symptoms to make a diagnosis. Most episodes of ischemia are painless ("silent" ischemia), and the presence of symptoms is not necessarily indicative of ischemia.

Prognostic Variables From Noninvasive Tests

In addition to data obtained from clinical assessment, several noninvasive tests appear to contribute important prognostic information. Exercise testing, for one, is a frequently used and widely studied measure of cardiac function. Maximal exercise capacity, increases in systolic BP, heart rate (HR) responses, and ST-segment displacement appear to be the most important prognostic variables provided by exercise tests (6-8). The usefulness of exercise testing for determining prognosis has also been supported by Pilote et al. (9), who found that treadmill exercise testing at 1 month post-MI was a significant predictor of death or reinfarction among patients with a low left ventricular ejection fraction (LVEF). This finding is also supported in a study by Kishida et al. (10), in which a reduced duration of exercise and asymptomatic ST-segment changes during low-level exercise testing helped determine short-term prognosis after MI. Although exercise testing appears to add important prognostic information to that gained in clinical assessment, it offers relatively little prognostic value compared with data obtained by cardiac catheterization (1).

Nuclear studies, such as radionuclide angiography (RNA) and thallium scintigraphy, represent another class of noninvasive testing procedures. The LVEF measured during RNA seems to be the single most important prognostic variable obtained. For example, in an investigation of the prognostic value of RNA in medically treated CAD patients compared with clinical and catheterization variables, Lee et al. (11) found that a low exercise LVEF was the most important RNA variable for predicting cardiovascular mortality in uni-

variate analysis and that exercise LVEF, change in HR with exercise, and end-diastolic volume index at rest were the most important RNA variables for mortality prediction in multivariate analysis. In addition, Lee et al. determined that RNA alone contributed 84% of the information provided by clinical and catheterization variables combined.

Because RNA studies characterize the functional significance of underlying coronary artery stenoses, RNA also contributes significant prognostic information beyond that of clinical assessment and catheterization. In studying the relative value of various testing techniques, de Belder et al. (12) compared clinical, exercise test, and angiographic variables. They found clinical and angiographic variables were more powerful predictors of mortality than submaximal exercise testing, but they emphasized the importance of exercise testing because it also is used to select patients for angiography.

Perfusion defects, degree of hypoperfusion, and lung thallium uptake are the most important prognostic variables in thallium scintigraphy (1). RNA and thallium scintigraphy appear to make similar contributions to prognosis. Miller et al. (13) found, however, that for patients with two-vessel disease, survival correlates with exercise thallium-201 uptake but was not predicted by MI or anginal history; resting left ventricular function (LVF); exercise BP response; angina or ST-segment depression; thallium-201 defect size, redistribution, or clearance; angiographic patterns; or the presence of proximal left anterior descending disease. Thus, there is some disagreement over the relative value of RNA and thallium scintigraphy for predicting prognosis in CAD patients.

Another noninvasive procedure, ambulatory electrocardiographic (ECG) monitoring, has been widely used with acute MI and angina patients to assess ST-segment depression and detect arrhythmias. Two large observational studies (14,15) show that frequent premature ventricular contractions (PVCs) in post-MI patients are predictive of worsened prognosis, independent of LVF. Cleland et al. (16) found a similar correlation in patients with CHF, but this correlation has not been found in patients with angina who underwent cardiac catheterization (17). Several studies have proposed that ventricular arrhythmia is the most powerful predictor of prognosis in patients with heart failure (18,19), but others disagree (20,21) finding that although ventricular arrhythmia may reflect the extent of left ventricular damage (15,19,22,23), it has little value as an independent predictor. It seems, therefore, that there is little consensus concerning the prognostic value of ambulatory ECG in cardiac patients.

Several other physiological measures, particularly silent ischemia, have been studied as they relate to prognosis in the post-MI patient (24). Erikssen (25), Yeung et al. (5), and Pryor et al. (26) have shown that silent myocardial ischemia, like symptomatic ischemia, is indicative of the presence of CAD and is associated with a worsened prognosis. Controversy remains, however, over the prognostic usefulness of this variable. Furthermore, indicators such as reduced HR variability (27), reduced baroreflex sensitivity (28), and signal-averaged ECG variables (29) seem to confer a worsened prognosis after MI, but they appear to provide little new information beyond that obtained from measures of cardiac performance during treadmill testing or cardiac catheterization.

Prognostic Variables From Cardiac Catheterization

Cardiac catheterization is a widely used invasive method of obtaining information about the severity and extent of CAD. LVF and coronary anatomy (degree of left main stenosis, number of diseased vessels, presence of proximal disease in the left anterior descending artery, mitral regurgitation, and left ventricular end-diastolic pressure) are the most important prognostic variables obtained from catheterization (1). When initial clinical assessment and catheterization variables were combined, LVF and coronary anatomy remained the most important. Lee et al. (11) suggest that RNA studies provide important prognostic information in addition to clinical and catheterization variables. In the Lee et al. study, prognosis was stratified by RNA exercise LVEF even when clinical and catheterization variables were known.

Post-Intervention Prognosis

Prognosis in CAD patients is improved in many cases as a result of various interventions, including medical therapy, coronary artery bypass graft (CABG) surgery, and percutaneous transluminal coronary angioplasty (PTCA).

Medical Therapy

Numerous studies of the effects of various pharmacological agents on prognosis in post-MI patients have been performed. Beta-blockers seem to be more beneficial in patients after an MI (30) than in patients with chronic stable angina (31). The early use of beta-blocking agents in the post-MI period has been associated with a decreased risk of sudden death and harmful ventricular arrhythmias, reduced anginal pain, and decreased use of analgesics (32,33). Furthermore, although Hjalmarson et al. (34) found that beta-blockers administered within 12 hours of an MI limited the size of infarct and lowered mortality at 2-year follow-up, Epstein and Palmeri (35) did not find a decrease in infarct size and suggest that beta-blocker therapy might have detrimental effects in some cases.

In general, anticoagulant medications have been found to effectively reduce platelet aggregation (36), while evidence of the usefulness of antiarrhythmics is controversial (37). The use of aspirin therapy in patients with unstable angina has been supported by two studies (38,39). Also, calcium-channel blockers have been used in post-MI patients, but their usefulness has yet to be consistently proven (40).

Several new medications for the acute treatment of post-MI patients have recently been developed. One of these, streptokinase, dissolves blood clots in the occluded artery and has been found to benefit approximately 80% to 90% of patients within the first 2 to 4 hours after an MI (41). Another relatively new medication, tissue-type plasminogen activator (t-PA), appears to confer the same (or possibly greater) benefits as streptokinase (42,43). However, more recent data show that t-PA increases the risk of stroke (44). Furthermore, t-PA therapy is considerably more expensive than streptokinase. Finally, new lipid-lowering drugs are effective in reducing cholesterol levels (45) and may improve prognosis. As mentioned previously, however, the influence of such traditional risk factors as elevated cholesterol levels appears greater with respect to initial coronary events than to recurrent events. The effectiveness of risk factor modification by medications on post-MI prognosis, therefore, has not yet been definitively demonstrated.

Surgical Therapy

Coronary artery bypass graft surgery has become a common surgical therapy for CAD. In the United States more than 332,000 such operations were performed in 1987 (46). The value of CABG surgery for improving prognosis has been the subject of many studies and reviews. Data have come from randomized trials, such as the Veterans Administration Cooperative Study, the European Coronary Surgery Study, and the Coronary Artery Surgery Study; from registries, such as the Duke University

Database and the Cleveland Clinic and Seattle Heart Watch registries; and from the personal registry of Dr. Cary Akin (47). Generally, patients with anatomically extensive disease (left main and triple-vessel disease) have the greatest improvement in prognosis. Furthermore, compared with medical therapy alone CABG surgery appears to prolong survival in patients judged to be at high risk according to clinical, functional, and anatomic characteristics (48). However, Robinson et al. (49) showed CABG surgery to be associated with cognitive deficits, and the long-term effects on quality of life are currently under investigation.

Percutaneous Transluminal Coronary Angioplasty

Another revascularization procedure, percutaneous transluminal coronary angioplasty, is an attractive alternative to CABG surgery because it does not require major surgery or general anesthesia. In a study of post-MI patients with unstable angina, DeFeyter et al. (50) suggest that for patients with predominantly single-vessel disease and well- maintained LVF, PTCA is relatively risk free and has a high initial success rate, despite a restenosis rate of more than 33% at 6 months after PTCA. Other studies confirm this high rate of early restenosis (51). Thus, the value of PTCA in modifying long-term prognosis is still unclear (52).

Biobehavioral Predictors of Prognosis in Patients With Coronary Artery Disease

The role of biobehavioral variables in the development of CAD and in determining prognosis for patients with established disease has received much attention. The most important of these variables are the Type A behavior pattern (TABP), hostility, vital exhaustion, and life stress and social resources. Other behavioral factors, including diet and smoking, will not be addressed here.

Type A Behavior Pattern

The *Type A behavior pattern*, a term coined by Friedman and Rosenman in the 1950s, has received more attention than any other behavioral or psychological variable as a risk factor for CAD. Individuals who exhibit TABP possess an intense, hard-driving competitiveness, a persistent sense of time urgency, and easily evoked hostility. A relative absence of this behavior characterizes the Type B behavior pattern. In 1981, a review panel assembled by the National Heart, Lung and Blood Institute concluded that TABP is an independent risk factor for CAD in employed, middle-aged U.S. citizens (53).

The conclusion of the review panel was based on the findings of a number of studies investigating the development of CAD in healthy subjects, as well as studies of individuals with documented CAD, prior MI, or cardiac risk factors. More recent studies, conducted in the past 10 years, have been inconsistent, however, raising questions about the value of TABP as a prognostic indicator.

Studies of Initially Healthy Subjects

The landmark study in Type A behavior and CAD was the Western Collaborative Group Study, which began in 1960 as a prospective, epidemiological investigation of CAD incidence in 3,524 employed white men 39 to 59 years of age who were recruited from 10 California business firms. All subjects were free from CAD at the beginning of the study. Behavior pattern was assessed by the Structured Interview. When 3,154 of the subjects were contacted for an 8.5-year follow-up, it was found that 13.2% of Type A men had CAD compared with only 5.9% of Type B men (54). Type A behavior was also strongly related to the incidence of recurring MI. Further, this positive association was independent of cholesterol, BP, and cigarette smoking.

The Framingham Study (55) measured Type A behavior by a self-report questionnaire (the Framingham Type A Scale) and reported TABP to be an independent predictor of the incidence of CAD in men and women 45 to 64 years old. For men, this relationship appeared only for those holding white-collar jobs, but the association appeared equally for women employed more than half their adult lives and for housewives. In another investigation, the French-Belgian Cooperative Heart Study (56), TABP was associated with an increased risk of CAD in healthy individuals. As measured by the Bortner Rating Scale, TABP significantly predicted total incidences of CAD, MI, and sudden death at a 5-year follow-up in healthy men from three European communities. As in the Framingham Study, this effect was independent of serum cholesterol, hypertension, smoking, and age.

Risk Factor Studies

As a secondary goal of the Multiple Risk Factor Intervention Trial (57), Type A behavior was assessed in 12,772 male subjects who were in the top decile of CAD risk due to high blood pressure and serum cholesterol levels and cigarette smoking. All subjects were asked to complete the Jenkins Activity Survey (JAS), a well-established self-report questionnaire concerning behavior patterns. One-fourth of the subjects also completed the Structured Interview. At an average follow-up of 7 years, Type A and Type B subjects identified by either the Jenkins Activity Survey or the Structured Interview did not differ in either the incidence of CAD or in rates of total mortality. Thus, TABP does not appear to be associated with increased morbidity or mortality in high-risk populations.

Studies of Individuals With CAD

Although the 8.5-year follow-up data of the Western Collaborative Group Study reported that Type A people had 5 times the rate of recurrent CAD as those with the Type B behavior pattern, the study's 22-year follow-up aimed to further investigate this relationship by continuing to track the 257 men who had CAD at the 8.5-year follow-up (58). For the 26 subjects who died within 24 hours of a coronary event, TABP was not related to mortality. However, for the 231 patients who survived for at least 24 hours, the long-term mortality rate associated with CAD was lower for Type A patients (24%) than for Type Bs (37%). Results did not differ for the younger and older subgroups, and the association was strongest among men whose first coronary event was a symptomatic MI. Thus, TABP was actually a better prognostic indicator post-MI.

Several explanations for these findings were offered. First, Type A people might cope more effectively with a coronary event than Type B individuals. However, there are no data to suggest that there were differences in their ability to successfully modify their lifestyles. Second, it was suggested that there could be a difference in disease identification rate between Type A and Type B subjects. For example, if Type A subjects pursued medical advice for their symptoms and Type B subjects ignored them, then the initial study group would have included Type A subjects with less severe initial disease and a more favorable prognosis. However, there is no evidence to suggest that behavior type affects a person's willingness to seek medical advice. It seems just as plausible that a Type A person would stoically resist pursuing

medical consultation while a Type B person would readily follow up on disturbing symptoms. Third, it is possible that behavior type might have altered spontaneously before the primary coronary event, have been changed by the event itself, or both. This explanation also appears unlikely, however.

In another study of TABP in cardiac patients, the Aspirin Myocardial Infarction Study (59), the Jenkins Activity Survey was administered to 2,314 patients (2,070 men and 244 women) from 18 clinical centers who had survived a previous MI. The Type A score from the survey was not significantly related to the risk of recurrent major coronary events for men or women or for a subgroup of 671 men who were employed in full-time professional, technical, or managerial jobs. Shekelle et al. (59) noted that the Jenkins Activity Survey was administered after randomization and that data were missing for 14% of the randomized patients, which may have affected the results. Furthermore, they noted that subjects who volunteer to participate in a clinical trial such as the Aspirin Myocardial Infarction Study could have different personality characteristics than individuals who participate in observational studies, and that these differences might account for the lack of association between behavior pattern and recurrent coronary events.

Negative findings were also reported in the Multicenter Post-Infarction Project (60). Behavior pattern was assessed by the JAS in male and female cardiac patients 2 weeks after they had suffered an acute MI. Of the 866 patients enrolled in the study, 548 completed the JAS, and Type A scores were obtained from 516 of them. Survey nonparticipants differed from participants in that there was a significantly higher percentage of female, older, unmarried, less well educated, and unemployed subjects among the nonparticipants. Nonparticipants also had more severe disease and a higher mortality rate at 1- to 3-year follow-up. However, a comparison of death rates among Type A and Type B JAS participants indicated no significant relationship between mortality and behavior type.

Because the Jenkins Activity Survey was developed in the Western Collaborative Group Study, the analysis by the Multicenter Post-Infarction Project was restricted to middle-aged men in order to approximate conditions under which the survey was developed. Even under this restricted analysis, however, no relationship between behavior type and the prognosis of CAD was observed.

Dimsdale and colleagues (61) followed for one year 189 male CAD patients 18 to 70 years of age to determine which risk factors or clinical findings predicted cardiac morbidity. Subjects who underwent cardiac catheterization because they showed symptoms of CAD were eligible for the study and completed a series of psychosocial measures including the Jenkins Activity Survey. The Type B behavior pattern emerged as a significant predictor of cardiac morbidity, which was interpreted as suggesting that in cardiac patients, Type B individuals' scores might reflect exhaustion and emotional depletion, which may predict poor prognosis (62). Thus, while evidence is mixed, there does not appear to be strong evidence that the TABP is an important prognostic variable in patients with CAD.

Angiography Studies

Investigators have also studied the possibility of Type A–CAD association by assessing the behavior pattern of individuals undergoing coronary angiography. Three early studies reported a positive association between TABP and the extent of CAD (63-65). However, subsequent studies have failed to find a relationship between TABP and CAD (66-68) or found only a small effect (69). Krantz et al. (70) found a nonsignificant trend for disease progression (defined as an increase in occlusion of more than 25% or a progression to total occlusion) in Type A patients classified by the Jenkins Activity Survey. These individuals had angiograms at a mean interval of 17 months. Thirty-one percent completed the JAS and the Structured Interview between angiograms, and 69% completed them after the repeat angiograms. This trend toward more severe occlusion was most apparent in individuals with extreme scores on the Jenkins Activity Survey. Patients with extreme Type A scores were more likely to exhibit disease progression, whereas those with extreme Type B scores were unlikely to show progression. However, there was little relationship between Structured Interview–assessed TABP and disease progression.

Williams et al. (71) reported a significant and positive association between Type A ratings from the Structured Interview and arteriographically documented CAD. Seventy-one percent of Type A patients had one or more significant ($\geq 75\%$) occlusions compared with 56% of Type B patients. In a subsequent study of more than 1,000 patients, Williams et al. (69) reported that TABP was a risk factor for young Type A patients, but not for older ones. Not unlike smoking and cholesterol, the declining prognostic significance of TABP is likely due to selective attrition; that is, individuals who are vulnerable to the effects of TABP (or smoking

or elevated cholesterol) die earlier in life, whereas the more hardy individuals (who presumably do not succumb to the effects of the risk factor) live longer.

In addition to the importance of age as a moderating factor, other reasons for the inconsistency of previous findings include different methods of assessing behavior patterns; identification of key components of TABP, such as hostility and mode of anger expression; and the presence of social support.

The use of different instruments to measure TABP is one important consideration in evaluating prior research. The Structured Interview, which detects not only self-reported attributes of TABP but also characteristic motor gestures and voice stylistics, is regarded as the "gold standard" for measuring TABP. Self-report instruments, including the Jenkins Activity Survey, the Bortner Rating Scale, the Type A Self-Rating Inventory, and the Framingham Type A Scale, are self-administered questionnaires that measure the extent to which individuals report they possess features of TABP. However, correlations among the Structured Interview and self-report measures are low. The inconsistent findings may in part reflect the use of different methods that assess different aspects of the behavior pattern.

Another explanation for the inconsistent findings about a possible association between TABP and CAD is that global Type A measures are too broad for identifying the significant components of TABP that are relevant to the disease. Just as not all components of cholesterol are detrimental and, indeed, some components (i.e., the high-density liproprotein [HDL] fraction) are actually beneficial, some aspects of Type A behavior may be irrelevant to CAD. What is regarded as the "toxic" component of TABP, however, is hostility. Indeed, there is accumulating evidence that high levels of anger and hostility are associated with CAD and other adverse health outcomes. In a reanalysis of the Western Collaborative Group Study data, Matthews et al. (72) noted that higher hostility and anger ratings from the Structured Interview differentiated CAD cases from controls. In addition, Williams et al. (71) showed that the Cook Medley Hostility Scale obtained from the Minnesota Multiphasic Personality Inventory was significantly related to angiographically documented CAD. Two prospective studies have also supported this association. In the Western Electric Study, Shekelle and colleagues (73) found that high hostility scores were associated with a 20-year CAD incidence. In a study of 255 medical students at the University of North Carolina, Barefoot et al. (74) determined that men with high hostility scores had 4 to 5 times the CAD incidence compared with men with low scores 20 years after they had taken the Minnesota Multiphasic Personality Inventory. Similarly, a reanalysis of data from a Massachusetts General Hospital sample (75) and a study of Finnish men with ischemic heart disease (76) reported hostility to be related to an increased risk of CAD. Although not all studies have supported the hostility-CAD relationship (77-80), the weight of the evidence strongly implicates hostility as a prognostic factor in the development of CAD.

Vital Exhaustion

Another factor that appears to be associated with CAD is a constellation of symptoms known as vital exhaustion. Vital exhaustion is characterized by excessive fatigue, decreased energy, feelings of dejection or defeat, loss of libido, and increased irritability. The proportion of individuals experiencing this syndrome prior to a cardiac event has been estimated to range from 30% to 50% (81,82).

Several studies have investigated the association of vital exhaustion and CAD. Appels and Mulder (83) studied 3,877 male city employees aged 39 to 65 years for a mean period of 4.2 years. Vital exhaustion, assessed by questionnaire, was positively associated with stable and unstable angina pectoris at the time of screening. Vital exhaustion was also associated with future angina pectoris and nonfatal MI.

Vital exhaustion may increase coronary risk by affecting normal sleep patterns. For example, Falger et al. (84) reported that sleep complaints (in particular, taking daytime naps and feeling exhausted upon waking in the morning) were significantly associated with MI, even after controlling for possible confounding effects of vital exhaustion, TABP, excessive coffee consumption, and smoking.

Depression has been reported to precede an MI in 33% to 50% of patients (85,86). Higher rates of MI have been reported among depressed psychiatric patients than among nondepressed psychiatric patients (87). Furthermore, depression in cardiac patients is associated with an increased mortality and medical morbidity after MI and cardiac surgery (88-91). Thus, vital exhaustion and depression appear to be indicators of poor prognosis.

Psychosocial Stress and Social Resources

Another factor relevant to prognosis in patients with CAD is psychosocial stress, including the degree of life stress experienced by an individual and the social resources available to cope with that stress.

Recently, the role of mental stress in the development of CAD has been studied in the laboratory. Rozanski and colleagues (92) assessed cardiac function during a series of mental tasks (arithmetic, Stroop Color-Word Task, simulated public speaking, and reading). Cardiac responses were compared with those recorded during exercise (cycle ergometry). Fifty-nine percent of the CAD patients had wall motion abnormalities during mental stress, and 36% had a decrease in LVEF of more than 5%. Eighty-three percent of the patients with wall motion abnormalities experienced silent, or asymptomatic, ischemia in response to mental stress, which also occurred at lower HRs than exercise-induced ischemia. Of all the mental tasks administered, the speaking task that was personally relevant and emotionally arousing led to more frequent and greater regional wall motion abnormalities.

Other studies also have shown ischemia to be provoked by stress. Freeman et al. (93) studied episodes of transient myocardial ischemia in 30 patients during a time of naturally occurring stress and uncertainty: the period during which patients were awaiting the results of coronary angiography. On two separate occasions subjects wore ambulatory Holter ST monitors, had urinary cortisol and catecholamine levels taken, and completed a questionnaire to assess psychological vulnerability. They also kept a diary that recorded times of chest pain, emotional upset, and activity. They were first evaluated before learning the results of angiography and the decision to perform surgery. The second evaluation period was a mean of 66 days later, after patients had had time to adjust to the decision-making process. There was a significantly greater number of silent ischemic events during the first time period. The assumption that the first time period was more stressful than the second was supported by the significantly higher cortisol and norepinephrine excretion levels on the first as compared with the second occasion in patients with more silent ischemia and longer total ischemic episodes. These data and others suggest a causal link between mental stress and episodes of symptomatic and asymptomatic myocardial ischemia.

As part of the Beta-Blocker Heart Attack Trial, Ruberman et al. (94) studied the prognostic value of education level and psychosocial characteristics (life stress, social isolation, TABP, and depression) in male post-MI patients. Among the psychosocial characteristics examined, life stress and social isolation showed pronounced inverse relationships to education level; high levels of life stress and social isolation were present in 35% of the least educated subjects (< 10 years of schooling) but in only 13% of the best educated subjects (> 12 years of schooling). Furthermore, there was a positive correlation between the levels of life stress and social isolation and the probability of death over a 3-year period. These associations help to explain the relationship of a low level of education with the high risk of death among survivors of MI. Neither TABP nor depression predicted mortality, however.

It has been hypothesized that social support and social networks protect against disease and aid in recovery by providing a buffer against stress (95-97). Two studies have examined the relationship of social support and TABP. Blumenthal et al. (98) evaluated patients undergoing coronary angiography and observed that Type A individuals with low levels of social support had more severe CAD than Type A persons with high levels of support; this relationship was not evident in Type B subjects. A similar interaction effect was found in a 10-year follow-up of middle-aged Swedish men, all of whom had CAD (99). Socially isolated Type A men experienced a 69% mortality rate compared with a 17% mortality rate among socially integrated Type A men. Social support and social isolation had little effect on mortality in Type B men. As mentioned above, these findings could suggest a mechanism through which TABP affects health and offer a possible explanation for inconsistencies in previous studies of associations between TABP and CAD.

Behavioral Interventions in Patients With CAD

Given the fact that the majority of CAD events are nonfatal, there is a great need to rehabilitate surviving cardiac patients. A variety of treatment programs have been developed in an effort to increase patients' life span as well as improve their quality of life.

Stress Management and Type A Behavior Modification

In an attempt to examine the efficacy of reduced Type A behavior on cardiac recurrences (nonfatal MI and cardiac deaths) in post-MI patients, Friedman et al. (100) conducted a randomized trial of TABP modification known as the Recurrent Coronary Prevention Project. A total of 1,013 patients who had experienced one or more MIs no less than 6 months earlier were followed for 4.5 years. At the beginning of the project, patients were randomly assigned to either a control group, which received group cardiac counseling, or a treatment group, which participated in both group cardiac and Type A behavioral counseling. A third group of patients, who volunteered to be assessed but not to participate in any counseling, formed a nonrandomized comparison group. TABP was assessed by a videotaped Structured Interview at entry and again at 3 and 4.5 years of follow-up.

Results showed that the Type A intervention was highly effective in reducing TABP. At the end of 4.5 years, 35.1% of patients in the treatment group exhibited a greatly reduced TABP compared with 9.8% of the control participants. The greatest decrease in TABP occurred at the end of the first year, but scores continued to fall throughout the 4.5-year study period. In addition, the treatment group experienced a significantly lower 4.5-year cardiac recurrence rate (12.9%) compared with the control group (21.2%) and the comparison group (28.2%). Between the treatment and control groups, this difference became and remained significant only after the second year of follow-up.

A second study, known as the Ischemic Heart Disease Life Stress Monitoring Program, also demonstrated the effectiveness of stress management in improving prognosis. Frasure-Smith and Prince (101) examined the effects of a brief stress management program on mortality and life stress in 461 male MI survivors. Patients were recruited while recovering in the hospital and randomized to a treatment or control group. Control participants received only standard medical follow-up from their physicians. Patients in the treatment group, however, received monthly phone calls from nurses in order to monitor 20 cognitive-behavioral symptoms of stress (assessed by the General Health Questionnaire). If the patient had five or more symptoms, or if he had been readmitted to the hospital, a nurse either called or visited his home to design a specific intervention to reduce those stresses through teaching, support, or referral. The program ended after 1 year, but patients' health statuses were followed for up to 7 years through their medical records.

At the end of the 1-year program, patients in the treatment group had significantly reduced symptoms of stress compared with controls. Also, controls were about twice as likely to die of cardiac problems as treatment group patients, although there were no significant differences in readmission rates or durations. Group differences in survival rates became apparent 4 months into the intervention and continued to increase through the end of the project year. These differences persisted for approximately 6 months after the end of the program, after which the survival rates for the two groups began to approach each other. Furthermore, while the rate of MI recurrence did not differ throughout the program duration, there was a significant group difference at the end of the follow-up period. Thus, the results of this project suggest that reducing life stress in post-MI patients has a significant beneficial effect on subsequent cardiac mortality.

A third study, the Lifestyle Heart Trial was a randomized, controlled clinical trial designed to study the impact of extensive lifestyle changes on the extent of coronary artery stenoses (102). Men and women with angiographically documented CAD who were not taking lipid-lowering drugs were randomly assigned to either a lifestyle change program (n = 22) or to a usual-care group (n = 19). Control group participants were free to make the lifestyle changes, although they were not asked to. Patients in the treatment group began the year-long intervention with a 1-week residential retreat during which they were taught the lifestyle changes, including a low-fat vegetarian diet, stress management training, moderate aerobic exercise, group support meetings, and smoking cessation (for 1 patient).

Compliance with the diet, exercise, and stress management parts of the intervention was excellent in the treatment group. Control group patients made lifestyle changes as well, but these were more moderate and in line with more conventional recommendations.

By the end of the program year, the experimental group had experienced a significant decrease in average percentage diameter stenosis from 40.0% to 37.8%, whereas the control group exhibited a significant progression from 42.7% to 46.1%. When analysis was restricted to only arteries with 50% or more stenosis, the average percentage diameter stenosis for the experimental group once again significantly regressed, this time from 61.1 to 55.8%, but it significantly progressed in the control group from 61.7% to 64.4%. The degree of adherence to the lifestyle change program was negatively correlated with changes in percentage diameter stenosis for the experimental group and the study group as a whole, such that participants with the most adherence had the largest decrease in percentage diameter stenosis.

Interestingly, the 5 women in the study did not fit the general pattern of results. Although these women made only moderate lifestyle changes, all had overall regression. The 4 control group women had more regression than any of the control group men, even though some of these men made greater lifestyle changes. Although the sample size was small, these data raise the possibility of gender effects on changes in coronary artery stenoses. Ornish et al. (102) conclude from the Lifestyle Heart Trial that conventional recommendations for CAD patients, such as a 30% fat diet, are not sufficient to bring about stenosis regression in most cases, and strongly suggest the need for a strict low-fat, vegetarian diet.

Exercise Interventions

Exercise is a well-established intervention for reducing risk factors, increasing functional capacity (103-105), and attenuating stress responses. Although exercise is a component of most cardiac rehabilitation programs, evidence that exercise prolongs life or decreases the risk of reinfarction remains equivocal.

In the National Exercise and Heart Disease Project, a randomized clinical trial, researchers assessed the effects of exercise on the physical and psychosocial rehabilitation of MI survivors (106). Six hundred and fifty-one men who had suffered an MI 2 to 36 months previously were assigned randomly to either an exercise or control group. The exercise group participants exercised three times weekly in the laboratory for 8 weeks. Thereafter, participants exercised three times a week (jogging, swimming, or cycling, as well as games) in a gymnasium. All participants had an interval history, physical examination, and treadmill test at 9 weeks, 6 months, and then semiannually after randomization.

Three years after the start of the project, the total mortality and recurrent MI rates for the two groups were not significantly different: Total mortality was 7.3% for the control group and 4.6% for the exercise group, and rates of recurrent MI were 7.0% and 5.3%, respectively. The authors concluded that exercise may reduce subsequent mortality in post-MI patients but that the evidence was not convincing. Adherence to the prescribed exercise regimen had dropped by 23% at the end of 2 years, at which time 31% of control group patients claimed to be exercising regularly. It is likely that these compliance problems significantly affected the study results.

Several recent reviews and a meta-analysis also explore the value of exercise in post-MI survival. May et al. (107) noted that in five of six studies there was a positive, though not statistically significant, trend toward the benefits of exercise. The six studies were prospective, randomized trials in which experimental group patients exercised two to four times per week for 20 to 40 minutes on each occasion. None of the studies alone showed significant differences in total mortality between the study groups, but pooling of the results indicated a 19% decrease in total mortality, which was significant. May et al. conclude from their review that the efficacy of exercise is not yet proven and that possible beneficial effects should be confirmed in studies with larger samples. Compliance was also a major problem with the supervised studies, with 40% to 60% of exercise group patients not adhering to the exercise schedule.

In another meta-analysis, Oldridge et al. (108) examined 10 randomized clinical trials (comprising 4,347 patients) of cardiac rehabilitation programs that included exercise. Pooled odds ratios indicated that the experimental-group patients experienced a significant reduction (24%) in all-cause death and a 25% decrease in cardiovascular mortality. There was no significant difference, however, for nonfatal reinfarctions. While recognizing the problems inherent in the meta-analytic approach, the authors conclude that their analysis reveals a substantial benefit, namely, a lower fatal cardiac event rate, for patients in a comprehensive cardiac rehabilitation program that includes exercise.

A similar debate exists over the value of exercise in improving psychosocial adjustment among post-MI patients. Exercise appears to improve psychological functioning in healthy subjects (109), and this association has been studied in cardiac patients. Several early studies reported reduced levels of depression (110) and an improved mood and sense of well-being in addition to decreased anxiety (111) in cardiac patients after they had participated in an exercise program. However, data from other studies are less conclusive.

In an analysis of the psychosocial measures administered to participants in the National Exercise and Heart Disease Project, Stern and Cleary (112) found virtually no differences between the exercise and control groups at 6-month, 1-year, or 2-year follow-up. This lack of group differences included measures of anxiety, depression, spouse-rated psychological and social behavior, and recent life stress.

Naughton et al. (113) failed to find any long-term benefit for cardiac patients from regular exercise.

Similarly, Mayou (114) found no significant differences among exercise, standard care, and advice groups after 18 months of participation. Along the same lines, Blumenthal et al. (115) found no differences in measures of anxiety, depression, stress, or TABP between low- and moderate-to-high-exercise group participants after 12 weeks of training, despite anecdotal reports that patients felt better. However, patients who were depressed at the beginning of the intervention showed a trend toward improvement at the end of the 12 weeks. It has been suggested that the low incidence of psychopathology among cardiac patients makes it difficult to measure any changes that might occur as a result of exercise and that this might explain the lack of consistent results.

Psychological Interventions

As described above, psychological factors such as depression, low morale, and distress can increase the risk of subsequent mortality in post-MI patients in addition to making a patient's adjustment to the illness more difficult. The effects of group and individual psychotherapy on the psychosocial adjustment of cardiac patients have been reported in several studies.

In one of the earliest studies, Adsett and Bruhn (116) exposed 6 post-MI male patients to nondirective group therapy (10 sessions) and assessed subsequent changes in their psychosocial adjustment. A similar therapy group was conducted with the patients' wives. The patients and their wives appeared to achieve improved psychosocial adaptation as a result of the therapy. A more extensive study by Rahe et al. (117) also investigated the effects of group therapy. Group therapy appeared to reduce some coronary-prone behaviors, but it had no effect on traditional risk factors such as smoking and obesity. In addition, lower morbidity and mortality rates were reported by group therapy patients than by controls. In a controlled clinical trial conducted by Ibrahim and colleagues (118), 118 post-MI patients were allocated to either a group psychotherapy condition or a control condition. The psychotherapy group met weekly for 1 year. No statistically significant differences emerged for either physiological or psychological variables, although the data suggested possible beneficial treatment effects for levels of social alienation and competitiveness, length of hospital stay, and favorable attitude toward the therapy experience. Despite this lack of hard findings, survival rates for the treatment patients tended to be higher, particularly for the most severely ill patients.

Individual psychotherapy has also been successfully conducted with cardiac patients. Gruen (119) treated 70 post-MI inpatients with individual supportive psychotherapy. These patients experienced significant improvement on a number of physical and psychological variables, such as time in an intensive care unit, length of hospital stay, occurrence of CHF, return to normal activity, depression, anxiety, and fear. Oldenburg et al. (120) compared the effects of educational and individual counseling interventions with routine medical care in a group of post-MI patients. Both intervention groups exhibited significant improvement on psychological and lifestyle measures, had fewer symptoms of heart disease, and were less dependent on treatment than patients who received only routine medical care when evaluated at 3-, 6-, and 12-month follow-up. More recently, Thompson (121) studied the effects of nurse counseling and education on first-time MI patients and their wives. Counseling was provided individually to couples during four separate 30-minute sessions: 24, 48, and 72 hours and 5 days after hospital admission. Beginning at 5 days after admission and continuing for 6 months after leaving the hospital, couples who received counseling reported significantly lower anxiety and depression scores compared with control group couples.

Summary

This chapter reviewed the importance of biobehavioral factors in the treatment and rehabilitation of patients with CAD. In addition to the traditional medical prognostic indicators, a number of behavioral and psychological factors—including TABP, hostility, vital exhaustion, stress, and social support—appear to offer potentially important prognostic information. Moreover, behavioral treatments, including dietary intervention, exercise, Type A behavior modification, and stress management, appear to offer considerable benefits in terms of both quality and, perhaps, quantity of life.

Acknowledgment

This chapter was supported in part by grants from the National Institutes of Health (HL30675 and HL43028).

References

1. Pryor, D.B.; Bruce, R.A.; Chaitman, B.R.; Fisher, L.; Gajewski, J.; Hammermeister, K.E.; Pauker, S.G.; Stokes, J. Task force I: Determination of prognosis in patients with ischemic heart disease. J. Am. Coll. Cardiol. 14:1016-1024; 1989.
2. Castello, R.; Alegria, E.; Merino, A.; Malpartida, F.; Martinez-Caro, D. Effect of age on long-term prognosis of patients with myocardial infarction. Int. J. Cardiol. 20:221-230; 1988.
3. Dittrich, H.; Gilpin, E.; Nicod, P.; Cali, G.; Henning, H.; Ross, J., Jr. Acute myocardial infarction in women: Influence of gender on mortality and prognostic variables. Am. J. Cardiol. 62:1-7;1988.
4. Wong, N.D.; Cupples, L.A.; Ostfeld, A.M.; Levy, D.; Kannel, W.B. Risk factors for long-term coronary prognosis after initial myocardial infarction: The Framingham study. Am. J. Epidemiol. 130:469-480; 1989.
5. Yeung, A.C.; Barry, J.; Selwyn, A.P. Silent ischemia after myocardial infarction. Prognosis, mechanism and intervention. Circulation. 82 [Suppl. 3]:143-148; 1990.
6. Fioretti, P.; Deckers, J.W.; Salm, E.; Baardman, T.; Roelandt, J.R. Four-year prognostic value of exercise-induced angina and painless ST segment depression early after myocardial infarction. Eur. Heart J. 9 [Suppl. N]:123-127; 1988.
7. Bruce, R.A.; Fisher, L.D.; Pettinger, M.; Weiner, D.A.; Chaitman, B.R. ST segment elevation with exercise: A marker for poor ventricular function and poor prognosis. Circulation. 77:897-905; 1988.
8. Mark, D.B.; Hlatky, M.A.; Harrell, F.E.; Lee, K.L.; Califf, R.M., Pryor, D.B. Exercise treadmill score for predicting prognosis in coronary artery disease. Ann. Intern. Med. 106:793-800; 1987.
9. Pilote, L.; Silberberg, J.; Lisbona, R.; Sniderman, A. Prognosis in patients with low left ventricular ejection fraction after myocardial infarction. Importance of exercise capacity. Circulation. 80:1636-1641; 1989.
10. Kishida, H.; Hata, N.; Kanazawa, M. Prognostic value of low-level exercise testing in patients with myocardial infarction. Jpn. Heart J. 30:275-285; 1989.
11. Lee, K.L.; Pryor, D.B.; Pieper, K.S.; Harrell, F.E.; Califf, R.M.; Mark, D.B.; Hlatky, M.A.; Coleman, R.E.; Cobb, F.R.; Jones, R.H. Prognostic value of radionuclide angiography in medically treated patients with coronary artery disease. Circulation. 82:1705-1717; 1990.
12. de Belder, M.; Skehan, D.; Pumphrey, C.; Khan, B.; Evans, S.; Rothman, M.; Mills, P. Identification of a high-risk subgroup of patients with silent ischaemia after myocardial infarction: A group for early therapeutic revascularisation? Br. Heart J. 63:145-150; 1990.

13. Miller, D.D.; Kaul, S.; Strauss, H.W.; Newell, J.B.; Okada, R.D.; Boucher, C.A. Increased exercise thallium-201 lung uptake: A noninvasive prognostic index in two-vessel coronary artery disease. Can. J. Cardiol. 4:270-276; 1988.

14. Mukharji, J.; Rude, R.E.; Poole, W.K. Risk factors for sudden cardiac death after acute myocardial infarction: Two-year follow-up. Am. J. Cardiol. 54:31-36; 1984.

15. Bigger, J.T.; Fleiss, J.L.; Miller, J.P.; Rolnitzky, L.M. Multicenter Post-Infarction Research Group. The relationships among ventricular arrhythmias, left ventricular dysfunction, and mortality in the 2 years after myocardial infarction. Circulation. 69:250-258; 1984.

16. Cleland, J.G.; Dargie, H.J.; Ford, I. Mortality in heart failure: Clinical variables of prognostic value. Br. Heart J. 58:572-582; 1987.

17. Califf, R.M.; McKinnis, R.A.; Burks, J. Prognostic implications of ventricular arrhythmias during 24 hour ambulatory monitoring in patients undergoing catheterization for coronary artery disease. Am. J. Cardiol. 50:23-31; 1982.

18. Meinertz, T.; Hoffmann, T.; Kasper, W.; Treese, N.; Bechtold, H.; Stienen, U.; Pop, T.; Leitner, E.V.; Andresen, D. Significance of ventricular arrhythmias as in idiopathic dilated cardiomyopathy. Am. J. Cardiol. 53:902-907; 1984.

19. Unverforth, D.V.; Magorien, R.D.; Moeschberger, M.L.; Baker, P.B.; Fetters, J.K.; Leier, C.V. Factors influencing the one-year mortality of dilated cardiomyopathy. Am. J. Cardiol. 54:147-152; 1984.

20. Shirey, E.K.; Proudfit, W.L.; Hawk, W.A. Primary myocardial disease. Correlations with clincial findings, angiographic and biopsy diagnoses. Follow up of 139 patients. Am. Heart J. 99:198-207; 1980.

21. Wilson, J.R.; Schwartz, J.S.; Sutton, M.S.J.; Ferraro, N.; Horowitz, L.M.; Reichek, N.; Josephson, M. Prognosis in severe heart failure: Relation to haemodynamic measurements and ventricular ectopic activity. J. Am. Coll. Cardiol. 2:403-410; 1983.

22. Glover, D.R.; Littler, W.A. Factors influencing survival and mode of death in severe chronic ischaemic heart disease. Br. Heart J. 57:125-132; 1987.

23. Von Olshausen, K.; Schafer, A.; Mehmel, H.C.; Schwartz, F.; Senges, J.; Kubler, W. Ventricular arrhythmias in idiopathic dilated cardiomyopathy. Br. Heart J. 51:195-201; 1984.

24. Rozanski, A.; Berman, D.S. Silent myocardial ischemia: II. Prognosis and implications for the clinical assessment of patients with coronary artery disease. Am. Heart J. 114:627-638; 1987.

25. Ekikssen, J. Prognostic importance of silent ischemia during long-term follow-up of patients with coronary artery disease. A short review based on own experience and current literature. Herz. 12:359-368; 1987.

26. Pryor, D.B.; Hindman, M.C.; Wagner, G.S.; Califf, R.M.; Rhoads, M.K.; Rosati, R.A. Early discharge after acute myocardial infarction. Ann. Intern. Med. 99:528-538; 1983.

27. Malik, M.; Camm, A.J. Heart rate variability. Clin. Cardiol. 13:570-576; 1990.

28. Bigger, J.T., Jr.; LaRovere, M.T.; Steinman, R.C.; Fleiss, L.; Rothman, J.N.; Rolnitzky, L.M.; Schwartz, P.J. Comparison of baroreflex sensitivity and heart period variability after myocardial infarction. J. Am. Coll. Cardiol. 14:1511-1518; 1989.

29. Seale, W.L.; Gang, E.S.; Peter, C.T. The use of signal-averaged electrocardiography in predicting patients at high risk for sudden death. PACE. 13:796-807; 1990.

30. Beta-Blocker Heart Attack Research Trial Group. A randomized trial of propranolol in patients with myocardial infarction. I. Mortality results. JAMA. 247:1707-1714; 1982.

31. Lambert, D.M.D. Beta blockers and life expectancy in ischemic heart disease. Lancet. 1:793; 1972.

32. Eckberg, D. Beta-adrenergic blockade may prolong life in post-infarction patients in part by increasing vagal cardiac inhibition. Med. Hypotheses. 15:421-432; 1984.

33. Hjalmarson, A. Early intervention with a beta-blocking drug after acute myocardial infarction. Am. J. Cardiol. 54:11E-13E; 1984.

34. Hjalmarson, A.; Herlitz, J.; Malek, I.; Ryden, L.; Vedin, A. Effect on mortality of metoprolol in acute myocardial infarction. A double-blind randomized trial. Lancet. 2:823-827; 1981.

35. Epstein, S.; Palmeri, A. Mechanisms contributing to precipitation of unstable angina and acute myocardial infarction: Implication regarding therapy. Am. J. Cardiol. 54:1245-1252; 1984.

36. Proceedings of the workshop on platelet-active drugs in the secondary prevention of cardiovascular events. Circulation. 60:1-135; 1981.

37. Myerberg, R.J.; Conde, C.; Sheps, D.S.; Appel, R.A.; Kiem, I.; Sung, R.J.; Castellanos, A. Antiarrhythmic drug therapy in survivals of prehospital cardiac arrest: Comparison of effects of chronic ventricular arrhythmias and recurrent cardiac arrest. Circulation. 59:855-863; 1979.

38. Lewis, H.D.; Davis, J.W.; Archibald, D.G.; Steinke, W.E.; Smitherman, T.C.; Doherty, J.E., III; Schnaper, H.W.; LeWinter, M.M.; Limares, E.; Pouget, J.M.; Sabharwal, S.C.; Chesler, E.; Demots, H. Protective effects of aspirin against acute myocardial infarction and death in men with unstable angina. N. Engl. J. Med. 309:396-402; 1983.

39. Cairns, J.A.; Gent, M.; Singer, J.; Finnie, K.J.; Froggatt, G.M.; Holder, D.A.; Jablonsky, G.; Kostuk, W.J.; Melendez, L.J.; Myers, M.G.; Sackett, D.L.; Sealey, B.J.; Tanser, P.H. Aspirin, sulfinpyrazone, or both in unstable angina. N. Engl. J. Med. 313:1369-1375; 1985.

40. Pearle, D. Nifedipine in acute myocardial infarction. Am. J. Cardiol. 54:21E-23E; 1984.

41. Vermeer, F.; Simoons, M.; Bar, F.; Tijssen, J.; van-Domburg, R.; Serruys, P.; Verheugt, F.; Res, J.; deZwaan, C.; Van der Laarse, A.; Krauss, X.; Lusen, J.;

Hugenholtz, P. Which patients benefit most from early thromboytic therapy with intracoronary streptokinase? Circulation. 74:1379-1389; 1986.

42. Graor, R.; Risius, B.; Lucas, F.; Young, J.; Ruschhaupt, W.; Beren, E.; Grossbard, E. Thrombosis with recombinant human tissue-type plasminogen activator in patients with peripheral artery and bypass graft occlusions. Circulation. 74 [Suppl. 1]:15-20; 1986.

43. Lyden, P.D.; Madden, K.P.; Clark, W.M.; Sasse, K.C.; Zivin, J.A. Incidence of cerebral hemorrhage after antifibrinolytic treatment for embolic strike in rabbits. Stroke. 21:1589-1593; 1990.

44. Kase, C.S.; O'Neal, A.M.; Fisher, M.; Girgis, G.N.; Ordia, J.I. Intracranial hemorrhage after use of tissue plasminogen activator for coronary thrombolysis. Ann. Intern. Med. 112:17-21; 1990.

45. Lees, A.; Stein, S.; Lees, R.; Therapy of hypercholesterolemia with mevinolin and other lipid-lowering drugs. Circulation. 74:200; 1986.

46. American Heart Association. 1990 heart and stroke facts. Dallas: American Heart Association; 1989.

47. Gersh, B.J.; Califf, R.M.; Loop, F.D.; Akins, C.W.; Pryor, D.B.; Takaro, T.C. Coronary bypass surgery in chronic stable angina. Circulation. 79 [Suppl. I]:I46-I59; 1989.

48. Califf, R.M.; Harrell, F.E., Jr.; Lee, K.L.; Rankin, J.S.; Hlatky, M.A.; Mark, D.B.; Jones, R.H.; Muhlbaier, L.H.; Oldham, H.N., Jr.; Pryor, D.B. The evolution of medical and surgical therapy for coronary artery disease. A 15-year perspective. JAMA. 261:2077-2086; 1989.

49. Robinson, M.; Blumenthal, J.A.; Burker, E.J.; Hlatky, M.; Reves, J.G. Coronary artery bypass grafting and cognitive function: A review. J. Cardiopul. Rehabil. 10:180-189; 1990.

50. DeFeyter, P.; Serruys, P.; Soward, A.; Van den Brand, M.; Bos, E.; Hugenholtz, P. Coronary angioplasty for early postinfarction unstable angina. Circulation. 74:1365-1370; 1986.

51. Schwartz, L.; Bourassa, M.G.; Lesperance, J.; Aldridge, H.E.; Kazim, F.; Salvatori, V.A.; Henderson, H.; Bonan, R.; David, P.R. Aspirin and diphyridamole in the prevention of restenosis after percutaneous transluminal coronary angioplasty. N. Engl. J. Med. 318:1714-1719; 1988.

52. Grueuntzig, A.R.; King, S.B., III.; Schlumpf, M.; Siegenthaler, W. Long-term follow-up after percutaneous transluminal coronary angioplasty: The early Zurich experience. N. Engl. J. Med. 316:1127-1132; 1987.

53. Review Panel. Coronary prone behavior and coronary heart disease: A critical review. Circulation. 19:583; 1981.

54. Rosenman, R.H.; Brand, R.J.; Jenkins, C.D.; Friedman, M.; Straus, R.; Wurm, M. Coronary heart disease in the western collaborative group study: Final follow-up experience of 8-1/2 years. JAMA. 233:872-877; 1975.

55. Haynes, S.G.; Feinleib, M.; Kannel, W.B. The relationship of psychosocial factors to coronary heart disease in the Framingham study: III. Eight-year incidence of coronary heart disease. Am. J. Epidemiol. 111:37-58; 1980.

56. French-Belgian Collaborative Group. Ischemic heart disease and psychosocial patterns: Prevalence and incidence studies in Belgium and France. Adv. Cardiol. 29:25-31; 1982.

57. Shekelle, R.B.; Hulley, S.B.; Jeaton, J.; Billings, J.H.; Borhani, N.O.; Gerace, T.A.; Jacobs, D.R.; Lasser, N.L.; Mittlemark, M.B.; Stamler, J. The MRFIT behavior pattern study. II: Type A behavior pattern and risk of coronary death in MRFIT. Am. J. Epidemiol. 122:559-570; 1985.

58. Ragland, D.R.; Brand, R.J. Type A behavior and mortality from coronary heart disease. N. Engl. J. Med. 318:65-70; 1988.

59. Shekelle, R.B.; Gale, M.; Norusis, M.; for the Aspirin Myocardial Infarction Study Research Group. Type A score (Jenkins activity survey) and risk of recurrent coronary heart disease in the aspirin myocardial infarction study. Am. J. Cardiol. 56:221-225; 1985.

60. Case, R.B.; Heller, S.S.; Case, N.B.; Moss, A.J.; the Multicenter Post-Infarction Research Group. Type A behavior and survival after acute myocardial infarction. N. Engl. J. Med. 312:737-741; 1985.

61. Dimsdale, J.E.; Gilbert, J.; Hutter, A.M.; Hackett, T.P.; Block, P.C. Predicting cardiac morbidity based on risk factors and coronary angiographic findings. Am. J. Cardiol. 47:73-76; 1981.

62. Bruhn, J.; McGrady, K.; duPlessis, A. Evidence of "Emotional Drain" preceding death from myocardial infarction. Psychiatry Digest. 29:34-40; 1968.

63. Zyzanski, S.J.; Jenkins, C.D.; Ryan, T.J.; Flessas, A.; Everist, M. Psychological correlates of coronary angiographic findings. Arch. Intern. Med. 136:1234-1237; 1976.

64. Blumenthal, J.A.; Williams, R.B.; Kong, Y.; Schanberg, S.M.; Thompson, L.W. Type A behavior and angiographically documented coronary disease. Circulation. 58:634-639; 1978.

65. Frank, K.A.; Heller, S.S.; Kornfeld, D.S.; Sporn, A.A.; Weiss, M.B. Type A behavior pattern and angiographic findings. JAMA. 240:761-763; 1978.

66. Dimsdale, J.E.; Hackett, T.P.; Hutter, A.M.; Block, P.C.; Catanzano, D.M.; White, P.J. Type A personality and extent of coronary atherosclerosis. Am. J. Cardiol. 43:583-586; 1978.

67. Krantz, D.S.; Schaeffer, M.A.; Davia, J.E.; Dembroski, T.M.; MacDougall, J.M.; Shaffer, R.T. Extent of coronary atherosclerosis, Type A behavior and cardiovascular response to social interaction. Psychophysiology. 18:654-664; 1981.

68. Kornitzer, M.; Magotteau, V.; Degre, C.; Kittel, F.; Struyven, J.; van Thiel, E. Angiographic findings and the Type A pattern assessed by means of the Bortner scale. J. Behav. Med. 5:313-320; 1982.

69. Williams, R.B.; Barefott, J.C.; Haney, T.L.; Harrel, F.E.; Blumenthal, J.A.; Pryor, D.B.; Peterson, B. Type A behavior and angiographically documented coronary atherosclerosis in a sample of 2,289 patients. Psychosom. Med. 50:139-152; 1988.

70. Krantz, D.S.; Sanmarco, M.I.; Selvester, R.H.; Matthews, K.A. Psychological correlates of progression of atherosclerosis in men. Psychosom. Med. 41:467-475; 1979.

71. Williams, R.B.; Haney, T.L.; Lee, K.L.; Kong, Y.; Blumenthal, J.A.; Whalen, R.E. Type A behavior, hostility, and coronary atherosclerosis. Psychosom. Med. 42:539-549; 1980.

72. Matthews, K.A.; Glass, D.C.; Rosenman, R.H.; Bortner, R.W. Competitive drive, pattern A, and coronary heart disease: A further analysis of some data from the western collaborative group study. J. Chronic Dis. 30:489-498; 1977.

73. Shekelle, R.B.; Gale, M.; Ostfeld, A.M.; Paul, O. Hostility, risk of coronary heart disease and mortality. Psychosom. Med. 45:109-114; 1983.

74. Barefoot, J.C.; Dahlstrom, W.G.; Williams, R.B. Hostility, CHD incidence, and total mortality: A 25-year follow-up study of 255 physicians. Psychosom. Med. 45:59-63; 1983.

75. MacDougall, J.M.; Dembroski, T.M.; Dimsdale, J.E.; Hackett, T.P. Components of Type A, hostility and anger-in: Further relationships to angiographic findings. Health Psychol. 4:137-152; 1985.

76. Koskenvuo, M.; Kaprio, J.; Rose, R.J.; Kesaniemi, A.; Sarna, A.; Heikkila, K.; Langinvainio, H. Hostility as a risk factor for mortality and ischemic heart disease in men. Psychosom. Med. 50:330-340; 1988.

77. McCranie, E.; Watkins, L.; Brandsma, J.; Sisson, B. Hostility, coronary heart disease incidence, and total mortality: Lack of association in a 25-year follow-up of 475 physicians. J. Behav. Med. 9:119-125; 1986.

78. Leon, G.R.; Finn, S.E.; Murray, D.; Bailey, J.M. Inability to predict cardiovascular disease from hostility scores or MMPI items related to type A behavior. J. Consult. Psychol. 56:597-600; 1988.

79. Hearn, M.D.; Murray, D.M.; Luepker, R.V. Hostility, coronary heart disease, and total mortality: A 33-year follow-up study of university students. J. Behav. Med. 12:105-121; 1989.

80. Helmer, D.C.; Ragland, D.R.; Syme, S.L. Hostility and coronary artery disease. Am. J. Epidemiol. 133:112-122; 1991.

81. Alonzo, A.A.; Simon, A.B.; Feinleib, M. Prodromata of myocardial infarction and sudden death. Circulation. 52:1056-1062; 1975.

82. Rissanen, V.; Romo, M.; Siltanen, P. Premonitory symptoms and stress factors preceding sudden death from ischemic heart disease. Acta Med. Scand. 20:389-396; 1978.

83. Appels, A.; Mulder, P.; Fatigue and heart disease. The association between "vital exhaustion" and past, present and future coronary heart disease. J. Psychosom. Res. 33:727-738; 1989.

84. Falger, P.; Schouten, E.; Appels, A.; de Vos, Y. Sleep complaints, behavioral characteristics and vital exhaustion in myocardial infarction cases. Psychol. Health. 2:231-258; 1988.

85. Lebovits, B.Z.; Shekelle, R.B.; Ostfeld, A.M.; Paul, O. Prospective and retrospective psychological studies of coronary heart disease. Psychosom. Med. 29:265-272; 1967.

86. Greene, S.W.; Goldstein, S.; Moss, A.J. Psychosocial aspects of sudden death. Arch. Intern. Med. 129:725-731; 1972.

87. Dreyfuss, F.; Dasberg, H.; Assael, M.I. The relationship of myocardial infarction to depressive illness. Psychother. Psychosom. 17:73-81; 1969.

88. Stern, J.J.; Pascale, L.; Ackerman, A. Life adjustment post myocardial infarction: Determining predictive variables. Arch. Intern. Med. 137:1680-1685; 1977.

89. Garrity, T.F.; Klein, R.F. Emotional response and clinical severity as early determinants of six-month mortality after myocardial infarction. Heart Lung. 4:730-737; 1975.

90. Kimball, C.P. Psychological responses to the experience of open heart surgery. I. Am. J. Psychiatry. 126:348-359; 1969.

91. Tufo, H.M.; Ostfeld, A.M. A prospective study of open-heart surgery. Psychosom. Med. 30:552-559; 1968.

92. Rozanski, A.; Bairey, C.N.; Krantz, D.S.; Friedman, J.; Resser, K.J.; Morell, M.; Hilton-Chalfen, S.; Hestrin, L.; Birtendorf, J.; Berman, D.S. Mental stress and the induction of silent myocardial ischemia in patients with coronary artery disease. N. Engl. J. Med. 318:1005-1112; 1988.

93. Freeman, L.J.; Nixon, P.G.; Sallabank, P.; Reaveley, D. Psychological stress and silent myocardial ischemia. Am. Heart. J. 114:477-482; 1987.

94. Ruberman, W.; Weinblatt, E.; Goldberg, J.D.; Chaudhary, B.S. Psychosocial influences on mortality after myocardial infarction. N. Engl. J. Med. 311:552-559; 1984.

95. Broadhead, W.E.; Kaplan, B.H.; James, S.A.; Wagner, E.H.; Schoenbach, V.J.; Grimson, R.; Heyden, S.; Tibblin, G.; Gehlbach, S.H. The epidemiological evidence for a relationship between social support and health. Am. J. Epidemiol. 117:521-537; 1983.

96. Cobb, S. Social support as a moderator of life stress. Psychosom. Med. 38:300-314; 1976.

97. Kaplan, B.H.; Cassel, J.C.; Gore, S. Social support and health. Med. Care. 15 [Suppl. 5]:47-57; 1977.

98. Blumenthal, J.A.; Burg, M.M.; Barefoot, J.; Williams, R.B.; Haney, T.; Zimet, G. Social support, Type A behavior, and coronary artery disease. Psychosom. Med. 49:331-340; 1987.

99. Orth-Gomer, K.; Unden, A. Type A behavior, social support, and coronary risk: Interaction and significance for mortality in cardiac patients. Psychosom. Med. 52:59-72; 1990.

100. Friedman, M.; Thoresen, C.E.; Gill, J.J.; Ulmer, D.; Powell, L.H.; Price, V.A.; Brown, B.; Thompson, L.;

Rabin, D.D.; Breall, W.S.; Bourg, E.; Levy, R.; Dixon, T. Alteration of type A behavior and its effects on cardiac recurrences in post myocardial infarction patients: Summary results of the recurrent coronary prevention project. Am. Heart J. 112:653-665; 1986.

101. Frasure-Smith, N.; Prince, R. Longterm follow-up of the ischemic heart disease life stress monitoring program. Psychosom. Med. 51:485-513; 1989.

102. Ornish, D.; Brown, S.E.; Scherwitz, L.W.; Billings, J.H.; Armstrong, W.T.; Ports, T.A.; McLanahan, S.M.; Kirkeeide, R.L.; Brand, R.J.; Gould, K.L. Can lifestyle changes reverse coronary heart disease? Lancet. 336:129-133; 1990.

103. Blumenthal, J.A.; Emery, C.F. Rehabilitation of patients following myocardial infarction. J. Consult. Clin. Psychol. 56:374-381; 1988.

104. Clausen, J.P.; Larsen, O.A.; Trap-Jensen, J. Physical training in the management of coronary artery disease. Circulation. 40:143-154; 1969.

105. Scheuer, J.; Tipton, C.M. Cardiovascular adjustments to physical training. Annu. Rev. Physiol. 39:221-251; 1977.

106. Shaw, L.W. Effects of a prescribed supervised exercise program on mortality and cardiovascular morbidity in patients after a myocardial infarction. Am. J. Cardiol. 48:39-46; 1981.

107. May, G.S.; Eberlein, K.A.; Furberg, C.D.; Passamani, E.R.; DeMets, D.L. Secondary prevention after myocardial infarction: A review of long-term trials. Prog. Cardiovasc. Dis. 24:331-352; 1982.

108. Oldridge, N.B.; Guyatt, G.H.; Fischer, M.E.; Rimm, A.A. Cardiac rehabilitation after myocardial infarction. JAMA. 260:945-950; 1988.

109. Plante, T.G.; Rodin, J. Physical fitness and enhanced psychological health. Curr. Psychol. Res. Rev. 9:3-24; 1990.

110. Hellerstein, H.K.; Hornsten, T.R.; Goldbarg, A.N.; Burlando, A.C.; Friedman, H.; Hirsch, E.Z.; Marik, S. The influence of active conditioning upon subjects with coronary artery disease: A progress report. Can. Med. Assoc. J. 96:901-903; 1967.

111. McPherson, B.; Paivio, A.; Yhasz, M.; Rechnitzer, P.; Pickard, H.; Lefcoe, N. Psychological effects of an exercise program for postinfarct and normal adult men. J. Sports Med. Phys. Fitness. 7:95-102; 1967.

112. Stern, M.J.; Cleary, P. The national exercise and heart disease project: Long-term psychosocial outcome. Arch. Intern. Med. 142:1093-1097; 1982.

113. Naughton, J.; Bruhn, J.; Lategola, M. Effects of physical training on physiologic and behavioral characteristics of cardiac patients. Arch. Phys. Med. Rehabil. 49:131-137; 1968.

114. Mayou, R.A. A controlled trial of early rehabilitation after myocardial infarction. J. Cardiac Rehabil. 3:397-402; 1983.

115. Blumenthal, J.A.; Emery, C.F.; Rejeski, W.J. The effects of exercise training on psychosocial functioning after myocardial infarction. J. Cardiopul. Rehabil. 8:183-193; 1988.

116. Adsett, C.A.; Bruhn, J.G.; Short-term group psychotherapy for post-myocardial infarction patients and their wives. Can. Med. Assoc. J. 99:577-584; 1968.

117. Rahe, R.H.; Ward, H.W.; Hayes, V. Brief group therapy in myocardial infarction rehabilitation: Three- to four-year follow-up of a controlled trial. Psychosom. Med. 41:229-242; 1979.

118. Ibrahim, M.A.; Feldman, J.G.; Sulz, H.A.; Staiman, M.G.; Young, L.J., Dean, D. Management after myocardial infarction: A controlled trial of the effect of group psychotherapy. Int. J. Psychiatry Med. 5: 253-268; 1974.

119. Gruen, W. Effects of brief psychotherapy during the hospitalization period on the recovery process in heart attacks. J. Consult. Clin. Psychol. 53:852-859; 1985.

120. Oldenburg, B.; Perkins, R.J.; Andrews, G. Controlled trial of psychological intervention in myocardial infarction. J. Consult. Psychol. 53:852-859; 1985.

121. Thompson, D.R. Counseling coronary patients and wives. Nurs. Times. 86(21):56; 1990.

Chapter 4

Exercise Testing: Clinical Applications

Victor F. Froelicher
Tianna M. Umann

In spite of technological advances in other cardiovascular testing modalities, exercise testing remains an important diagnostic tool because of its widespread availability and its yield of clinically useful functional information. Thus, improvements in the modality's performance have extensive impact in health care. A joint paper from the American College of Cardiology (ACC) and the American Heart Association (AHA) (1) assessed the appropriateness of the exercise test for applications (Table 4.1). The most common clinical applications for exercise testing are the diagnosis of chest pain and the prognostication and estimation of coronary artery disease (CAD) severity. This chapter—on the clinical application of exercise testing—will therefore focus on the diagnostic and prognostic uses of exercise testing.

Diagnostic Use of Exercise Testing

The probability of diagnosing CAD from an exercise test depends upon the clinical characteristics of the patients tested and the test's sensitivity (the percentage of times the test gives an abnormal result when those with disease are tested) and specificity (the percentage of times the test gives a normal result when those without disease are tested) (2). Sensitivity and specificity can be affected by the population tested but in most clinical situations, the patient mix averages out such influence. Combining sensitivity and specificity values provides the predictive accuracy, which is the percentage of responses, both positive (associated with disease) and negative (not associated with disease) that are correct. Predictive value is the percentage of either positive or negative responses that are correct.

A basic step in applying any test for separating patients with and without disease is to determine a value measured by the test that best separates the two groups, i.e., a discriminant value, or cut point. Cut points cannot discriminate absolutely because people with and without disease have overlapping values. This explains why sensitivity and specificity are inversely related; that is, if you increase one by using a certain cut point, you decrease the other.

Although other electrocardiographic (ECG) responses (such as R-wave amplitude, QT or QRS duration, or ST elevation) have been reported as useful in analyzing ECG results to identify people with disease (3), ST-segment depression has received the most attention. Experts agree concerning the importance of ST depression in the diagnosis of CAD; however, there is disagreement as to how to make ST measurements. Furthermore, differences occur as to the number and type of leads used, the type of exercise employed, computerization scoring methods, and the treatment of equivocal results.

Gianrossi et al. recently investigated the variability of the reported diagnostic accuracy of exercise ECG by applying a meta-analysis of 147 consecutively published reports involving 24,074 patients who underwent both coronary angiography and exercise testing (4). Details regarding population characteristics and methods were entered, including publication year, number of ECG leads, exercise protocol, preexercise hyperventilation, definition of an abnormal ST response, exclusion of certain subgroups, and blinding of test interpretation. Wide variability in sensitivity and specificity was found among the reports: the mean sensitivity was 68% with a range of 23% to 100% and a standard deviation of ± 16 percentage points; the mean specificity was 77% with a range of 17% to 100% and a standard deviation of ± 17 percentage points.

Sensitivity was found to be significantly and independently related to four study characteristics:

1. The method of dealing with equivocal or nondiagnostic tests: Sensitivity decreased when these tests were considered normal.

Table 4.1   American College of Cardiology/American Heart Association Task Force on Assessment of Cardiovascular Procedures: Guidelines for Use of Exercise Tesing

Exercise testing used	Class I: General consensus that exercise testing is justified	Class II: Exercise testing is frequently used but there is a divergence of opinion regarding justification	Class III: General agreement regarding little or no value, inappropriate contraindications
—in patients with signs and symptoms of coronary artery disease (CAD) or with known CAD	To diagnose male patients with atypical signs or symptoms of CAD To assess functional capacity For prognosis To evaluate patients with symptoms consistent with recurrent exercise-induced arrhythmias	To diagnose women with chest pain To diagnose patients on digoxin, with right bundle branch block To evaluate functional capacity and response to therapy with drugs in CAD or congestive heart failure To evaluate variant angina To serially follow (1 year or longer) patients with CAD	To evaluate patients with single premature ventricular contractions To serially evaluate patients in rehabilitation To diagnose CAD in patients with Wolf-Parkinson-White Syndrome or left bundle branch block
—in screening of apparently healthy people	None	To evaluate asymptomatic males over 40: • in special occupations • with two or more risk factors (cholesterol > 240, high blood pressure, cigarettes, diabetes mellitus, family history of CAD, age less than 55 years) • who are sedentary and plan to enter a vigorous exercise program	To evaluate asymptomatic men and women: • with no risk factors • with chest discomfort not thought to be cardiac
—soon after myocardial infarction	To evaluate prognosis and functional capacity in uncomplicated myocardial infarctions	To evaluate those with baseline electrocardiograms or medical problems that affect responses To evaluate those with complicated myocardial infarctions	To evaluate acute ischemia To evaluate patients who are unstable or have complicating illnesses
—after specific procedures	To evaluate coronary artery bypass graft surgery and percutaneous transluminal coronary angioplasty patients	To follow asymptomatic patients with coronary artery bypass graft surgery or percutaneous transluminal coronary angioplasty yearly	
—in patients with valvular heart disease	Not used	To evaluate functional capacity	To evaluate symptomatic critical aortic stenosis or asymmetrical septal hypertrophy
—in the management of patients with high blood pressure or cardiac pacemakers	Not used	To evaluate blood pressure response in patients treated for high blood pressure who wish to exercise vigorously	To evaluate patients with severe high blood pressure, high–blood pressure patients who do not plan to exercise, and pacemaker function

Note. From the subcommittee on Exercise Testing. A report of the American College of Cardiology/American Heart Association Task Force on Assessment of Cardiovascular Procedures. *J. Am. Coll. Cardiol.* 8:725-738; 1986. Reprinted by permission.

2. Comparison with a "better" test (i.e., thallium scintigraphy): The sensitivity of the exercise ECG was lower when the study compared it with another testing method reported as "superior."
3. Exclusion of patients on digitalis: Excluding patients taking digitalis was associated with improved sensitivity.
4. Publication year: An increase in sensitivity and a decrease in specificity were noted over the years the exercise test has been used. This may be due to the possibility that clinicians allow a test's results to influence their decision to proceed to angiography as they become more familiar with the test and increasingly trust its results.

Specificity was also found to be significantly and independently related to four variables:

1. Treatment of upsloping ST depression: When upsloping ST depression was classified as abnormal, specificity was lowered significantly (73% versus 80%).
2. Exclusion or inclusion of subjects with prior myocardial infarction (MI): The exclusion of patients with a prior MI was associated with a decreased specificity.
3. Exclusion or inclusion of patients with left bundle branch block: The specificity increased when patients with left bundle branch block were excluded.
4. Preexercise hyperventilation: The use of preexercise hyperventilation was associated with a decreased specificity.

Stepwise linear regression explained less than 35% of the variance in sensitivities and specificities reported in the 147 papers. This wide variability in the reported accuracy of the exercise ECG is not explained by the information available in the published reports. Though this could be explained by unsuspected technical, methodological, or clinical variables that affect test performance by poorly understood mechanisms, it is more likely that the authors of the 147 reports did not disclose important information, did not consider the key points that are known to affect test performance when performing and analyzing their studies, or both.

This wide variability in test performance makes it important for clinicians to control rigorously the methods they use for testing and analysis. Individuals with truly nondiagnostic or equivocal tests should be retested or offered other testing methods, and standard ST-segment criteria should not be used to make a diagnosis in patients who are receiving digoxin or have left ventricular hypertrophy (LVH) or resting ST depression. Upsloping ST depression should be considered borderline or negative, and hyperventilation should not be performed prior to testing.

Prognostic Use of Exercise Testing

There are two principal reasons for estimating prognosis. The first is to provide accurate answers to a patient's questions regarding the probable outcome of his or her illness. This is inherently delicate, and probability statements can be misunderstood; however, most patients find this information useful in planning their futures. The second reason is to identify those patients in whom interventions might improve their outcome.

Patients with responses associated with a high risk for CAD are frequently evaluated further by coronary angiography. A study evaluating the appropriateness of the performance of coronary angiography in clinical practice considered angiography to be inappropriate 17% of the time, mainly because of the failure to obtain an exercise test (5). Why not perform coronary angiography on everyone? It is quite natural that when a physician sees a significant lesion on angiography, there is a tendency to want to do something. Even though observational studies (6) suggest a wider benefit of coronary artery bypass grafting (CABG) surgery, the available randomized trials have demonstrated improved survival only in CABG patients with certain anatomic patterns. These patterns include moderately depressed left ventricular function (LVF) (ejection fraction between 30% and 50%), left main occlusion, and triple-vessel disease or left main equivalent. Since only patients with these anatomic subsets can expect improved survival, it is important to select patients carefully for catheterization in whom interventions can improve the length and quality of life.

The prognostic value of the exercise test will be presented by reviewing studies of patients after MI, patients with stable CAD (including silent ischemia), and patients who become symptomatic after CABG surgery.

Post–Myocardial Infarction Exercise Testing

In patients who have had an MI, an exercise test prior to discharge is important for providing activity guidelines, giving reassurance regarding physical status, optimizing medications, and determining the risk of complications. It provides a safe basis for advising patients to resume or increase their activity levels and return to work. Using the following guidelines, a submaximal test is clinically appropriate at the time of discharge:

- For patients younger then 40 years, a heart rate (HR) limit of 140 beats/min and a MET (metabolic equivalent) level of 7
- For patients over 40 years, a HR limit of 130 beats/min and a MET level of 5

Particularly for patients taking beta-blockers, a rating perceived exertion (RPE) level of 15 on the category scale (see Table 17.7) can be used to end the test. Three weeks or more after an MI, when a patient is ready to return to full activities, a symptom-limited graded exercise test (SL-GXT) is recommended.

Of the 24 institutions with articles published before 1987 that present results of exercise testing in post-MI patients with follow up, 10 reported the mortality in patients selected for and those rejected from exercise testing (7). Exclusion from testing was based on clinical criteria. In each of the studies, mortality was much higher in patients excluded from exercise testing than in those who underwent testing. This shows the importance of clinical criteria for identifying high-risk patients.

The results of a meta-analysis for various exercise test responses that occurred in post-MI patients in the studies are presented in Table 4.2 (7). Only 11 institutions out of the 24 found that an ST segment shift induced by exercise was associated with an increased risk. However, only 18 of the 24 studies actually considered the ST-segment response. None of the exercise test responses were predictive more frequently, than by chance alone, if all 24 studies were considered. Only an abnormal systolic blood pressure (BP) response and an abnormal exercise capacity were associated with an increased risk when studies that considered each

response were considered in the denominator. This is rather surprising, since position papers have included the recommendation that patients with abnormal ST-segment depression should undergo cardiac catheterization (8).

The failure of exercise-induced ST-segment depression to be associated consistently with increased risk in patients after MI was hard to explain until recently. A study using thallium scintigraphy demonstrated that ST-segment shifts in patients with anterior Q-wave patterns were not associated with perfusion defects (9). These findings led to the hypothesis that the failure of exercise-induced ST-segment depression to consistently predict prognosis in post-MI patients could be a result of population differences and the resting ECG. This hypothesis was tested by studying 198 males who survived an MI, underwent a submaximal predischarge treadmill test, and were followed for cardiac events for 2 years (10). During this time, 29 deaths, 19 reinfarctions, and 28 revascularization procedures occurred. Abnormal ST-segment depression on a predischarge submaximal treadmill exercise test was associated with twice the risk for death in the first 2 years after MI. The risk increased to 11 times in a subgroup of 55 patients without diagnostic Q waves on the resting ECG recorded at the time of their exercise test. Similar results were obtained by Krone et al. (11) from the Multicenter Post–Myocardial Infarction Research Group, which studied 111 patients with an initial non–Q wave MI. Their results suggest that the difference in the prognostic value of the post-MI exercise ECG between studies is due to variations in the prevalence of the patterns of the rest ECG among study populations. Future studies should consider a more complete classification of the ECG as well as its interaction with exercise-induced ST-segment changes. Angiographic studies, however, have demonstrated that exercise-induced ST depression is associated with severe CAD whether

Table 4.2   Meta-Analysis of 24 Post–Myocardial Infarction Exercise Test Studies

	Systolic blood pressure	Premature ventricular contractions	Decreased exercise capacity	Angina	ST-segment changes
Number of studies that reported results relative to the symptom shown	14	19	12	15	18
Number with positive results[a]	12	13	12	11	11

[a]Exercise test response associated with an increased risk ratio for predicting cardiac events.

or not Q waves are present (12). The conflicting results from follow-up and angiographic studies in patients after MI most probably relate to the fact that early mortality is strongly associated with left ventricular damage while later mortality is associated with ischemia and severe CAD. A resting ECG that exhibits ST depression without Q waves also generates an increased risk immediately after an MI (13).

Prognosis in Patients With Stable Coronary Artery Disease

Various exercise test responses have been used with varying results for predicting prognosis and the presence of left main or triple-vessel disease. ST depression correlates rather closely with the extent of angiographic coronary occlusions (14). A surprising observation is that exercise capacity is extremely important for predicting prognosis (i.e., prognosis is extremely good if exercise capacity exceeds 10 METs and poor if less than 5 METs) but does not appear to distinguish the severity of angiographic disease (15). This could be due to a selection bias for cardiac catheterization. The following paragraphs and Table 4.3 summarize the eight major follow-up studies that have required both coronary angiography and exercise testing with the goal of comparing the prognostic value of various clinical, exercise test, and catheterization variables. The most important clinical variable is a history of congestive heart failure (CHF), and evidence of a prior MI is the next most important. Surprisingly, ST depression was not chosen by a Cox regression model in most of the studies, while exercise capacity was.

Since the pioneering studies at the University of Alabama (16), numerous investigators have utilized clinical, exercise test, and catheterization data to predict prognosis in patients with CAD. Implicit in these studies has been the issue of which variables are predictive and whether exercise testing and coronary angiography improve prediction sufficiently to merit their performance despite their expense and risk.

Using discriminant function analysis, Reeves et al. (16) found that cardiac enlargement on plain films and a history of CHF were the two most predictive independent clinical variables and that angiography improved the prediction of death. They did not consider exercise test results because of incomplete data, but found that patients unable to perform the test had a poorer prognosis. Ellestad

and Wan (17) reported the predictive implications of maximal exercise testing in 2,700 individuals followed from 6 months to 9 years. ST depression and prior MI were both associated with subsequent mortality. This study did not require coronary angiography and so is not comparable.

From the Seattle Heart Watch, Hammermeister et al. (18) assessed 733 medically treated patients by first going stepwise through clinical markers and then having the patients perform the exercise test. CHF was the most important clinical variable, and maximal double product was the most important exercise variable. Maximal systolic BP, HR, and exercise capacity were far less important. Cox's regression analysis showed ejection fraction, age, number of diseased vessels, and resting ventricular arrhythmias, in that order, to be most predictive. From Bad Krozingen, Germany, Gohke et al. (19) followed 1,034 patients with CAD specifically to answer the question, Can exercise testing provide additional prognostic information when angiographic information is available? They found exercise capacity, angina during the exercise test, and maximal HR (HR max) to predict independently the risk of death. Exercise-induced ST depression was only independently predictive in the subgroup with triple-vessel disease and normal LVF.

From the Italian Multicenter Study, Brunelli et al. (20) reported their findings in 1,083 patients less than 65 years of age followed for a mean period of 66 months. They found that clinical markers stratified risk and that coronary angiography added prognostic information only in patients with moderately severe disease. A Q-wave presence and a history of MI were the most important clinical predictors (CHF was not considered). Exercise-induced ST depression was not considered independently but was combined with angina and exercise capacity to create a marker associated with cardiovascular death.

From the Coronary Artery Surgery Study, Weiner et al. (21) analyzed 30 exercise test, coronary angiographic, and clinical variables in 4,083 patients to identify predictors of mortality in medically treated patients with symptomatic CAD. When multivariate stepwise Cox regression was used, nearly the same clinical and exercise test variables were chosen as in our study: CHF, exercise capacity, and prior MI in descending order of importance. ST depression was barely included as the weakest significant variable. When including catheterization variables, LVF was far more important than the number of diseased vessels, and the ST response was no longer significant. Using

Table 4.3 Population Descriptors From Studies of Multivariate Prediction of Cardiac Events

	Seattle	German	Italian	CASS	Duke	VA CABG	Buenos Aires	LBVAMC
Clinical								
Years entered	1971-1974	1975-1978	1976-1979	1974-1979	1969-1981	1970-1974	1972-1982	1984-1990
Population size	733	1,034	1,083	4,083	2,842	245	180	592
Age	52 (mean)	50 (mean)	50	50	49 (median)	51 (mean)	51	59 (mean)
Males	80%	90%	—	80%	70%	100%	96%	100%
Congestive heart failure	13%	—	—	8%	4%	9%	—	8%
MI	—	—	42%	40%	29%	54%	64%	45%
Q waves (at least one)	45%	—	37%	—	22%	38%	—	37%
Digoxin	18%	—	—	14%	11%	NA	—	8%
Beta-blockers	—	—	—	—	54%	14%	—	35%
Typical angina	—	—	95%	—	100%	100%	71%	52%
Exercise test								
% with 1 mm ST depression	—	—	—	44%	35%	72%	65%	58%
% Angina	—	—	—	—	50%	66%	60%	35%
HRmax beats/min	—	—	—	—	—	125	—	124
Max. SBP (mm Hg)	—	—	—	—	—	156	—	159
METs	—	—	—	—	—	5.7	5.5	6.6
PVCs	—	—	—	—	—	19%	13%	12%

Cardiac catheterization findings							
Triple-vessel disease	12%	45%	5%	23%	27%	55%	14%
Left main	—	0%	15%	—	—	13%	7%
No significant lesion	39%	0%	26%	34%	39%	0%	26%
Ejection fraction	—	—	—	—	60 (median)	—	60 (mean)
Significant lesion criteria	70%	50%	75%	70%	75%	50%	70%
Follow-up							
Years	3.5	5	5.5	5	5	7	5
CABG	—	—	15%	36%	24%	24%	20%
Annual CV mortality	—	—	1.54%	1.0%	—	NA	2.7%
Total annual mortality	—	—	2.0%	1.6%	—	4.0%	3.5%
Independent predictors of mortality	CHF	Exercise capacity	Q wave	CHF	ST depression	Exercise-induced	Max. SBP
	Max. DP	Angina	Prior MI	Treadmill stage	Angina index	PVCs	< 130
	Max. SBP	Max. HR	Effort ischemia	ST depression	Treadmill time	HRmax 140 beats/min	ST elevation
	Angina frequency		Poor exercise capacity			>2mm ST depression	< 4 METs
	Resting ST depression						CHF
							Q waves
							< 5 METs

Note. Studies are as follows: Seattle = Seattle Heart Watch; German = results of Gohke et al. (19); Italian = Italian Multicenter Study; CASS = Coronary Artery Surgery Study; Duke = Duke University Database; VA CABG = Veterans Administration, coronary artery bypass grafting trial; Buenos Aires = results of Lerman et al. (24); LBVAMC = Long Beach VA Medical Center. Other abbreviations are as follows: CABG = coronary artery bypass graft; CHF = congestive heart failure; HRmax = maximal heart rate; Max. DP = maximal double product; Max. SPB = maximal systolic blood pressure; MET = metabolic equivalent; MI = myocardial infarction; PVC = premature ventricular contraction.

univariate analysis, 2 mm ST depression generated a modest risk ratio of 1:4.

From the Duke University Database, Mark et al. (22) reported on 2,842 consecutive patients with chest pain who had both a treadmill test and coronary angiography. During the mean follow-up of 5 years (10% followed for 10 years), 24% underwent CABG surgery and were censored at this time. Ranking treadmill variables by relative prognostic importance for predicting cardiovascular death or cardiovascular death and MI, ST depression came first, angina index (0 = none, 1 = occurred during test, 2 = stopped test) next, and treadmill time last. These were chosen by the Cox model, and coefficients from the model were used to derive weights for a score.

From the Veterans Affairs randomized trial of CABG, Peduzzi et al. (23) reported on a 7-year follow-up of 245 patients randomized with regard to medical management who had a baseline treadmill test. Using univariate analysis and a Cox analysis, the study found that ST depression (≥ 2 mm), exercise-induced premature ventricular contractions (PVCs), and a final HR greater than 140 beats/min were significant predictors. These results are in marked contrast to our and other studies, since PVCs have not been shown to have independent predictive power, high HRs have been protective rather than associated with risk, and poor exercise capacity was not found to be predictive.

In Buenos Aires, Lerman et al. (24) reported on 190 patients with exercise tests and coronary angiograms who were followed for 6 years. Their patients had a high annual mortality rate and a low rate of interventions, yet exercise-induced ST depression failed to predict prognosis. A maximal systolic BP of less than 130 mm Hg was the strongest predictor.

Again from the Duke University Database, Califf et al. (25) applied clinical measures of ischemia (exercise test results were not considered) to predict infarct-free survival in 5,896 patients with angina and angiographically documented (> 75% lesions) CAD. The Cox regression model chose the following variables in descending order: more than 1 mm of resting ST depression or T-wave inversion, frequency of angina, unstable angina, typical angina, and duration of symptoms. An angina score was derived from the Cox coefficients, and, when entered into a model with catheterization data, the following variables were chosen in descending order for predicting survival: ejection fraction, number of diseased vessels, left main stenosis, angina score, and age and sex. This score helped predict

prognosis even when the catheterization data were considered.

Because of the differences in the variables chosen to have independent predictive power in the reported studies, we have presented their key characteristics in Table 4.3. Other than the fact that the Duke population and the Veterans Administration CABG study patients appeared to be more "ischemic," no obvious population, methodological, or test characteristics explain the different results. All had to deal with interventions that alter the natural history but censored on them.

One explanation that immediately comes to mind for the failure of ST depression to predict prognosis in our and other studies is that the clinical process was highly adept at selecting high-risk patients with exercise-induced ST depression for interventions. However, this explanation can be excluded for the following reasons: (1) all patients were censored at the time of their CABG surgery or percutaneous transluminal coronary angioplasty (PTCA), (2) the same variables were chosen when patients who received these interventions during follow-up were excluded, and (3) examining and contrasting the characteristics of patients with exercise-induced ST-segment depression who did or did not receive interventions failed to detect any consistent differences. Also, four of the eight comparable studies did not find ST-segment depression to be predictive, and this did not appear to be related to intervention rates.

A paradox exists in that while exercise-induced ST-segment depression best predicts severe CAD in our patients (14), it fails to predict prognosis. In contrast, while exercise capacity predicts prognosis (15), it is a poor predictor of severe angiographic disease. Part of this may be due to a work-up bias (26); that is, patients with excellent exercise capacities are not directed to the cardiac catheterization laboratory, and thus no high–exercise capacity cut point associated with minor or no angiographic disease is observed. On the other hand, a low–exercise capacity cut point that is associated with multiple factors is observed, both causally and secondarily related to CAD, and this cut point predicts a poor outcome.

Ischemic exercise test variables clearly are related to ischemic events during follow-up (i.e., nonfatal MI, CABG surgery, PTCA). In addition, these variables are associated with subsequent hospitalization for unstable angina and to rule out MI. This is logical but of little help in clinical decision making, since, given the established symptomatic benefit from interventions, the clinician has no trouble in justifying these procedures for patients with accelerating symptoms after adequate medical management. Also, surgical intervention has not been shown to prevent subsequent MIs.

The problem lies in justifying intervention to improve survival for patients whose symptoms are satisfactorily managed medically. Simple clinical indicators can stratify these patients with stable CAD into high- or low-risk groups. Cardiac catheterization is not needed to do so in the majority of such patients. Surprisingly, exercise-induced ischemic variables commonly thought by physicians to identify high risk did not do so in four of the eight studies in Table 4.3.

Cardiac death occurs along a spectrum of patients from those with myocardial damage who die of CHF (or pump failure) to those with normal ventricles in whom ischemia precipitates death. Ventricular arrhythmias are usually a secondary event, although they are most often the final cause of death. The clinical and test markers would thus be expected to be quite different for patients who die at the extremes of this spectrum. While markers of myocardial damage (history of CHF, Q waves) track the former, markers of ischemia (angina, ST-segment depression) better track the latter (and arrhythmias are associated with both). Other studies have suggested that markers of myocardial damage predict short-term deaths, while ischemic markers predict deaths occurring 2 or more years later (27).

Given this etiological milieu, associating clinical and test markers with death as an outcome becomes quite difficult. Other ischemic events (i.e., unstable angina, hospitalization for chest pain) are too soft for consideration. In addition, interventions, even if considered an end point only when they occur months after testing, are clearly related to the test response (i.e., patients are referred for interventions because of abnormal tests). Since a nonfatal MI is most likely an ischemic event, infarct-free survival is another way of including more ischemic end points, but we had similar results considering it as the end point in the Cox model.

Different populations may favor a particular type of mortality (pump failure vs. ischemia), which might explain why ischemic variables are more predictive in one population and myocardial-damage variables in another. Arguably, our population included a majority of patients who died secondary to CHF; however, the same results were obtained after removing 75 patients who either carried that diagnosis or were taking digoxin at the time of entry into our study. (Most other studies had a similar proportion of such patients.)

The results of our study and others raise an interesting question: Can we disregard marked amounts of ST-segment depression in patients who do not have other clinical and exercise indicators of high risk? Certainly this is not done in clinical practice. But considering the potential savings of money and morbidity through identifying a low-risk subgroup, we should not catheterize every patient with ST-segment depression. Clearly, exercise-induced ST-segment depression is indicative of ischemia and not necessarily of prognosis. Just as we are often tempted to pursue spurious laboratory results or chemistry panel tests, so do we still subject a large number of patients to CABG surgery or PTCA intervention merely on the basis of anatomy without regard to functional status and without evidence of an impact on their mortality.

Thus, on the basis of clinical and exercise test data, we can classify patients as low- or high-risk. High-risk patients clearly need to proceed to cardiac catheterization, while low-risk ones need not, unless otherwise indicated by their symptoms or response to medications. The presence of CHF, the involvement of two or more Q-wave areas, and an exercise capacity of less than 5 METs appear to be the most important predictors of risk. Ejection fraction, as determined by noninvasive methods rather than by cardiac catheterization, can be added when needed.

Enthusiasm for a new technique (i.e., cardiac catheterization) may well have led to an acceptance of invasive measurements as being superior to clinical variables for prognostication in patients with CAD. Though clinical variables were mentioned in the early studies, key variables were often not considered, nor were they considered together or defined as accurately as they are today. It was assumed that laboratory methods and images were more accurate and more precise than simple clinical data. Also, the importance of clinical data could have been underestimated because of the unavailability of modern survival analysis techniques. A further consideration is that the decline in mortality in patients categorized by vessel score (28) is not actually due to disease treatment but rather to patient selection (i.e., excluding patients with CHF because of a better recognition of it).

Comparison With Radionuclide Techniques

Skeptics may say that the standard exercise test must be augmented by either radionuclide ventriculography (RNV) or thallium scintigraphy. However, most of the studies that examine these techniques have not compared them with clinical and routine exercise test results. Simari et al. (29) evaluated the ability of supine exercise ECG and RNV to predict subsequent cardiac events in 265 patients who had a normal resting ECG, were not receiving digoxin and had undergone cardiac catheterization. The Cox regression model chose ST depression, exercise HR, and gender as being equivalent to the RNV data. They concluded that exercise RNV was not justified for use over standard exercise testing variables. This is countered by Lee et al. (30) who evaluated 571 patients, among whom RNV provided more prognostic information than did clinical variables. In an elegant review by Brown (31), the prognostic value of thallium imaging was presented. Of the studies reviewed, the most comparable is that by Kaul et al. (32), who concluded that a change in HR and other exercise test variables was superior to the presence of thallium defects for prognostication.

Exertional Hypotension

Although exertional hypotension (EIH) has been related to a poor prognosis in patients with CAD, various criteria have been used to define it and little consideration has been given to the measurement difficulties or to its reproducibility. To determine the cut point, or discriminant value, for EIH (33), we applied the following criteria: (1) a drop in systolic BP of 20 mm Hg or more after an initial rise but without a fall below rest and (2) a drop of the systolic BP below the standing rest value. The first criterion was chosen to avoid the technical and reproducibility limitations of BP measurements taken during exercise. EIH is best defined as a drop of systolic BP during exercise below the standing preexercise value, which occurs in about 6% of patients tested, and indicates a significantly increased risk for cardiac events (three times) when associated with myocardial ischemia or damage. As in other studies, more than half of the patients tested who exhibited EIH had left main or triple-vessel disease.

Silent Ischemia During Exercise Testing

The prognostic implication of ST depression unaccompanied by angina is controversial. It has been suggested that those with silent ischemia are at greater risk for cardiac death because they do not have an intact warning system. Because of the increased reliability of ST segment recording during exercise testing compared with ambulatory monitoring, we performed a study to determine the prognosis of patients with silent ischemia in an unselected population referred for exercise testing

(34). A second objective was to determine whether the presence of an old or recent MI, diabetes mellitus, or age influenced the prevalence of silent myocardial ischemia. The study population was predominantly male veterans (1,747 male and 26 female patients, mean age 58 years) excluding those with resting ST depression or LVH and those receiving digoxin. In approximately 60% of our patients with exercise-induced ST-segment depression, the ischemia was silent. Mean maximal ST-segment depression was significantly greater among patients with both angina and ST depression than among patients with silent ischemia. Exercise-induced ST-segment depression conferred an adverse 2-year prognosis, and there was a trend toward better survival in those with silent ischemia compared with those with angina and ST depression. The prevalence of silent ischemia was not altered by the presence or absence of a previous MI, nor by diabetes mellitus, but it was directly related to age.

A more rigorous follow-up study performed at Duke (35) and a Canadian study (36) have definitively demonstrated the trend in our study for silent ischemia to have a better prognosis when ST depression is accompanied by angina. An angiographic study of 586 patients (37) at our institution was in agreement, demonstrating milder disease in patients with silent myocardial ischemia. This was even the case in those with true silent ischemia, that is, those without a prior history of angina. Thus, therapy should not be more aggressive for patients with silent ischemia than for patients who have angina and ST-segment depression. Since antianginal medication has not been demonstrated to improve survival, there is no indication to treat silent ischemia. However, if such patients have exercise test markers of severe disease (i.e., poor exercise capacity or marked or prolonged amounts of ST depression), then catheterization and revascularization should be considered, as for patients with symptomatic disease.

At times, we may be frustrated with our patients' symptoms and complaints, but evidence supports the clinicians' concerns and direction of therapy for angina pectoris. This is supported by the Duke Angina Score (25). Perhaps silent ischemia is beneficial, since ischemia is the best producer of collaterals, and when it is painless people are able to achieve higher levels of exercise and accelerate collateral development. This is hypothetical but perhaps more logical than the exaggerated dangers of silent ischemia.

Prognosis in Patients Who Become Symptomatic After Coronary Artery Bypass Graft Surgery

Predicting the outcome of patients who become symptomatic after CABG surgery is an important issue, given that more than 200,000 patients undergo this surgical procedure in the United States each year. These patients experience an annual 2% to 3% recurrence rate for angina (38), reoperations are associated with an increased mortality (39), and the role of PTCA for dilating occluded grafts is uncertain (40). Studies have evaluated graft occlusion and recurrence of symptoms, but none has addressed the use of exercise testing to predict the outcome after CABG surgery. Therefore, we performed a mean 2-year follow-up on 298 patients who had undergone CABG surgery and had then undergone an exercise test to check for recurrence of symptoms or to assess functional capacity (41). Signs and symptoms of ischemia during the treadmill test did not predict an increased risk either in the total population or in those with either typical or atypical angina. The ST-segment response may not be predictive in this group of patients, because left ventricular dysfunction (LVD) is the dominant predictor. Those with events had a lower exercise capacity and other hemodynamic responses, but these variables were not powerful enough to predict the outcome. However, the ability to exceed 9 METs had a protective effect. The inability of the

exercise ECG to predict cardiac events in post-CABG patients suggests that other modes of testing should be investigated, such as nuclear exercise testing or exercise echocardiographic studies (42).

Heart Rate Adjustment of the ST Segment

Several investigators have shown an improvement in the diagnostic accuracy of ST-segment depression using a variety of HR adjustment schemes. Figure 4.1 illustrates the differences between the ST/HR slope and the ST/HR index. The index is a simple approach to HR adjustment and, as demonstrated by Kligfield et al. (43), functions as well as the more time-consuming method of computing the ST/HR slope. Hoping to validate the diagnostic accuracy of the index, we studied 328 patients who had undergone cardiac catheterization (44). Unfortunately, this technique failed to exhibit any improvement in diagnostic accuracy over the standard analysis, nor was it a better means of identifying triple-vessel or left main disease. Its performance characteristics were no different in patients receiving beta-blockers, patients with Q waves on their resting ECGs or patients who had prior MIs. Until population characteristics are identified that are associated with an improvement in exercise test characteristics when using the index, it cannot be recommended for general application. Herbert

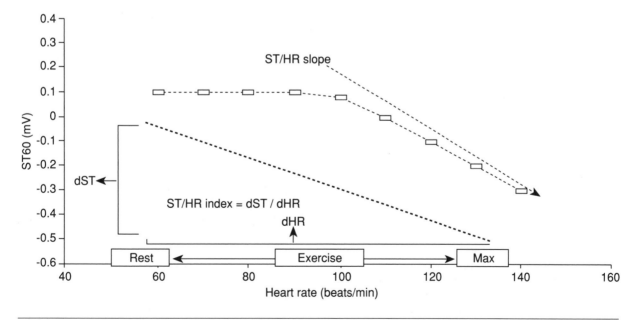

Figure 4.1 Difference between the ST/HR (heart rate) slope and ST/HR index. The ST/HR slope is calculated by dividing the total ST-segment shift by the change in heart rate during exercise; the ST/HR index = dST/dHR.

et al. (45) have also shown the index not to improve the diagnostic value of the test in patients on beta-blockers. In fact, beta-blockers appeared to improve the test characteristics using the standard ST measures as well.

ST Changes Occurring During Recovery From the Exercise Test

Due to technical limitations, the first diagnostic use of the exercise ECG involved observations made only after exercise. After the development of modern techniques that could accurately record the ECG during activity, the emphasis in testing shifted to changes occurring during the exercise period itself. The diagnostic accuracy of ST changes limited to the postexercise period has been controversial. It has been proposed that such changes are more likely to represent false positives or be due to coronary artery spasm. Studies comparing nuclear procedures to the exercise ECG often do not even include postexercise ECG evaluation so as to facilitate imaging as soon as possible during recovery (46). In addition, most of the exercise test scores consider only ST segment changes that occur during exercise, thereby excluding changes that occur during recovery alone (3). Also, a cool-down walk, which is known to delay or obscure recovery changes (47), is frequently used for reasons of safety (48) and patient comfort.

ST Depression

We performed a study to determine whether ST-segment depression limited to the recovery period increased the diagnostic yield of the exercise test or whether these changes should be disregarded (49). Three hundred twenty-eight male patients who had undergone an SL-GXT and coronary angiography made up the study population. Abnormal ST-segment depression in "recovery only" occurred in 16% of the total abnormal group of 168. "Recovery only" ST depression had a predictive value for significant angiographic disease of 84%, which was not statistically different from the predictive value of ST depression occurring during exercise (87%). Taking into account ST depression during recovery significantly increased the sensitivity, from 50% to 59%, without a change in predictive value. ST-segment depression occurring only in recovery is not a "false positive," and taking into account data from the recovery period increases the diagnostic yield of the exercise test.

Most exercise test scores and exercise ECG analyses performed in conjunction with scintigraphy or with the use of a cool-down walk have a falsely lowered sensitivity that could be increased by considering ST-segment changes that occur in recovery.

ST Elevation

Exercise-induced ST elevation differs in prevalence and meaning from ST depression, depending upon the status of the baseline ECG (50,51). When the baseline ECG does not exhibit diagnostic Q waves, then ST elevation is very rare (< 2%) and is associated with severe transmural ischemia. This is usually due to a tight proximal lesion in a major coronary artery or to coronary spasm. The test should be stopped immediately upon observing such ST elevation, since it is arrhythmogenic, and the individual should be considered for coronary angiography. If diagnostic Q waves are present on the resting ECG, then the elevation in such leads is a more common finding and does not indicate myocardial ischemia.

Computer Analysis of the Exercise Electrocardiograph and Treadmill Scores

Computer signal averaging is now available in the routine clinical exercise laboratory thanks to microprocessor technology. Manufacturers have utilized software research to filter and average ECG signals with the aim of making exercise ECG analysis more reproducible and accurate. However, since researchers utilized large mainframe computers and were not concerned with on-line analysis, manufacturers have had to alter these programs for the real-time exercise laboratory environment. This has led to problems with the fidelity of the computer-processed ECG wave forms. Though these computer averages are very attractive, they can be distorted and may not represent the raw data. It is extremely important that physicians carefully observe the raw ECG data that are used to generate the averaged wave forms. Distortion can be caused by noise, baseline wander, aberrant beats, and changes in conduction. The numerical measurements are dependent upon the average wave forms and therefore may also be erroneous. The measurements are particularly problematic because even with good averages it may be difficult for the algorithms to find the ST-segment onset. We recommend using the averages by first looking at the raw data to see that they are not grossly distorted, make measurements over at least 3 consecutive beats, and then see if the averages agree. The averages can be used as a summary of the results if they agree with the raw data. All too frequently we have seen healthy people with normal raw data that have clearly abnormal averaged complexes due to the inaccuracies of the ECG algorithms (52). Skin preparation is critical to obtaining adequate raw ECG data—do not rely on filtering or averaging.

Numerous computer scores have been recommended, most of which are very laborious and require computerization. Unfortunately, none of these have been validated, and all are still recommended by only the investigators who first evaluated them. Consequently, none of the scores is currently appropriate for clinical utilization. The multivariate approach of Detry et al. (53) has been demonstrated by Decker et al. (54) to be more accurate than the ST/HR index (43), the Hollenberg Score (55), and Simoons's method (56). Though experts disagree, most studies have demonstrated that multivariate approaches for predicting outcome are more robust than Bayesian methods (57).

Exercise Testing in Asymptomatic, Apparently Healthy Populations

Though more than 10 follow-up studies have been completed to address the issue of exercising in apparently health populations, none has demonstrated that the exercise test is effective in screening asymptomatic individuals for purposes of preventing cardiac events. In fact, the ACC-AHA Guidelines (1) state that the exercise test should not be used in this group unless a patient has two or more of the standard risk factors (i.e., cigarette smoking, hypercholesterolemia, hypertension, family history). Sox et al. (58) suggested that screening exercise tests might be justifiable in asymptomatic individuals who have at least one clinical risk factor or a total cholesterol–high-density lipoprotein (HDL) ratio greater than 6.0. However, Ekelund et al. (59) recently reported the results of exercise testing in a population with elevated blood cholesterol levels, which still found a very low predictive value for an abnormal test. The first eight screening studies included angina pectoris as an end point, while later studies only used hard end points (i.e., MI or death) (Table 4.4). These later studies were more valid and demonstrated a much lower predictive value for an abnormal response. Only 1 in 20 people with an abnormal ST response will have a hard cardiac event within 5 to 8 years after the test. This leaves 19 out of 20 to deal with the psychological, sociological, and financial problems of a false-positive test.

When Is Expired Gas Analysis Necessary?

Recent technical advances have lessened the difficulty with which expired-gas analysis can be performed during exercise (60). Such measurements allow an accurate assessment of the maximal oxygen uptake ($\dot{V}O_2max$) as compared with estimating it from treadmill speed and grade. $\dot{V}O_2max$ is directly related to maximal cardiac output and gives the best measurement of cardiac performance during exercise. In addition, gas exchange parameters allow assessment of the anaerobic threshold. This submaximal measurement may be of more importance clinically than $\dot{V}O_2max$, since it defines a person's limitations at submaximal levels, which are common to daily activities. Currently, the clinical application of gas exchange variables is limited

Table 4.4 Screening of Asymptomatic, Apparently Healthy Individuals for Silent Ischemia (ST Depression) With Exercise Testing

	N	Sensitivity (%)	Specificity (%)	Positive predictive value (%)	Risk ratio
Including angina pectoris as endpoint	8	48	90	26	9
Only hard endpoints	4	27	91	6	4

Note. "Hard" = documented myocardial infarction, death.

to evaluating treatments that determine whether lung or cardiac disease predominates, to sports medicine, and to documenting disability. In regard to the latter, many physicians have the impression that gas exchange variables identify patients who are malingering during disability evaluations and are not giving a maximal performance. Such judgements should be made cautiously, since many of the parameters used to quantify maximal performance, such as plateauing, exceeding the anaerobic threshold, or a respiratory exchange of unity, have considerable measurement error and intersubject variability (61).

Exercise-Induced Ventricular Tachycardia: Risk and Prognosis

Exercise-induced ventricular tachycardia is believed to increase risk during testing; it has also been thought to confer a poor prognosis, though whether this is true or not has not been specifically studied. In a retrospective view of 3,351 patients who had undergone routine clinical exercise testing between September 1984 and June 1989, we identified 55 patients with exercise-induced ventricular tachycardia (62). *Nonsustained ventricular*

tachycardia was defined as ventricular ectopic beats greater than or equal to 3 consecutive beats (range = 3 to 12 beats). *Sustained ventricular tachycardia* was defined as tachycardia longer than 30 s or requiring intervention. Mean follow-up was 26 months (range = 2 to 58 months). Fifty patients had nonsustained ventricular tachycardia during exercise testing, and only 1 patient died due to CHF during the follow-up period. Five patients had sustained ventricular tachycardia during exercise testing, and only 1 died of sudden death 7 months after the test. Exercise-induced ventricular tachycardia was reproduced in only 2 of the 29 patients who underwent repeat testing. Thus, this phenomenon was rare, with a prevalence of 1.6%, and was not associated with complications during testing. Annual mortality in the exercise-induced ventricular tachycardia group (1.7%) was not significantly different from the mortality in the entire test population (2.5%) (Figure 4.2).

Exercise Test Protocols

Protocols suitable for clinical exercise testing should include a low-intensity warm-up phase and progressive exercise of a continuous nature in

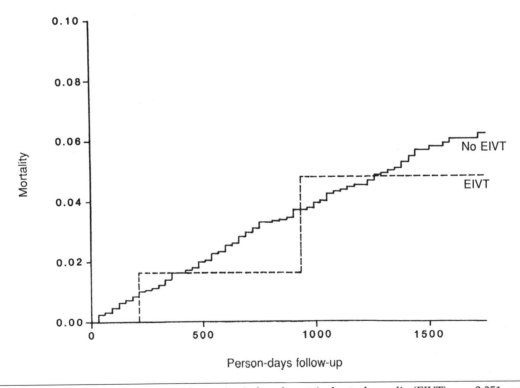

Figure 4.2 Follow-up data on patients with exercise-induced ventricular tachycardia (EIVT): n = 3,351 men; nonsustained ventricular tachycardia (VT) = 50; sustained VT = 5; prevalence of EIVT = 1.5%.

which the demand is elevated to a patient's maximal level within a total duration of 8 to 10 min. It is important to report exercise capacity in METs and not in minutes so that the protocol used does not make comparing results difficult. METs can be estimated from any protocol using Figure 4.3. Today, the most widely used treadmill test employed in clinical settings is the Bruce protocol. Unfortunately, this protocol has significant disadvantages for functional testing, especially among patients with low exercise capacities or orthopedic problems. The Bruce protocol has been modified in recent years for testing low-functional capacity patients by adding two preliminary stages of lower intensities. Nevertheless, because the MET increments in the Bruce protocol are large and uneven, and because it severely limits the number of submaximal responses that may be observed in relation to exercise stages, we do not recommend its use. The U.S. Air Force San Antonio modification of the Balke-Ware protocol is a particularly attractive alternative because of its constant treadmill speed of either 2.0 mph or 3.3 mph and grade increments of 5% applied every 2 or 3 min. This protocol provides good flexibility so that an optimal exercise time to maximum can be achieved, thereby allowing an examination of patient responses across four or five stages (Figure 4.4).

One recent advance in test methodology that overcomes many of the limitations of multistage exercise tests is the ramp protocol (63). The ramp involves a nearly continuous and uniform increase in metabolic demand that replaces the staging used in conventional exercise tests (Figure 4.5). With ramping, the uniform increase in demand allows for a steady rise in cardiopulmonary responses and permits a more accurate prediction of oxygen uptake ($\dot{V}O_2$). Protocols have been developed that provide for ramping rates appropriate for patients with different functional capacities, for use both with a cycle ergometer and a treadmill.

Deciding on an exercise protocol that will optimize test duration for each patient is important, whether the approach is ramping or staging. Errors in this step can advance the patient toward the maximum too rapidly or too slowly. The consequence of early test termination is an inadequate opportunity to observe clinically important responses. The consequence of a prolonged procedure is muscular fatigue, which may limit performance before a myocardial challenge adequate for diagnosis is obtained. Thus, the protocol should be individualized to accommodate the patient's limitations. When no exercise test has previously been performed by the patient, as is most often the case, consulting tables that show normal values in METs for functional capacity and are graded by age, sex, and habitual physical activity level can prove helpful. The Califf approach, published by Hlatky et al. (64), may be particularly helpful in guiding the selection of the exercise test protocol (Table 4.5). It is easily completed as a self-administered questionnaire and demonstrates reasonable validity when correlated with measured $\dot{V}O_2$ max.

Conclusion

Despite newer cardiovascular testing technologies, the use of exercise testing continues to increase. The last survey by the American College of Physicians (ACP) (65) indicated that 50% of internists now perform the test in the office, using it as a gatekeeper in the decision-making process of who should be referred to a cardiologist. Critical to appropriate and timely referral for therapeutic interventions is an up-to-date application of exercise testing methods and interpretation. Some of the newer concepts are summarized here:

1. Ischemic ST depression normally occurs mainly in the lateral leads (1, V4, V5, V6). However, when the ECG changes are affected by Q-wave presence, isolated ST depression can occur in other areas (i.e., V2 or limb lead II). When there is severe ischemia, changes in the lateral leads are often accompanied by changes in the inferior and anterior leads as well (i.e., V2 and AVF, 11). Otherwise, ST changes isolated to the interior or anterior leads are usually false-positive responses.
2. ST depression *does not localize* ischemia to an area of myocardium.
3. Silent ischemia (ST depression without angina) indicates milder forms of coronary disease and has a lower risk than ST depression accompanied by angina pectoris.
4. ST depression indicates neither ischemia in patients with left bundle branch block nor increased risk in patients after Q-wave MIs or CABG surgery.
5. ST elevation means different things, depending upon the baseline ECG:
   over Q-wave areas = myocardial damage;
   over non–Q-wave areas = localized area of transmural ischemia that is arrhythmogenic.

TREADMILL PROTOCOLS

FUNCTIONAL CLASS	CLINICAL STATUS	O_2 COST ml/kg/min	METS	BICYCLE ERGOMETER (1 WATT = 6 KPDS) FOR 70 KG BODY WEIGHT KPDS	BRUCE 3 MIN STAGES MPH	BRUCE %GR	KATTUS MPH	KATTUS %GR	BALKE-WARE % GRADE AT 3.3 MPH 1-MIN STAGES	ELLESTAD 3/2/3 MIN STAGES MPH	ELLESTAD %GR	USAFSAM MPH	USAFSAM %GR	"SLOW" USAFSAM MPH	"SLOW" %GR	McHENRY MPH	McHENRY %GR	STANFORD % GRADE AT 3 MPH	STANFORD % GRADE AT 2 MPH	METS
NORMAL AND I (HEALTHY, DEPENDENT ON AGE, ACTIVITY)			16						26											16
		56.0	16						25											15
		52.5	15		5.5	20			24	6	15	3.3	25							14
		49.0	14				4	22	23							3.3	21			13
		45.5	13	1500	5.0	18	4	18	22	5	15	3.3	20			3.3	18			12
	SEDENTARY HEALTHY	42.0	12	1350	4.2	16			21							3.3	15	22.5		11
		38.5	11	1200			4	14	20	5	10	3.3	15	2	25			20.0		10
		35.0	10	1050	3.4	14	4	10	19					2	20	3.3	12	17.5		9
		31.5	9	900					18									15.0		8
		28.0	8	750	2.5	12			17	4	10	3.3	10	2	15	3.3	9	12.5		7
II	LIMITED	24.5	7	600			3	10	16	3	10							10.0	17.5	6
		21.0	6	450			2	10	15			3.3	5	2	10	3.3	6	7.5	14	5
		17.5	5	300	1.7	10			14	1.7	10			2	5			5.0	10.5	4
III	SYMPTOMATIC	14.0	4	150					13			3.3	0			2.0	3	2.5	7	3
		10.5	3		1.7	5			12					2	0			0.0	3.5	2
IV		7.0	2		1.7	0			11			2.0	0							1
		3.5	1						10 9 8 7 6 5 4 3 2 1											

Figure 4.3   METs for cycle ergometer and various treadmill protocols.

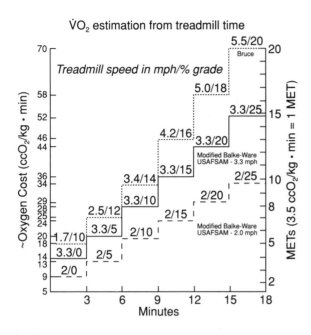

Figure 4.4 Bruce protocol versus U.S. Air Force San Antonio modification treadmill protocol.

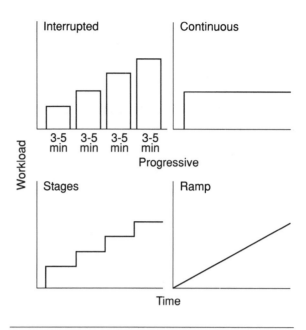

Figure 4.5 Types of exercise protocols.

6. Do not rely on computer averages or new scores (e.g., ST/HR index, ST/HR slope, Hollenberg Index).
7. Report exercise capacity as the MET level achieved, not total exercise time ("METs not minutes"). Avoid overestimation of exercise capacity due to insufficient time (< 1 min) in peak test stages.
8. Exertional hypotension is best defined as a drop in systolic BP below preexercise values and indicates three-fold higher risk.
9. ST depression (subendocardial ischemia) is not as arrhythmogenic as ST elevation (transmural ischemia).
10. Markers of severe disease include exertional hypotension; angina that limits the exercise test; poor exercise capacity (< 5 METs); downsloping ST depression, particularly in recovery; ST depression beginning at a low double product (< 15,000); ST depression in multiple leads; and ST depression that persists late into recovery.

The key values for METs are as follows:

1 MET = basal = 3.5 ml $O_2 \cdot kg^{-1} \cdot min^{-1}$
2 to 5 mph, mph = METs
< 5 METs: poor prognosis
5 METs: minimal activities of daily living, post-MI limit for 1 month

Table 4.5 The Duke Activity Status Index

Activity: Can you . . .	Weight
Take care of yourself (eat, dress, bathe, and use the toilet)?	2.75
Walk indoors, such as around your house?	1.75
Walk a block or two on level ground?	2.75
Climb a flight of stairs or walk up a hill?	5.50
Run a short distance?	8.00
Do light work around the house, like dusting or washing dishes?	2.70
Do moderate work around the house like vacuuming, sweeping floors, or carrying in groceries?	3.50
Do heavy work around the house, like scrubbing floors or lifting or moving heavy furniture?	8.00
Do yard work, like raking leaves, weeding, or pushing a power mower?	4.50
Have sexual relations?	5.25
Participation in moderate recreational activities, like golf, bowling, dancing, doubles tennis, or throwing a basketball or football?	6.00
Participate in strenuous sports, like swimming, singles tennis, football, basketball or skiing?	7.50

Note. The Duke Activity Status Index (DASI) = the sum of the weights for "yes" replies; oxygen uptake (VO₂) = (0.43 × DASI) + 9.6.

10 METS: fit, no benefit in terms of survival from CABG surgery compared with medial management

13 METs: good prognosis regardless of treadmill test results

20 METs: aerobic master athlete

24 METs: aerobic athlete

Though books such as this are sure to help in this regard, the exercise statement from the AHA provides this information in a widely available format (66).

Summary

Proper methodology must be applied during the exercise test to insure patient safety and the acquisition of accurate test results. The criteria that defines proper methodology includes preparing the patient physically and emotionally for the exercise test. A brief physical examination serves to rule out significant valvular disease, specifically aortic valve disease. During this exam a patient interview allows the physician to screen for exclusion criteria and factors leading to early termination of the exercise test. Of no less importance, the interview encourages physician-patient interaction. Physically preparing the patient for testing requires standard 12 lead ECG's in both the supine and standing positions. To obtain accurate readings and avoid artifact, good skin preparation must be performed, which may cause some patient discomfort. In addition, inaccurate electrode placement can lead to artifactual ECG recordings. To avoid these changes, the arm electrodes should be placed on the shoulder (rather than on the chest) while in the supine position. This modified exercise limb lead placement can serve well as the reference resting ECG to compare to prior tracings. The standing ECG however, should be used for determining the baseline ST segment level for comparison with changes that occur during the exercise test. Finally, access to the appropriate emergency equipment is essential for safe exercise testing in all individuals.

Few studies have correctly evaluated the relative yield or sensitivity and specificity of different electrode placements for exercise-induced ST segment shifts. Traditionally, physicians have looked closely at V5 for ST segment changes. Studies show that using other leads in addition to V5 will increase the sensitivity but decrease the specificity, leading to an increase in the number of false positives. Particularly, ST segment changes isolated to the inferior leads often are false positive responses.

Lastly, vectorcardiographic and body surface mapping lead systems do not appear to offer any advantage over simpler approaches for clinical purposes.

The exercise protocol for testing various individuals should be progressive with even increments in speed and grade whenever possible. Smaller, even, and more frequent work increments are preferable to larger, uneven, and less frequent increases. The clinical importance of the former approach has been demonstrated in several studies through a yield of more accurate estimates of exercise capacity. Rather than using the same protocol for every patient, the value of individualizing the exercise protocol, such as with the ramp protocol, has recently been emphasized by many investigators. These researchers suggest an optimal test duration is from eight to 12 minutes; thus, the protocol workloads for each patient should be adjusted to permit this duration. Because ramp testing uses small increments, it permits a more accurate estimation of exercise capacity, and can be individualized for every patient to yield a targeted test duration. As of yet, however, only a few equipment companies manufacture a controller which performs such tests using a treadmill.

When predicting maximum exercise, target heart rates based on age should not be used because the relationship between maximal heart rate and age is poor, and has a wide scatter around many different proposed regression lines. Consequently, predicted heart rate targets can result in a submaximal test for some individuals, a maximal test for others, and an unrealistic goal for still others. An alternative to the predicted maximal heart rate as a predictor of maximal exercise are the Borg perceived exertion scales (both linear and nonlinear) which accurately quantify an individual's exercise effort.

Throughout the exercise test, blood pressure should be measured with a standard stethoscope and sphygmomanometer; the available automated devices are a tempting alternative to the manual approach, but are not reliable for detection of exertional hypotension, an important clinical finding when observed during an exercise test. When interpreting test results, exercise capacity should not be reported in total time but rather as oxygen uptake ($\dot{V}O_2$) or MET equivalents of the workload achieved. The use of METs instead of total exercise time allows one to compare the results of many different exercise testing protocols.

It is worth noting that hyperventilation should no longer be used prior to exercise testing. Subjects with and without disease may or may not exhibit

ST segment changes with hyperventilation, and thus the value of this procedure in lessening the number of false positive responders is no longer considered useful by most researchers. A more recent and critical diagnostic development has been the analysis of the postexercise period. The patient should be placed in the supine position immediately after testing without a cool-down walk to allow for the capture of any electrocardiographic changes that may be too subtle or absent when a cool-down walk is performed.

Summary of Exercise ECG Interpretation

ST-segment depression has long been recognized as a predictor of coronary artery disease. It represents global subendocardial ischemia, except when found in the inferior leads (II, AVF) where it can be a result of atrial repolarization. Atrial repolarization begins in the PR segment and can extend to the beginning of the ST segment. With subendocardial ischemia, the direction of the vector is determined largely by the placement of the heart in the chest. Furthermore, ST depression does not localize coronary artery lesions. It is becoming increasingly clear that ST segment depression found only in the recovery period does not generally represent a "false positive" response. Inclusion of analysis during this time period increases the diagnostic yield of the exercise test.

ST elevation, on the other hand, is associated with severe transmural ischemia as a result of wall motion abnormalities. These abnormalities cause a shift of the vector in the direction of the wall motion abnormality. However, pre-existing areas of wall motion abnormality (i.e., scar) usually indicated by a Q wave, can also cause such a shift, resulting in ST elevation without ischemia being present. Q-waves appearing in a resting ECG (indicating an old MI) can indicate ischemia or wall motion abnormalities or both, whereas accompanying ST depression can be due to a second area of ischemia or reciprocal changes. When the resting ECG is normal (absent of Q waves), ST elevation is due to severe ischemia (spasm or a critical lesion), and the accompanying ST depression is a reciprocal phenomena. Such ST elevation is uncommon, very arrhythmogenic and localizes the area of ischemia. Exercise-induced R-wave and S-wave amplitude changes do not correlate well with changes in left ventricular volume, ejection fraction, or ischemia. The consensus of many studies

is that these changes do not have diagnostic value. Additionally, performing exercise ECG analysis in conjunction with scintigraphy, or performing a cool-down walk can falsely lower the sensitivity of the exercise ECG, since they obscure ST segment changes occurring in recovery, and result in a number of false negatives. Other criteria for diagnosis that improve test performance include downsloping ST changes in recovery and prolongation of ST depression. An alternative diagnostic method that has been investigated is the use of exercise test scores. These scores have not been adequately validated, however, and should be used with caution.

As with resting ventricular arrhythmias, the significance of exercise induced ventricular arrhythmias are related to the disease processes with which they are associated (history of syncope, sudden death, physical exam with a large heart, murmurs; ECG showing prolonged QT, preexcitation, Q waves). If there are no signs or symptoms of associated diseases, then exercise induced ventricular arrhythmias can be viewed as benign (you don't behave like you are in a CCU). Exercise induced ventricular arrhythmias rarely have an independent association with death in most patients with coronary disease; that is, you can get better prediction from other variables. However, it is probable that there are a small percentage of patients in whom exercise induced ventricular arrhythmias are independently predictive of death. In summary, nonsustained ventricular tachycardia is uncommon during routine clinical treadmill testing, is well tolerated, and is associated with a relatively good prognosis. Outcome of the exercise test in reference to the patients state of disease is primarily determined by concomitant clinical features, such as ventricular function, ischemia, and the presence or absence of symptoms. Treatment should be directed toward these signs and symptoms rather than the episode of arrhythmia.

The same exercise test responses can have different meanings from one population or clinical subset to another thus, interpretation of the exercise test depends upon the application of the test. The interpretation of the exercise test is not simple, but requires the understanding of physiology and pathophysiology. One should not accept that all medical professionals can adequately interpret an exercise test. Certification in performing and evaluating the exercise test is extremely important now that this technology is rapidly spreading beyond the subspecialty of Cardiology. Training and experience are required for exercise testing as they are in all other diagnostic procedures. In part for these reasons, the American College of Physicians has recently published guidelines on clinical competence for physicians performing exercise testing. All of the results of the test must be considered. Attempts should be made to make the interpretation reliable by using appropriate methods and following the above suggestions. When properly interpreted, the exercise test is one of the most important diagnostic and clinically helpful tests in medicine.

In studies that have attempted to predict the number of occluded coronary arteries through evaluation of the exercise test, increased sensitivity of the test was found as more diseased vessels were identified, resulting in a higher percentage of true positives. The most false negatives have been reported among patients with single vessel disease, particularly if the diseased vessel was not the left anterior descending artery. Regardless of the techniques used, there is a reciprocal relationship between sensitivity and specificity. The more specific a test is (i.e., the more able it is to determine who is disease free), the less sensitive it is and vice versa. The values for sensitivity and specificity can be altered by adjusting the criterion used for abnormal. For instance, when the criterion for an abnormal exercise-induced ST-segment response is altered to 0.2 mV depression, making it more specific for coronary artery disease, the sensitivity of the test will be reduced by half. For unknown reasons, the specificity of the ST-segment response is decreased when the exercise test is used in women, in patients who have ST-segment depression at rest, left ventricular hypertrophy, vasoregulatory abnormalities, mitral valve prolapse, and when ST depression is isolated to the inferior leads. Moreover, standard criteria of exercise-induced ST-segment depression fails to distinguish between patients with or without coronary artery disease if they are taking digoxin at the time of exercise testing. Interestingly, the persistence of exercise-induced ST-segment depression > 4 minutes into recovery or the development of downsloping ST-segment depression during recovery are better markers for coronary artery disease in these same patients. Patients who have resting ST-segment depression on their baseline electrocardiogram, which is not due to left ventricular hypertrophy, conduction defects, or drug effects, have a higher prevalence of severe coronary artery disease and a poorer long-term prognosis than patients without resting ST-segment depression.

Exercise-induced ST-segment depression continues to have discriminatory power for the diagnosis of coronary artery disease in these patients.

For the diagnosis of coronary artery disease in patients without a prior myocardial infarction, the criteria of 2 millimeters of additional exercise-induced ST-segment depression and the appearance of downsloping ST-segment depression during recovery are particularly effective. For the diagnosis of severe coronary disease in patients who have survived a prior myocardial infarction, the criteria of 2 mm of additional exercise-induced ST-segment depression and prolonged recovery ST-segment depression are better markers than standard criteria. An understanding of predictive modeling (the effect of disease prevalence or positive predictive value) and Bayesian statistics (pre and post test probability and likelihood ratios) is important for the clinician. In addition, the rules by Philbrick, Horwitz, and Feinstein (68) are important for assessing new diagnostic techniques which are possible valuable additions to the standard exercise test (i.e., thallium, echo).

Why do the various prognostic studies fail to get the same results? The most likely explanation lies in the fact that cardiac patients die in a pathophysiological spectrum ranging from those that die due to CHF (little myocardium remaining) to those that die from an ischemic related event (ample myocardium remaining). The clinical and exercise test variables most likely associated with CHF deaths (CHF markers) include a history or symptoms of CHF, prior MI, Q waves, and other indicators of LV dysfunction. Variables most likely associated with ischemic deaths (ischemic markers) are angina, and rest and exercise ST depression. Certain variables are associated with either extremes of the type of CV death; these include exercise capacity, maximal heart rate, and maximal systolic blood pressure. These variables' dual association may explain why they are consistently reported in published studies. Another problem is that ischemic deaths occur later in follow up and are more likely to occur in those lost to follow up whereas CHF deaths are more likely to occur early (within 2 years) and are more likely to be classified. Work-up bias probably explains why exercise-induced ST depression fails to be a predictor in most of the follow-up studies that require an angiogram.

Rather than focusing on the differences, it is better to stress the consistencies. Risk can be assessed by considering simple clinical variables. An exercise capacity of greater than 5 METs, no evidence or history of CHF or ventricular damage (Q waves, etc.), no ST depression or only one of these clinical findings are associated with a very low risk. These patients are low risk for participation in exercise programs and need not be considered for CABG to prolong their life. High-risk patients can be identified by two or more of the clinical markers or by using the scores. Exertional hypotension is particularly ominous. Identification of high risk implies that such patients in exercise training programs should have lower goals and should be monitored. Such patients should also be considered for CABG to improve their longevity. Intervention may not always be feasible but it should at least be considered.

The mathematical models for determining prognosis are usually more complex than those used for identifying severe angiographic disease. As shown by Stone, LaFollette, & Cohn (67), the status of the right coronary artery greatly affects the hemodynamic and ST segment responses to exercise testing in patients with multivessel coronary disease. For instance, left main or left main equivalents cannot be distinguished from two-vessel disease when the right coronary is not diseased. Diagnostic testing can utilize multivariate discriminant function analysis to determine the probability of severe angiographic disease being present or not.

On the other hand, prognostic testing must utilize survival analysis which includes censoring for patients with uneven follow-up end points due to "lost to follow up" or other cardiac events (i.e., CABG, PTCA). Furthermore, one must account for time-person units of exposure. In addition, survival curves must be developed and the Cox proportional hazards model is often preferred. How to test these models for confidence, accuracy, reproducibility, and power is controversial.

From this perspective, it is obvious that there is much information supporting the use of exercise testing as the first non-invasive step after the history, physical exam, and resting ECG has been obtained for the prognostic evaluation of coronary artery disease patients. The data collected from the exercise test accomplishes both of the purposes of prognostic testing: to provide information regarding the patient's status and to help make recommendations for their optimal management. Thus, the exercise test results help us make reasonable decisions for selection of patients who should undergo coronary angiography. Perhaps some of the newer computerized ST segment scoring techniques will enable an even more accurate prediction of high risk patients. Since the exercise test can be performed in the doctor's office and provides valuable information for clinical management in regard to activity levels, response to therapy, and disability, the exercise test remains the reasonable first choice for prognostic assessment.

Simple clinical and exercise test scores can be used to decide which patients need interventions in order to improve their prognosis; these scores frequently obviate the need for cardiac catheterization. The VA score is recommended for the male veteran population and the Duke score for the general population including women. Patients can be given estimates of their relative annual mortality with medical versus surgical therapy using scores and case mix data. It is important to note that quality of life issues cannot be resolved with such scores; these issues require an understanding physician and an informed patient. In general, physicians overestimate the danger of ischemia; perhaps if given accurate mortality estimates, the practice of medicine would be more conservative.

References

1. Subcommittee on Exercise Testing. Guidelines for exercise testing. A report of the American College of Cardiology/American Heart Association task force on assessment of cardiovascular procedures. J. Am. Coll. Cardiol. 8:725-738; 1986.
2. Froelicher, V.F.; Marcondes, G. A manual of exercise testing. Chicago: Year Book Medical Publishers; 1989.
3. Froelicher, V.F. Exercise and the heart. Clinical concepts. Chicago: Year Book Medical Publishers; 1987.
4. Gianrossi, R.; Detrano, R.; Mulvihill, D.; Lehmann, K.; Dubach, P.; Colombo, A.; McArthur, D.; Froelicher, V.F. Exercise-induced ST depression in the diagnosis of coronary artery disease. A meta-analysis. Circulation. 80:87-98; 1989.
5. Chassin, M.R.; Kosecoff, J.; Solomon, D.H.; Brook, R.H. How coronary angiography is used. Clinical determinants of appropriateness. JAMA. 258:2543-2547; 1987.
6. Califf, R.M.; Harrell, F.E.; Lee, K.L.; Rankin, J.S.; Hlatky, M.A.; Mark, D.B.; Jones, R.H.; Muhlbaier, L.H.; Oldham, H.N.; Pryor, D.B. The evolution of medical and surgical therapy for coronary artery disease. A 15 year perspective. JAMA. 261:2077-2086; 1989.
7. Froelicher, V.F.; Perdue, S.; Pewen, W.; Risch, M. Application of meta-analysis using an electronic spread sheet to exercise testing in patients after myocardial infarction. Am. J. Med. 83:1045-1054; 1987.
8. DeBusk, R.F. Evaluation of patients after acute myocardial infarction. Annals Int. Med. 110:485-488; 1989.
9. Ahnve, S.; Savvides, M.; Abouantoun, S.; Atwood, J.E.; Froelicher, V.F. Can myocardial ischemia be recognized by the exercise electrocardiogram in coronary disease patients with abnormal resting Q waves? Am. Heart J. 111:909-916; 1986.

10. Klein, J.; Froelicher, V.F.; Detrano, R.; Dubach, P.; Yen, R. Does the rest electrocardiogram after myocardial infarction determine the predictive value of exercise-induced ST depression? A 2 year follow-up study of a veteran population. J. Am. Coll. Cardiol. 14:305-311; 1989.

11. Krone, R.J.; Dwyer, E.M.; Greenberg, H.; Miller, J.P.; Gillespie, J.A. Risk stratification in patients with first non-Q wave infarction: Limited value of the early low level exercise test after uncomplicated infarcts. J. Am. Coll. Cardiol. 14:31-37; 1989.

12. Miranda, C.P.; Herbert, W.; Dubach, P.; Lehmann, K.G.; Froelicher, V.F. Post-myocardial infarction exercise testing: Non Q-wave versus Q-wave, correlation with coronary angiography and long-term prognosis. Circulation. 84:2357-2365; 1991.

13. Schwartz, D.J.; Roberts, R.; Young, P.M.; Boden, W.E. Risk stratification of patients with non-Q wave myocardial infarction. The critical role of ST segment depression. Circulation. 90:1148-1158; 1989.

14. Ribisl, P.M.; Morris, C.K.; Kawaguchi, T.; Ueshima, K.; Froelicher, V.F. Angiographic patterns and severe coronary artery disease: Exercise test correlates. Arch. Intern. Med. 152:1618-1624; 1992.

15. Morris, C.K.; Ueshima, K.; Kawaguchi, T.; Hedig, A.; Froelicher, V.F. The prognostic value of exercise capacity: A review of the literature. Am. Heart J. 122:1423-1430; 1991.

16. Reeves, T.J.; Oberman, A.; Jones, W.B.; Sheffield, L.T. Natural history of angina pectoris. Am. J. Cardiol. 33:423-430; 1974.

17. Ellestad, M.; Wan, M. Prediction implications of stress testing. Circulation. 51:363-369; 1975.

18. Hammermeister, K.E.; DeRouen, T.A.; Dodge, H.T. Variables predictive of survival in patients with coronary disease. Selection by univariate and multivariate analyses from the clinical, electrocardiographic, exercise, arteriographic, and quantitative angiographic evaluation. Circulation. 59:421-430; 1979.

19. Gohke, H.; Samek, L.; Betz, P.; Roskamm, H. Exercise testing provides additional prognostic information in angiographically defined subgroups of patients with coronary artery disease. Circulation. 68:979-985; 1983.

20. Brunelli, C.; Cristofani, R.; L'Abbate, A., for the ODI Study Group. Long-term survival in medically treated patients with ischemic heart disease and prognostic importance of clinical and electrocardiographic data. (The Italian CNR multicenter prospective study OD1). Eur. Heart J. 10:292-303; 1989.

21. Weiner, D.A.; Ryan, T.; McCabe, C.H.; Chaitman, B.R.; Sheffield, T.; Ferguson, J.C.; Fisher, L.D.; Tristani, F. Prognostic importance of a clinical profile and exercise test in medically treated patients with coronary artery disease. J. Am. Coll. Cardiol. 3:772-779; 1984.

22. Mark, D.B.; Hlatky, M.A.; Harrell, F.E.; Lee, K.L.; Califf, R.M.; Pryor, D.B. Exercise treadmill score for predicting prognosis in coronary artery disease. Ann. Intern. Med. 106:793-800; 1987.

23. Peduzzi, P.; Hultgren, H.; Thomsen, J.; Angell, W. Prognostic value of baseline exercise tests. Prog. Cardiovasc. Dis. 28:285-292; 1986.

24. Lerman, J.; Svetlize, H.; Capris, T.; Perosio, A. Follow-up of patients after exercise test and catheterization. Medicina (B. Aires). 46:201-211; 1986.

25. Califf, R.M.; Mark, D.B.; Hlatky, M.A.; Pryor, D.B. Importance of clinical measures of ischemia in the prognosis of patients with documented coronary artery disease. J. Am. Coll. Cardiol. 11:20-26; 1988.

26. Philbrick, J.T.; Horwitz, R.J.; Feinstein, A.R.; Langou, R.A.; Chandler, J.P. The limited spectrum of patients studied in exercise test research. Analyzing the tip of the iceberg. JAMA. 248:2467-2470; 1982.

27. Froelicher, V.F.; Perdue, S.; Pewen, W.; Risch, M. Application of meta-analysis using an electronic spread sheet to exercise testing in patients after myocardial infarction. Am. J. Med. 83:1045-1054; 1987.

28. Deering, T.F.; Weiner, D.A. Prognosis of patients with coronary artery disease. J. Cardiopulmonary Rehabil. 5:325-331; 1985.

29. Simari, R.D.; Miller, T.D.; Zinsmeister, A.R.; Gibbons, R.J. Capabilities of supine exercise electrocardiography versus exercise radionuclide angiography in predicting coronary events. Am. J. Cardiol. 67:573-577; 1991.

30. Lee, K.L.; Pryor, D.B.; Pieper, K.S.; Harrell, F.E.; Califf, R.M.; Mark, D.B.; Hlatky, M.A.; Coleman, R.E.; Cobb, F.R.; Jones, R.H. Prognostic value of radionuclide angiography in medically treated patients with coronary artery disease. A comparison with clinical and catheterization variables. Circulation. 82:1705-1717; 1990.

31. Brown, K.A. Prognostic value of thallium-201 myocardial perfusion imaging. A diagnostic tool comes of age. Circulation. 83:363-381; 1991.

32. Kaul, S.; Lilly, D.R.; Gasho, J.A.; Watson, D.D.; Gibson, R.S.; Oliner, C.A.; Ryan, J.M.; Beller, G.A. Prognostic utility of the exercise thallium-201 test in ambulatory patients with chest pain. Circulation. 77:745-748; 1988.

33. Dubach, P.; Froelicher, V.F.; Klein, J.; Oakes, D.; Grover-McKay, M.; Friis, R. Exercise-induced hypotension in a male population. Criteria, causes, and prognosis. Circulation. 78:1380-1387; 1988.

34. Callaham, P.R.; Froelicher, V.F.; Klein, J.; Risch, M.; Dubach, P.; Friis, R. Exercise-induced silent ischemia: Age, diabetes mellitus, previous myocardial infarction and prognosis. J. Am. Coll. Cardiol. 14:1175-1180; 1989.

35. Mark, D.B.; Hlatky, M.A.; Califf, R.M.; Morris, J.J.; Sisson, S.D.; McCants, C.B.; Lee, K.L.; Harrell, F.E.; Pryor, D.B. Painless exercise ST deviation on the treadmill: Long-term prognosis. J. Am. Coll. Cardiol. 14:885-892; 1989.

36. Bogaty, P.; Dagenais, G.; Cantin, B.; Alain, P.; Rouleau, J.R. Prognosis in patients with a strongly positive exercise electrocardiogram. Am. J. Cardiol. 64:1284-1288; 1989.

37. Miranda, C.P.; Lehmann, K.G.; Lachterman, B.; Coodley, E.M.; Froelicher, V.F. Comparison of silent and symptomatic ischemia during exercise testing in men. Ann. Intern. Med. 114:649-656; 1991.

38. Grondin, C.M.; Campeau, L.; Thornton, J.C.; Engle, J.C.; Cross, F.S.; Schreiber, H. Coronary artery bypass grafting with saphenous vein. Circulation. 79:I24-I29; 1989.

39. Parsonnet, V.; Dean, D.; Bernstein, A.D. A method of uniform stratification of risk for evaluating the results of surgery in acquired adult heart disease. Circulation. 79:I3-I12; 1989.

40. Platko, W.; Hollman, J. Percutaneous transluminal coronary angiography of saphenous vein graft stenosis. J. Am. Coll. Cardiol. 14:1645-1650; 1989.

41. Dubach, P.; Froelicher, V.F.; Klein, J.; Detrano, R. Use of the exercise test to predict prognosis after coronary artery bypass grafting. Am. J. Cardiol. 63:530-533; 1989.

42. Sawada, S.G.; Judson, W.E.; Ryan, T.; Armstrong, W.F.; Feigenbaum, H. Upright bicycle exercise echocardiography after coronary artery bypass surgery. Am. J. Cardiol. 64:1123-1129; 1989.

43. Kligfield, P.; Ameisen, O.; Okin, P.M. Heart rate adjustment of ST segment depression for improved detection of coronary artery disease. Circulation. 79:245-255; 1989.

44. Lachterman, B.; Lehmann, K.G.; Neutel, J.; Froelicher, V.F. Comparison of the ST/heart rate index to standard ST criteria for analysis of the exercise ECG: Diagnosis of any and recognition of severe coronary artery disease. Circulation. 83:44-50; 1991.

45. Herbert, W.; Froelicher, V.F. The effect of beta blockade on the diagnostic performances of the exercise test. Am. Heart J. 122:993-1000; 1991.

46. Detrano, R.; Janosi, A.; Lyons, K.P.; Marcondes, G.; Abbassi, N.; Froelicher, V.F. Factors affecting sensitivity and specificity of a diagnostic test: The exercise thallium scintigram. Am. J. Med. 84:699-709; 1988.

47. Gutman, R.A.; Alexander, E.R.; Li, Y.T.; Bruce, R.A. Delay of ST depression after maximal exercise by walking for 2 minutes. Circulation. 42:229; 1970.

48. Gibbons, L.; Blair, S.N.; Kohl, H.W.; Cooper, K. The safety of maximal exercise testing. Circulation. 80:846-852; 1989.

49. Lachterman, B.; Lehmann, K.G.; Abrahamson, D.; Froelicher, V.F. "Recovery only" ST segment depression and the predictive accuracy of the exercise test. Ann. Intern. Med. 112:11-16; 1990.

50. Nosratian, F.; Froelicher, V.F. ST elevation during exercise testing: A review. Am. J. Cardiol. 63:986-988; 1989.

51. Nosratian, F.; Froelicher, V.F. ST elevation during exercise testing: Two case reports. Chest. 96:653-654; 1989.

52. Milliken, J.A.; Abdollah, H.; Burggraf, G.W. False-positive treadmill exercise tests due to computer signal averaging. Am. J. Cardiol. 65:946-948; 1990.

53. Detry, J.M.R.; Luwaert, R.J.; Rousseau, M.F.; Brasseur, L.A.; Melin, J.A.; Brohet, C.R.; Derwael-Barchy, C.; Fesler, R. Diagnostic value of computerized exercise testing in men without previous myocardial infarction. A multivariate, compartmental and probabilistic approach. Eur. Heart J. 6:227-238; 1985.

54. Deckers, J.W.; Rensing, B.J.; Tijssen, J.G.; Vinke, R.V.; Azar, A.J.; Simoons, M.L. A comparison of methods of analysing exercise tests for diagnosis of coronary artery disease. Br. Heart J. 62:438-444; 1989.

55. Hollenberg, M.; Zoltick, M.J.; Go, M., Jr.; Yaney, S.F.; Daniels, W.; Davis, R.C., Jr.; Bedynek, J.L. Comparison of a quantitative treadmill exercise score with standard electrocardiographic criteria in screening asymptomatic young men for coronary artery disease. N. Engl. J. Med. 313:600-606; 1985.

56. Simoons, M.L. Optimal measurements for detection of coronary artery disease by exercise ECG. Comput. Biomed. Res. 10:483-489; 1977.

57. Morise, A.P.; Duval, R.D. Comparison of three Bayesian methods to estimate posttest probability in patients undergoing exercise stress testing. Am. J. Cardiol. 64:1117-1122; 1989.

58. Sox, H.C.; Littenberg, B.; Garber, A.M. The role of exercise testing in screening for coronary artery disease. Ann. Intern. Med. 110:456-469; 1989.

59. Ekelund, L.G.; Suchindran, C.M.; McMahon, R.P.; Heiss, G.; Leon, A.S.; Romhilt, D.W.; Rubenstein, C.L.; Probstfield, J.L.; Ruwitch, J.F. Coronary heart disease morbidity and mortality in hypercholesterolemic men predicted from an exercise test: The lipid research clinics coronary primary prevention trial. J. Am. Coll. Cardiol. 14:556-563; 1989.

60. Myers, J.; Froelicher, V.F. Optimizing the exercise test for pharmacologic investigations. Circulation. 82:1839-1846; 1990.

61. Myers, J.; Walsh, D.; Froelicher, V.F. Can maximal cardiopulmonary capacity be recognized by a plateau of oxygen uptake? Chest. 96:1312-1316; 1989.

62. Yang, J.C.; Wesley, R.; Froelicher, V.F. Ventricular tachycardia during routine treadmill testing. Risk and prognosis. Arch. Intern. Med. 151:349-353; 1991.

63. Myers, J.; Buchanan, N.; Walsh, D.; Kraemer, M.; McAuley, P.; Hamilton-Wessler, H.; Froelicher, V.F. Comparison of the ramp versus standard exercise protocols. J. Am. Coll. Cardiol. 17:1334-1342; 1991.

64. Hlatky, M.A.; Boineau, R.E.; Higginbotham, M.B.; Lee, K.L.; Mark, D.B.; Califf, R.M.; Cobb, F.R.; Pryor, D.B. A brief self-administered questionnaire to determine functional capacity (the Duke activity status index). Am. J. Cardiol. 64:651-654; 1989.

65. Wigton, R.S.; Nicholas, J.A.; Blank, L.L. Procedural skills of the general internist. A survey of 2500 physicians. Ann. Intern. Med. 111:1023-1034; 1989.

66. Fletcher, G.F.; Froelicher, V.F.; Hartley, H.; Haskell, W.L.; Pollock, M.L. Exercise standards. A statement for health professionals from the American Heart Association. Circulation. 82:2286-2322; 1990.

67. Stone, P.H.; LaFollette, L.; Cohn, P. Patterns of exercise treadmill test performance in patients with left main coronary disease: Detection dependent on left coronary dominance or coexistent dominant right coronary artery. Am. Heart J. 104:13-19; 1982.

68. Philbrick, J.T.; Horwitz, R.I.; Feinstein, A.R. Methodologic problems of exercise testing for coronary artery disease: Groups analysis and bias. Am. J. Cardiol. 46:807-816; 1980.

Chapter 5

Nuclear Cardiology and Echocardiography: Noninvasive Tests for Diagnosing Patients With Coronary Artery Disease

Donald H. Schmidt

Steven C. Port

Rami A. Gal

Since the second edition of this book was published in 1986 there have been many exciting developments in the field of noninvasive testing for diagnosing coronary artery disease (CAD). New technology has improved the quality of cardiovascular images and the accuracy of quantitated results. Likewise, new pharmacologic agents and radiopharmaceuticals have broadened the spectrum of the diagnostic procedures that can be performed and have expanded the patient populations that can be studied.

This chapter will describe the different techniques and applications of the most commonly performed noninvasive tests: nuclear cardiology and echocardiography.

Nuclear Cardiology

The primary objectives of nuclear cardiology testing continue to be the assessment of myocardial perfusion and ventricular function. Qualitative and quantitative evaluations of myocardial perfusion and function assist physicians in diagnosing the presence and clinical significance of CAD, in selecting the method of treatment that will best affect long-term prognosis, and in longitudinally following the results of that treatment. These procedures play an important role in all aspects of managing patients with CAD.

Blood Pool Imaging

The technique called "blood pool imaging" involves a scintillation camera placed over the patient's chest to detect a radioactive substance that has been injected into the bloodstream via an antecubital or jugular vein; this creates a picture of how blood is being pumped through the heart at rest and during exercise or other interventions.

In addition to the scintigraphic data, the clinician obtains and records the following information from a graded exercise test (GXT) on either a treadmill or a cycle ergometer: heart rate (HR) and blood pressure (BP) responses, workload achieved, symptoms experienced, and electrocardiographic (ECG) changes. By applying quantitative formulas to the image data, left and right ventricular ejection fractions, left ventricular volumes, and cardiac output can be calculated. Finally, cine-display techniques show the beating heart, so that global and regional wall motion abnormalities can be detected. Similar data can be obtained using pharmacologic stress.

Techniques of Blood Pool Imaging

Blood pool imaging can be performed by either of two methods. The *equilibrium method* requires a stable blood pool tag so that imaging can be performed over an extended period of time. This tag is most commonly created by a modified in vivo red blood cell–labeling technique (1). To accomplish this, nonradioactive stannous pyrophosphate is injected intravenously; 20 to 30 min later 10 ml of blood is withdrawn from the patient into a syringe containing 20 to 30 mCi of technetium-99m-pertechnetate (Tc-99m). The stannous ion causes binding of the Tc-99m within the red blood cells. When reinjected into the patient, this provides a blood pool tag that is relatively stable for several hours. Imaging can then be performed as often and in as many views as necessary during that period of time.

The equilibrium method uses an ECG "gate," or trigger, to identify the beginning of each cardiac cycle. Data from hundreds of cycles are then combined to provide counting statistics that are sufficient for high-resolution image display and quantitative data processing. Consequently, data must be acquired for a period of 3 to 8 min in each view. Because the entire blood pool is labeled, the left anterior oblique view is the only view that can be used to quantify ventricular function. In this view, the interventricular septum spatially separates the left and right ventricles (Figure 5.1).

The other method of blood pool imaging is the *first-pass method*. With this method, no blood cell labeling is required; rather, all data are acquired during the "first pass," or first transit, of the radionuclide through the central circulation. Using a 15 to 20 mCi bolus injection of Tc-99m or Tc-99m-DPTA (diethylene triamine pentaacetic acid) provides adequate counting statistics for image display and quantitative data processing in 5 to 30 s—less than one-tenth of the time needed for the equilibrium acquisition.

The rapidity of this method makes it particularly suitable for imaging during peak exercise and for evaluating short-duration phenomenon or rapidly changing physiological states. Because the transit of the tracer bolus is routinely imaged with the first-pass method (Figure 5.2), it is also possible to determine chamber-to-chamber transit times, to delineate abnormal routes of tracer transit (as might occur in congenital heart disease), and quantitate intracardiac left-to-right shunts. Figure 5.3 compares the end-diastolic and end-systolic images of patients with normal and abnormal ventricular function obtained at rest and during peak exercise using the first-pass technique.

Analysis of the Data

Either of the blood pool imaging methods is useful to quantitatively analyze global and regional ventricular function. By combining data from several hundred cardiac cycles for the equilibrium method or from 5 to 8 cardiac cycles for the first-pass method, time-activity curves for the different cardiac chambers or for portions of these chambers can be generated. These curves are identical to the left ventricular volume curves obtained from frame-by-frame analysis of contrast angiograms, where the peak of the curve represents end-diastole and the nadir represents end-systole. In blood pool analysis, after subtracting background counts, the left ventricular ejection fraction (LVEF) can be calculated as end-diastolic counts minus end-systolic counts divided by end-diastolic counts. The ejection fraction represents the percentage of end-diastolic volume that is ejected with each heart beat.

Ventricular volumes can then be measured using either geometric or count-based methods. The *geometric method* evaluates the nuclear data in the same way as a contrast angiogram—using a modification of the Sandler-Dodge approach (2) to calculate end-diastolic volume. End-diastolic volume is calculated using the end-diastolic area and the long axis of the ventricle. Stroke volume (SV), end-systolic volume, and cardiac output ($\dot{Q}$) are then derived from established formulas.

Count-based methods can also be used to calculate left ventricular volume. In contrast to the geometric method, count-based methods are less dependent on precise spatial resolution of the ventricle, since they are based on the fact that radioactivity in a chamber is directly proportional to the blood volume of that chamber after adequate mixing has occurred. Using the count-based method, volume can be calculated either by comparing the radioactivity from the chamber with the radioactivity of a reference sample of blood (3,4) or by determining the ratio of total radioactivity counts to the

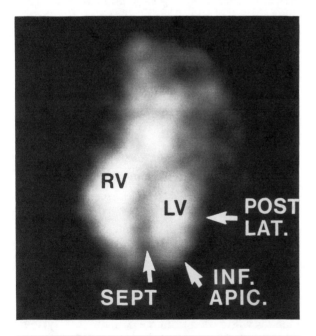

Figure 5.1 Equilibrium blood pool image, left anterior oblique (best septal) view, showing the right (RV) and left ventricular (LV) chambers. The arrows indicate the posterolateral (POST LAT.) and the inferoapical (INF APIC.) walls of the left ventricle and the septum (SEPT).

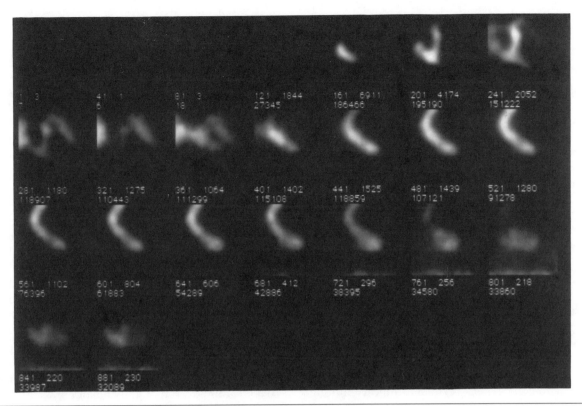

Figure 5.2   Serial images of a first-pass blood pool study showing the tracer transit through the heart. The bolus travels from the superior vena cava (upper left) to the aorta (bottom right).

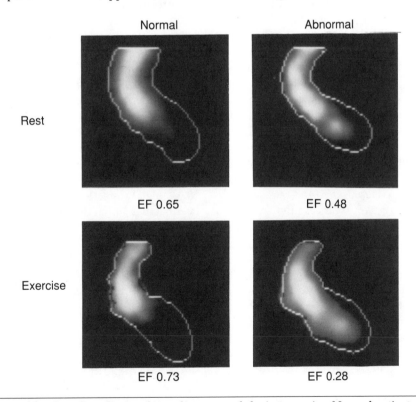

Figure 5.3   First-pass blood pool studies performed at rest and during exercise. Normal patient: the resting left ventricular ejection fraction (EF) of 0.65 increases with exercise to 0.73. Abnormal patient: the resting ventricular ejection fraction is mildly decreased, and there is inferior hypokinesis of 0.48. During exercise, left ventricular function deteriorates with global hypokinesis and an ejection fraction of 0.28.

maximum pixel count within the chamber. Using the latter method, we have developed count-based methods for calculating the end-diastolic volume for both the equilibrium (5) and the first-pass techniques (6). Once end-diastolic volume is calculated, end-systolic volume, SV, and cardiac output can be computed.

We noted above that the major advantage of high–count rate first-pass studies is their short data acquisition time, but in some ways this has also been a limiting factor. Because only data obtained with the first transit of the tracer are used for analysis, a radionuclide bolus must be injected for each measurement. Due to limits on radiation exposure, a maximum of three to five injections can be made. With equilibrium imaging, numerous measurements can be made in the 4- to 6-h life-span of the blood pool tag. Consequently, some investigators have used such short-lived radionuclides as iridium and gold-195m with first-pass imaging because they result in much lower exposure than with Tc-99m. Using these agents, rapid sequential studies can be obtained (7-9). However, these radionuclides are expensive, their technical handling is complicated, and they have not been approved for clinical use in the United States.

In addition to the standard analysis of systolic ventricular function using a cinematic display of the beating ventricle, blood pool data can be used to generate a variety of so-called functional images, that is, parametric images that are used to analyze the amplitude, timing, and regional contraction sequences of the ventricles. In particular, phase analysis (which uses a Fourier transform) may be very useful for characterizing such time-related phenomena as arrhythmias and preexcitation. Blood pool imaging is also well suited for analyzing diastolic filling patterns of the ventricles. Delays in the onset and decreases in the rate of ventricular rapid filling, as well as the relative contributions of early and late (atrial) filling, can be readily displayed and quantified. These changes can be seen in the absence of systolic abnormalities in patients with CAD (10).

An exciting development for blood pool imaging is the recent market approval (in 1991) of two technetium-based perfusion agents. When used for myocardial perfusion testing, these agents allow the clinician to obtain a first-pass blood pool scan at the same time without the need for an additional radionuclide injection. (This is discussed later in this chapter under "Myocardial Perfusion Imaging.") Technetium perfusion studies can also be gated, which allows visualization of wall motion and wall thickening.

Another new development in first-pass imaging is the ability to acquire data while the patient exercises on a treadmill. Previously, only exercise on a cycle ergometer (performed either upright or supine) allowed enough stabilization of the patient's chest directly against the camera head for blood pool imaging. Now, by using a multicrystal camera with simultaneous dual energy capacity and a point source placed on the patient's chest, each frame of data can be corrected for motion (11).

Clinical Applications of Blood Pool Imaging

By analyzing LVEF, volume data, and regional wall motion, blood pool imaging provides a diagnostic sensitivity of 80% to 90% for CAD. Likewise, exercise data are predictive of the likelihood of death (12-14). Study results can also be used to select the most appropriate treatment, and serial studies can be used to assess treatment results. For screening applications, rest and exercise blood pool imaging studies are best used in high-risk patients, such as those with chronic hypertension, diabetes, and a strong family history of CAD, who do not otherwise have symptoms associated with CAD.

Information on ventricular size, systolic function, and valvular regurgitation can be used to diagnose and assess treatment results for patients with valvular heart disease. Information on ventricular size and function, ejection fraction, and regional wall motion can also be used to diagnose patients with cardiomyopathy; and serial resting studies in these patients can be used to evaluate the effects of therapy. Finally, first-pass studies can delineate abnormal routes of tracer transit and allow the quantitation of intracardiac left-to-right shunts in patients with congenital heart disease (e.g., atrial defect) or acquired heart disease (e.g., ventricular septal defect as a complication of acute myocardial infarction [MI]).

Myocardial Perfusion Imaging

The majority of new developments in the field of nuclear cardiology testing have taken place in the area of myocardial perfusion imaging. In the first two editions of this book, we noted that a major limitation of perfusion imaging was an inability to quantitate the data. At that time, data interpretation consisted primarily of the qualitative evaluation of planar images, which can vary widely among interpreters. Another limitation was the use of thallium-201 as an imaging agent.

Since then, numerous technological changes that have improved the ability to quantitate data have taken place, and, in January 1991, two new technetium-based perfusion agents that may prove to be superior to thallium were approved for clinical use. In addition, in December 1990, intravenous dipyridamole, which had been used experimentally for more than 10 years as a pharmacologic alternative to exercise, was approved for clinical use, thus expanding the patient population that can be studied.

Thallium Myocardial Perfusion Imaging

Thallium imaging is still the most commonly performed perfusion scan. Thallium-201, a potassium analog, is taken up avidly by myocardial tissue. After its intravenous administration, thallium's myocardial concentration is directly related to regional myocardial blood flow over a wide range of coronary flow, but its concentration is not directly proportional at very high flow rates.

Although it is an excellent physiologic marker of flow, thallium-201 is not an ideal imaging agent because of the low energy (70 keV) of its predominant photopeak, which results in photon scatter and attenuation—both of which degrade images and can lead to image artifacts. In addition, thallium-201 begins to wash out of the heart when its concentration in the myocardium equilibrates within the potassium space; therefore, imaging must be started within 10 to 15 min after completing an exercise test. Another disadvantage is that, because thallium-201 is a cyclotron by-product, it must be delivered to the laboratory on a daily basis. Finally, the long half-life of thallium-201 (72 h) markedly limits the amount that can be injected.

Despite these disadvantages, thallium perfusion imaging has been used extensively for diagnosing CAD—the hallmark of which is the regional nonhomogeneity of coronary flow. Because this regional nonhomogeneity is greatest during high flow states, and because the ratio of myocardial-to-background counts is most favorable during states of high coronary flow, thallium is most often injected during exercise. Imaging is then begun about 10 to 15 min later and repeated 3 to 4 h later. Myocardial regions that receive less coronary flow than other regions will have lower thallium concentrations. If regional disparity in thallium concentrations is sufficient, and if the size of the tracer-deficient area is within the spatial resolution of the gamma camera, then a "defect" will appear on the images.

Because defects due to ischemia are transient, whereas those due to infarction are persistent, delayed images (those taken at 3 to 4 h) are used to detect any redistribution of thallium. The presence of redistribution (or a "filling in" of defects seen on the immediate postexercise images) indicates that transient, exercise-induced ischemia was present at the time of the thallium injection (Figure 5.4). If no redistribution occurs, or the defect persists, then the myocardium in that area is suspected to be nonviable. Delayed images are also acquired to quantify thallium washout, which may be of further help in diagnosing ischemia.

However, the assumption that fixed thallium defects always indicate infarction was challenged by studies (15,16) documenting that up to 50% of the defects (thought to be irreversible, based on delayed perfusion imaging results) showed functional improvement after revascularization. One new and more accurate method to assess myocardial viability is positron emission tomography (PET). Regional uptake of 18F-fluorodeoxyglucose (FDC) in the myocardium is used as a marker of intact metabolic activity. A pattern of enhanced FDG uptake in a myocardial region showing decreased blood flow on perfusion imaging studies indicates that this area is still metabolizing glucose and is, therefore, viable. The function of such segments within the myocardium has

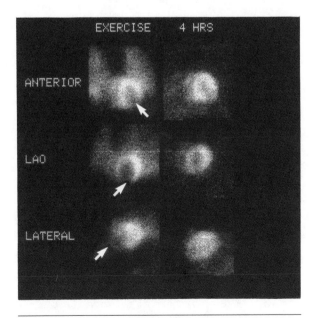

Figure 5.4 Thallium myocardial perfusion planar scans. (Left) Immediately after exercise, perfusion defects (arrows) are seen in all three views. Four hours later, redistribution images show markedly improved perfusion. (LAO = left anterior oblique.)

been shown to improve after revascularization (17).

Recently, though, delayed thallium perfusion imaging (performed from 8 to 72 h after initial postexercise study) or repeat imaging (performed after a second injection of a smaller dose of thallium [usually 1 mCi]) has been shown to predict myocardial viability with results that are similar to PET imaging. Some investigators have found that ostensibly nonreversible defects, seen on 3- to 4-h postexercise thallium images, often reversed by 24 h (15,16). Because perfusion imaging is more readily available and is less expensive than PET imaging, 8- to 72-h delayed imaging or reinjection thallium imaging may be the methods of choice for evaluating myocardial viability.

Tomographic Imaging

While conventional planar imaging provides adequate images of thallium-201 distribution in the myocardium, it suffers from the inherent problem of providing a two-dimensional depiction of a three-dimensional distribution of radionuclide. Levels of radionuclide activity at varying depths in the myocardial muscle are superimposed and recorded as a two-dimensional display, with the result that areas of normal myocardium can mask areas where there is diminished perfusion. Consequently, much work has been done with single-photon emission computerized tomography (SPECT) for myocardial perfusion imaging to provide three-dimensional tomographic slices of the heart and better separation of normal and abnormal areas of myocardium from background.

In SPECT, 30-60 planar images are obtained over a 180-degree arc. The arc typically extends from the 45-degree right anterior oblique projection to the 45-degree left posterior oblique projection. Tomographic slices are then reconstructed and the apex and the base of the left ventricle are defined (Figure 5.5, top). Quantitative techniques are subsequently applied to the short-axis slices from the apex to the base of the ventricle. This generates a circumferential profile of the maximum count per pixel for each of the slices. To facilitate analysis of the SPECT images, these circumferential profiles are then arranged from apex to base in a polar ("bull's-eye") map, with the apex at the center and the base at the periphery of the map (Figure 5.5, bottom). Identically reconstructed tomographic images and bull's-eye maps are obtained from the immediate postexercise images and the redistribution images. The presence and location of perfusion defects can be determined by carefully evaluating the radionuclide distribution on the tomographic slices and the bull's-eye maps and by comparing these images with those compiled in a normal SPECT database.

Intravenous Dipyridamole Perfusion Imaging

As mentioned previously, because the regional nonhomogeneity of coronary blood flow is greatest during high-flow states, perfusion imaging is usually performed after exercise. However, many patients may need pharmacologic "stress" testing because they are unable to either exercise or to exercise long enough for an adequate GXT to be performed. Intravenous dipyridamole perfusion imaging can be used with these patients. This subgroup of patients includes those particularly at high risk for CAD, such as chronic smokers or those with peripheral vascular disease (PVD), those with deforming or painful rheumatologic or orthopedic problems or with certain neurologic impairments, those who are not in condition or who are poorly motivated to exercise, and those who are being treated with medications that inhibit maximal exercise effect, such as beta-blockers and some calcium channel blockers.

Dipyridamole elevates endogenous adenosine levels, resulting in coronary arteriolar vasodilation (due to a decrease in coronary resistance) and increased coronary blood flow. These effects are inhibited by aminophylline, which acts as a receptor antagonist of adenosine.

After dipyridamole administration, coronary vascular beds supplied by vessels that are free of significant stenoses will show a maximum decrease in resistance and, hence, a maximum increase in blood flow. However, vascular beds supplied by stenotic vessels have an already-reduced coronary resistance to maintain a normal level of blood flow at rest. Therefore, the vasodilatory effect of dipyridamole is attenuated, and there will be a much smaller change in resistance and a proportionately smaller increase in blood flow in these vessels. These differences in blood flow between normal and stenotic vessels can be detected on perfusion images. Hemodynamically, dipyridamole causes a much smaller increase in HR and actually decreases BP compared to exercise. Clinical evidence of ischemia (i.e., ST-segment depression and angina) also occurs less frequently with dipyridamole than with exercise.

Intravenous dipyridamole perfusion imaging has been proven to be reliable and safe and to have levels of sensitivity and specificity comparable to

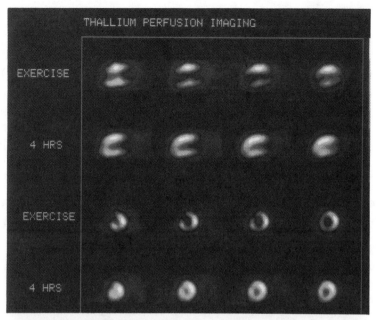

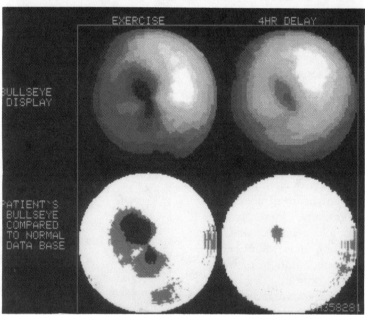

Figure 5.5 SPECT perfusion scan showing (top) tomographic slices of the myocardium (postexercise and 4-hour redistribution images) and (bottom) the bull's-eye display for the same patient. The bottom row compares these results with those compiled from a database of normal volunteers.

those of exercise-thallium imaging (18). Procedures for safety and efficacy were determined by investigators who evaluated approximately 4,000 patients during the experimental evaluation of dipyridamole. Side effects were found to be usually minor and easily reversed with the use of intravenous aminophylline, as mentioned above; the overall incidence of drug-related, serious, nonfatal complications and mortality is low (19). In addition to its important application in evaluating myo-

cardial perfusion in patients who are unable to exercise to diagnostically adequate levels, intravenous dipyridamole perfusion imaging has prognostic value in patients who have PVD (20-22), a recent MI (23), or a normal scan (24).

Because most, if not all, of the effects of dipyridamole are mediated by increased tissue levels of adenosine, some investigators are also evaluating the use of a direct infusion of exogenous adenosine to induce coronary vasodilation (25). The main advantage of adenosine is its extremely short half-life (< 10 s), which may make it especially desirable for patients with CAD, since symptoms and side effects dissipate rapidly after discontinuing the infusion. This drug has also been accepted for clinical use (26); considerable experience suggests that it is as diagnostically accurate as dipyridamole imaging, although side effects are more frequent.

Technetium-Based Perfusion Agents

In contrast to the disadvantages we noted with thallium-201, the photopeak energy of Tc-99m is 140 keV—twice that of thallium. This makes it less likely to scatter and attenuate in the body; consequently, it produces images of better quality. Because it is a generator-produced radionuclide, rather than cyclotron-produced, it is more widely available and does not require daily delivery to the laboratory. Its shorter half-life of only 6 h (compared to 72 h for thallium) allows higher doses to be injected, yielding a higher photon flux and the possibility for shorter imaging sequences.

Two new perfusion agents are available that use Tc-99m. One comes from a family of compounds known as isonitriles and is called sestamibi (methoxyisobutyl isonitrile). The other is from the so-called boronic acid adducts of technetium dioximes (BATO) family of compounds and is called teboroxime. Both agents are efficiently taken up by the myocardium and, as with thallium, their uptakes are proportional to myocardial blood flow.

Tc-99m sestamibi behaves quite differently from either thallium-201 or Tc-99m teboroxime. Once taken up by the myocardium, the sestamibi compound demonstrates a minimal amount of washout and no significant redistribution. The lack of redistribution is both advantageous and disadvantageous compared with other agents. The advantage is that the distribution of the radionuclide at the time of injection will remain constant for hours, allowing for greater flexibility in imaging times. The major disadvantage is that a second injection is required for the second set of images.

So, if a rest-and-exercise or rest-and-pharmacologic stimulation study is to be performed on the same day, the second injection must be given when the myocardial activity from the first is still present and quite visible. To reduce the effect of this activity on the appearance of the second set of images, the dose of the second injection must be significantly higher than that of the first. At present, a dose three times higher is recommended (27). Ideally, it would be best to acquire rest and intervention studies on separate days. Whether a 1-day

or 2-day protocol is used, the sequence of acquisitions is optional; either the rest or the intervention study may be performed first.

A major advantage of the higher photon flux of Tc-99m sestamibi is that high-resolution collimation can be used; this is, in fact, recommended for both planar and tomographic acquisitions. In addition to reduced photon scatter, this high-resolution collimation results in much sharper images compared to those that use thallium (Figure 5.6).

In marked contrast to the myocardial kinetics of the sestamibi compound, Tc-99m teboroxime has an extremely fast rate of washout from the myocardium, so rapid that imaging must be completed within a few minutes, placing a premium on speed. For the same reason, a separate injection must be given for the second set of images, and tomographic imaging cannot be reliably performed unless a multiheaded detector is used. The major advantage of teboroxime is that a second injection can be given very shortly after the first without concern for background, as noted with Tc-99m sestamibi. It is therefore possible to perform a complete exercise-and-rest study in about 1 h (28).

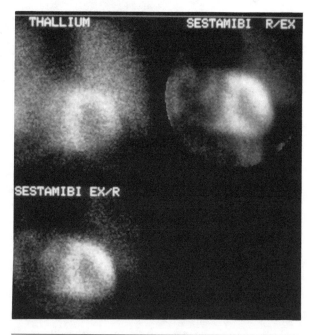

Figure 5.6 Three exercise perfusion images from the same patient: (upper left) thallium-201; (upper right) Tc-99m sestamibi (22 mCi) using rest-exercise (R/EX) same-day protocol; and (lower left) Tc-99m sestamibi (8 mCi) using an exercise-rest (EX/R) same-day protocol. The sestamibi images show less background activity and sharper myocardial borders than in the thallium-201 image.

Combined Perfusion-Function Imaging. Because the technetium-based agents can be injected in sufficiently large doses, it is now possible to acquire technically adequate ventricular function images using the first-pass approach, at peak exercise and at rest, and then to acquire perfusion images 10 to 60 min later. Thus, with a single injection of a radiopharmaceutical, regional wall motion, right and left ventricular ejection fractions, and myocardial perfusion can all be evaluated. This combined imaging provides an exciting potential for improved diagnosis and better prognostication. Another possible approach to function-perfusion imaging is to gate the acquisition of the perfusion images to permit analysis of wall thickening at rest, which may enhance the assessment of myocardial viability.

Acute Myocardial Infarction and Unstable Angina. Tc-99m sestamibi is also used to assess the benefit of thrombolysis or angioplasty in treating an acute MI (29). Prior to receiving any therapy, these patients are injected with sestamibi; thrombolytic therapy or angioplasty is then performed and the patient is stabilized. Next, perfusion imaging takes place; the images acquired show the myocardial distribution of the radionuclide before treatment. Subsequently, another injection of sestamibi is given and repeat imaging is performed. Now the images illustrate the radionuclide distribution after therapy. By comparing the two sets of images, the size of the initial perfusion defect and the improvement due to therapy can be quantified. Sestamibi can also be injected into hospitalized patients who have spontaneous chest pain; they can then be treated without delay and imaged later to determine whether the pain represented ischemia.

Echocardiography

Echocardiography is widely accepted as a useful technique for diagnosing and managing various forms of congenital and acquired heart disease, in part because it alone can provide spatial information on cardiac structure and function noninvasively without the use of radioactive tracers. In addition, echocardiography offers the advantage of immediate results—unlike newer modalities such as magnetic resonance imaging (MRI) and computerized tomography (CT). These advantages of echocardiography make it the second most frequently used modality (after ECG) for diagnosing cardiac disorders.

Transthoracic Echocardiography

A state-of-the-art echocardiographic procedure currently consists of a two-dimensional, M-mode, and Doppler echocardiogram.

A *two-dimensional echocardiogram* is usually performed with the patient supine and at rest. A probe, or transducer, is placed on the surface of the chest and oriented toward the heart. The transducer sends out a wide ultrasonic beam that reflects off the heart and is received by another part of the probe, then relayed to a computer, which creates and displays real-time images of the heart on the screen and records them on a videocassette recorder.

In contrast to the two-dimensional technique, *M-mode echocardiography* utilizes a narrow ultrasonic beam that crosses one specific section of the heart and records changes over time for that section.

Doppler echocardiography techniques analyze blood flow in the heart and in the blood vessels. There are two types of Doppler echocardiography: continuous-wave and pulsed-wave. *Continuous-wave* Doppler echocardiography detects and displays average blood flow along the course of the ultrasonic beam. Since no depth selection or special filters are used, it can resolve very high velocities, such as those seen in severely stenotic lesions. *Pulsed-wave* Doppler echocardiography uses a range-gated mode that is able to select and examine a specific area along the ultrasonic beam. Since it cannot display high velocity flows, it is used primarily to map atria and ventricles for estimating valvular insufficiency.

Color-coded flow Doppler echocardiography uses pulsed Doppler properties to display blood flow in colors that are determined by the direction of flow and flow velocity. Its primary advantage over standard pulsed Doppler is its ability to provide a bidimensional display of blood flow in real-time. Color-coded flow Doppler is used primarily to assess regurgitant lesions and shunts.

Transesophageal Echocardiography

In certain patients, conventional transthoracic echocardiography may produce images and Doppler recordings of compromised quality. This is particularly true in patients who are obese or who have chronic pulmonary disease, chest wall deformities, or prosthetic valves. In these patients, transesophageal echocardiography offers a means by which important diagnostic information may still be obtained.

As the name implies, transesophageal echocardiography is performed by means of a transducer placed in the patient's esophagus. The patient's oropharynx is locally anesthetized, and a vagolytic agent may be given to reduce secretions along with a short-acting sedative. The probe is inserted into the patient's mouth and the patient is asked to swallow it when it reaches the oropharynx. Once the probe is in the esophagus, the gag reflex diminishes in most patients and the echocardiogram can begin. Including both imaging and color-coded Doppler flow, the complete investigation of the heart and lungs takes between 10 and 20 min.

With this approach, signal-to-noise ratio improves because the chest wall is circumvented, and a higher-frequency transducer can be used because of the shorter distance between the probe and the heart. This results in highly detailed images, better resolution of cardiac structures, and better visualization of structures poorly displayed by the standard echocardiographic approach, including the atrial appendages, the left main coronary artery and its proximal branches, and the descending thoracic aorta.

Transesophageal echocardiography is used for evaluating prosthetic valves and for interrogating the native valves, e.g., to rule out flail mitral valve and to assess the severity of mitral valve regurgitation. It is useful in cases of infective endocarditis and in the assessment of cardiovascular sources of emboli and cardiovascular tumors. It is also useful interoperatively for patients who are at high risk for ischemic events (30). During surgery, it can be used to monitor left ventricular function (LVF) by detecting changes in wall motion and wall thickening that may precede ECG changes, without interrupting the sterile surgical field.

Clinical Applications

In the past, echocardiography procedures were indicated primarily for imaging cardiac anatomy in the evaluation of patients with valvular heart disease (e.g., stenosis, regurgitation, mitral valve prolapse) as well as for evaluating prosthetic valves. Cardiac anatomy was also typically studied echocardiographically in cases of congenital heart disease, cardiomyopathy, cardiac masses and thrombi, infective endocarditis, myocarditis, pericardial diseases, and aortic diseases. Now, through Doppler echocardiography, physiological parameters can also be analyzed, including the evaluation of blood flow through the cardiovascular system and the calculation of pressures in the various heart chambers.

As for CAD applications—the focus of this chapter—echocardiography can detect abnormalities in global systolic and diastolic function and in regional wall motion and wall thickening—all indicators of reduced myocardial perfusion due to coronary artery stenoses. Also detectable and quantitatable are such complications of ischemia and MI as mitral regurgitation, ventricular septal defect, right ventricular infarction, and pericardial effusion. Other diseases of the chest that may present as CAD, such as dissecting aortic aneurysm and mitral valve prolapse, can be unmasked or excluded. Currently there are a number of stress echocardiography techniques that may further increase this procedure's utility for evaluating CAD. Some are mentioned below.

Exercise Echocardiography

As with nuclear cardiology procedures, the presence of ischemia can be detected echocardiographically by evaluating the changes in the heart induced by stress. Placing the transducer directly on the patient's chest during exercise provides a beat-to-beat analysis of myocardial function. Since the images are tomographic, it is necessary to obtain several views so that the different walls affected by different coronary arteries are represented.

For greater technical ease and improved image resolution, exercise echocardiography can also be performed immediately after exercise. Although some functional changes that occur during exercise may be missed, postexercise imaging is thought to provide data comparable with a typical exercise equilibrium blood pool imaging study, in which data are collected over a 2-min period and the average results are reported. Some investigators have shown that the presence of exercise-induced mitral regurgitation (31) and a change in the mean velocity of mitral flow of less than 50% (32) are also indicators of ischemia. Their presence increases the sensitivity of exercise echocardiography for diagnosing CAD. In the literature, the sensitivity of exercise echocardiography for diagnosing CAD ranges between 66% and 91% and the specificity ranges between 69% and 100%. These ranges are quite broad because the studies included different patient populations and different ultrasound technologies.

The main advantages of using exercise echocardiography in diagnosing CAD are that it is truly noninvasive and does not involve radiation. The equipment is less expensive, more readily available, and usually adaptable to exercise laboratories. However, about 20% of patients must be excluded from this means of study (and therefore studied using pharmacologic stress) due to body habitus, respiratory interference, positioning problems, or inability to exercise.

Exercise echocardiography is best used in patients who have ECG changes at rest and ambiguous responses to treadmill GXT, as well as those requiring an evaluation of the functional significance of lesions seen on contrast angiography. This technique has also been used to assess post-MI prognosis (33-35). It is not warranted as a screening procedure in asymptomatic patients, because the sensitivity of detecting CAD in these patients is relatively low.

Echocardiography Combined with Pharmacologic Stress

As noted with nuclear cardiology procedures, patients who cannot exercise to diagnostically adequate levels may be studied using pharmacologic stress. Both intravenous dipyridamole (described in the section on "Nuclear Cardiology") and intravenous dobutamine have been used for this purpose. Of those who use dipyridamole for echocardiographic testing, Picano et al. (36,37) use it most frequently. They claim that the procedure provides

good results for assessing coronary angioplasty and for determining the prognosis of patients with CAD. Either dipyridamole or dobutamine can be used to diagnose and evaluate the presence and significance of CAD through rest-to-stress changes in global and regional wall motion and wall thickening. According to the literature, both dipyridamole and dobutamine echocardiography provide sensitivity and specificity values in the range of 80% to 90% for diagnosing CAD (38,39).

In contrast to dipyridamole, dobutamine increases HR, BP, and myocardial contractility, all of which increase myocardial oxygen demand—in patients with CAD, this may provoke ischemia. Intravenous administration of dobutamine begins at the rate of 5 μg · kg · min and increases to a rate of 40 μg · kg · min.

Currently, dobutamine is commonly used for stress echocardiography because it tends to provoke ischemia, whereas dipyridamole causes nonhomogeneous blood flow but rarely causes ischemia. Since echocardiography detects only wall motion abnormalities and not changes in coronary artery blood flow, dobutamine is preferred. Figures 5.7 and 5.8 illustrate ischemic changes not seen at rest that were caused by dobutamine in

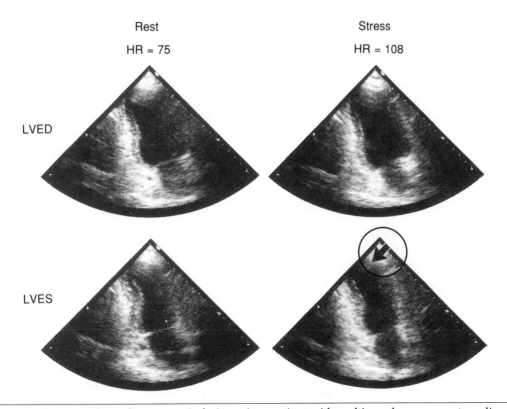

Rest	Stress
HR = 75	HR = 108

LVED

LVES

Figure 5.7 Transthoracic echocardiogram, apical views, in a patient with multivessel coronary artery disease. Images are normal at rest, but show severe apical hypokinesis (arrow) with dobutamine stress. (HR = heart rate, LVED = left ventricular end-diastole, LVES = left ventricular end-systole.)

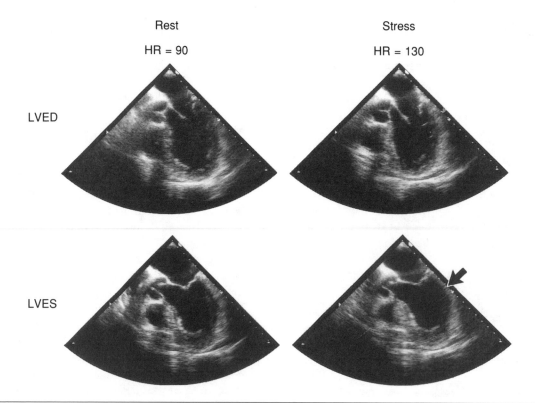

Figure 5.8   Transesophageal echocardiogram, basal long-axis views, in a patient with severe proximal right coronary artery disease. Images are normal at rest, but show inferoposterior wall akinesis (arrow) with dobutamine stress. (HR = heart rate, LVED = left ventricular end-diastole, LVES = left ventricular end-systole.)

two patients with CAD. In patients with MI, dobutamine stress echocardiography has high sensitivity for detecting the extent and location of CAD (39,40) and for determining the viability of the myocardium after thrombolytic therapy (41). This procedure is also useful for predicting perioperative cardiac events (42).

Summary

Within the broad areas of nuclear cardiology and echocardiography, there are a variety of procedures used in current clinical practice to diagnose CAD noninvasively. As we have discussed in this chapter, all the procedures are used to evaluate myocardial perfusion and performance (or ventricular function), which themselves are indicators of ischemia and which allow the clinician to evaluate the significance of coronary stenoses.

Particularly when there is an intermediate pretest likelihood of disease, the procedures provide high sensitivity and specificity values. In addition to diagnosing CAD, they are vital in managing and in serially following the treatment of patients

with disease, as well as in providing valuable prognostic information in many subsets of patients. For specific applications, a particular procedure may be indicated; for others, user biases will play a larger role.

For all of these modalities, technological advances, as well as new imaging and pharmacologic agents, have improved the usefulness and applicability of all of these procedures and should continue to do so in the future.

References

1. Pavel, D.G.; Zimmer, A.M.; Patterson, V.N. In vivo labeling of red blood cells with 99Tc: A new approach to blood pool visualization. J. Nucl. Med. 18:305-308; 1977.
2. Kennedy, J.W.; Trenholme, S.E.; Kasser, I.S. Left ventricular volume and mass from single-plane angiocardiogram. A comparison of anteroposterior and right anterior oblique methods. Am. Heart J. 80:343-352; 1970.
3. Slutsky, R.; Karliner, J.; Ricci, D.; Kaiser, R.; Pfisterer, M.; Gordon, D.; Peterson, K.; Ashburn, W. Left ventricular volumes by gated equilibrium radionuclide

angiocardiography: A new method. Circulation. 60:556-564; 1979.

4. Dehmer, G.J.; Lewis, S.E.; Hillis, L.D.; Twieg, D.; Falkoff, M.; Parkey, R.W.; Willerson, J.T. Nongeometric determination of left ventricular volumes from equilibrium blood pool scans. Am. J. Cardiol. 45:293-300; 1980.

5. Massardo, T.; Gal, R.A.; Grenier, R.P.; Schmidt, D.H.; Port, S.C. Left ventricular volume calculation using a count-based ratio method applied to multigated radionuclide angiography. J. Nucl. Med. 31:450-456; 1990.

6. Gal, R.A.; Grenier, R.P.; Schmidt, D.H.; Port, S.C. Count-based left ventricular volume measurement without blood sampling or attenuation correction from first-pass radionuclide angiography. J. Nucl. Med. [Abstract]. 27:912; 1986.

7. Dymond, D.S.; Elliott, A.T.; Flatman, W.; Stone, D.; Bett, R.; Cuninghame, G.; Sims, H. The clinical validation of gold-195m: A new short half-life radiopharmaceutical for rapid, sequential, first-pass radionuclide angiography in patients. J. Am. Coll. Cardiol. 2:85-92; 1983.

8. Mena, I.; Narahara, K.A.; deJong, R.; Maublant, J. Gold-195m, an ultra-short-lived generator-produced radionuclide: Clinical application in first-pass ventriculography. J. Nucl. Med. 24:139-144; 1983.

9. Wackers, F.J.T.; Stein, R.; Pytlik, L.; Plankey, M.W.; Lange, R.; Hoffer, P.B.; Sands, M.J.; Zaret, B.L.; Berger, H.J. Gold-195m for serial first-pass radionuclide angiography during upright exercise in patients with coronary artery disease. J. Am. Coll. Cardiol. 2:497-505; 1983.

10. Bonow, R.O.; Kent, K.M.; Rosing, D.R.; Lipson, L.C.; Bacharach, S.L.; Green, M.V.; Epstein, S.E. Improved left ventricular diastolic filling in patients with coronary artery disease after percutaneous transluminal coronary angioplasty. Circulation. 66:1159-1167; 1982.

11. Port, S.C.; Gal, R.A.; Grenier, R.P.; Acharya, K.; Shen, Y.; Skrade, B. First-pass radionuclide angiography during treadmill exercise: Evaluation of patient motion and a method for motion correction. J. Nucl. Med. [Abstract]. 30:770; 1989.

12. Jones, R.H.; Floyd, R.D.; Austin, E.H.; Sabiston, D.C., Jr. The role of radionuclide angiocardiography in the preoperative prediction of pain relief and prolonged survival following coronary artery bypass grafting. Ann. Surg. 197:743-754; 1983.

13. Lee, K.L.; Pryor, D.B.; Pieper, K.S.; Harrell, F.E., Jr.; Califf, R.M.; Mark, D.B.; Hlatky, M.A.; Coleman, R.E.; Cobb, F.R.; Jones, R.H. Prognostic value of radionuclide angiography in medically treated patients with coronary artery disease. A comparison with clinical and catheterization variables. Circulation. 82:1705-1717; 1990.

14. Johnson, S.H.; Bigelow, C.; Lee, K.L.; Pryor, D.B.; Jones, R.H. Prediction of death and myocardial infarction by radionuclide angiocardiography in patients with suspected coronary artery disease. Am. J. Cardiol. 67:919-926; 1991.

15. Kiat, H.; Berman, D.S.; Maddahi, J.; Yang, L.D.; Van Train, K.; Rozanski, A.; Friedman, J. Late reversibility of tomographic myocardial thallium-201 defects: An accurate marker of myocardial viability. J. Am. Coll. Cardiol. 12:1456-1463; 1988.

16. Dilsizian, V.; Rocco, T.P.; Freedman, N.M.T.; Leon, M.B.; Bonow, R.O. Enhanced detection of ischemic but viable myocardium by the reinjection of thallium after stress-redistribution imaging. N. Engl. J. Med. 323:141-146; 1990.

17. Tillisch, J.; Brunken, R.; Marshall, R.; Schwaiger, M.; Mandelkern, M.; Phelps, M.; Schelbert, H. Reversibility of cardiac wall-motion abnormalities predicted by positron tomography. N. Engl. J. Med. 314:884-888; 1986.

18. Albro, P.C.; Gould, K.L.; Westcott, R.J.; Hamilton, G.W.; Ritchie, J.L.; Williams, D.L. Noninvasive assessment of coronary stenoses by myocardial imaging during pharmacologic coronary vasodilatation. III. Clinical trial. Am. J. Cardiol. 42:751-760; 1978.

19. Ranhosky, A.; Kempthorne-Rawson, J. Intravenous dipyridamole thallium imaging study group: The safety of intravenous dipyridamole thallium myocardial perfusion imaging. Circulation. 81:1205-1209; 1990.

20. Boucher, C.A.; Brewster, D.C.; Darling, R.C.; Okada, R.D.; Strauss, H.W.; Pohost, G.M. Determination of cardiac risk by dipyridamole-thallium imaging before peripheral vascular surgery. N. Engl. J. Med. 312:389-394; 1985.

21. Leppo, J.A.; Plaja, J.; Gionet, M.; Tumulo, J.; Paraskos, J.A.; Culter, B.S. Noninvasive evaluation of cardiac risk before elective vascular surgery. J. Am. Coll. Cardiol. 9:269-276; 1987.

22. Eagle, K.A.; Singer, D.E.; Brewster, D.C.; Darling, R.C.; Mulley, A.G.; Boucher, C.A. Dipyridamole-thallium scanning in patients undergoing vascular surgery; Optimizing preoperative evaluation of cardiac risk. JAMA. 257:2185-2189; 1987.

23. Leppo, J.A.; O'Brien, J.; Rothendler, J.A.; Getchell, J.D.; Lee, V.W. Dipyridamole-thallium-201 scintigraphy in the prediction of future cardiac events after acute myocardial infarction. N. Engl. J. Med. 310:1014-1018; 1984.

24. Gal, R.A.; Gunasekera, J.; Massardo, T.; Shalev, Y.; Port, S.C. Long-term prognostic value of a normal dipyridamole thallium-201 scan. Clin. Cardiol. 14:971-974; 1991.

25. Verani, M.S.; Mahmarian, J.J.; Hixson, J.B.; Boyce, T.M.; Staudacher, R.A. Diagnosis of coronary artery disease by controlled vasodilation with adenosine and thallium-201 scintigraphy in patients unable to exercise. Circulation. 82:80-87; 1990.

26. Gupta, N.C.; Esterbrooks, D.J.; Hilleman, D.E.; Mohiuddin, S.M. Comparison of adenosine and exercise thallium-201 single-photon emission computed tomography (SPECT) myocardial perfusion imaging. J. Am. Coll. Cardiol. 19:248-267; 1992.

27. Taillefer, R.; Gagnon, A.; Laflamme, L.; Grégoire, J.; Léveillé, J.; Phaneuf, D.C. Same day injections of

Tc-99m methoxyisobutyl isonitrile (hexamibi) for myocardial tomographic imaging: Comparison between rest-stress injection sequences. Eur. J. Nucl. Med. 15:113-117; 1989.

28. Zielonka, J.S.; Cannon, P.; Johnson, L.; Seldin, D.; Bellinger, R.L.; Chua, E.; Coleman, R.E.; Reba, R.C.; Wasserman, A.; Drane, W.; Williams, C.; Coris, M.L.; Leppo, J.A.; Akhtar, R.; Bamrah, V.S.; Krubsack, A.J. Multicenter trial of Tc-99m teboroxime (Cardiotec): A new myocardial perfusion agent. J. Nucl. Med. [Abstract]. 31:827; 1990.

29. Gibbons, R.J. Perfusion imaging with 99m-sestamibi for the assessment of myocardial area at risk and the efficacy of acute treatment of myocardial infarction. Circulation. 84 [Suppl. I]:137-142; 1991.

30. Matsumoto, M.; Oka, Y.; Strom, J.; Frishman, W.; Kadish, A.; Becker, R.M.; Frater, R.W.; Sonnenblick, E.H. Application of transesophageal echocardiography to continuous intraoperative monitoring of left ventricular performance. Am. J. Cardiol. 46:95-105; 1980.

31. Zachariah, Z.P.; Hsiung, M.C.; Nanda, N.C.; Kan, M.; Gatewood, R.P., Jr. Color Doppler assessment of mitral regurgitation induced by supine exercise in patients with coronary artery disease. Am. J. Cardiol. 59:1266-1270; 1987.

32. Mitchell, G.D.; Brunken, R.C.; Schwaiger, M.; Donohue, B.C.; Krivokapich, J.; Child, J.S. Assessment of mitral flow velocity with exercise by an index of stress-induced left ventricular ischemia in coronary artery disease. Am. J. Cardiol. 61:536-540; 1988.

33. Jaarsma, W.; Visser, C.A.; Kupper, A.J.F.; Res, J.C.J.; VanEenige, M.J.; Roos, J.P. Usefulness of two-dimensional exercise echocardiography shortly after myocardial infarction. Am. J. Cardiol. 57:86-90; 1986.

34. Ryan, T.; Armstrong, W.F.; O'Donnell, J.A.; Feigenbaum, H. Risk stratification after acute myocardial infarction by means of exercise two-dimensional echocardiography. Am. Heart J. 114:1305-1316; 1987.

35. Applegate, R.J.; Dell'Italia, L.J.; Crawford, M.H. Usefulness of two-dimensional echocardiography during low-level exercise testing early after uncomplicated acute myocardial infarction. Am. J. Cardiol. 60:10-14; 1987.

36. Picano, E.; Pirelli, S.; Marzilli, M.; Faletra, F.; Lattanzi, F.; Campolo, L.; Massa, D.; Alberti, A.; Gara, E.; Distante, A.; L'Abbate, A. Usefulness of high-dose dipyridamole echocardiography test in coronary angioplasty. Circulation. 80:807-815; 1989.

37. Picano, E.; Severi, S.; Michelassi, C.; Lattanzi, F.; Masini, M.; Orsini, E.; Distante, A.; L'Abbate, A. Prognostic importance of dipyridamole-echocardiography test in coronary artery disease. Circulation. 80:450-457; 1989.

38. Picano, E.; Lattanzi, F.; Orlandini, A.; Marini, C.; L'Abbate, A. Stress echocardiography and the human factor: The importance of being expert. J. Am. Coll. Cardiol. 17:666-669; 1991.

39. Sawada, S.G.; Seger, D.S.; Ryan, T.; Brown, S.E.; Dohan, A.M.; Williams, R.; Fineberg, N.S.; Armstrong, W.F.; Feigenbaum, H. Echocardiographic detection of coronary artery disease during dobutamine infusion. Circulation. 83:1605-1614; 1991.

40. Berthe, C.; Piérard, L.A.; Hiernaux, M.; Trotteur, G.; Lempereur, P.; Carlier, J., Kulbertus, H.E. Predicting the extent and location of coronary artery disease in acute myocardial infarction by echocardiography during dobutamine infusion. Am. J. Cardiol. 58: 1167-1172; 1986.

41. Piérard, L.A.; Delandsheere, C.M., Berthe, C.; Rigo, P.; Kulbertus, H.E. Identification of viable myocardium by echocardiography during dobutamine infusion in patients with myocardial infarction after thrombolytic therapy: Comparison with positron emission tomography. J. Am. Coll. Cardiol. 15:1021-1031; 1990.

42. Lane, R.T.; Sawada, S.G.; Ryan, T.; Armstrong, W.F.; Feigenbaum, H. Dobutamine echocardiography as a predictor of perioperative cardiac events. Circulation. 80:[Suppl. II]:67; 1989.

Chapter 6

Coronary Angiography and Interventional Techniques in the Management of Patients With Coronary Artery Disease

Douglass A. Morrison
Stephen T. Crowley

Coronary angiography, or the production of X-ray pictures of the human heart circulation (coronary arteries), has revolutionized the practice of cardiology. It has allowed physicians and scientists to characterize the nature of atherosclerotic coronary artery disease (CAD), or hardening of the arteries. In addition, obtaining a map of the human heart circulation was a necessary step in the development of revascularization strategies. Both coronary artery bypass graft surgery (CABG) and percutaneous transluminal coronary angioplasty (PTCA) require that an angiogram or road map be obtained first.

This chapter reviews first the history of the development of heart catheterization and coronary angiography. Then a review of the reasons doctors recommend an angiogram will be obtained from a recent American College of Cardiology and American Heart Association published guideline. Considerations important to protecting patient safety will be outlined. X-ray views or projections necessary to separate and identify the separate heart arteries and their most important branches are summarized. Although the most common clinical problems involve atherosclerosis, there are also some congenital abnormalities of the heart arteries, and these are reviewed. We include a brief discussion of balloon dilatation, or PTCA, and other new techniques used in the catheter laboratory for the treatment of heart artery problems. The chapter ends with a summary of coronary angiography and PTCA procedures that were performed on approximately 1,000,000 and 300,000 Americans, respectively, in 1990.

Historical Background

Werner Forssman passed the first catheter into the human vascular system in 1926 (1). He used a urologic catheter, which he inserted into his own vein and advanced into the right side of his heart. His objective was to obtain direct cardiac access for administering drugs. His experiment precipitated the development of diagnostic right and left heart catheterization and advanced cardiac life support (ACLS) (1,2).

Cournand and Richards used right heart catheterization to measure intracardiac pressures and measure cardiac output (3). They and other researchers described the rest and exercise hemodynamics of patients who had a variety of cardiac and pulmonary disorders (3,4). Based on these seminal works, Forssman, Cournand, and Richards received the Nobel Prize for Medicine and Physiology in 1956.

The use of contrast agents to opacify and film the human circulatory system was pioneered by other physicians, including Seldinger, Radner, Ricketts, Abrams, and Sones (5-8). The first selective cannulation and opacification of a human coronary artery was accomplished by Sones at the Cleveland Clinic in 1956 (9). Quick to capitalize on this novel idea and supported by the development of a successful revascularization strategy or coronary artery bypass grafting (CABG), Sones and his colleagues went on to record films of human coronary arteries from more than 50,000 patients. The development of CABG surgery was pioneered by Favolaro, also at the Cleveland Clinic (10).

Later, Judkins used Seldinger's percutaneous approach and designed catheters to be used performing coronary angiography from the groin (11,12). This greatly simplified matters, as the Sones approach required arterial cutdown and arterial repair for the catheter introduction (13,14). Besides recording the coronary anatomy of thousands of human subjects, Judkins and Sones combined forces to organize the Society for Cardiac

Angiography (now known as the Society for Cardiac Angiography and Interventions) into an international organization dedicated to excellence in the performance of cardiac catheterization procedures.

Dotter, a colleague of Judkins, was the first to attempt an interventional technique in human arteries (15). He used a series of dilators to enlarge the lumen of human leg arteries and successfully improved limb flow in a number of patients considered to be inoperable. Nevertheless, his idea was not taken seriously within the American radiological or vascular communities. A German physician, Zeitler, was intrigued by Dotter's work and began further study. In turn, his student, Gruntzig, pursued the idea of interventional work in human cardiac circulation. Gruntzig performed the first dilatation of a coronary artery in a conscious patient in 1977 (16). He called his procedure *percutaneous transluminal coronary angioplasty*. His first case was not only angiographically successful but led to the resolution of the patient's angina. Follow-up angiography of this first patient showed continued patency after 10 years.

Since Gruntzig's first dilatation, use of the percutaneous transluminal coronary angioplasty (PTCA) method has grown exponentially. However, despite technical improvements, PTCA is limited by two major problems; restenosis of a successfully dilated artery at 6 months follow-up in approximately 30% of cases and acute occlusion of the artery due to coronary dissection or thrombus formation in as many as 5% of procedures (17). These limitations, as well as the need to improve clinical outcomes in more complex coronary lesions, have led to the rapid development of new technologies, such as coronary stents, lasers, and atherectomy catheters. Although the restenosis rates with these new coronary interventions are not dramatically different from conventional balloon angioplasty, in some patients the new techniques have certain advantages. Directional coronary atherectomy of proximal left anterior descending artery and ostial vein graft stenoses have been shown to decrease restenosis rates slightly, albeit at greater complications and costs (18). Coronary stents have been proven to restore vessel patency following failed PTCA and may improve restenosis rates in native coronaries and vein grafts (19). Lasers and mechanical rotational atherectomy catheters may ultimately prove useful for total coronary occlusion and complex, elongated lesions, which are not highly favorable for conventional balloon angioplasty.

PTCA has joined CABG surgery as a means of revascularizing patients with obstructive coronary artery disease (CAD). With these two options available, the need for a road map, that is, a coronary angiogram, is apparent. Accordingly, the growth in the use of cardiac catheterization generally (including valve and pump assessment, which are required for such operative procedures as valve replacement, aneurysmectomy, and cardiac transplantation), and coronary angiography in particular, have also been exponential (14,20,21).

In 1991 there were over 1,100 cardiac catheterization laboratories in the United States and more than 2,000 worldwide. In 1990, more than 300,000 catheter therapeutic procedures were performed in the United States. The largest registry of these procedures is maintained by the Society for Cardiac Angiography and Interventions, currently located in Breckenridge, Colorado. Reports from previous Society Registries in Seattle, Washington, and Syracuse, New York, are among the largest data bases of coronary angiography in the world (22,23).

Current Indications for Coronary Angiography

Coronary angiography is a means of outlining the coronary arteries with contrast and recording these outlines on cine film or digital data storage. The outline may be used to

1. establish the diagnosis of CAD (usually agreed upon as one or more narrowings of greater than 70% of the luminal diameter of a major epicardial coronary artery except for the left main artery, where a narrowing of greater than 50% is used),
2. make inferences regarding a patient's prognosis (usually based upon the number of vessels involved, severity of the stenoses, and extent of ventricular dysfunction), and
3. plan a revascularization strategy (CABG surgery or PTCA).

A task force of the American College of Cardiology (ACC) and the American Heart Association (AHA) has carefully reviewed the medical literature and current practice patterns and has made specific recommendations regarding patient categories for whom coronary angiography is recommended (Class I), debatable (Class II), or clearly not indicated (Class III) (14). These recommendations are summarized here:

Indications for Coronary Angiography
[Adapted from
ACC/AHA Task Force Recommendations (14)]

Class I. Patients for whom there is general agreement that coronary angiography is justified

A. Asymptomatic patients
Evidence from exercise testing, thallium scintigraphy or radionuclide ventriculography (RNV) of "high risk," i.e., reduced life expectancy secondary to CAD

B. Symptomatic patients
   1. with angina that is inadequately responsive to therapy
   2. with unstable angina
   3. with variant angina
   4. with angina and various high-risk factors
   5. with angina before vascular surgery
   6. after resuscitation from a cardiac arrest

C. Patients having atypical chest pain of uncertain etiology but high-risk factors, including left ventricular dysfunction (LVD)

D. Patients with angina occurring more than 8 weeks after an acute MI

E. Patients who are within the early period after an MI experience recurrent episodes of pain with changes in electrocardiogram (ECG) or the suspicion of a ruptured interventricular septum, acute mitral regurgitation, or a pseudoaneurysm (free-wall rupture)

F. Patients who are being prepared for surgery for valvular heart disease or congenital heart disease and who have signs or symptoms suggesting concomitant CAD

Class II. Patients with conditions for which coronary angiography is frequently performed but about which there is considerable debate regarding its value and appropriateness.

A. Asymptomatic patients who have more than mildly positive exercise tests, multiple risk factors for CAD, silent ischemia, or prior revascularization procedures (PTCA or CABG surgery) or who are being tested as part of a heart transplantation follow-up

B. Mildly symptomatic patients (Canadian Class I or II) who are either female or young (< 40 years), who require major nonvascular surgery, or who cannot be risk-stratified noninvasively (for example, because they cannot exercise)

C. Patients with atypical chest pain in whom noninvasive studies are equivocal or cannot be performed

D. Patients in the convalescent phase of infarction (< 8 weeks) if angina is occurring; patients who have had electrical or pump instability

E. Patients in the early phase after a myocardial infarction (MI) if the course has been complicated by ventricular tachycardia, shock, or failure

F. Patients being prepared for surgery for valvular or congenital heart disease who are suspected of having coronary anomalies or endocarditis or who are at moderate risk

Class III. Patients with conditions for which there is general agreement that coronary angiography is not justified

A. Asymptomatic patients being "screened" for CAD without first undergoing noninvasive testing (exercise tests, thallium scintigraphy, RNV)

B. Symptomatic patients who are well controlled medically, who are at low risk for CAD, and, in particular, who have comorbid conditions

C. Patients with atypical chest pain who have previously had a normal coronary angiogram

D. Patients convalescing from MI who are of advanced age and have comorbid conditions, very severe pump dysfunction (left ventricular ejection fraction [LVEF] < 20%) and only mild arrhythmia with no ischemia

E. Patients in the early post-MI stages for whom no revascularization strategy is contemplated

F. Very young patients who are being prepared for valvular or congenital heart disease surgery and in whom no congenital anomalies or coronary emboli are suspected

A recent editorial by Ambrose emphasized that coronary angiography was debatable if used (1) to look for lesions amenable to angioplasty in patients who are not being considered for CABG surgery, (2) in asymptomatic or minimally symptomatic patients (either post MI or not), (3) in survivors of sudden death, and (4) in post-CABG patients (24).

Complications of Coronary Angiography

Risk factors for catheterization-related mortality include left main stenosis of greater than 50%, unstable angina of functional Class IV, congestive heart failure, and advanced age. The major potential complications from coronary angiography include death in up to 0.1% of cases, MI in up to 0.1% of cases, and cerebrovascular accident in up to 0.1% of cases (22,23). Arterial access complications and major arrhythmia problems occur in approximately 0.5% of cases. Renal failure and allergic reactions to contrast can also occur (22,23,25-30). Renal failure is largely dependent upon the patient's level of renal function going into the catheterization (i.e., creatinine > 2.0 mg%), state of hydration, total contrast dose used (> 125 ml), and the presence of concomitant hypertension, diabetes, or congestive heart failure (29,30).

Patient Safety in Coronary Angiography

The single highest priority in any catheterization procedure should be the safe completion of the procedure. To this end, the clinician must pay attention to seven safety aspects, outlined here.

Patient Safety in the Catheterization Laboratory

I. Monitor the patient's vital signs

A. Real-time oscilloscopic tracing of the patient's heart rate (HR) and rhythm

B. Either oscilloscopic tracing of intraarterial blood pressure (BP) or regular sphygmomanometer recordings or both

C. Frequent talking to the patient, to observe changes in character or content of speech

Comments: Although not continuously the primary focus, the patient's vital signs (including mentation) should remain within the primary operator's awareness throughout the procedure. Bringing the vital signs into focus should require nothing more than a glance at the ECG and pressures on the monitoring oscilloscope and a brief question or two to the patient.

II. Intravenous access

Comments: An intravenous access should be obtained on the patient; if nothing else is available, a femoral or brachial venous sheath (5F or 6F) can be placed next to the arterial access site. This access can be used for a temporary pacemaker or right heart hemodynamic monitoring, but, most importantly, it provides a means to give atropine, epinephrine, or other emergency medication.

III. Support and monitoring of patient's oxygenation

A. Have a low threshold for using supplemental oxygen

B. Monitor oxygenation by means of finger or ear oximetry or checking oxygen in arterial blood sample

Comments: Any laboratory that provides diagnostic or interventional coronary procedures should have not only the full range of means of giving supplemental oxygen (masks, cannulae, airways), but also the means of assessing adequacy of oxygenation (finger or ear oximetry and blood oxygen saturation or tension analyzers).

IV. Rapid access to cardioversion

Comments: Ready availability of cardioversion means not only a functional device, but someone assigned to use it. The time from onset of ventricular fibrillation to successful cardioversion to normal sinus rhythm should not ordinarily exceed 10 sec. Cardioverters need to be regularly tested by the hospital biomedical department for grounding and adequacy of "dose" on discharge.

V. Staff training in basic life support (BLS) and ACLS

Comments: All catheterization laboratory staff should be trained and certified in BLS and preferably ACLS. AHA courses are ideal for keeping staff current on resuscitative techniques in general and on pharmacological and adjunctive mechanical supports in particular (31).

VI. Pharmacological support

A. For pain

1. Local anesthetic agents (subcutaneous)
2. Morphine IV
3. Demoral IV

B. For bradycardia

1. Atropine IV
2. Isoproterenol IV

C. For tachycardia

1. Digoxin IV
2. Verapamil IV
3. Lidocaine IV
4. Procainamide IV
5. Adenosine IV

D. For hypertension

1. Nitroprusside IV
2. Nitroglycerin IV

3. Nifedipine SL

4. Captopril

E. Hypotension IV fluid

1. Dopamine IV

2. Epinephrine IV

3. Calcium IV

F. For pulmonary congestion

1. Lasix IV

2. Morphine IV

G. For reaction to contrast medium

1. Corticosteroids IV

2. Antihistamines IV

H. For acute thrombosis or embolism

1. Urokinase IV

2. Streptokinase IV

3. Heparin IV

Comments: The pharmacology and use of most of these agents is well described in the ACLS manual (31,32).

VII. Mechanical support availability (31,32)

A. Temporary transvenous and external pacemakers

B. Perfusion catheters

C. Intraaortic balloon counterpulsation equipment

D. Intubation and airway adjuncts

E. Percutaneous cardiopulmonary bypass

Comments: It is difficult to predict which technologies, such as lasers and stents, will be "required" for patient safety in future interventional cardiology (32).

Angiographic Views

After patient safety, the next highest priority in the performance of a coronary angiographic study is obtaining information adequate to answer the clinical questions regarding presence of stenoses and lesions that a coronary angiogram should answer. The development of percutaneous coronary interventions has increased the need for views adequate to separate side branches of vessels and to determine the exact course of arteries and the extent of lesions. A simple but crude estimate of the adequacy of catheter studies is the proportion of patients brought back for restudy because of inadequate data. The better the laboratory and angiographer, the less frequently this should occur.

The clinical questions, in order of importance, and the views most suited to answering them (for most patients) are summarized here (35-50). Refer to Figures 6.1-6.4 for the views described.

1. Is there a left main artery stenosis (> 50% narrowing in luminal diameter)?

Best views: straight anterior-posterior (AP); shallow right anterior oblique (RAO); shallow left anterior oblique (LAO). These views should be highly magnified and well collimated. LAO caudal ("weeping willow" or "spider" view) (35-37) and LAO cranial (hemiaxial or "head-up" view) are also possibly helpful.

2. Is there a proximal left anterior descending artery stenosis?

Best views: LAO cranial (38-42); LAO caudal—for obese patients with a horizontal heart, whose left anterior descending artery is foreshortened in the

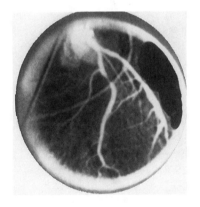

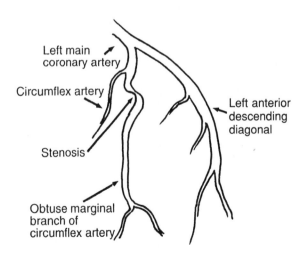

Figure 6.1 Right anterior oblique view, caudal angulation, of the left coronary artery. The circumflex and its obtuse marginal branches are usually best seen in this view.

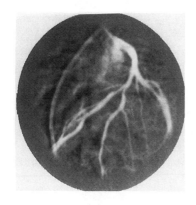

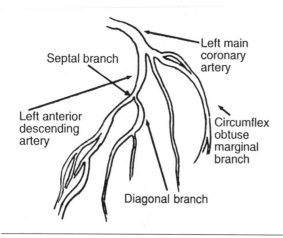

Figure 6.2 Left anterior oblique view with cranial angulation of the left coronary artery. This view is frequently useful for visualizing the proximal left anterior descending artery, including the take-off of the septal and diagonal branches.

cranial view (35-37); RAO cranial—frequently separates the left anterior descending artery from its septal and diagonal branches (43); left lateral, with or without angulation—can frequently open the proximal left anterior descending artery (38-41,45).

3a. Is there a mid left anterior descending artery stenosis?
Best views: LAO cranial; RAO cranial.

3b. Is there a stenosis in the left anterior descending of the diagonal branches (39-44)?
Best views: LAO cranial; left lateral; lateral with cranial angulation; RAO cranial.

4. Is there a proximal circumflex artery stenosis (42-49)?
Best views: RAO caudal; LAO caudal. Also try left lateral view.

5. Is there a stenosis of the obtuse marginal branches of the circumflex (42-49)?
Best views: RAO caudal; LAO caudal; left lateral.

6. Is there a proximal right coronary lesion (50)?
Best views: straight LAO; shallow RAO.

7. Is there a mid right coronary lesion (50)?
Best views: straight LAO; shallow RAO.

8. Is there a distal right coronary lesion?
Best views: RAO cranial and caudal—useful because of overlap of the posterior descending and posterolateral branches of the right coronary artery or left ventricular extension branches (45,50); LAO cranial—best for seeing the crux.

Congenital Anomalies of the Coronary Arteries

Congenital anomalies of the coronary arteries are uncommon (found in less than 1% of adult angiograms) but important from the viewpoint of technically achieving selective cannulation and an adequate study. They are also important because several types are potentially significant hemodynamically even in the absence of atherosclerosis. Finally, atherosclerosis can involve anomalous segments that may be amenable to angioplasty or bypass revascularization, or both. The various possible congenital anomalies are outlined here.

I. Hemodynamically significant (51-62)
   A. Coronary fistulae (53,57-62)
   B. Origin of the left coronary artery from the pulmonary artery (51,52)
   C. Congenital coronary stenosis or atresia (54)
   D. Origin of the left coronary artery from the right sinus of Valsalva with passage between the aorta and the pulmonary artery (51)
   E. Origin of the right coronary artery from the left sinus with a passage between the great vessels (55).

II. Hemodynamically insignificant (course is either anterior or posterior to both great vessels)
   A. Circumflex artery originates from a separate ostium in the right sinus of Valsalva (52-54)
   B. Circumflex artery originates as a branch of the right coronary artery (52,53)
   C. Origin of the right coronary artery from the left sinus of Valsalva (52,53)
   D. Anomalous origin of the left anterior descending artery from the right sinus of Valsalva (52,53)

Pre PTCA   Post PTCA

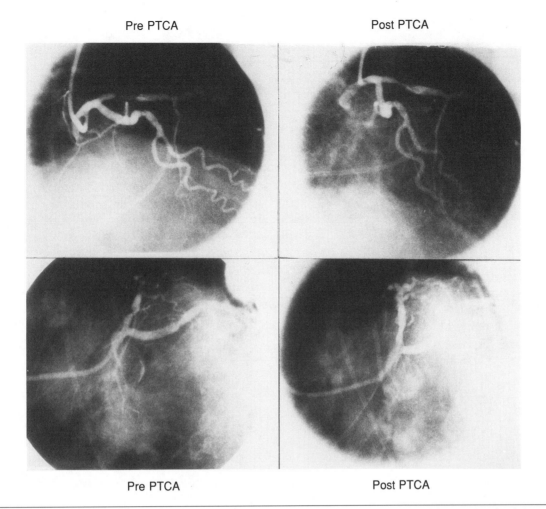

Pre PTCA   Post PTCA

Figure 6.3 Angioplasty of left anterior descending artery. The shallow right anterior oblique view (top) is a good view for assessing the left main coronary artery and the proximal left anterior descending artery, as in this patient. The left anterior oblique caudal view (bottom) is also useful for visualizing the left main coronary artery and, in many patients, the proximal left anterior descending artery. The photos on the left show the arteries prior to a percutaneous transluminal coronary angioplasty; those on the right were taken after this procedure.

E. Anomalous origin of the left main artery from the right sinus of Valsalva (52,53,54)

F. Anomalous origin of the left main artery from the posterior (noncoronary) sinus of Valsalva (52,53,54)

Catheter Interventions for Coronary Artery Disease

PTCA provides an alternative revascularization strategy to CABG surgery for selected patients with significant coronary atherosclerosis (14,16,33, 34). The primary clinical indication is ischemia that is refractory to medication and that might otherwise warrant CABG surgery if the patient is without prohibitive risk for untoward events. The un-

toward events that can accompany PTCA have been discussed earlier (14). The probability of angioplasty success and the risks of associated untoward events have both been predicated, in part, on the coronary anatomy. Table 1 in reference 34 summarizes a clinically useful anatomic scheme for characterizing angioplasty lesions and for predicting success versus complications. Type A lesions include short, straight, noncalcified native artery segments; type B lesions have greater length (10 to 20 mm), angulation (45° to 90°), or calcium; type C lesions are greater than 20 mm in length or greater than 90 degrees in angulation, or total occlusions or found in old vein grafts.

More than a decade of experience with PTCA has demonstrated its potential to improve anatomic narrowings with relief of both rest and exertional ischemia and symptoms. Although the

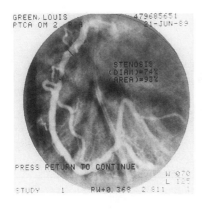

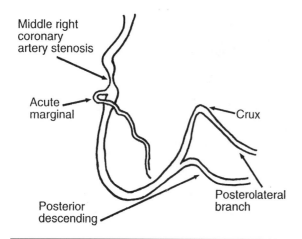

Middle right
coronary
artery stenosis

Acute
marginal

Crux

Posterior
descending

Posterolateral
branch

Figure 6.4   Left anterior oblique view of a mid right coronary artery lesion.

growth in usage of angioplasty during this period of time has been logarithmic, it would likely have been even greater and have resulted in some diminution in CABG surgery (which it has not) were it not for two major problems: acute occlusive syndromes and restenosis. A variety of new technologies, including stents, lasers, atherectomy devices, perfusion catheters, oxygen-carrying solutions, percutaneous bypass, and an array of pharmacologic adjuncts have all been used to try to extend the anatomic range of angioplasty and to solve these two problems.

Summary

The early achievements of Sones, Judkins, Favolaro, Dotter, and Gruntzig have led to further advances in cardiac catheterization and catheter-based interventional techniques. Accordingly,

more effective treatment of acute coronary syndromes have helped reduce the mortality and morbidity of patients with CAD.

References

1. Forssman, W. Die sondierung des rechten Herzens. Klin Wochenschr. 8:2085; 1929.
2. Forssman, W. Experiments on myself. Memoirs of a surgeon in Germany. New York: St. Martin's Press; 1974.
3. Cournand, A.F.; Riley, R.L.; Breen, E.S.; de Baldwin, E.; Richards, D.W., Jr. Measurement of cardiac output in man using the technique of catheterization of the right auricle or ventricle. J. Clin. Invest. 24: 106; 1945.
4. Dexter, L.; Haynes, F.W.; Burwell, C.S.; Eppinger, E.C.; Sagerson R.P.; Evans; J.M. Studies of congenital heart disease II. The pressure and oxygen content of blood in the right auricle, right ventricle, and pulmonary artery in control patients with observations on the oxygen saturation and source of pulmonary "capillary" blood. J. Clin. Invest. 26:554; 1947.
5. Zimmerman, H.A.; Scott, R.W.; Becker, N.D. Catheterization of the left side of the heart in man. Circulation. 1:357; 1950.
6. Seldinger, S.I. Catheter placement of the needle in percutaneous arteriography: A new technique. Acta Radiol. 39:368; 1953.
7. Radner, S. An attempt at roentgenologic visualization of coronary blood vessels in man. Acta Radiol. 26:492; 1945.
8. Ricketts, J.H.; Abrams, H.L. Percutaneous selective coronary cine arteriography, JAMA. 181:620; 1962.
9. Sones, F.M.; Shirey, E.K. Cine coronary arteriography. Modern Concepts in Cardiovasc. Dis. 31:735; 1962.
10. Favolaro, R.G. Saphenous vein autograft replacement of severe segmental coronary artery occlusion-operative technique. Ann. Thorcac. Surg. 5:334-339; 1968.
11. Judkins, M.P. Selective coronary arteriography I. A percutaneous transfemoral technique. Radiology. 89:815-824; 1967.
12. Judkins, M.P. Percutaneous transfemoral selective coronary arteriography. Radiol. Clin. North Am. 6:467-492; 1968.
13. Amplatz, K.; Formanek, G.; Stanger, P.; and Wilson, W. Mechanics of selective coronary artery catheterization via femoral approach. Radiology. 89:1040-1047; 1967.
14. ACC/AHA Task Force on Assessment of Diagnostic and Therapeutic Cardiovascular Procedures (subcommittee on coronary angiography). Guidelines for coronary angiography. J. Am. Coll. Cardiol. 10:935-950; 1987.

15. Dotter, C.T.; Gruntzig, A.R.; Schoop, W.; Zeitler, E. Percutaneous transluminal angioplasty. Berlin: Springer-Verlag; 1983.

16. Gruntzig, A.R.; Senning, A.; Siegenthaler, W.E. Non-operative dilation of coronary-artery stenosis: Percutaneous transluminal coronary angioplasty. N. Engl. J. Med. 301:61-68; 1979.

17. Topol, E.J.; Leys, F.; Pinkerton, C.A. A comparison of directional atherectomy with coronary angioplasty in patients with coronary artery disease. N. Engl. J. Med. 329:221-227; 1993.

18. Caveat II Investigators: Coronary angioplasty versus excisional atherectomy trial. Circulation. 88:I-594; 1993.

19. Sigwart, U.; Puel, J.; Mirkovitch, V.; Joffre, F.; Kappenberger, L. Intravascular stents to prevent occlusion and restonosis after transluminal angioplasty. N. Engl. J. Med. 316:701-706; 1987.

20. Inter-society commission for Heart Disease Resources. Optimal resources for examination of the heart and lungs: Cardiac catheterization and radiographic facilities. Circulation. 68:893A-930A; 1983.

21. Health and Public Policy Committee, American College of Physicians. The safety and efficacy of ambulatory cardiac catheterization in the hospital and free standing setting. Ann. Intern. Med. 103:294-298; 1985.

22. Kennedy, J.W. Symposium on catheterization complications associated with cardiac catheterization and angiography. Cathet. Cardiovasc. Diagon. 8:5-11; 1982.

23. Johnson, L.W.; Lozner, E.C.; Johnson, S.; Krene, R.; Pichard, A.D.; Vetrovec, G.W.; Noto, T.J.; Registry Committee of the Society for Cardiac Angiography and Interventions. Coronary arteriography 1984-1987. Cathet. Cardiovasc. Diagn. 17:5-10; 1989.

24. Ambrose, J.A. Unsettled indications for coronary angiography. J. Am. Coll. Cardiol. 3:1575-1580; 1984.

25. Adams, D.F.; Fraser, D.B.; Abrams, A.L. The complications of coronary arteriography. Circulation. 48:609-618; 1973.

26. Davis, K.; Kennedy, J.W.; Kemp, H.G., Jr.; Judkins, M.P.; Gosselin, A.J. Complications of coronary arteriography from the collaborative study of coronary artery surgery (CASS). Circulation. 59:1105-1112; 1979.

27. Cabin, H.S.; Roberts, W.C. Fatal cardiac arrest during cardiac catheterization for angina pectoris: Analysis of 10 necropsy patients. Am. J. Cardiol. 48:1-8; 1981.

28. Drost, H.; Buis, B.; Haan, D.; Hillers, J.A. Cholesterol embolism as a complication of left heart catheterization. Br. Heart J. 52:339-343; 1984.

29. Parfrey, P.S.; Griffiths, S.M.; Barrett, B.J.; et al. Contrast material induced renal failure in patients with diabetes mellitus, renal insufficiency, or both. N. Engl. J. Med. 320:143-149; 1989.

30. Talierco, C.P.; Vlietstra, R.E.; Fisher, L.D.; Barnett, J.C. Risks for renal dysfunction with cardiac angiography. Ann. Intern. Med. 104:501-504; 1986.

31. AHA Standards Committee. 1985 national conference on standards and guidelines for cardiopulmonary resuscitation and emergency cardiac care. JAMA. 255:2843-2989; 1986.

32. AHA Committee. Textbook of advanced cardiac life support. American Heart Association; 1987.

33. ACC/AHA Task Force Report. Guidelines for percutaneous transluminal coronary angioplasty. J. Am. Coll. Cardiol. 22:2033-2054; 1993.

34. Waller, B.F. "Crackers, breakers, stretchers, drillers, scrapers, shavers, burners, selders, and melters"—the future treatment of atherosclerotic coronary artery disease? A clinical-morphologic assessment. J. Am. Coll. Cardiol. 13:969-987; 1989.

35. Nath, P.H.; Velasquez, G.; Castaneda-Zuniga, W.R.; Zollikofer, C.; Formanek, A.; Amplatz, K. An essential view in coronary arteriography. Circulation. 60:101-106; 1979.

36. Isner, J.M.; Kishel, J.; Kent, K.M.; Ronan, J.A., Jr.; Ross, A.M.; Roberts, W.C. Accuracy of angiographic determination of left main coronary arterial narrowing. Circulation. 63:1056-1064; 1981.

37. Elliott, L.P.; Bream, P.R.; Soto, B.; Russell, R.O., Jr.; Rogers, W.J.; Mantle, J.A.; Hood, W.P., Jr. Significance of the caudal left-anterior oblique view in analyzing the left main coronary artery and its major branches. Radiology. 139:39-43; 1981.

38. Arani, D.T.; Bunnell, I.L.; Greene, D.G. Lordotic right posterior oblique projection of the left coronary artery. Circulation. 52:504-508; 1975.

39. Sus, T.A.; Lee, J.G.; Levin, D.C.; Baltane, H.A. New Lordotic projection for improved visualization of the left coronary artery and its branches. Am. J. Roentgen. 121:575-582; 1974.

40. Bunnell, I.L.; Greene, D.G.; Tandon, R.N.; Arani, D.T. The half-axial projection a new look at the proximal left coronary artery. Circulation. 48:1151-1156; 1973.

41. Eldh, P.; Silverman, J.F. Methods of studying the proximal left anterior descending coronary artery. Radiology. 113:738-740; 1974.

42. Miller, R.A.; Warkentin, D.L.; Felix, W.G.; Hashenian, M.; Leighton, R.F. Angulated views in coronary angiography. Am. J. Radiol. 134:407-412; 1980.

43. Frederick, P.R.; Fry, W.A.; Russell, J.G.; Marshall, H.W. Longitudinal angulation in coronary arteriography. Cathet. and Cardiovasc. Diag. 3:305-311; 1977.

44. Sos, T.A.; Galtaxe, H.A. Cranial and caudal angulation for coronary angiography revisited. Circulation. 56:119-123; 1977.

45. Elliott, L.P.; Green, C.E.; Rogers, W.J.; Mantle. J.A.; Papapietro, S.E.; Hood, W.P., Jr.; Russell, R.O., Jr. Advantage of the cranial right anterior oblique view in diagnosing mid left anterior descending and distal right coronary artery disease. Am. J. Cardiol. 48:754-764; 1981.

46. Taylor, K.W.; McLoughlin, M.J.; Aldridge, H.E. Specification of angulated projections in coronary arteriography. Cathet. and Cardiovasc. Diag. 3:367-374; 1977.

47. Lesperance, J.; Saltiel, J.; Petitclerc, R.; Bourassa, M.G. Angulated views in the sagittal plane for improved accuracy of cinecoronary angiography. Am. J. Roentgen. Published by American Roentgen Ray Society 1891, Preston White Dr., Reston, VA 22091.

48. Aldridge, H.E.; McLoughlin, M.J.; Taylor, K.W. Improved diagnosis in coronary cinearteriography with routine use of 110° oblique views and cranial and caudal angulations. Am. J. Cardiol. 36:468-473; 1975.

49. Aldridge, H.E. Better visualization of the asymmetric lesion in coronary arteriography utilizing cranial and caudal angulated projections. Chest. 71:502-507; 1977.

50. Gomes, A.S.; Esposito, V.A.; Grollman, J.H., Jr.; O'Reilly, R.J. Angled views in the evaluation of the right coronary artery. Cathet. and Cardiovasc. Diag. 8:71-82; 1982.

51. Levin, D.C.; Fellows, K.E.; Abrams, H.L. Hemodynamically significant primary anomalies of the coronary arteries. Circulation. 58:25-34; 1978.

52. Click, R.L.; Holmes, D.R., Jr.; Vlietstra, R.E.; Kosinski, A.J.; Kronmal, R.A., and participants of CASS. Anomalous coronary arteries: Location, degree of atherosclerosis and effect on survival. J. Am. Coll. Cardiol. 13:531-537; 1989.

53. Liberthson, R.R.; Dinsmore, R.E.; Fallon, J.T. Aberrant coronary artery origin from the aorta. Circulation. 59:748-754; 1979.

54. Koops, B.; Kerber, R.E.; Wexler, L.; Greene, R.A. Congenital coronary artery anomalies. JAMA. 226:1425-1429; 1973.

55. Roberts, W.C.; Siegel, R.J.; Zipes, D.P. Origin of the right coronary artery from the left sinus of valsalva and its functional consequences: Analysis of 10 necropsy patients. Am. J. Cardiol. 49:863-868; 1982.

56. Barth, C.W. III; Roberts, W.C. Left main coronary artery originating from the right sinus of valsalva and coursing between the aorta and pulmonary trunk. J. Am. Coll. Cardiol. 7:366-373; 1986.

57. Swaye, P.S.; Fisher, L.D.; Litwin, P.; et al. Aneurysmal coronary artery disease. Circulation. 67:134-138; 1983.

58. Robinson, F.C. Aneurysms of the coronary arteries. Am. Heart J. 109:129-134; 1985.

59. Markis, J.E.; Joffee, C.D.; Cohn, P.F. Clinical significances of coronary artery ectasia. Am. J. Cardiol. 37:217-222; 1976.

60. Dawd, A.S.; Rankin, D.; Tulgan, H.; Florentin, R.A. Aneurysms of the coronary artery. Am. J. Cardiol. 11:228-237; 1963.

61. Aintablian, A.; Hmby, R.I.; Hoffman, I.; Kramer, R.J. Coronary ectasia: Incidence and results of coronary bypass surgery. Am. Heart J. 96:309-315; 1978.

62. Befeler, B.; Arando, J.M.; Embi, A. Coronary artery aneurysms. Am. J. Med. 672:597-607; 1977.

63. Wilson, C.S.; Werner, W.F.; Forker, A.D. Bilateral arteriosclerotic coronary arterial aneurysms successfully treated with saphenous vein bypass grafting. Am. J. Cardiol. 35:315-318; 1975.

64. Mattern. Congenital coronary aneurysms with angina pectoris and myocardial infarction treated with saphenous vein bypass graft. Am. J. Cardiol. 30:906-909; 1972.

Chapter 7

Medical Versus Surgical Management of the Cardiac Patient

Donald A. Weiner

Most patients who have stable angina pectoris or who are asymptomatic following a myocardial infarction (MI) can be managed without coronary artery bypass graft (CABG) surgery. Selective antianginal agents and vigilant coronary risk factor reduction have extended the time period during which patients with coronary artery disease (CAD) can be managed medically.

The major indicator for revascularization with CABG surgery is the presence of disabling anginal symptoms, despite adequate antianginal treatment, in patients in whom coronary angioplasty is not indicated or cannot be successfully accomplished (1). Other subgroups of patients with CAD, that is, those who have certain characteristics associated with poorer outcomes, may also live longer if CABG is performed (2,3). My review focuses on the studies that have evaluated the risk stratification of patients with CAD (4) and looks at the major controlled trials that have compared medical and surgical therapy.

The Natural History of Coronary Artery Disease

We can best evaluate the role of CABG surgery among patients with CAD by reviewing studies that evaluate the natural history of CAD (5). These studies involve the long-term follow-up of medically treated patients either with a clinical diagnosis of angina but without coronary angiographic confirmation of disease (6-10) or with anatomically defined CAD (11-14). These natural-history studies, performed 8 to 30 years ago, revealed a 4% overall average annual mortality rate among patients with CAD, but this varied between 2% and 15% according to the number of diseased coronary vessels and left ventricular function (LVF) (6-14).

More recently, three major multicenter clinical trials of CABG surgery have shown improved survival of medically treated patients with CAD. The Veterans Administration Cooperative Study (15), the European Coronary Surgery Study (16), and the Coronary Artery Surgery Study (17) revealed that the annual mortality rate of the medically assigned patients were 3.9%, 2.8%, and 2.1%, respectively, 11, 12, and 10 years later. Various factors, including more vigorous antianginal therapy and exclusion of certain high-risk patients, have contributed to the improved survival rate. Nevertheless, the annual medical mortality rate of about 2% in the Coronary Artery Surgery Study population, which was randomized to medical therapy, can realistically be applied to patients without left main coronary stenosis, disabling angina, or severe congestive heart failure (CHF) (5).

Means of Risk Stratification

Three general (and non–mutually exclusive) means of risk stratification—clinical factors, exercise testing, and radionuclide testing—will be examined.

Risk Stratification by Clinical Factors

Early studies evaluating clinical characteristics associated with poorer outcomes identified age, gender, prior MI, baseline electrocardiographic (ECG) abnormalities, and heart failure as predictive variables (4). Different results were found by more recent studies using statistical techniques designed to identify clinical characteristics that contain independent prognostic information:

Duke University, large population study (18)
These clinical or ECG variables independently predicted survival:

- History of peripheral vascular disease (PVD)
- Class IV heart failure
- Premature ventricular contractions (PVCs) on the resting ECG
- Nonspecific interventricular conduction defects
- Progressive chest pain
- Nocturnal chest pain
- Left bundle branch block

Duke University study (19)

Higher anginal scores, among the following group of patients, indicated greater likelihood for adverse outcome:

- Frequent daily angina
- Unstable or variant angina
- Progressive angina with nocturnal episodes
- Ischemic ST-T abnormalities on the resting 12-lead ECG

Coronary Artery Surgery Study (20)

These clinical factors best predicted cardiac mortality:

- Cardiac enlargement
- Prior MI
- CHF score

Patients with no or minimal heart failure had a 4-year survival rate of 90%; those with moderate heart failure, 62%; those with severe heart failure, 18%.

Seattle Heart Watch (21)

These were independent predictors of survival:

- Functional state of left ventricle (most important predictor)
- Cardiac enlargement
- Use of diuretics
- S3 gallop
- CHF

The following summaries appear to be the best clinical predictors of outcome among patients with angina pectoris:

Clinical variables

- Presence and severity of CHF
- Severity of angina
- Prior MI
- Other atherosclerotic disease

ECG

- Left bundle branch block
- Ischemic ST-segment and T-wave abnormalities
- Left ventricular hypertrophy (LVH)

Echocardiography or radionuclide angiography (RNA)

- Abnormal LVF

Risk Stratification by Exercise Testing

Risk stratification by exercise testing in patients with stable angina pectoris is useful for predicting prognosis and for identifying patients who might have an improved survival following CABG surgery (4).

Exercise Testing in Predicting Prognosis

Results of several large studies that have used exercise testing in this way are summarized in Table 7.1 and listed in more detail here:

Seattle Heart Watch (21,22)

a. High-risk group had left ventricular dysfunction (LVD) manifested by at least two of the following three criteria:
   - Cardiomegaly
   - Ability to exercise less than 3 min on the Bruce protocol
   - Peak systolic blood pressure (SBP) of less than 130 mm Hg during exercise testing
   Annual mortality rate was 5.6%.

Table 7.1 Studies Evaluating the Prognostic Significance of Exercise Testing

Study	n	Follow up (years)	Annual mortality rate (%)		
			High-risk	Moderate-risk	Low-risk
Seattle Heart Watch (22)	2,001	4.1	5.6	2.2	1.2
Duke University Database (23)	1,472	4	10.0	—	2.0
Coronary Artery Surgery Study (20)	5,303	5	5.3	2.0	0.8
Duke University (24)	2,842	5	5.6	1.8	0.6

Note. From Weiner, 1991 (4). Reprinted with permission.

b. Low-risk group had none of the above criteria and a mortality rate of 1.2%.
c. Intermediate-risk group had exertional myocardial ischemia alone and an annual mortality rate of 2.2%.

Conclusion: Patients with preserved ventricular function and exercise tolerance, even with ischemia, have a good prognosis with medial therapy.

Duke University (23)

a. High-risk group had a positive result in Stage I or II of the Bruce protocol, with a 12-month survival rate of 85%, a 48-month survival rate of 63%, and an average annual mortality rate of 10%.
b. Low-risk group exhibited the following in any combination:

  • Negative result on the exercise test
  • Exercise duration greater than or equal to Stage IV of the Bruce protocol
  • Maximal heart rate (HRmax) ≥ 160 beats/min

The 12-month survival rate was 99%; the 48-month survival rate, 93%; and the average annual mortality rate, 2%.

Conclusion: Presence of ischemia at an early workload is associated with a poorer outcome.

Coronary Artery Surgery Study (20)

a. The high-risk group exhibited

  • relatively significant ischemia (≥ 1-mm ST depression) and
  • extremely limited exercise tolerance (ability to reach, at most, Stage 1 of the standard Bruce protocol).

  Annual mortality rate exceeded 5%.
b. The low-risk group exhibited

  • no ischemia (< 1-mm ST-depression) and
  • moderate exercise tolerance (ability to reach Stage 3 or greater of the Bruce protocol).

  Annual mortality rate was less than 1%.
c. The intermediate risk group exhibited

  • relatively significant ischemia (≥ 1-mm ST depression) and
  • moderate exercise tolerance (ability to reach Stage 3 or greater of the Bruce protocol).

  Annual mortality rate was 2%.

Conclusion: Patients with ischemia and poor exercise tolerance constitute a high-risk group.

A later study at Duke University (24) looked at the prognostic value of treadmill exercise testing in patients who complained of chest pain. A score based on total exercise duration, ST-segment deviation during testing, and a treadmill angina index yielded 5-year survival rates ranging from 72% to 97%. This score added independent prognostic information to that provided by clinical data, coronary anatomy, and LVF. Subset analysis revealed that among patients with triple-vessel CAD, patients with an abnormal exercise score had a 5-year survival rate of 67% compared with 93% for those with a more normal exercise score.

The following summarizes the exercise test variables that, either alone or in combination, have been associated with increased risk of an adverse outcome in patients with angina pectoris:

  • Poor exercise capacity (< 5 METs [metabolic equivalents])
  • ≥ 2 mm ischemic ST depression at a low workload (≤ Stage 2 of Bruce protocol or heart rate [HR] ≤ 130 beats/min)
  • Early onset (Stage 1) or prolonged duration (> 5 min) of ST depression
  • Multiple leads (≥ 5) with ST depression
  • ST-segment elevation
  • Abnormally low peak SBP (< 130 mm Hg) or a fall in the SBP during exercise
  • Inability to attain the target HR (off medications)
  • Exercise-induced angina
  • Ventricular couplets or tachycardia at a low workload
  • ST/HR slope ≥ 6 $\mu V \cdot beat^{-1} \cdot min^{-1}$

Exercise Testing in Predicting Improved Post-Revascularization Survival

An improved survival following CABG surgery has been shown in patients with abnormal exercise test results in four studies (23-27) (Table 7.2). It will be noted that in the Seattle Heart Watch Study (22), surgical versus medical survival rates were virtually the same when the original condition was only exertional myocardial ischemia. Similarly, in the Coronary Artery Surgery Study (26), survival was not different between surgical and medical therapy among patients without ischemic ST depression who could exercise into Stage 3 or greater. When broken down by disease type, however, a significant difference in survival among patients with early positive exercise test results was found in the subset with triple-vessel CAD, in whom the 7-year survival was 81% for the surgical group and 58% for the medical group.

Table 7.2   Studies Evaluating Survival Rates Following Surgical and Medical Intervention

Study or researcher	Symptoms indicating need for intervention	No. years at which survival rate was measured	Survival rate (%) with:	
			CABG surgery	Medical intervention
Seattle Heart Watch (22)	At least two from among • cardiomegaly • < Stage 1 in Bruce protocol • systolic blood pressure < 130 mm Hg	5	94	67
	Exertional myocardial ischemia	5	92	91
Varnauskas et al. (16)	≥ 1.5-mm ST-segment depression	10	75	62
European Coronary Surgery Study (25)	At least two from among • ≥ 2-mm ST-segment depression • premature ventricular contractions during exercise • peak heart rate ≥ 140 at a low exercise level	11	67	31
Coronary Artery Surgery Study (26)	≥ 1-mm segment depression ≤ Stage 1 in Bruce protocol (see also Figure 7.1)	7	82	72
	Nonischemic ST depression ≥ Stage 3 in Bruce protocol Breakdown of these patients by disease type (see also Figure 7.2):	7		
	—Single-vessel CAD		83	79
	—Double-vessel CAD		80	74
	—Triple-vessel CAD		81	58

Note. CABG = coronary artery bypass graft; CAD = coronary artery disease. From Weiner, 1991 (4). Reprinted with permission.

Risk Stratification by Exercise Radionuclide Testing

For patients whose coronary risk is not adequately defined by exercise testing, other noninvasive tests have been used to predict outcome. These would include exercise imaging studies such as exercise thallium testing and exercise radionuclide ventriculography.

Thallium-201 Imaging

Various exercise thallium-201 parameters have been associated with a greater chance of an adverse outcome among patients with chest pain. When these abnormal parameters are combined with an abnormal clinical profile or exercise test response, the prediction of risk is even better (4). At least two parameters have proven useful. One is the presence and extent of thallium defects and their reversibility which have been found to be an excellent predictor of outcome. The ratio of lung to heart thallium uptake is another potent predictor of risk (Table 7.3). Transient ischemic left ventricular dilatation immediately after exercise also has been found to be helpful in identifying patients with multivessel CAD even in the absence of multiple reversible thallium defects. In one study this parameter had a sensitivity of 60% and a specificity of 95% for identifying patients with multivessel critical coronary stenoses (32).

In summary, the following variables relative to thallium-201 imaging have important prognostic significance:

- Multiple severe initial thallium defects
- Multiple areas showing thallium redistribution
- Increased lung-heart thallium uptake ratio
- Transient ischemic left ventricular dilatation

Table 7.3   Predictive Value of Thallium-201 Testing

Researchers	Findings
Thallium defects and their reversibility	
Staniloff et al. (27)	Annual event rate of patients with • normal thallium exercise test was 0.1%; • multiple thallium defects on initial scan was 16%; • severe initial thallium defects was 21%.
Brown et al. (28)	Number of myocardial segments showing thallium redistribution was the only significant predictor of future events among 100 patients without prior MI (patients followed 3-5 years).
Kaul et al. (29)	Event-free survival at 5 years for patients • without thallium distribution was 82%; • with thallium distribution was 60%.
Ladenheim et al. (30)	Extent and severity of thallium defects were exponentially correlated with outcome. Event rate for patients who • were able to exercise adequately without developing thallium hypoperfusion was 0.4%; • developed severe and extensive hypoperfusion at a low heart rate was 78%.
Ratio of lung to heart thallium uptake	
Kaul et al. (29)	Lung-heart ratio is the most important predictor of cardiac events among patients followed for 5 years. Increased thallium-201 lung uptake is thought to indicate the presence of left ventricular dysfunction usually resulting from severe ischemia.
Gill et al. (31)	Lung-heart ratio is the most important predictor of outcome among patients followed for 5 years, at which time the cardiac event rate for patients with • normal thallium scan was 5%; • abnormal thallium scan but normal thallium activity in lungs was 25%; • increased thallium uptake by the lungs was 67%.

Exercise Radionuclide Angiography

RNA at rest and during exercise can evaluate both regional and global LVF and thus help estimate the extent of reversibly ischemic and irreversibly scarred myocardium, both of which determine prognosis (33). In three independent studies, both the peak left ventricular ejection fraction (LVEF) and the change in the LVEF from rest to exercise were correlated with future coronary events (34-36). Using a multivariate discriminant analysis of 42 clinical and exercise test variables, Gibbons et al. (37) found that four independent variables were able to predict left main or triple-vessel CAD: magnitude of exercise ST-segment depression, exercise LVEF, peak rate–pressure product (RPP), and patient's gender. Thus, exercise RNA also can help risk stratify patients with CAD.

Medical Versus Surgical Therapy

Although the majority of patients undergoing CABG surgery have disabling angina, some patients with milder symptoms may have increased survival following revascularization. Three major multicenter randomized trials (15-17) compared the outcome after CABG surgery with that after medical therapy (Table 7.4). All three trials randomized patients who had chronic stable angina or who were asymptomatic at least 2 months after an MI. The trials were designed to exclude elderly patients (over the age of 67), as well as patients with disabling or unstable angina, recent MI (< 2 months), severe left ventricular impairment, and prior CABG surgery. Thus, the results could not be considered applicable to a great segment of the population with CAD. Although none of the studies showed an overall survival advantage of one or the other treatment at the time of

Table 7.4   Surgical Versus Medical Survival Rates (%) in Three Major Controlled Trials

	VACT (15) (11 years)	ECSS (16) (12 years)	CASS (17) (10 years)
Overall			
Medicine	57	67	79
Surgery	58	71	82
Single-vessel CAD			
Medicine	65	—	82
Surgery	70	—	85
Double-vessel CAD			
Medicine	69	71	79
Surgery	55	67	83
Triple-vessel CAD			
Medicine	50	66	75
Surgery	56	74	76

Note. VACT = Veterans Administration Cooperative Trial; ECSS = European Cooperative Surgical Study; CASS = Coronary Artery Surgery Study; CAD = coronary artery disease.

the last follow up, the results did indicate certain subgroups of patients who showed a survival advantage after CABG surgery:

Veterans Administration Cooperative Study (15)

- Left main CAD (survival at 5 years)
- Triple-vessel CAD and impaired LVF (survival at 7 years)
- Patients with two of the following (survival at 7 years):

    Resting ST depression on ECG
    History of MI
    History of hypertension

Note: The benefits of surgery started to diminish at 7 years, possibly due to saphenous vein graft occlusion.

European Coronary Surgery Study (16)

- Triple-vessel CAD, especially with proximal left anterior descending artery stenosis
- Double-vessel CAD with only proximal left anterior descending artery disease
- Age over 53 years
- Abnormal baseline ECG
- Markedly positive exercise test
- Peripheral arterial disease

Coronary Artery Surgery Study (17)

- Triple-vessel CAD and a resting LVEF between 0.35 and 0.50

The three trials all showed that CABG surgery did not reduce the rate of subsequent MI compared with medical therapy (1). However, the patients randomly assigned to surgery had greater improvement of symptoms and more enhanced exercise tolerance than the medically treated patients.

Conclusions Regarding Revascularization

The indications for revascularization with CABG surgery in an individual patient depend on many factors, including symptoms and functional limitation, age, gender, coronary anatomy, LVF, objective evidence of ischemia, and other medical conditions (38). The survival benefit for surgical treatment is greatest for patients whose mortality risk is highest if medical therapy alone were undertaken (3). The following characteristics favor one form of therapy or the other:

Medical intervention

- Single- or double-vessel CAD without proximal left anterior descending artery stenosis
- LVEF > 0.50
- No history of CHF
- Normal baseline ECG
- Negative exercise test at Stage 3 of Bruce protocol or equivalent

Surgical intervention

- Left main CAD
- Triple-vessel CAD ($\geq$ 70% stenosis)
- Double-vessel CAD including proximal left anterior descending artery stenosis
- LVEF < 0.50
- History of CHF or MI
- Abnormal baseline ECG
- Early positive exercise test

The primary indication for CABG surgery is to relieve symptoms in patients with severe angina in whom an adequate antianginal treatment plan is either ineffective or not well tolerated and in whom coronary angioplasty cannot be performed (39). Similarly, CABG surgery is recommended for patients with unstable angina whose symptoms cannot be easily controlled with medications. In both cases, cardiac catheterization would be performed to determine the feasibility of surgery.

For patients with mild angina whose symptoms are controlled with medications or who are asymptomatic following an MI, the initial work-up should include an exercise test to estimate the extent of CAD and the degree of functional limitation, and a resting echocardiogram or RNA to measure LVF, especially for patients with prior MI. Patients who demonstrate substantial ST-segment depression at an early work load have an overall annual mortality rate ranging from 5.3% to 10% and thus constitute a higher-risk subset (5). The mortality rate is even higher if the patient has LVD. Cardiac catheterization would be recommended in this subset of patients, and CABG surgery would be indicated if left main or triple-vessel CAD is found. For patients with double-vessel CAD in whom coronary angioplasty is not feasible, CABG surgery likely would be indicated if any two of the following are present: significant proximal left anterior descending artery disease, substantially abnormal exercise test results, and LVD.

For the mildly symptomatic patient who has borderline abnormal or equivocal exercise test results, risk stratification using exercise thallium testing or RNA would be indicated. If the exercise nuclear tests demonstrated substantial abnormalities, cardiac catheterization would be indicated, and the guidelines for CABG surgery mentioned in the previous paragraph would be followed.

For the mildly symptomatic or asymptomatic patient who has normal LVF and the absence of ischemic ST depression at a high work load (Stage 3 of the Bruce protocol or equivalent), the prognosis is excellent with medical therapy. These patients should receive specific instructions regarding risk factor reduction, but cardiac catheterization would not ordinarily be indicated unless increasing anginal symptoms occur (40).

Summary

The objectives of performing CABG surgery on patients with angina are to relieve symptoms and to prolong survival. Risk stratification of patients with mild angina is important because the survival benefit for CABG surgery is greatest for patients who are at high risk on medical therapy alone. This assessment usually begins with the clinical history, physical examination, and resting and exercise ECGs. In selected patients, an exercise radionuclide test or cardiac catheterization may help further stratify the risk and identify which patients are candidates for CABG surgery.

References

1. Killip, T.K.; Ryan, T.J. Randomized trials in coronary bypass surgery. Circulation. 71:418-421; 1985.
2. Bolli, R. Bypass surgery in patients with coronary artery disease. Indications based on the multicenter randomized trials. Chest. 91:760-764; 1987.
3. Nwasokwa, O.N.; Koss, J.H.; Friedman, G.H.; Grunwald, A.M.; Bodenheimer, M.M. Bypass surgery for chronic stable angina: Predictors of survival benefit and strategy for patient selection. Ann. Intern. Med. 114:1035-1049; 1991.
4. Weiner, D.A. Risk stratification in angina pectoris. In: Abrams, J., ed. Cardiology clinics. Angina pectoris: Mechanisms, diagnosis, and therapy. Philadelphia: Saunders; 1991:39-47.
5. Deering, T.F.; Weiner, D.A. Prognosis of patients with coronary artery disease. J. Cardiopulm. Rehab. 5:325-331; 1985.
6. Block, W.; Crumpacker, E.; Day, T.; Gage, R. Prognosis of angina pectoris: Observations in 6,882 cases. JAMA. 150:239-264; 1952.
7. Richards, D.W.; Bland, E.F.; White, P.D. A completed twenty-five year follow-up study of 456 patients with angina pectoris. J. Chronic Dis. 4:423-433; 1956.
8. Frank, C.W.; Weinblatt, E.; Shapiro, S. Angina pectoris in men: Prognostic significance of selected medical factors. Circulation. 47:509-517; 1973.
9. Graham, I.; Mulcahy, R.; Hickey, N.; O'Neill, W.; Daly, L. Natural history of coronary heart disease: A study of 586 men surviving an initial acute attack. Am. Heart J. 105:249-257; 1983.
10. Kannel, W.B.; Feinleib, M. Natural history of angina pectoris in the Framingham study: Prognosis and survival. Am. J. Cardiol. 29:154-163; 1972.
11. Moberg, C.H.; Webster, J.S.; Sones, F.M., Jr. Natural history of severe proximal coronary artery disease as defined by cineangiography (200 patients, 7 year follow-up). Am. J. Cardiol. 29:282; 1972.
12. Oberman, A.; Jones, W.B.; Riley, C.P.; Reeves, T.J.; Sheffield, L.T.; Turner, M.E. Natural history of coronary artery disease. Bull. NY Acad. Med. 48:1109-1125; 1972.
13. Burggraff, G.W.; Parker, J.O. Prognosis in coronary artery disease: Angiographic, hemodynamic, and clinical factors. Circulation. 51:146-156; 1975.
14. Proudfit, W.L.; Bruschke, A.V.G.; Sones, F.M., Jr. Natural history of obstructive coronary artery disease: Ten-year study of 601 nonsurgical cases. Prog. Cardiovasc. Dis. 21:53-78; 1978.
15. The Veterans Administration Coronary Artery Bypass Surgery Study Group. Eleven-year survival in the Veterans Administration randomized trial of coronary bypass surgery for stable angina. N. Engl. J. Med. 311:1333-1339; 1984.
16. Varnauskas, E.; the European Coronary Surgery Study Group. Twelve-year follow-up of survival in the randomized European coronary surgery study. N. Engl. J. Med. 319:332-337; 1988.
17. Alderman, E.L.; Bourassa, M.G.; Cohen, L.S.; Davis, K.B.; Kaiser, G.G.; Killip, T.; Mock, M.B.; Pettinger, M.; Robertson, T.L. Ten-year follow-up of survival and myocardial infarction in the randomized coronary artery surgery study. Circulation. 82:1629-1646; 1990.
18. Harris, P.J.; Harrell, F.E., Jr.; Lee, K.L.; Behar, V.S.; Rosati, R.A. Survival in medically treated coronary artery disease. Circulation. 60:1259-1267; 1979.
19. Califf, R.M.; Mark, D.M.; Harrell, F.E., Jr.; Hlatky, M.A.; Lee, K.L.; Rosati, R.A.; Pryor, D.B. Importance of clinical measures of ischemia in the prognosis of patients with documented coronary artery disease. J. Am. Coll. Cardiol. 11:20-26; 1988.
20. Weiner, D.A.; Ryan, T.J.; McCabe, C.H.; Chaitman, B.R.; Sheffield, L.J.; Ferguson, J.C.; Fisher, L.D.; Tristani, F. Prognostic importance of a clinical profile and exercise test in medically treated patients with coronary artery disease. J. Am. Coll. Cardiol. 3:772-779; 1984.
21. Hammermeister, K.E.; DeRouen, T.A.; Dodge, H.T. Variables predictive of survival in patients with coronary disease: Selection by univariate and multivariate analyses from the clinical, electrocardiographic, exercise, arteriographic, and quantitative

angiographic evaluation. Circulation. 59:421-430; 1979.

22. Bruce, R.A.; DeRouen, T.A.; Hammermeister, K.E. Noninvasive screening for enhanced 4-year survival after aortocoronary bypass surgery. Circulation. 60:638-646; 1979.

23. McNeer, J.F.; Margolis, J.R.; Lee, K.L.; Kisslo, J.A.; Peter, R.H.; Kong, Y.; Behar, V.S.; Wallace, A.G.; McCants, C.B.; Rosati, R.A. The role of the exercise test in the evaluation of patients for ischemic heart disease. Circulation. 57:64-70; 1979.

24. Mark, D.B.; Hlatky, M.A.; Harrell, F.E., Jr.; Lee, K.L.; Califf, R.M.; Pryor, D.B. Exercise treadmill score for predicting prognosis in coronary artery disease. Ann. Intern. Med. 106:793-800; 1987.

25. Peduzzi, P.; Hultgren, H.; Thomsen, J.; Angell, W. Prognostic value of baseline exercise tests. Prog. Cardiovasc. Dis. 28:285-292; 1986.

26. Weiner, D.A.; Ryan, T.J.; McCabe, C.H.; Chaitman, B.R.; Sheffield, L.J.; Fisher, L.D.; Tristani, F. The role of exercise testing in identifying patients with improved survival after coronary artery bypass surgery. J. Am. Coll. Cardiol. 8:741-748; 1986.

27. Staniloff, H.M.; Forrester, J.S.; Berman, D.S.; Swan, H.J.C. Prediction of death, myocardial infarction, and worsening chest pain using thallium scintigraphy and exercise electrocardiography. J. Nucl. Med. 27:1842-1848; 1982.

28. Brown, K.A.; Boucher, C.A.; Okada, R.D.; Guiney, T.E.; Newell, J.B., Strauss, H.W. Pohost, G.M. Prognostic value of exercise thallium-201 imaging in patients presenting for evaluation of chest pain. J. Am. Coll. Cardiol. 1:994-1001; 1984.

29. Kaul, S.; Finkelstein, D.M.; Homma, S.; Leavitt, M.; Okada, R.D.; Boucher, C.A. Superiority of quantitative exercise thallium-201 variables in determining long-term prognosis in ambulatory patients with chest pain: A comparison with cardiac catheterization. J. Am. Coll. Cardiol. 12:25-34; 1988.

30. Ladenheim, M.L.; Pollock, B.H.; Rozanski, A.; Berman, D.S., Staniloff, H.M.; Forrester, J.S.; Diamond, G.A. Extent and severity of myocardial hypoperfusion as predictors of prognosis in patients with suspected coronary artery disease. J. Am. Coll. Cardiol. 7:464-471; 1986.

31. Gill, G.; Ruddy, T.D.; Newell, J.B.; Finkelstein, D.M.; Strauss, H.W.; Boucher, C.A. Prognostic importance of thallium uptake by the lungs during exercise in coronary artery disease. N. Engl. J. Med. 317:1485-1489; 1987.

32. Weiss, A.T.; Berman, D.S.; Lew, A.S.; Nielsen, J.; Potkin, B.; Swan, H.J.C.; Waxman, A.; Maddahi, J. Transient ischemic dilation of the left ventricle on stress thallium-201 scintigraphy: A marker of severe and extensive coronary artery disease. J. Am. Coll. Cardiol. 9:752-759; 1987.

33. Bonow, R.O. Prognostic implications of exercise radionuclide angiography in patients with coronary artery disease. Mayo Clin. Proc. 63:630-634; 1988.

34. Bonow, R.O.; Kent, K.M.; Rosing, D.R.; Lan, K.K.G.; Lakatos, E.; Borer, J.S.; Bacharach, S.L.; Green, M.V.; Epstein, S.E. Exercise-induced ischemia in mildly symptomatic patients with coronary artery disease and preserved left ventricular function: Identification of subgroups at risk of death during medical therapy. N. Engl. J. Med. 311:1339-1345; 1984.

35. Pryor, D.B.; Harrell, F.E., Jr.; Lee, K.L.; Rosati, R.A.; Coleman, R.E.; Cobb, F.R.; Califf, R.M.; Jones, R.H. Prognostic indicators from radionuclide angiography in medically treated patients with coronary artery disease. Am. J. Cardiol. 53:18-22; 1984.

36. Iskandrian, A.S.; Hakki, A.-H.; Goel, I.P. The use of rest and exercise radionuclide ventriculography in risk stratification in patients with suspected coronary disease. Am. Heart J. 110:864-872; 1985.

37. Gibbons, R.J.; Fyke, F.E.; Clements, I.P.; Lapegre, A.C.; Zinsmeister, A.R.; Brown, M.L. Noninvasive identification of severe coronary artery disease using radionuclide angiography. J. Am. Coll. Cardiol. 11: 28-34; 1988.

38. Kannel, W.B. Coronary artery surgery study revisited. Limitation of the intent-to-treat principle. Circulation. 82:1859-1862; 1990.

39. Kirklin, J.W.; Akins, C.W.; Blackstone, E.H.; Booth, D.C.; Califf, R.M.; Cohen, L.S.; Hall, R.J.; Harrell, F.E., Jr.; Kouchoukos, N.T.; McCallister, B.D.; Naftel, D.C.; Parker, J.O.; Sheldon, W.C.; Smith, H.C.; Wechsler, A.S.; Williams, J.F., Jr. ACC/AHA guidelines and indications for coronary artery bypass graft surgery. A report of the American College of Cardiology/American Heart Association task force on assessment of diagnostic and therapeutic cardiovascular procedures (subcommittee on coronary artery bypass graft surgery). Circulation. 83:1125-1173; 1991.

40. Weiner, D.A.; Kannel, W.B. A comparison of surgical and medical therapy for coronary artery disease. Cardiovasc. Review & Reports. 8:43-46; 1987.

PART III

Risk Factor Modification

Chapter 8

Scientific Rationale for Preventive Practices in Atherosclerotic and Hypertensive Cardiovascular Disease

Arthur S. Leon

This chapter will review the scientific rationale for targeting major risk factors as a strategy for the primary and secondary prevention of atherosclerotic and hypertensive cardiovascular disease (CVD). Although there has been a substantial reduction in the death rate attributed to CVD over the past 30 years, CVD remains the leading cause of premature death and disability in the United States and other economically developed, Westernized countries, with coronary artery disease (CAD) being the principal contributor (1). In addition, about half of all CAD victims are under 65 years of age (including 5% under age 40)—people usually at the height of their careers. Moreover, sudden death is the initial manifestation of CAD in 30% of new victims, and CAD contributes toward half of the secondary CVD events in myocardial infarction (MI) survivors.

Clinical manifestations of atherosclerosis of the cerebral arteries generally occur later in life than CAD manifestations. Most of the 500,000 strokes experienced by Americans each year are atherogenic in origin (1). The resulting mortality of about 150,000 deaths per year makes stroke the third-leading cause of death, behind only CAD and cancer. In addition, 28% of the 2 million stroke survivors in the United States are under 65 years of age.

The national economic impact of CVD in 1990—including medical, hospital, and convalescent care services; prescription medications; and lost productivity—was estimated at $94.5 billion (1), or about 15% of total U.S. health care expenditures. These facts and figures emphasize the need for continued research on the causes of CVD and for primary and secondary preventive strategies.

During the past 50 years, multiple research approaches have been applied to elucidate the pathophysiology of CVD. These approaches include systematic epidemiological observations of populations, clinical pathological studies, basic laboratory and animal research, and, more recently, controlled intervention trials. An explosion of knowledge of underlying etiologic mechanisms is the result.

As is true with most chronic diseases, atherosclerotic CVD has a multifactorial etiology. Both hereditary and environmental factors contribute to a host of underlying pathophysiological processes, including injury to endothelial linings of large and middle-sized arteries; interactions with blood-borne cells (monocytes, neutrophils, and platelets); artery smooth muscle migration and proliferation; lipid alterations, insudation, and deposition; plaque formation and subsequent damage with progressive obstruction of blood flow; hemostatic disturbances contributing to thrombosis; and factors increasing myocardial oxygen demands, predisposing to fatal arrhythmias (2). People generally remain asymptomatic during the early stages of atherosclerosis, and the functional effects of the full-blown disease process vary a great deal in clinical impact and severity.

Although we have much to learn about the etiology and pathogenesis of the underlying atherosclerotic process, multiple factors have been identified that appear to play causative roles. Furthermore, many of these factors are modifiable and serve as targets for preventive medical and public health strategies. In fact, it has been estimated that as much as 90% of symptomatic CAD in the United States is associated with modifiable risk factors (3). In addition, even when rigorous scientific proof of cause for some of the risk factors is absent, sufficient circumstantial evidence often suggests that intervention should substantially reduce the risk of CVD morbidity and mortality.

115

Atherosclerotic CVD, as indicated in chapter 1, does not strike people at random as they age. Susceptible individuals in a population can be identified in advance of clinical manifestations by the presence of risk factors that in longitudinal epidemiologic studies have been associated with a statistical increased probability of future CVD development. Approximately 300 possible risk factors for CAD have been identified (3). However, most of these factors represent secondary associations that are not causally related to CAD; that is, the factor in question and the disease are statistically associated because both are related to another factor, which is the causative one.

How to Distinguish Causative From Noncausative Associations

Before reviewing the individual risk factors, it is important to outline the "rules of evidence" that have evolved for establishing causality with associations identified by observational studies. These include the following (4):

1. **Time sequence.** Either the causative characteristic must precede the disease in time, or the change in the outcome is a consequence of a change in the factor in question.
2. **Strength of the association.** In general, the stronger an association is in its predictive power, the less likely that it is spurious and the more likely that it represents a cause-and-effect relationship. The strength of an association is usually expressed in terms of the relative risk: that is, the ratio of the disease rate in persons with the risk factor in question to the disease rate in those who do not possess this factor. If the suspected cause is a quantitative variable, the demonstration of a *dose-response linkage* strengthens the possibility of a causal relationship.
3. **Consistency among studies.** Finding the same association in observational studies from different populations—that is, its replicability and predictability—increases the possibility that the association is real and not an artifact based on study design; however, consistency does not guarantee a cause-and-effect relationship. The possibility of causality is further strengthened if the association from observational studies is confirmed by other research approaches, such as clinical pathological studies and laboratory experiments.

4. **Biological plausibility.** A plausible hypothesis compatible with available biological knowledge should exist between the factor in question and disease pathophysiology. The identification of an association, however, may initiate research efforts that may reveal new pathophysiological mechanisms for the disease.

Even if a risk factor meets all of these criteria, this still provides only circumstantial evidence of causation. The ultimate scientific proof requires controlled, randomized primary and secondary intervention trials in which the elimination or attenuation of the risk factor in question results in a statistically significant reduction in disease morbidity or mortality. Unfortunately, such trials require large cohorts of high-risk people and long-term management and follow-up, making them expensive and logistically difficult. Thus, this final step in proving causation has been obtained only for a small number of the multiple risk factors identified as probably causative for atherosclerotic CVD; namely, elevated blood total and low-density lipoprotein (LDL) cholesterol levels and hypertension. Nevertheless, there exists extremely strong evidence for many other risk factors, which is generally considered sufficient for the purposes of medical practice, public health action, and development of preventive clinical and community programs. The positive relationship of most of the risk factors discussed in this chapter to CVD are independent and additive or synergistic in their contributions to primary and secondary CVD morbidity and mortality.

Considering the available data and the considerations just noted, the following propositions provide the basis for current prevention strategies with CAD and other atherosclerotic complications (5):

1. Individuals, and indeed entire populations, vary immensely in their risk of atherosclerotic CVD.
2. The probability of severity of atherosclerosis and its clinical manifestations, particularly CAD and stroke, are strongly and consistently associated with levels of major risk factors.
3. Some of these risk factors are considered causal, even in the absence of definitive clinical trials, because of their strong predictive value, their strength and consistency, congruence of evidence by multiple research approaches, and plausible biological mechanisms for their potential roles in initiating

or promoting atherosclerosis, or in precipitating acute clinical events in the presence of atherosclerosis.

4. Most modifiable risk characteristics are behavioral or sociocultural in origin.

5. Risk factor identification, education, and modification, including altering associated risk behaviors, provide the rational basis for prevention of atherosclerotic manifestations.

Classification of Risk Factors

Conceptual models have been proposed as a means of classifying the plethora of risk factors statistically associated with CVD in epidemiologic studies (6,7). Risk indicators may be classified as follows:

Biological determinants or factors

- Aging
- Gender
- Menopause
- Circadian rhythms
- Genetic factors contributing to dyslipidemias, hypertension, glucose intolerance/diabetes mellitus, and obesity

Anatomical, physiological, and metabolic (biochemical) traits

- Dyslipidemias
- Hypertension
- Obesity and fat distribution
- Disorders of glucose-insulin dynamics
- Hematologic, rheologic, and blood-clotting factors
- Left ventricular hypertrophy (LVH)
- Physical fitness (aerobic power)

Behavioral factors

- Dietary habits
- Cigarette smoking
- Physical activity
- Alcohol consumption
- Coronary-prone behavior
- Oral contraceptive and noncontraceptive estrogen use
- Cocaine abuse

Note that there is some overlap among the categories. The probability of CAD and other CVD increases additively or synergistically with increasing number and magnitude of these risk factors.

In the remainder of this chapter we present evidence for the contributions to risk of CAD from biological risk factors and major modifiable physiological and metabolic risk factors, with discussion of relevant behavioral risk factors interspersed as appropriate. The association of a sedentary lifestyle and poor physical fitness to the risk of initial and recurrent CAD events is discussed in chapters 11 and 12; the relationship of psychological stress and so-called coronary-prone behavioral characteristics to CAD is discussed in chapter 3.

Biological Factors

The biological determinants of CAD—aging, gender differences, genetic factors, and circadian rhythms—are discussed in the sections that follow.

Aging

It is well documented that the atherosclerotic process is initiated during childhood in populations with a high incidence of atherosclerotic CVD (8). Cross-sectional postmortem studies confirm that the severity of atherosclerosis then progressively increases with age. Already by the age of 35, CAD is one of the 10 leading causes of death in the United States (6), and 1 man in 5 can expect to have a heart attack by age 60. Between 55 and 64 years of age, 10% of all deaths among men are due to CAD. The incidence of stroke is even more strongly related to advanced age. In fact, the incidence doubles for each successive decade after age 55; however, about 29% of people who develop a stroke in a given year are less than 65 years of age (1).

Evidence that aging is independently related to the risk of atherosclerotic CVD is the observation from prospective observational studies that risk increases with age even when other risk factors remain in the "normal" range (6). Nevertheless, it also is clear that much of the increased risk of CAD and stroke with aging is related to modifiable risk factors acting over time. For example, a 55-year-old man with a high composite level of risk factors for CAD has a 55% probability of developing clinical CAD in 6 years as compared with a probability of less than 4% for a similar-aged man with a low composite risk level (6). Evidence is also accumulating that modification of major risk factors at any age will reduce the probability of morbidity and mortality from initial or recurrent atherosclerotic

CVD events. There also is increasing attention being paid to risk factor modification during childhood to minimize the early development of atherosclerosis and to reduce the "tracking" of risk factors into adult life (8).

Gender, Menopause, Oral Contraceptive Use, and Estrogen Use

A gender gap favoring women clearly exists in the rate of the development of atherosclerosis and associated CVD events. In general, the severity of coronary atherosclerosis and the CAD rate for women lag behind the figures for men by 10 years for Caucasians and 7 years for African-Americans (9). However, CAD still accounts for one third of all deaths in American women, and CVD is the predominant cause of death in older women (10). In addition, while death from CAD remains relatively stable at 60% in men after 50 years of age, in women it continues to increase steadily with age. Furthermore, women are less likely than men to survive an initial or recurrent MI or coronary artery bypass graft surgery (CABG surgery). It is now strongly suspected that this may be related to a sex bias by physicians in managing women with CAD. Recent studies show that women hospitalized with suspected or diagnosed ischemic chest pain undergo fewer diagnostic and therapeutic procedures than men (11,12). Thus, women in general may have more advanced CAD than men by the time an adequate diagnosis is made and their symptoms are treated.

The same major risk factors are associated with an increased risk of CAD in both sexes. The gender gap in CAD rates that favors younger women appears to be at least partially explained by differences in risk-factor levels between men and women (10). For example, before 50 years of age (about the usual time of the natural menopause), the prevalence of hypertension is lower in women than in men; however, above this age the reverse is true. Younger women also generally have more favorable levels of blood lipids and lipoproteins than men. Plasma total and LDL cholesterol and triglyceride levels are generally lower in women than men until about age 50, after which the reverse gradually becomes true. Furthermore, antiatherogenic plasma high-density lipoprotein (HDL) cholesterol levels are generally significantly higher in women than in men without any age-related trends.

Although the proportion of cigarette smokers has increased among women in the United States and other industrialized countries, the cigarette-smoking rate in women traditionally has been lower than for men. In addition, recent data suggest that women who smoke newer brands of cigarettes with reduced yields of nicotine and carbon monoxide do not have a lower risk of initial MI than those who smoke higher yield brands (13).

The presence of diabetes mellitus eliminates the advantage that women under the age of 50 have over men in terms of lower rates of CVD. Use of oral contraceptives substantially increases the risk of CAD, as well as of nonhemorrhagic strokes and thrombophlebitis in women, particularly if their use is accompanied by cigarette smoking (10). This is especially true for women who use oral contraceptive preparations containing 50 mcg or more of estrogen. Proposed mechanisms for an excess risk of CAD among users of the pill include impaired glucose tolerance, hyperinsulinemia, increased plasma triglyceride and total cholesterol levels, and a variable effect on HDL cholesterol levels related to the relative content of estrogen and progesterone. In general, HDL cholesterol levels appear to be directly related to the estrogen content and inversely related to the progesterone content, with formulations that contain both steroids resulting in an intermediate level of HDL cholesterol (10,14).

On the other hand, most studies have shown that noncontraceptive estrogen replacement therapy prescribed after natural or surgical menopause either has no effect or reduces the risk of CAD and atherosclerotic vascular diseases as well as all-cause mortality (10,15,16). A much smaller dose of estrogen is generally employed as replacement therapy as compared with oral contraceptive use (i.e., 0.3 mg/day versus 0.625 mg/day of conjugated estrogen). However, a few studies, including the Framingham Study, report an increased risk of CVD or venous thromboembolism in women using replacement estrogens (10). A clinical trial with postmenopausal women that employs a design including assignment to estrogen alone or in combination with progestational agents versus placebo is required before physicians can routinely recommend replacement estrogen therapy for the prevention of atherosclerotic CVD in postmenopausal women. Safety considerations include the potential direct effect of estrogen on the risk of endometrial and breast cancer (17).

The consequences of menopause on the risk for CVD have been studied in both postsurgical and spontaneous menopausal women. An increased frequency of atherosclerotic CVD has been seen after both types of menopause in a majority of the studies (10). For example, in one study, the relative risk of nonfatal MI between women who had a bilateral oopherectomy at an early age was 2.9 as compared to menstruating women of similar age, with the highest risk found in women who were less than 35 years old at the time of the surgery (18). In the Framingham Study, no premenopausal women experienced a fatal or nonfatal MI during the first 24 years of follow-up, with uncomplicated angina pectoris being the most common CAD manifestation in women less than 54 years of age (10,19).

A worsening of the CAD risk profile with the transition from premenopausal to the menopausal status appears to contribute significantly to increased CVD rates (10). Women with a natural menopause are generally reported in observational studies as experiencing greater increases in plasma levels of LDL cholesterol and triglyceride levels and greater decreases in HDL cholesterol as compared with age-matched premenopausal control subjects (10,20). An associated increase in body weight appears to contribute substantially to the magnitude of changes in these CAD risk factors. This gives rise to the hope that preventing such weight gain would prevent or attenuate these potentially adverse changes in CAD risk factors and thereby reduce the risk of CVD (20).

Genetic Factors

The fact that CAD clinical events cluster in families is well documented. Individuals who have first-degree family members (i.e., parents or siblings) with symptomatic CAD have an increased risk of developing heart disease. The associated increase in relative risk is quite variable, but may be as much as five times higher compared with matched people with negative family histories (8). Excess risk is particularly high if a first-degree relative experienced a CAD event prior to 55 years of age. Inherited factors, as yet poorly understood, include those that contribute to dyslipidemias, hypertension, diabetes mellitus, obesity, and perhaps behavioral patterns (7,8).

Apart from sharing such genetic determinants, there are environmental and learned health risk behaviors that are concentrated in families (8). For example, families usually eat many meals from a common kitchen and share food preferences. Overeating and physical underactivity often make obesity a "family affair." Parents who smoke also tend to have children who smoke. Because of these environmental influences, many epidemiologists question whether a strong family history of CAD remains an independent risk factor of CAD when

statistical adjustments are made for other risk factors. However, data from the Framingham Study show that parental death from CAD remains an independent predictor of future CAD events for men, but not for women, when a multiple logistic analytical model is employed that includes age, gender, systolic blood pressure (SBP), serum total cholesterol, glucose intolerance, relative body weight, and other risk factors (7). The failure of family history to have a statistically significant independent effect on CAD events in women in the Framingham Study is believed to stem from the lower incidence of CAD events in women as compared with men—at least until women experience menopause.

Circadian Rhythms

Circadian rhythms affect many physiological functions of the body, including those of the neuroendocrine and cardiovascular systems (21). They result in substantial fluctuations throughout the 24-hour cycle in plasma concentrations of hormones that affect body temperature, blood volume, and cardiovascular performance; these hormones include catecholamines, renin-angiotensin-aldosterone, corticosteroids, and atrial naturetic hormone. Cardiovascular functions showing rhythmic changes include heart rate (HR), BP, stroke volume (SV), vascular smooth muscle tone (including that of the coronary arteries), blood flow, and capillary resistance. Rhythmic changes also occur in the viscosity, coagulability, and fibrinolytic activity of the blood.

Recent evidence from both observational and clinical research that these endogenous, cyclic, and temporal fluctuations in physiological functions influence profoundly the time of appearance of ischemic manifestations associated with CAD and cerebrovascular atherosclerotic disease (21-23). For example, the total ischemic burden of CAD appears to increase within the first few hours of awakening, generally between 6 a.m. and noon. This includes a peak incidence of angina pectoris, symptomatic or asymptomatic ischemic ECG changes during ambulatory monitoring, a lower HR threshold before myocardial ischemia during exercise testing, MI, and sudden cardiac death. Some studies also detected a secondary peak of such events in the evening hours. Cerebral infarction, presumably usually associated with thrombosis, also has been reported to be more frequent either in the early- or late-morning hours.

A number of well-characterized daily endogenous rhythms may contribute to the peak incidence of ischemic manifestations in the morning hours. Sympathetic nervous system activity rises during arousal from sleep as a result of a progressive increase in plasma catecholamine levels from 6 a.m. to noon. This is accompanied by a rise in HR, arterial pressure, and left ventricular contractility, and, thus, myocardial oxygen requirements; an excess of oxygen demand over supply can precipitate myocardial ischemia. Increased adrenergic activity may also be responsible for inducing coronary artery, as well as systemic, vasoconstriction (21-23).

Cyclic prothrombogenic factors may also contribute to the peak incidence of acute MI and atherothrombolic stroke in the morning hours (21). These include an elevated tendency for platelets to aggregate in the morning hours (to be expected during a period of peak levels of plasma catecholamines); in addition, there is an associated trough in the fibrinolytic activity of the blood.

It is interesting that beta-adrenergic blockade therapy appears to eliminate the significant morning peak in the onset of MI (21), which may help explain the well-documented reduction by beta-blockade therapy in the risk of fatal and nonfatal recurrent MIs after an initial MI. A blunting by beta-blocker drugs of the increased myocardial demand for oxygen and of other catecholamine-related changes that occur in the morning may be the protective mechanisms involved (21).

There also is evidence that circadian BP patterns in patients with essential hypertension contribute to the development of left ventricular hypertrophy (LVH), an important predictor of CVD morbidity and mortality to be discussed in more detail later in this chapter. Verdecchia et al. (24) found that increased left ventricular mass seen in echocardiography was more strongly related to nighttime systolic and diastolic BP levels than to daytime levels in hypertensive patients. Further, hypertensive patients whose systolic and diastolic BP levels declined during the night by more than 10% were less likely to develop LVH.

It is concluded that there is strong scientific evidence that biological factors, including male gender, a premature menopause, aging, and a positive family history of CAD, appear to be independent contributors to the risk of CAD and other atherosclerotic CVD. The presence of these biological risk factors should alert the clinician to a magnified need for screening and intervening on modifiable risk factors. The judicious use of low doses of estrogen in postmenopausal women needs to be further investigated for its possible role in CVD prevention. In addition, individuals identified as being at increased risk for CAD must be vigilant during the morning hours or the first few hours after awakening to minimize factors that can precipitate CAD events or a stroke. For example, they should avoid physical exertion and emotional confrontations and perhaps should be started on such drugs as beta-blockers, which improve the balance between myocardial oxygen demands and supply, or on such agents as aspirin, which reduce the risk of thrombosis.

Major Modifiable Risk Factors

The major modifiable physiological and metabolic (biochemical) risk factors for which there is strong evidence of a causative relationship with atherosclerotic CVD are dyslipidemias, elevated BP, obesity, and diabetes mellitus. Cigarette smoking is the most important of the behavioral risk factors for CAD. The three other major risk factors for CAD are serum total cholesterol, BP, and physical inactivity, the last mentioned recently upgraded to this status by the American Heart Association (AHA) (25). Dietary and physical activity habits contribute to the blood lipid-lipoprotein and BP levels and risk of diabetes mellitus. In addition, habitual physical activity and associated level of physical fitness appear to be independently, inversely related to the risk of CAD morbidity and mortality (6,26). There also is inconsistent evidence that the behavioral response to self-imposed or environmentally induced stress also contributes to the risk of CAD, but these latter factors are topics of other chapters. The evidence supporting the causative relationship and effect of intervention on the major modifiable risk factors for atherosclerotic CVD follows.

Relationship of Blood Lipid and Lipoprotein Levels and Associated Dietary Factors to Coronary Heart Disease

Blood lipid and lipoprotein levels and associated dietary factors related to coronary heart disease are discussed in sections that follow.

Blood Total and Low-Density Lipoprotein Cholesterol Levels and Risk of Coronary Artery Disease

Of all the potentially modifiable atherogenic traits, the evidence is strongest and the mechanisms are best understood for the contributions of blood total cholesterol and LDLs, which normally transport

60% to 70% of blood cholesterol. In addition, conclusive evidence is now available that a substantial reduction in the LDL cholesterol level can halt or even reverse the atherosclerotic process and thereby reduce the rate of initial or recurrent CVD events. While LDL or modified LDL appears to be the actual principal atherogenic culprit (2), total blood cholesterol, because of its close correlation with the concentration of LDL cholesterol, commonly serves as its surrogate in observational studies and is generally measured in place of LDL cholesterol, at least in the initial stages of evaluating a patient's blood lipid profile. Related predictors of CAD are the levels of small LDL particles (LDL-III) and the principal apolipoprotein component of LDL, apoB-100. Health experts agree that the severity of atherosclerosis and the risk of CAD increase with increased levels of plasma total and LDL cholesterol, and these are often associated with a high saturated fat–high cholesterol dietary pattern (27-29). This consensus is based on a strong chain of evidence and the congruence of results from a wide variety of research approaches, as outlined below.

Epidemiological Studies. A large body of observational epidemiological data from more than 20 major prospective studies in many countries supports the direct relationship between levels of blood total and LDL cholesterol and the rate of CAD events. These include pooled data from eight cohort studies involving initially healthy middle-aged men, comprising the United States National Cooperative Pooling Project (30); the Seven Countries Study, a long-term study involving 12,763 subjects in 16 cohorts in six western countries and Japan (31,32); a 7-year mortality follow-up of a cohort of 361,662 men screened for the Multiple Risk Factor Intervention Trial (33); a 10-year mortality follow-up of 2,541 men participating in the Lipid Research Clinics Prevalence Mortality Follow-up Study (34); and a 5-year follow-up of 4,916 men participating in the Physicians Health Study (35). In general, these prospective studies show that within populations the risk of CAD clinical events increases continuously throughout the range of blood cholesterol levels, and particularly for those whose total cholesterol level is above 200 mg/dL or whose LDL cholesterol level is above 130 mg/dL. The probability of CAD events over 6 years increases about 2% for each 1% increase in total cholesterol above 200 mg/dL. For persons in the top 10% of the population distribution of total cholesterol, the risk of CAD mortality is four to seven times as high as the risk in the bottom 10%

of the population. Among people with preexisting CVD, total and LDL cholesterol levels are even stronger predictors of CVD mortality when compared with those without preexisting CVD (34).

Comparisons among various populations throughout the world also reveal a strong relationship between serum total cholesterol level and population rate of CVD. This was best documented by the landmark Seven Countries Study, which also was the first large-scale study to demonstrate convincingly that diet is the principal contributor to population differences in serum cholesterol levels (31,32). The saturated fat and accompanying cholesterol intake was found to account for about 90% of the variability in mean serum cholesterol levels among the 16 study populations.

Migration Studies. Additional evidence that population differences in blood cholesterol levels and CAD rates are primarily related to dietary habits rather than genetic differences comes from migration studies. When groups of middle-aged men from countries with a low dietary intake of saturated fat and cholesterol, mean serum cholesterol levels less than 200 mg/dL, and low CAD rates emigrated to countries with high rates of CAD, they assumed blood cholesterol levels and rates of CAD similar to men in their adopted countries (29) as their dietary habits changed. This was most elegantly demonstrated in the Ni-Hon-San Study, in which thousands of men in Japan were compared with matched Japanese emigrants in Honolulu and San Francisco (36). Similar observations have been made in Jews who emigrated from Yemen to Israel, Italians from Naples to Boston, Polynesians from small Pacific islands to New Zealand, and Indians from Asia to South Africa.

Postmortem Studies. Additional confirmation of the blood cholesterol–CAD relationship comes from postmortem examination of arteries of people of all ages in many regions of the world (29,37,38). Such studies, and in particular the International Atherosclerosis Project, which involved autopsies on 31,000 individuals in 15 countries worldwide (37), documented a marked variability in the extent of atherosclerosis at autopsy in the coronary arteries, aortas, and other arteries among diverse populations. The extent and severity of atherosclerotic lesions were positively correlated with antemortem blood total cholesterol levels and other risk factors. The extent and severity of coronary atherosclerotic (CAD) lesions were also considerably greater in populations with a high intake of saturated fat and cholesterol as compared with populations in which intake of these dietary lipids was lower. Significant differences among populations in severity of CAD were generally already apparent in adolescents and young adults. Furthermore, the extent of atherosclerosis at autopsy paralleled the CAD mortality rates among populations. Similarly, within populations in different regions of the world a linear relationship has been observed between antemortem serum total and LDL cholesterol levels and the severity of postmortem coronary atherosclerosis (29). In addition, postmortem studies have demonstrated progressive reductions in atherosclerotic lesions in Europeans during severe war-related dietary deprivations, particularly in fat intake, presumably associated with reductions in blood total and LDL cholesterol levels (39). Reduced severity of atherosclerosis in these studies was associated with a substantial reduction in the CAD mortality rates.

Clinical and Genetic Associations.   Further proof of the blood cholesterol–CAD connection is the well-documented relationship between diseases causing secondary hypercholesterolemia (such as hypothyroidism and the nephrotic syndrome) and accelerated atherosclerosis. In addition, genetic dyslipidemias characterized by severe hypercholesterolemia, such as Type II hyperlipoproteinemia or familial hypercholesterolemia, are invariably associated with advanced atherosclerosis early in life and with premature CAD clinical manifestations. Familial hypercholesterolemia was demonstrated by Goldstein and Brown (40) to be caused by a defect in the genes that encode for the LDL-apoB receptor, which is responsible for removing LDL from the circulation and control of cell cholesterol synthesis. Approximately 1% of individuals at increased risk of CAD because of elevated blood cholesterol levels are believed to have some clearly definable genetic disorder (40).

Animal Research.   Counterparts of familial hypercholesterolemia have also been identified in rabbits and more recently in a rhesus monkey family (41). These animals mimic the human condition by having extremely high plasma concentrations of total and LDL cholesterol and accelerated atherosclerosis. Many other animal models of human atherosclerosis, employing a wide variety of animal species, including nonhuman primates, have been developed (42). Almost all the nongenetic animal models involve as their principal etiologic agent the induction of chronic hypercholesterolemia by a diet high in cholesterol and saturated fat. Severe coronary atherosclerosis so induced in monkeys regresses when the blood total and LDL cholesterol levels are substantially reduced by diet

or lipid-lowering drugs, confirming the reversibility of atherosclerosis. In addition to animal research, a considerable body of in vitro experiments have identified cellular and molecular mechanisms demonstrating how LDL is involved in atherogenesis (29).

Human Feeding Experiments.   Controlled isocaloric human feeding experiments, most of which were performed in the 1950s and 1960s, provided quantitative evidence of the effects of different types of dietary lipids on blood cholesterol levels (29,43–46). The percentage of food energy from medium-chain saturated fatty acids (C12 to C16) was found to have the greatest measurable effect in raising total and LDL cholesterol levels. The percentage of energy intake from medium-chain omega-6 polyunsaturated fatty acids (mainly linoleic and linolenic acid), found in large quantities in certain vegetable oils, depresses blood cholesterol levels to half the extent that an equivalent quantity of saturated fatty acids raises these levels. Replacing the percentage of food energy from saturated fatty acids with an equivalent quantity of oleic acid, a monounsaturated fatty acid, either has no effect on serum cholesterol level (43,46) or a cholesterol-lowering effect equivalent to omega-6 polyunsaturated fatty acids (47); however, the substitution of oleic acid does not depress HDL cholesterol, as often occurs with the substitution of omega-6 polyunsaturated fatty acids (29). Dietary cholesterol has less of an effect on serum cholesterol level than do fatty acids, and its intake directly affects it in a curvilinear fashion. The curvilinear relationship indicates that in situations in which initial cholesterol intake is very low, the effect of additional dietary cholesterol will be greater than if the baseline diet contains large amounts of cholesterol. Keys and colleagues (43,44) summarized the results of their many feeding studies in a now-famous equation, which resembles what Hegsted independently derived (45):

Expected change in serum cholesterol in

$$mg/dL = 1.35(2S - P) + 1.5\sqrt{1000\ DC/E},$$

where S is the change in percentage of energy from saturated fatty acids, P is the change in percentage of energy from polyunsaturated fatty acids, DC is the change in dietary cholesterol in mg/day, and E is the total energy of the diet in kcal/day.

The current prudent dietary recommendations of the AHA and the National Academy of Sciences (NAS) Expert Panel are to reduce the percentage of energy (i.e., caloric intake) from total fat to 30% or less, with no more than 10% derived from saturated fatty acids, and to restrict dietary cholesterol to at most 300 mg per day (29).

Other dietary factors that subsequently have been shown to reduce total and LDL cholesterol levels are loss of excess weight (48) and the consumption of certain water-soluble dietary-fiber components that promote the fecal elimination of cholesterol in the form of bile salts and neutral steroids and thereby increase LDL removal from the body by the liver (49). Total intake of two long-chain omega-3 polyunsaturated fatty acids, eicosa-pentaenoic acid and decosahexaenoic acid, found in fish oils and other marine products, reduces plasma triglycerides levels substantially, but has a variable effect on LDL cholesterol levels; these oils cause no change or lower or even raise LDL cholesterol levels (50). It has been postulated that omega-3 polyunsaturated fatty acids reduce the risk of CAD, based on studies of their lipid effects as well as their antithrombotic properties. This is based on epidemiological observations that populations regularly consuming marine products (including Eskimos, Japanese, and Dutch men) have reduced rates of CAD events and also on some supporting animal research (50,51). After reviewing the available evidence, the AHA recommends consumption of fish several times a week in place of red meat.

In addition, boiled coffee appears to contain a lipid-soluble fraction that raises blood total and LDL cholesterol levels; however, this fraction is eliminated by filtering the coffee (52,53). There exists some inconsistent epidemiologic evidence, recently reviewed (54), of an independent, positive association between heavy coffee consumption (> 4 to 6 cups/day) and increased risk of heart disease.

Clinical Intervention Trials. Despite the strong circumstantial evidence provided by epidemiologic, postmortem, clinical, and genetic studies, as well as evidence from basic laboratory, animal, and feeding research, skeptics remained reluctant to make broad populationwide recommendations for widespread dietary and lipid-lowering drug therapy prior to clinical trial demonstrations that cholesterol reduction safely reduces the rate of atherosclerotic CVD events. A number of dietary interventions performed in the 1960s, including the National Diet Heart Study in the U.S., demonstrated the feasibility and safety of reducing blood cholesterol by dietary changes (55). Although favorable trends were noted in reducing the CAD rate with blood cholesterol lowering, these trials lacked sufficient sample size and design to provide the statistical power to prove conclusively the value of cholesterol reduction. The final link in the chain of evidence proving that reducing levels of blood total and LDL cholesterol can reduce the incidence of CAD events has come from a number of primary and secondary clinical intervention trials.

The Oslo Diet-Antismoking Trial (56) in the 1970s involved 1,232 hypercholesterolemic, normotensive men aged 40 to 49 years. Simultaneous dietary and smoking intervention resulted in a 46% reduction in CAD events in the intervention group, which was shown by multivariate analysis to be primarily due to a dietary-induced reduction in serum total cholesterol level of 13% as compared with the control group.

The Multiple Risk Factor Intervention Trial was a multicenter, randomized, controlled study designed to test whether simultaneous interventions, including dietary treatment of hypercholesterolemia, hypertension management, and cigarette-smoking cessation would protect against CAD mortality in a large cohort of high-risk middle-aged men (57,58). A subgroup of the cohort similar in composition to the Oslo Study population had a 49% reduction in CAD mortality, confirming the findings from that study.

The most notable intervention trial to test the cholesterol-CAD hypothesis was the Lipid Research Clinics Coronary Primary Prevention Trial (59,60). Almost 4,000 middle-aged men with hypercholesterolemia were randomly assigned in a double-blind fashion to one of two groups, which received the same AHA dietary advice for lowering blood cholesterol levels. In addition, one group received cholestyramine, a cholesterol-lowering drug, and the other (control) group received a placebo. A significant 19% reduction in initial major CAD events over a 7.4-year period was noted in the active drug intervention group. For every 1% reduction in blood cholesterol level there was a 2% reduction in heart disease risk, a trend that confirmed the observational data. A subgroup that attained a 25% decrease in blood cholesterol level had a 50% decline in CAD event rate.

The Helsinki Heart Study was another large-scale double-blind, randomized, controlled primary prevention trial. Involving over 4,000 middle-aged men with various types of dyslipidemias, this study compared the effects on CAD event rate of another lipid-lowering drug, gemfibrozil, with placebo (61). A 34% reduction in the 5-year rate of fatal and nonfatal major CAD events was associated with a 9% reduction in plasma total and LDL cholesterol, a 35% reduction in triglycerides, and an 8% increase in HDL cholesterol levels. However, neither the Helsinki Heart Study nor the Lipid Research Clinics Coronary Primary Prevention Trial observed a significant reduction in total mortality. Furthermore, both had higher rates of deaths due to homicides, suicides, and accidents in the groups receiving cholesterol-lowering drugs when compared with the control group, although the relative number of cases were small and the differences between experimental and placebo groups were not statistically significant. These deaths in the active-treatment groups for both trials were recently reexamined to determine if the changes noted were related to blood cholesterol reduction (61). It was concluded that when dropouts and prior risk factors for violent behavior, such as alcohol abuse or previous psychiatric histories, were taken into consideration, there was no evidence to support the hypothesis that cholesterol-lowering agents are causally related to violent deaths. Further, a literature review by the authors failed to uncover evidence for a causal association between lower-than-average serum cholesterol levels and adverse social behavior (62).

The earlier Cooperative Clofibrate Trial of the World Health Organization (WHO), begun in 1965, was a large-scale randomized, controlled primary prevention trial that involved over 15,000 healthy European men, 50% of whom had serum cholesterol levels in the upper third of the normal population distribution (63). A 9% reduction in plasma total cholesterol level was accompanied by a 25% reduction in first nonfatal MIs at 5-year follow-up in hypercholesterolemic men assigned to clofibrate treatment as compared with those receiving placebo; however, no reduction in fatal CAD events was noted in the clofibrate group. In addition, the death rate from all causes in the clofibrate group was 28% higher than that of the control group, a statistically significant difference. The excess in total mortality appeared nonspecific and was not associated with excess cancer mortality.

In addition to these primary prevention trials involving lipid-lowering drugs, there have been a number of secondary cholesterol-lowering CAD prevention trials in the United States and Europe. In the Coronary Drug Project initiated in the United States in the late 1960s, 8,341 men, unselected by cholesterol levels, who had experienced a documented MI were randomly assigned to a number of cholesterol-lowering drugs, including clofibrate and niacin, or placebo (64). At 6-year follow-up the only significant difference seen in

CAD events was between the niacin and placebo groups; relative to the placebo group, the active group showed a 27% reduction in nonfatal MIs associated with a 10% reduction in serum total cholesterol levels. Furthermore, 9 years later the niacin group had a nonsignificantly lower rate of CAD events and a significantly lower rate (11%) of overall mortality (65).

The Program on Surgical Control of Hyperlipidemias was a recent multicenter, randomized secondary prevention trial that employed a partial ileal bypass surgical procedure to lower blood total and LDL cholesterol levels (66). The study population consisted of 838 men and women who had survived a first MI and had a mean baseline total cholesterol level of 251 mg/dL. At 10-year follow-up a significant 35% reduction in combined fatal and nonfatal CAD events was noted in the intervention group as compared with the control group. This was associated with a 23% reduction in total cholesterol and a 38% reduction in LDL cholesterol levels. Mortality due to CAD and overall mortality for the intervention group was also reduced (28% and 22%, respectively), but did not achieve statistical significance. However, overall mortality was significantly (36%) lower in a surgical subgroup with initially good left ventricular function. Further, serial coronary arteriograms consistently showed either less progression or regression of atherosclerosis in the treatment group as compared with the control group.

Table 8.1, adapted and updated from Superko (67), summarizes the results of the major primary and secondary prevention trials designed specifically to evaluate the effect of cholesterol-lowering therapy on the risk of CAD. It appears from this table that every 1% reduction in serum total and LDL cholesterol results in a 2% to 3% reduction in major CAD events, particularly nonfatal MI. Again, these findings are consistent with associations previously described in epidemiologic observational studies.

The pilot phase of another major controlled multicenter cholesterol-lowering primary CAD prevention primary drug trial, the Cholesterol Reduction in Seniors Program, is under way in the United States to determine the value of vigorous cholesterol management in people over 60 years of age. The drug being employed in this study is lovastatin, a potent inhibitor of HMG-CoA reductase that increases receptor-mediated LDL removal from the plasma by the liver. The efficacy and safety of this agent along with a cholesterol-lowering diet was recently demonstrated in the

Table 8.1 Summary of Results of Major Primary and Secondary Prevention Trials to Determine the Effect of Total Cholesterol Reduction on the Incidence of Coronary Artery Disease

Study (reference) (agent)	n	Exposure (years)	Mean TC reduction (%)	End point	Reduction in end point (%)
WHO (62) (clofibrate)	15,745	5.0	9.0	Nonfatal MI	25
CDP (63)[a] (niacin)	8,341	6.0	10.0	Nonfatal MI	26
CDP (64) (niacin)		15.0		All-cause mortality	11
Helsinki (60) (gemfibrozil)	4,081	5.0	9.0	Fatal and nonfatal MI	34
LRC-CPPT (58,59) (cholestyramine)	3,806	7.4	8.5	Nonfatal MI CAD deaths	19 24
POSCH (65)[a] (partial ileal bypass)	838	9.7	23.0	Fatal and nonfatal MI	35

Note. WHO = World Health Organization; CDP = Coronary Drug Project; Helsinki = Helsinki Heart Study; LRC-CPPT = Lipid Research Clinics Coronary Primary Prevention Trial; POSCH = Program on Surgical Control of Hyperlipidemias; MI = myocardial infarction; TC = total cholesterol. Adapted and updated from Superko, 1989 (67).

[a]Secondary prevention trials

placebo-controlled, double-blind Expanded Clinical Evaluation of Lovastatin Study, which involved over 8,000 patients with hypercholesterolemia (68). In this study, daily doses of 20 mg of lovastatin resulted in a 24% to 40% reduction in plasma LDL cholesterol with an associated 6.6% to 9.5% elevation in HDL cholesterol levels.

A number of smaller studies have also confirmed that the progression of CAD (as documented quantitatively by angiography) can be attenuated or even reversed by a substantial reduction in plasma LDL cholesterol levels attained through dietary changes or drugs within a therapy period as short as 1 to 2 years (67,69-71). For example, the Cholesterol Lowering Atherosclerotic Study (70) involved 162 CABG surgery patients randomly assigned to a combination of diet and drugs (cholestyramine and niacin) or diet and placebo. After 2 years of therapy, the drug-treated group exhibited significantly fewer coronary atherosclerotic lesions that had progressed, fewer subjects with new atheroma in native coronary arteries, and fewer adverse changes in bypass grafts. Furthermore, atherosclerosis regressed in 16% of the drug-treated group as compared with 2% in the control group. The associated blood lipid changes in the treatment group included a 43% reduction in LDL cholesterol and a 37% increase in HDL cholesterol levels. More recently, Ornish et al. (71) performed a controlled study involving 48 patients with CAD. Comprehensive lifestyle changes, including a substantial reduction in plasma total and LDL cholesterol levels by a low-fat vegetarian diet associated with a mean 10-kg

weight loss, moderate exercise, smoking cessation, and stress management training, resulted in an average of 1% regression of angiographically documented coronary artery lesions at 1-year follow-up in 82% of the subjects in the intervention group, while the control group generally showed progression of lesions. A large number of additional angiographic investigations are currently in progress.

Blood Total and Low-Density Lipoprotein Cholesterol Levels and Risk of Stroke

The relationship of blood total cholesterol and LDL cholesterol to stroke has been reviewed (72). Epidemiological cross-sectional, case-control, cohort, angiographic, and ultrasonographic studies have failed to find a consistent association between blood total or LDL cholesterol levels and clinical manifestations of stroke. For example, in the Framingham Study a U-shaped relationship was noted between plasma total and LDL cholesterol levels and stroke risk (73). The highest risk of stroke and acute brain infarction was observed at total serum cholesterol levels above 295 mg/dL and below 190 mg/dL. A U-shaped relationship has also been observed in several other prospective studies (72). In more recent studies (73,74), in which discrimination was made between intracerebral hemorrhagic and cerebral thrombotic atherosclerotic-thrombotic strokes, a clearer epidemiologic picture has emerged. A positive linear association definitely exists between total cholesterol level and death from thrombotic-atherosclerotic stroke, explaining the right side of the U-shaped total cholesterol–stroke risk curve. Further, a strong negative linear relationship appears to exist between total cholesterol level and deaths due to cerebral hemorrhage, explaining the left side of the curve. However, the latter finding appears to be limited to people with serum cholesterol levels under 160 mg/dL in combination with elevated diastolic BP (74). Blood total and LDL cholesterol levels are also weaker predictors of angiographically demonstrated carotid artery atherosclerosis than cigarette smoking and hypertension are (75,76). A paucity of data exists on the value of blood cholesterol lowering for the prevention of stroke, which perhaps will be remedied by the Cholesterol Reduction in Seniors Program, mentioned previously.

High-Density Lipoprotein Cholesterol and Risk of Coronary Heart Disease

High-Density Lipoprotein Cholesterol Levels. HDL is generally reputed to play a protective role against atherogenesis (29,77), a phenomenon thought to be related to its role in the reverse cholesterol transport system. This system involves the removal of cholesterol from tissues (including artery wall foam cells) by HDL. The cholesterol is esterfied and trapped within the core of the HDL particle and transported to the liver, where it is taken up via receptors and excreted into the gastrointestinal tract either directly or in the form of bile salts. However, as was recently reviewed in detail elsewhere (29,77), the evidence that low levels of plasma HDL cholesterol independently enhance, or that increased levels of HDL cholesterol protect against, the atherosclerotic process is considerably weaker than the evidence supporting the direct atherogenic contribution of LDL cholesterol. Further, no clinical intervention trials have examined the effects of modification of low levels of plasma HDL cholesterol alone on the risk of CAD.

An inverse association of plasma HDL cholesterol to CAD was first suggested by a number of prospective and cross-sectional epidemiological studies reviewed elsewhere (29,77) and was recently confirmed by the Lipid Research Clinics Mortality Follow-up Study (78) and the Physicians Health Study (35). In the United States most observational cohort studies show that CVD and CAD mortality rates are inversely associated with levels of plasma HDL cholesterol, and this association persists after adjusting for other risk factors (35,77-80). For example, in the Framingham Study, an increment of 1 mg/dL in HDL cholesterol was independently associated with a 3.1% lower rate

of CAD events (80). This is consistent with the findings in the recent Physicians Health Study (35) of a 3.5% reduction in the risk of MI associated with each 1 mg/dL increment in the HDL cholesterol level. However, the results of epidemiological studies within some populations have been mixed, with some failing to find an inverse association and others, such as the Finnish cohort in the Seven Countries Study (29,81), finding accelerated atherosclerosis with elevated HDL cholesterol levels. Furthermore, HDL cholesterol levels failed to predict CAD events rates among countries in this latter study.

A widely held misconception that the anti-atherogenic properties of HDL are solely associated with the HDL-2 subfraction has scant supporting evidence. Most observational studies measuring HDL subfractions have found that both principal subfractions, HDL-2 and HDL-3, are inversely related to the risk of CAD events (35,82).

The possible connection between plasma HDL cholesterol levels and the severity of atherosclerosis has general support from clinical investigations. Several coronary angiographic studies have shown an inverse relationship between plasma HDL cholesterol levels and the extent and severity of angiographically defined atherosclerosis (29). Additional, indirect clinical support for an HDL-CAD inverse relationship is the finding of a high CAD event rate in medical conditions that exhibit low plasma HDL cholesterol levels. These include diabetes mellitus, obesity, and dyslipidemias associated with hypertriglyceridemia. The lower heart disease rate in women prior to menopause as compared with men of a similar age may also be at least partially attributable to higher plasma HDL cholesterol levels in women. Similarly, the lower CAD event rate associated with moderate alcohol use and with regular endurance exercise observed in most epidemiological studies has been attributed at least in part to increased HDL cholesterol levels. Further, cigarette smoking is associated with reduced HDL cholesterol levels.

On the other hand, clinical observations of genetic disorders causing altered HDL cholesterol levels reveal exceptions to the general inverse association of HDL to the risk of CAD events. Gwynne (77) noted that several genetically related conditions that manifested low HDL cholesterol levels were not associated with premature heart disease, while in other genetic disorders increased HDL cholesterol levels were not associated with a reduced risk of heart attacks. Furthermore, fat-restricted diets, particularly those enriched in omega-6 polyunsaturated fatty acids, appear to reduce both LDL and HDL cholesterol levels yet apparently contribute to reduced risk of CAD (77).

Although there have not been any clinical trials specifically designed to evaluate the health impact of raising plasma HDL cholesterol levels, some pharmacological intervention trials to lower plasma LDL cholesterol levels, such as the Helsinki Heart Study involving gemfibrozil (61) have observed a greater-than-expected reduction in CAD rate attributable to lowering LDL cholesterol, apparently related to a simultaneous increase in HDL cholesterol levels. This also appeared to be true in the Lipid Research Clinics Coronary Primary Prevention Trial (83), the Coronary Drug Project (64), and the Cholesterol Lowering Atherosclerotic Study (70). Other lipid-lowering agents that, in addition to lowering LDL cholesterol increase HDL cholesterol levels, include fibric acid derivatives other than gemfibrozil, niacin, estrogen, and, to a lesser extent, lovastatin and cholestyramine. Furthermore, commonly employed, nonpharmacologic CAD prevention strategies, including cessation of cigarette smoking, regular endurance exercise, and loss of excess weight, are reported to raise HDL cholesterol levels, particularly in men.

Ratio of Total Cholesterol to High-Density Lipoprotein Cholesterol.

Although the ratio of total cholesterol or LDL cholesterol to HDL cholesterol is a strong predictor of future CAD risk in the American population (29,35,77), the NAS Expert Panel (29), the National Cholesterol Education Program Panel (28), and other experts (84) advise against using this ratio as the basis of estimating the risk of CAD or as a key factor in decisions regarding treatment of elevated LDL cholesterol levels. The reasons for this opinion are that the measurement of HDL cholesterol is not as accurate as total or LDL cholesterol and that both lipoproteins are independent risk factors with different determinants; thus combining them into a single number may conceal information that can be useful to the clinician.

Lipoprotein (a) and
Risk of Cardiovascular Disease

There is growing interest in the apparent role of lipoprotein (a) [lp(a)] in atherosclerotic CVD. Lp(a) is structurally related to LDL in that both contain apoB-100. In lp(a), apoB-100 is linked to the unique apolipoprotein (a), which structurally resembles plasminogen and interferes with its fibrinolytic function through competitive inhibition. Based on these structural and functional properties, lp(a) is commonly believed to be involved both in athero-

genesis and thrombogenesis (29,85,86). Lp(a) is present in small concentrations in the plasma, vessel wall linings, and atherosclerotic plaques. Elevated levels (> 30 mg/dL) are genetically determined as a Mendalian trait and are found in 10% to 15% of the white population and in a higher percentage of the black population in the United States. Diabetic people appear more likely to have elevated levels of lp(a) than nondiabetic people. A strong association has been found between plasma levels of lp(a) and both coronary heart disease events and severity of coronary artery atherosclerosis in case-control epidemiologic studies. High levels of lp(a) are more frequent in survivors of MI (87,88) and in the presence of severe coronary atherosclerosis as assessed by angiography (89) than in comparison groups. Lp(a) does not appear to be affected by diet or exercise, but large doses of niacin may reduce levels of lp(a), although not in all subjects (86). The influence of this reduction on risk of CAD events is unknown. Obviously, much remains to be learned about the apparent contribution of lp(a) to the risk of CAD and more effective approaches to reducing elevated levels.

Apolipoproteins and
Risk of Cardiovascular Disease

Of the 14 major identified apolipoproteins, 2 (apoAI and apoB-100) have been associated with premature heart disease and severity of CAD atherosclerosis in observational epidemiological studies. Mean plasma levels of these apolipoproteins in adults are 80 and 140 mg/dL, respectively (87). ApoB-100, the major structural apolipoprotein of LDL, binds to cell surfaces, allowing the uptake and incorporation of LDL cholesterol by these cells (87). ApoAI is the principal apolipoprotein of HDL and activates lecithin:cholesterol acyltransferase (LCAT) (87). LCAT esterifies free cholesterol, allowing it to be incorporated into the core of HDL molecules. Controversy exists as to whether measurement of the blood level of apoB provides a better indicator of CAD risk than measurement of total or LDL cholesterol and whether the same is true for apoAI as opposed to HDL cholesterol. A number of case-control epidemiological studies suggest that both apolipoproteins have a strong association with heart attacks and severity of coronary atherosclerosis—that is, a direct association with apoB levels and an inverse association with apoAI levels—as would be expected from similar associations with their parent lipoproteins (90,91). However, a recent large-scale prospective study failed to find any predictive value for levels of these apolipoproteins after conventional risk factors were statistically adjusted for (35). Further, there remain standardization problems in obtaining these measurements. Nonpharmacological and pharmacological interventions previously described, which favorably alter LDL- and HDL cholesterol levels, appear to impact the apolipoproteins in similar directions (87).

Triglycerides and Risk of Cardiovascular Disease

After more than three decades of research, it remains controversial and unclear as to whether or not triglyceride levels are independently related to the severity of atherosclerosis and the risk of CVD (29,92). Although most epidemiological studies reveal a positive association between blood triglyceride levels and heart disease by univariate analysis, this association usually does not persist after statistical adjustments are made for confounding variables, notably the inverse relation between triglyceride level and HDL cholesterol (29,93-95). In addition, positive associations often exist between serum triglyceride levels and total cholesterol, fasting blood glucose, insulin, age, obesity, physical inactivity, cigarette smoking, and alcohol intake (93). However, measuring triglycerides is indicated, since this may have some independent predictive value for coronary events in women and its measurement is required along with total and HDL cholesterol, to estimate LDL cholesterol levels (94,95).

Hypertension and Risk of Left Ventricular Hypertrophy

High BP is a common medical problem worldwide. In the United States, 15% to 20% of adult men and women (some 50 million people) have elevated levels of diastolic (≥ 90 mm Hg) and/or systolic (≥ 140 mm Hg) BP (96). The vast majority of these people are classified as having mild, or stage 1, hypertension (diastolic BP of 90 to 104 mm Hg). The prevalence of hypertension is much higher in African-American populations than in Caucasian populations, and the disparity increases with age. Less than 10% of hypertension can be attributed to such secondary causes as endocrine, renal parenchymal, or renovascular diseases; the remainder is classified as primary, or essential, hypertension.

Multiple factors, both genetic and environmental, interact to contribute to underlying dysfunction in arterial BP regulation involved in the etiology of essential hypertension (97). The common end result is a chronic increase in total peripheral vascular resistance due to exaggerated arterial smooth muscle tone. In at least some people with essential hypertension, this may be preceded during childhood or adolescence by an increase in cardiac output ($\dot{Q}$) from overactivity of the sympathoadrenomedullary system with an accompanying overstimulation of the renin-angiotensin-aldosterone system (98).

Risk factors for essential hypertension include a positive family history, aging, overweight, excess dietary intake of sodium (> 3 g/day) and perhaps a low intake of potassium, calcium, and magnesium salts; excess alcohol (≥ 2 oz/day) intake; a low ratio of intake of polyunsaturated fatty acids to intake of saturated fatty acids, physical inactivity, and psychological stresses (96-98). Isolated systolic hypertension (systolic BP ≥ 160 mm Hg with diastolic BP ≤ 90 mm Hg) is primarily found in elderly or diabetic individuals and is usually due to a loss of aortic elasticity associated with atherosclerosis.

Irrespective of the etiology, both elevated levels of systolic and diastolic BP have consistently been demonstrated to have independent causative relationships to the future development of CVD complications (30-32,96). These complications include not only fatal and nonfatal coronary events but also transient ischemic attacks (so-called "small" strokes), atherosclerotic and hemorrhagic stroke, occlusive peripheral vascular disease (PVD), dissecting aortic aneurysms, nephropathy, LVH, and congestive heart failure (CHF). Substantial evidence now exists that drug treatment of even mild diastolic hypertension and of isolated systolic hypertension in the elderly significantly reduces the risk of these complications.

LVH represents an adaptive increase in myocardial mass in response to a chronic physiological or pathological augmentation in the work load of the heart. Hypertension is the most commonly observed cause of LVH. A symmetrical thickening of the left ventricular walls without chamber dilatation ("concentric LVH") results as a consequence of the chronic increase in total peripheral resistance associated with a persistent elevation of arterial BP, particularly of its systolic component (99). The sympathetic nervous system and angiotensin II activity are believed to contribute to the pathogenesis of LVH in people with hypertension. Myocardial changes associated with aging and the coexistence of obesity have a synergistic influence on the severity of LVH associated with hypertension (99,100). In addition, African-American populations appear more susceptible to LVH than Caucasian populations.

Based on experimental animal work, the following biochemical sequence of events appears to be associated with the development of LVH in the pressure-overloaded heart in response to a chronic increase in wall stress: (1) increased myocardial energy requirements, (2) depletion of high-energy phosphate stores, (3) increased messenger RNA synthesis and ribosomal RNA concentration, (4) stimulation of contractile and mitochondrial protein synthesis and sarcomere formation, (5) increased DNA synthesis, and (6) increased deposition of collagen and fibrous tissue in the heart (101). Initially this adaptive process is well tolerated and appears beneficial, since it reduces myocardial wall stress by normalizing the ratio of chamber radius to wall thickness. However, at some critical level of myocardial mass, ventricular functional reserve and coronary flow reserve are impaired, and ventricular ectopic activity and CHF may develop (99,101-103).

LVH may be diagnosed according to echocardiographic, ECG, or chest x-ray criteria (104). The echocardiagraph provides by far the most sensitive of these indicators of LVH, while ECG criteria are the least sensitive. However, longitudinal epidemiologic studies on the relationship of LVH to the risk of CVD have primarily relied on ECG criteria. In the Framingham Study, 20% of the men and 13% of the women with hypertension had coexisting ECG criteria for LVH (105). The prevalence of ECG criteria for LVH in populations of hypertensive people increases with the level of BP and the age of the subjects. At systolic BP of 180 mm Hg or more, the incidence of ECG evidence of LVH is about 50% within 12 years (106). As is discussed in more detail in a later section, ECG criteria for LVH substantially and independently increase the risk of heart attacks, sudden death, transient ischemic attacks, strokes, and CHF, irrespective of levels of other major risk factors (105,106). The presence of ECG repolarization ST-T wave depression—the so-called LV strain pattern—carries a particularly bad prognosis.

Epidemiological Studies

Major prospective observational studies have consistently noted a strongly positive, continuous, independent contribution in both men and women of systolic and diastolic BP levels to atherosclerotic CVD sequelae (107). The relationship between BP and the risk of CVD is log linear; that is, the percent change in risk of heart disease associated with BP

level is similar at all levels within the range studied and no threshold exists below which there is no risk of stroke and CAD events (108). For example, in the Framingham Study the 18-year relative risk for both CAD death and stroke for men aged 45 to 74 years at entry with diastolic BP of 80 to 89 mm Hg was about double that of men whose diastolic BP was less than 80 mm Hg (108). For men whose BP was 105 mm Hg or more at entry, the relative risk for CAD death was more than four times higher, and for stroke five times higher, as compared with those whose baseline diastolic BP was less than 80 mm Hg.

It also is evident from prospective observational studies, including those in children, that an increase in BP over time is positively related to the initial value, that is, BP "feeds on itself" (109). This emphasizes the need for early intervention for primary prevention of hypertension and for preventing CVD complications in persons with borderline and stage 1 hypertension.

ECG evidence of LVH in a man or woman with hypertension at any age substantially further escalates the risk of CVD events (106). For example, in the Framingham Study, 30% of individuals with LVH on the ECG at baseline had a major CVD event within 5 years, and the age-adjusted relative risk of any CVD event was about 4 for men and 6 for women at 20-year follow-up; risk of stroke, CHF, occlusive peripheral vascular disease (PVD) and every clinical manifestation of CAD, including sudden death, also increased. The presence of a left ventricular strain pattern on the ECG is a particularly grave prognostic sign, since it is associated with twice the risk of LVH, as defined by ECG QRS amplitude criteria (110). The adverse prognostic implications of LVH by ECG criteria after an MI have also been demonstrated (99,107). Chest x-ray evidence of cardiac enlargement is associated with half of the extent of increased risk of CVD as compared with LVH documented by an ECG (104,107).

Migrant Studies

A number of migrant studies have documented environmental influence on BP levels in populations. For example, South Pacific Polynesian islanders, who traditionally have a low prevalence of hypertension and CAD and no significant changes in BP levels with age, experience an increase in BP levels at all ages along with an increased risk of CVD complications after they migrate to areas that have high hypertension and

CVD rates, such as New Zealand (109). The obvious conclusion is that there are strong environmental influences on BP levels, which indicates the potential value of lifestyle measures for preventing and treating hypertension.

Postmortem Findings

Autopsies of people with a history of prolonged hypertension almost always turn up evidence of advanced atherosclerosis in the coronary and other major systemic arteries (110,111). In addition, in a classic study of 500 consecutive cases of fatal MI, Master et al. (112) reported a history of hypertension in 50% of the male cases and 80% of the female cases. The International Atherosclerosis Project allowed pathologists to compare the severity of coronary and aortic atherosclerosis among multiple racial and ethnic groups in 14 countries. In each population studied, the prevalence and extent of raised fibrous atherosclerotic plaques and complicated, calcified lesions were greater in hypertensive than in nonhypertensive cases (111). In addition, the mean heart weight of persons coded as having hypertension consistently exceeded the mean heart weight of age- and sex-matched nonhypertensive persons. In population and race groups with high death rates from atherosclerotic CVD, hypertension appeared to aggravate the severity of atherosclerosis at all stages of the disease and to promote heart failure in hearts damaged by MI. In populations with a low prevalence of atherosclerotic lesions and clinical CVD, hypertension appeared to worsen the arterial intimal disease. At autopsy, the severity of cerebral atherosclerosis also has consistently been reported to be greater in hypertensive than nonhypertensive cases (113). However, from the available postmortem data it appears that while hypertension is a potent contributor to the severity of atherosclerosis, it is not an essential factor, nor is it responsible for the major differences in the severity of atherosclerosis among geographic locations and racial groups.

Animal Research

There are a number of animal models available for evaluating arterial hypertension, including strains of rats bred for hypertension that is either spontaneous or environmentally induced (by "salt loading," stress, or excess protein intake) (114,115). The genetic spontaneous hypertensive rat (SHR) model most closely resembles the pathophysiology of essential hypertension in humans (115). Overactivity of the sympathetic nervous system appears to play a role in the initiation of hypertension in the SHR, as do biomembrane abnormalities, commonly detected in erythrocytes. Similar abnormalities are postulated to occur in human essential hypertension. In addition, the principal hemodynamic alteration contributing to hypertension in the SHR is arterial vasoconstriction, causing increased total peripheral vascular resistance, similar to the human condition. Vascular smooth muscle hypertrophy and LVH also develop early in the SHR, as is the situation in human children and young adults with borderline or stage 1 hypertension. The elevated BP in the SHR and other animal models of hypertension results in arterial wall damage (arterionecrosis) and thrombosis, which in some strains of the SHR can precipitate a stroke by either cerebral hemorrhage or infarction. However, inducing coronary atherosclerosis and MI in the SHR or other animal models of hypertension requires the simultaneous induction of hypercholesterolemia, usually by dietary means (114). These findings appear to confirm data from autopsy studies indicating that hypertension is an accelerating, rather than an initiating, factor for coronary atherosclerosis.

Biological Plausibility and Mechanisms for Increased Risk of Cardiovascular Disease

There are a number of plausible potential biological mechanisms that help explain the increased risk of CVD in hypertensive individuals, particularly in those with LVH. Severe hypertension damages the endothelium of the medium-sized and large arteries, including the coronary and cerebral vessels. As a consequence of this damage, the formation and release of endothelium-derived vasoactive substances, including endothelial-derived relaxing factor is believed to be impaired. In addition, an increase may result in the formation and release of endothelin, which may contribute to coronary and cerebral artery vasoconstriction. In fact, it is postulated that such endothelial changes contribute to the acceleration of atherosclerosis in the presence of hypercholesterolemia, as well as to myocardial collagen deposition and fibrosis frequently associated with hypertension-induced LVH (99). Furthermore, vascular smooth muscle hypertrophy and increased tone in smaller resistance coronary arteries associated with hypertension may reduce vasomotion and the coronary flow adaptive reserve; that is, the ratio of maximal flow to resting flow. In addition, both hypertension and LVH increase myocardial oxygen demands and consumption, which helps explain why angina pectoris or silent ischemia may be present in patients with hypertension even in the absence of gross coronary atherosclerosis. Relative or absolute coronary artery insufficiency and myocardial fibrosis in patients with hypertension and LVH also are believed to provide the milieu for ventricular dysarrhythmias and sudden cardiac death (116). In fact, a reduced threshold for ventricular fibrillation (117) in the SHR with cardiac hypertrophy has been demonstrated experimentally.

Intervention Trials

Based on pooled data from nine major prospective observational epidemiologic studies involving 37,000 people, a 5 to 6 mm Hg reduction in usual diastolic BP should reduce the incidence of fatal stroke and fatal CAD by 20% to 30% (108,118,119). Since the landmark Veterans Administration Cooperative Trial in the 1960s (120) there have been at least 13 additional major randomized trials of antihypertensive therapy for the primary prevention of CVD in patients with essential hypertension. These include the Hypertension Detection and Follow-up Program (121), the Multiple Risk Factor Intervention Trial (57,58), and the U.S. Public Health Service Hospitals Cooperative Trial (122), in the United States; the Medical Research Council Trial, in Great Britain (123); the Australian Therapeutic Trial (124); and the Oslo (Heart) Study, in Norway (125). An intensive stepped-care approach, generally starting with hydrochlorothiazide or chlorothalidone, was employed in the active intervention group in most of these trials. Only the Veterans Administration Cooperative Trial (120) and the Australian study (124) employed a placebo control group for comparison purposes. In the other studies, the control group received "referred" or "usual care" by community physicians. In the Multiple Risk Factor Intervention Trial (57,58), the active treatment group also received dietary modifications to lower blood cholesterol levels and smoking modification programs.

These clinical trials unequivocally demonstrated the value of lowering BP in reducing the risk of morbid events directly associated with hypertension, including progression of the severity of hypertension, advanced retinopathy, renal failure, CHF, and fatal and nonfatal strokes. However, only the Hypertension Detection and Follow-up Program showed a statistically significant reduction in the death rate from acute MI over a 5-year follow-up period (121). The rate of MI deaths in this program was 28% lower in the stepped-care group as compared with the referred-care group.

However, because of the absence of difference in deaths associated with other CAD events, the overall difference in CAD deaths between the two groups was only 12%. There also was an overall statistically significant reduction in death rate (17%) from all causes for the stepped-care group as compared with the referred-care group.

In the Multiple Risk Factor Intervention Trial, however, at 7-year follow-up there were essentially no differences between the special intervention and usual care groups for either CAD deaths or all causes of mortality (57). Furthermore a subgroup of men with hypertension and abnormal resting ECGs (including LVH or ST-T–wave changes) was identified in which death rates (particularly sudden death) were sizably higher in the special intervention, apparently related to therapy with high doses of hydrochorothiazide.

Recently, data from all the major randomized, controlled CAD prevention trials employing antihypertensive drugs have been pooled using meta-analysis (118,119). Collins et al. (118) reviewed 14 such randomized trials involving over 37,000 men and women in which the average diastolic BP was 5.8 mm Hg lower in the intensive intervention as compared with control groups over a mean treatment period of 5 years. Intensive intervention was associated with a 42% reduction ($p < 0.0001$) in fatal and nonfatal strokes, which is consistent with the reduction estimated from pooled data from prospective epidemiologic studies cited previously. However, for CAD events, the effect of BP reduction in these trials was just over half of that estimated from the pooled epidemiological data; that is, only a 14% reduction in coronary disease events ($p < 0.01$). It has been postulated that the metabolic side effects of hydrochlorothiazide and chlorothalidone diuretics, the initial drugs in the stepped-care approach—in particular, an increase in plasma total and LDL cholesterol levels—may have offset some of the benefits of BP reduction on risk of CAD (118,119). Some of the other antihypertensive drugs used in some clinical trials, namely propranolol (123) and methyldopa (57,121), significantly lowered plasma HDL cholesterol levels. In addition, large doses of thiazide diuretics and chlorothalidone can reduce serum and total body levels of potassium and magnesium and increase catecholamine secretion and renin-angiotensin activity, which may result in an increased risk of ventricular arrhythmias and sudden death (96). The value of nonpharmacologic measures (reductions in excess body weight, salt intake, alcohol consumption, and increased physical activity) for preventing the progression of BP levels in people with borderline elevated BP has been demonstrated by a controlled clinical trial (126). In addition, these hygienic measures may provide an opportunity for reducing the dosage of antihypertensive medications, and even eventual drug withdrawal in selected patients with well-controlled and carefully monitored mild hypertension (127).

Controversy has long existed as to the safety and effectiveness of pharmacological intervention in isolated systolic hypertension in the elderly, a condition that contributes up to two thirds of all cases of hypertension between the ages of 65 and 89 (128). Results of the double-blind, placebo-controlled Systolic Hypertension in the Elderly Program, which involved 4,737 men and women aged 60 years and older (mean age = 72 years) were recently reported (129). In this 5-year clinical trial, in which low-dose chlorothiazide was used as the initial antihypertensive medication, the incidence of fatal and nonfatal stroke was reduced by 36%. The absolute reduction in all major CVD events in the active-intervention group was 55 per 1,000.

Reversal of Left Ventricular Hypertrophy With Antihypertensive Treatment

In light of the marked increase in risk of CVD complications and death associated with LVH, one of the important aims of antihypertensive therapy should be reversal of LVH (as well as of the associated hypertrophic changes in arteriolar smooth muscle). Although a general relationship exists between a reduction in BP and LVH reversal, not all antihypertensive agents appear to be equally effective in this respect. Recent reviews (99,130) of this issue report that antihypertensive medications that reduce sympathetic nervous system activity, such as beta-blocking agents, methyldopa, and possibly clonidine, and those that do not elicit a reflex adrenergic stimulation, such as the angiotensin-converting enzyme (ACE) inhibitors and calcium antagonists, have been shown in animal models and clinical studies to reverse or reduce LVH concomitantly with their lowering of arterial BP. On the other hand, such direct-acting vasodilating agents as hydralizine and minoxidil, although effectively lowering elevated BP levels, have been found not to reverse LVH or may actually exacerbate ventricular mass, probably because of reflex adrenergic stimulation (130,131). Thiazide diuretics also have been reported to have no effect on left ventricular mass in hypertensive patients (99). Furthermore, there appear to be differences

in reversibility of vascular smooth-muscle hypertrophy by the various antihypertensive drugs (130). However, it remains to be proven whether antihypertensive drugs that reverse LVH and vascular muscle hypertrophy can reduce CVD morbidity and mortality beyond that produced by BP control alone. Although one would assume that this would be the case, animal experiments have shown that some antihypertensive drugs that cause regression of LVH leave behind an increased concentration of myocardial collagen, which may reduce LVF (132). Further, a strikingly greater reduction in myocardial mass than in BP could theoretically be harmful, since this might increase wall stress.

Comment

We may conclude from this review of available data that there is strong consistent evidence that hypertension accelerates the severity of atherosclerosis and is a potent causative factor of CVD, particularly when hypertension is accompanied by LVH. The ability to prevent cardiovascular complications, particularly stroke, by antihypertensive therapy has been conclusively proven with both essential hypertension and isolated systolic hypertension in the elderly. Possible adverse effects of antihypertensive therapy appear to diminish the expected effectiveness of BP lowering in reducing major CAD events. This has led to an increased interest in nonpharmacologic means of preventing and managing hypertension in order to minimize drug requirements. In addition there is a growing appreciation of the need for a flexible, individualized approach toward the drug treatment of hypertension that takes into consideration patient characteristics, coexisting medical conditions, blood lipid profile, presence of LVH, and factors affecting quality of life (96).

Cigarette Smoking and Risk of Cardiovascular Disease

A general consensus exists, based primarily on observational epidemiological data, that cigarette smoking ranks with dietary and blood lipids and hypertension as a major causative factor for CVD, including risk of CAD deaths, nonfatal MIs, angina pectoris, atherosclerotic aortic and PVD, and atherosclerotic and hemorrhagic stroke. In addition, observational evidence indicates that smoking cessation reduces the risk of CVD. A number of plausible mechanisms have been defined from experimental studies supporting the causative relationship of smoking to CVD.

In 1989, 25 years after the first Surgeon General's report on smoking and health, a progress report from the Surgeon General indicated a decline in the prevalence of smoking among adults in the United States from 40% in 1965 to 29% in 1987 (133). The smoking rates in men and women are now much closer to one another than previously, because fewer women smokers have quit than men and because of an increase in the prevalence of adolescent and young women smokers. Approximately 789,000 smoking-related deaths were believed to have been avoided or postponed over the 22-year period from 1965 to 1987 because of smoking cessation and reduced initiation of smoking. However, smoking remains responsible for more than one in every six deaths in the United States, or over 400,000 annually. Because of the relatively large number of people who still smoke and the associated increased health risks, smoking is generally considered to be the single most preventable contributor to premature death in the United States. In addition to CVD, health hazards associated with smoking include a substantial increase in the risk of various forms of cancer (of the lungs, larynx, mouth, esophagus, bladder, and elsewhere) and of chronic obstructive lung disease. There is also a growing awareness of the adverse health consequences of involuntary, or passive, smoking; that is, nonsmoker exposure to smokers' smoke (134).

Epidemiological Studies

Major intrapopulation cross-sectional and cohort observational studies have consistently demonstrated a strong dose-related relationship between cigarette smoking and morbidity and mortality from CAD, particularly in populations with a high intake of dietary saturated fat and cholesterol (9,135). These include the studies within the National Cooperative Pooling Project in the United States (30), as well as similar studies in Canada, continental Europe, Great Britain, New Zealand, and Israel. On the other hand, in populations such as those of Japan and southern Europe that have a relatively low dietary intake of cholesterol and low saturated-fat and serum cholesterol levels, the relationship between smoking and CAD events is either weak or nonexistent (32,135).

In high-risk populations, such as those in the Framingham Study, people who smoke 20 or more cigarettes a day experience twice the incidence of heart attacks, a 70% greater rate of CAD mortality, and a threefold increase in the rate of sudden death as compared with nonsmokers (133,135). Furthermore, heavy smokers (those who consume two or more packs of cigarettes daily) show an incidence of coronary events four times that of nonsmokers and a CAD mortality rate twice as high. CAD event rates increase with increasing cigarette smoke exposure as measured by the usual number of cigarettes smoked daily, total years of smoking, and depth of inhalation. Similarly, the risk of both thromboembolic and hemorrhagic stroke increases with the number of cigarettes smoked daily (133,136). The relative risk for thromboembolic stroke is 1.5 to 3 times higher and for hemorrhagic stroke 3 to 4 times higher, respectively, for heavy smokers as compared with nonsmokers. Statistical adjustments for other risk factors for CVD do not significantly impact the increase in relative risk with smoking, illustrating its independent contribution. Cigarette smoking also acts synergistically with other physiological and behavioral risk factors to substantially increase the risk of CVD. However, persons whose smoking habits have been limited to pipes or cigars appear to be at a risk level for CVD similar to that of nonsmokers.

The cessation of smoking in observational studies results in a substantial reduction in CAD event rates as compared with participants who continue to smoke. Although within 5 years of quitting the risk level approaches that of nonsmokers, the persistence in increased residual risk is proportional to the total lifetime exposure to cigarette smoke (134,135). In addition, individuals with known heart disease who continue to smoke have over twice the mortality rate of that of persons who quit smoking.

The health consequences of involuntary or passive smoking, including its relationship to CVD, have been reviewed by the Surgeon General (134). Approximately 85% of involuntary smoking exposure comes from side-stream smoke that emanates from the lit end of the cigarette between puffs. Side-stream particles are smaller than mainstream particles and are more likely to penetrate deeper into distal alveoli. In addition, the concentration of carbon monoxide is 2.5 times higher in side-stream smoke than in mainstream smoke.

The relationship of involuntary smoking to CVD has been the subject of a number of epidemiological studies. Among participants in the Multiple Risk Factor Intervention Trial, male nonsmokers whose wives smoked had twice the risk of fatal and nonfatal CAD events as compared with nonsmokers with nonsmoking wives after statistical adjustment for other risk factors (137). These findings were in agreement with those of a cohort study by Garland et al. (138) involving men and women aged 50 to 79 years. After multivariate adjustment for possible confounding variables, the relative risk of death due to CAD was 2.7 for women married to smokers or former smokers in this study. The Framingham Study (139) also observed excess CAD deaths in nonsmoking women married to men who quit, demonstrating the sustained adverse effects of involuntary smoking. In a follow-up study in Scotland, rates of death for nonsmoking men and women exposed to secondary smoke were significantly higher when compared with nonexposed nonsmokers (140). However, in the Scottish study, other risk factors were not adjusted for in the analysis and the difference was not tested for statistical significance. In a Japanese cohort study, Hirayama (141) observed an elevated risk for CAD in nonsmoking women married to smokers (relative risk of 1.3), but he also did not adjust for other risk factors. More research is clearly needed in this area. Involuntary smoking also has been shown to exacerbate angina pectoris (142). In contrast, in a case-controlled study Lee et al. (143) found no significant difference between subjects with clinically evident heart disease and matched controls in their exposure to involuntary smoking, based on smoking habits of spouses or on an index of total exposure to secondary smoking at work, home, or during travel or leisure activities.

Despite the strong link between smoking and CAD in observational studies within populations, smoking rates among countries do not parallel heart disease rates. For example, no association was evident between cigarette smoking and the 10-year incidence of coronary events in the Seven Countries Study (32). In this study the Japanese cohorts were the heaviest smokers but had the lowest risk of CAD events. Furthermore, within individual cohorts, the influence of smoking on the risk of CAD events was most evident in persons in whom CAD incidence was highest; that is, in cohorts in whom the mean serum cholesterol levels and associated dietary intake of saturated fat and cholesterol were high. Thus, it appears that the risk of CAD associated with smoking depends on the serum cholesterol level, which implies an interactive effect (135). Based on these findings, it appears again from observational-study data that diet and serum cholesterol play an essential role in the coronary atherogenesis process and that cigarette smoking, like elevated BP, serves as an accelerating factor.

Strong positive associations between cigarette smoking and occlusive atherosclerotic PVD or intermittent claudication have been well documented by observational studies since the early 1900s (135). People with PVD have a 10-fold greater risk of abdominal aneurysms as compared with matched control subjects.

Autopsy Studies

A large body of evidence from autopsy studies, based on both retrospective and cohort smoking data, confirms the positive association of smoking with the severity of atherosclerosis. The contribution of smoking to atherosclerosis appears to be more pronounced in the aorta than in the coronary arteries (136,144). In a review article Solberg and Strong (144) identified five retrospective autopsy studies and three prospective studies with autopsy follow-ups that all showed positive associations between cigarette smoking and quantitative measures of the severity of aortic atherosclerosis. The retrospective studies included autopsy findings in deceased men in New Orleans from the International Atherosclerosis Project (145). Raised atherosclerotic lesions in the abdominal aorta were more extensive in heavier smokers than in nonsmokers, with a definitive trend for more extensive and severe lesions with increasing levels of smoking. In addition, aortic aneurysms at autopsy were about eight times more frequent in smokers than nonsmokers.

Most of the autopsy studies showed a positive association between smoking and coronary atherosclerotic lesions (136,144). Retrospective studies showing a progressive increase in the extent of CAD atherosclerosis with increasing amounts of smoking included American male veterans who came to autopsy (146) and deceased men in New Orleans (145). In addition, one cohort study, the Honolulu Heart Study, revealed significant positive associations between cigarette smoking and measures of the severity of atherosclerosis in both the coronary arteries and aortas in Japanese-American men (147). However, two other major prospective studies failed to find an association between cigarette smoking and the extent of coronary atherosclerosis (136).

The association between cigarette smoking and the extent of cerebral atherosclerosis at autopsy has not been as fully investigated. One small-scale study in Sweden found more extensive atherosclerotic lesions in the basilar arteries of smokers than nonsmokers, and the Oslo Heart Study showed a positive trend, although it did not achieve statistical significance (136). A recent study involving patients who underwent carotid arteriography at the Mayo Clinic found that cigarette smoking was an independent predictor of the severity of extracranial carotid artery atherosclerosis (75).

Reduction in Risk of Coronary Artery Disease After Smoking Cessation

As previously indicated, observational studies have clearly and consistently demonstrated a substantial reduction in the risk of initial or recurrent MI and CAD deaths among ex-smokers within the first few years of smoking cessation (135,136). However, these findings are weakened by self-selection of those who quit smoking. Even after controlling for other risk factors, it remains uncertain whether other characteristics of quitters and of those who continue to smoke contributed to the differences in future CAD event rates.

The few clinical trials that randomized subjects to either a smoking cessation program or control group reduced but did not completely eliminate potential biases. Obviously, such trials cannot be blinded nor ethically require those in the control group to continue smoking; furthermore, there are major compliance problems involved. The interpretation of the results of the limited number of such trials therefore depends not only on the efficacy of smoking cessation in reducing the risk of CAD events but also on the percentage of those who quit smoking in both the intervention and comparison groups and the lag phase between smoking cessation and the reduction of CAD events risk (135).

Three major randomized primary prevention trials involving high-risk individuals have included smoking intervention: The Oslo Diet–Smoking Cessation Study (56), which involved hypercholesterolemic normotensive individuals, had only a 24% smoking quit rate in the intervention group as compared with a 18% quit rate in the control group. Multivariate analysis suggested that the observed significant reduction in fatal and nonfatal MIs in the intervention group in this study was due primarily to a reduction in serum total cholesterol level rather than smoking cessation. The Multiple Risk Factor Intervention Trial observed a statistically nonsignificant 7% reduction in the 7-year CAD mortality rate among men in the intervention group as compared with the controls (57). However, men who quit smoking in both study groups had half the 7-year CAD mortality as those who continued to smoke. The Whitehall

Study, in Great Britain, the only major CAD prevention trial that was limited to smoking intervention, observed a 21% reduction in major CAD events in the intervention group as compared with the control group (135,136).

An additional study, the WHO Collaborative Trial, was a multifactorial CAD primary prevention trial that randomized factories in four European countries into intervention and control groups (148). In this study, a mean reduction of 9 cigarettes per day in men in intervention factories was associated with an 8% reduction in the CAD death rate over 6 years.

After an MI, individuals who quit smoking clearly have a much more favorable survival rate than those who continue to smoke (135). The increased survival rate observed in several epidemiological studies was greater than that attributed to beta-blocking agents or exercise training in other secondary prevention trials. However, there have been no secondary CAD prevention trials specifically limited to smoking cessation. In a comprehensive, post-MI, rehabilitation–health education study in Finland, men and women MI survivors were randomized to an intervention or control group and then followed for 3 years (149). Health education included antismoking strategies, dietary advice, and a self-administered physical activity program. Although there was a significant reduction (36%) in CAD deaths in the intervention group as compared with the control group, this could not be attributed to smoking cessation, since cigarette smoking was reduced 50% in both the intervention and control groups. There have as yet been no major studies to study the impact of smoking cessation on prognosis following CABG surgery or angioplasty.

Plausible Mechanisms

Cigarette smoke contains over 4,000 chemical constituents. Of these, nicotine and carbon monoxide appear to be the principal contributors to the adverse cardiovascular effects of smoking. Proposed mechanisms of the increased risk are outlined here.

a. Adrenergic stimulating effects of nicotine:
   - Increase myocardial oxygen requirements
   - Increased dysrhythmias and reduced ventricular fibrillation threshold

b. Carbon monoxide toxicity
   - Reduces oxygen-carrying capacity of the blood and oxygen delivery to the heart due to carboxyhemoglobin formation

- Interferes with myocardial aerobic metabolism
- Has a negative ionotropic effect
- Reduces ventricular fibrillation threshold

c. Direct and indirect synergistic effects of nicotine and carbon monoxide on progression and severity of atherosclerosis

- Reduces plasma HDL cholesterol levels
- Increases platelet adhesiveness and tendency for thrombosis

Nicotine. Nicotine in cigarette smoke is rapidly absorbed from the lungs, with almost the same efficacy as intravenous administration, with peak plasma concentrations after a cigarette of 25 to 50 ng/ml is smoked (150). Its elimination half-life in a chronic smoker is about 2 h. The circulating nicotine results in vasoconstriction, tachycardia, and elevated resting systolic and diastolic BP that are characteristically most marked with the first cigarette of the day. These cardiovascular responses to nicotine are the result of catecholamine release through stimulation of the sympathetic nervous system and adrenal medulla, and activation of chemoreceptors of the aortic and carotid bodies (150). These hemodynamic changes increase myocardial oxygen demand, which theoretically could induce myocardial ischemia, angina pectoris, ventricular dysrhythmias, and sudden death in the presence of severe coronary arteriosclerosis. Coronary artery spasm due to alpha-adrenergic stimulation is another possibility. In a classic experimental study, a 30% to 40% decrease in ventricular fibrillation threshold from an electrical stimulus was demonstrated both in healthy dogs and in dogs with experimentally induced MI created through inhalation of cigarette smoke, confirming the increased risk of sudden death with cigarette smoking following one MI (151).

However, tolerance to chronic nicotine exposure in smokers may include a small reduction in the basal BP level. This, in turn, may lead to a small rebound increase (< 5 mm Hg) in systolic and diastolic BP levels upon quitting smoking (152), a phenomenon that appears to be independent of the concomitant weight gain prevalent in people who quit smoking. To minimize the anticipated increase in BP, a combination of weight maintenance, reduced salt and alcohol intake, and increased physical activity is recommended for people about to quit smoking.

Carbon Monoxide. Considerable evidence also supports the role of carbon monoxide as a major contributing factor to CAD events in cigarette smokers (135,136,153). Incomplete combustion of organic materials in cigarettes gives rise to carbon monoxide, which is inhaled along with other volatile components of smoke. Typically, the pulmonary capillary blood is exposed to at least 400 ppm of carbon monoxide during the smoking of one cigarette (153). Since the affinity of hemoglobin for carbon monoxide is about 245 times greater than its affinity for oxygen, carbon monoxide displaces oxygen from hemoglobin, decreasing the amount of oxygen available to the myocardium. A rise in venous carboxyhemoglobin levels also causes a leftward shift in the oxyhemoglobin dissociation curve, resulting in tighter binding of oxygen to hemoglobin. This further reduces the availability of oxygen to the myocardium. In addition, carbon monoxide binds to myoglobin, impairing the diffusion of oxygen to mitochondria in heart muscle fibers. Aerobic metabolism in the heart is further impaired by carbon monoxide binding to cytochrome oxidase.

Increased carboxyhemoglobin levels, even from the relatively small amounts of carbon monoxide inhaled after exposure to passive smoking, can decrease the ischemic threshold for the onset of angina pectoris (142,153). This reflects the decrease in myocardial oxygen supply. Furthermore, venous carboxyhemoglobin levels correlate well in smokers with the initial development of angina pectoris, MI, and intermittent claudication.

Like nicotine, carbon monoxide has been shown experimentally in animals to reduce the ventricular fibrillation threshold (153). Carbon monoxide exposure also can cause an impairment in LVF.

Further, as previously mentioned, both nicotine and carbon monoxide appear to accelerate the atherosclerotic process in the presence of hypercholesterolemia by promoting coronary endothelial injury and lipid insudation. Indirectly, smoking further enhances atherogenesis by reducing plasma HDL cholesterol levels and perhaps by increasing LDL cholesterol concentration (135). Further, nicotine and carboxyhemoglobin increase platelet adhesiveness and thereby increase the possibility of coronary artery thrombosis (133,153).

Comment

The evidence is strong that both nicotine and carbon monoxide contribute to the increase in nonfatal and fatal MI and sudden cardiac death in cigarette smokers by acting synergistically with other major risk factors to promote atherosclerosis. In addition, nicotine increases myocardial oxygen demands, and carboxyhemoglobin reduces myocardial supply and myocardial function. Furthermore, both chemicals promote tendencies for coronary thrombosis and lower the threshold for ventricular fibrillation in the presence of myocardial ischemia. Limited clinical evidence also supports the probability that smoking cessation can reduce the risk of initial or recurrent CVD events.

Obesity and Risk of Cardiovascular Disease

Overweight and associated obesity (excess fat) are prevalent conditions in the United States. Obesity is generally considered a contributor to many major health problems, including non–insulin-dependent diabetes mellitus and some forms of cancer (29,154). However, its contribution to the etiology of atherosclerotic CVD, particularly CAD, is the source of considerable controversy and remains an enigma. Although studies clearly show that excess weight increases the risk of a number of metabolic and physiological risk factors related to atherosclerosis, widely divergent results have been reported in observational studies between the association of overweight or measures of body fatness and severity of atherosclerosis and incidence of CAD (155). Confounding factors, such as a lower incidence of obesity in cigarette smokers, may contribute to the discrepancies among epidemiological studies but are not the entire explanation. The distribution of body fat and related different phenotypes of obesity and associated metabolic characteristics have emerged as important predictors of health hazards related to obesity (156). So-called upper-body obesity (also called male, or android, obesity), characterized by excessive fat concentrated in the abdominal region, is now generally believed to be the most atherogenic form of obesity with the strongest relationship to CVD. Not distinguishing different obesity phenotypes in epidemiological studies may contribute to the confusion regarding the role of obesity in the etiology of atherosclerosis and heart disease. In addition, a recent observational study suggests that wide fluctuations in body weight, which commonly occur with the so-called yo-yo diet syndrome, may increase risk of atherosclerotic CVD and contribute to the confusion in this area (157).

Weight Standards

The most frequently employed standards for body weight relative to height and gender are those derived from the Metropolitan Life Insurance Co.'s Actuarial Mortality Follow-up Study data, initially published in 1959 and updated in 1984 (158,159). The tables generated by these studies are based on body weight associated with the lowest mortality rate among insured adults in the United States. Unfortunately, these height-weight tables are flawed by well-recognized conceptual and methodological limitations:

a. the population sample is not representative;
b. age is not taken into consideration;
c. the technical quality of the data is suspect because of nonstandardized or self-reported height and weight measurements, the subjective nature of frame-size determinations in the 1959 data set, and a nonvalidated method for frame-size determinations (elbow width) reflected in the 1984 tables;
d. the data fail to adjust statistically for confounding factors that affect mortality rate, such as cigarette smoking; and
e. the expression of relative weight as a percentage of standard weight for height does not accurately reflect body fat levels or distribution (although relative weight is significantly correlated with direct measurements or estimates of body fatness, the association is not strong, leaving a considerable percentage of the variance in body fatness unexplained) (155,160,161).

Nevertheless, the use of these height-weight tables for determining relative weight is entrenched in both medical and lay culture, and they are commonly employed as a surrogate for fatness, which is more difficult to measure than body weight.

A Consensus Development Conference on the Health Implications of Obesity sponsored by the National Institutes of Health in 1985 recommended using the 1959 Metropolitan Life tables as standards rather than the 1984 tables because of concerns about the higher standard weight, particularly for the shortest stature groups, in the latter tables (160). In addition, the conference recommended that the midpoint of the weight range for the middle frame size for a given height be used as the optimal, or standard, weight. Using this criterion, a person is considered "significantly overweight" (and probably excessively fat) if he or she weighs at least 20% more than the standard weight (160).

As an alternative to the life insurance tables, Keys et al. (161) proposed the use of a weight-height squared ratio called the body mass index

(BMI) and is commonly expressed as kg/m². The BMI has a stronger relationship to body fatness than percent of standard weight; however, it still accounts for only 43% to 66% of the variance in body fatness. Nevertheless, the National Center for Health Statistics in the United States has proposed weight standards based on BMI data derived from a survey of a representative sample of the non-institutionalized, civilian American population in 1976 to 1980; these data are derived from the 1976-1980 Second National Health and Nutrition Examination Survey (NHANES II) (154). In these proposed standards *overweight* is defined as a BMI in the 85th percentile for men and women aged 20 to 29 years in the NHANES II population sample. This is based on the assumption that weight gain after 29 years of age is most likely due to fat accumulation (i.e., people over 29 years would still use the data for ages 20 to 29 to determine if they are overweight). *Severe overweight* is defined as a BMI at the 95th percentile for the same age group. The BMI values for men are 27.8 or greater and 31.1 or greater for "overweight" and "severely overweight," respectively. The corresponding cut-off values for women are 27.3 and 32.3.

Prevalence of Overweight in the United States

Based on the NHANES II data and the BMI standards just mentioned, it was estimated that about 34 million, or 26%, of noninstitutionalized civilian Americans aged 20 to 74 were overweight and 12.4 million were severely overweight as of the late 1970s (154). This represents an 18% increase in prevalence of overweight persons and a 48% increase in severely overweight persons relative to results of NHANES II's predecessor, NHANES I, which covered 1971 to 1975. The prevalence of overweight is consistently higher for men above the poverty line, but the reverse is true for women, particularly African-American women.

Epidemiological Studies

Since 1930, studies of mortality rates among insured persons have consistently observed an association between relative weight and rate of mortality. According to 1979 insurance company mortality studies, the lowest mortality rate in men under 50 was that of subjects whose weights fell between 5% and 15% below standard weight for height (158,162). In men aged 50 or older, the optimal weight lay closer to the standard weight. Among women, the optimal weight was in the range of 5% to 15% below standard at virtually all ages. In both sexes, the relative mortality rate rose progressively with increasing overweight: the relative risks of mortality for men 20%, 40%, and 60% overweight were 1.2, 1.4, and 1.9, respectively, and for women were 1.1, 1.2, and 1.4. Medical conditions contributing to excess mortality rates were heart and circulatory diseases, diabetes, digestive disorders, strokes, and cancer (the latter in women 50% or more overweight only). The American Cancer Society also observed a weak linear association between self-reported body weight and subsequent mortality in a cohort of volunteers (162).

In contrast to these results, cohort studies from more representative populations of North American and European men and women have failed to consistently confirm an association between relative weight, BMI, or skinfold estimates of body fatness and all-cause mortality or morbidity and mortality from CAD. In an extensive review of cross-sectional and prospective epidemiological studies on this topic, Larsson et al. (163) observed in 10 reports U- or J-shaped associations of over-weight with total mortality; that is, the death rates were higher at both the upper and lower extremes of body weight. In two reports, a monotonic increase in mortality was found with increasing weight, but two other reports failed to find such an association. In seven studies evaluating the relationship between weight and CAD mortality, four showed a positive association while three showed no association. Similarly, in seven studies of relative weight and the incidence of CAD events, three showed a positive association and four found no association. More recently Hubert (164) reviewed 10 prospective studies and concluded that only 6 of them observed an independent association of some measure of overweight or obesity in men with a subsequent incidence of CAD events.

The 10-year follow-up to the Seven Countries Study failed to find a significant positive relationship between either relative weight, BMI, or skinfold thickness and CAD death in any of the 16 cohorts of men aged 40 to 59 years at entry (32). In fact, in most cohorts the probability of death appeared to be lowest for men who were above average in terms of relative weight or fatness. In Finland, where CAD event rates were the highest, the lowest frequency of "hard" fatal and nonfatal CAD end points was seen in men in the upper decile of relative weight. Furthermore, relative weight was inversely related to CAD death in Southern European populations who were at relatively low risk for CAD.

The eight cohort studies making up the U.S. National Cooperative Pooling Project also found discrepant results, with either a U-shaped relationship, a positive relationship, or no relationship of overweight with CAD (30,155). However, the Framingham Study and pooled data from five of its eight cohorts in the Pooling Project showed statistically significant linear relationships between relative weight and CAD events (155). In the Framingham Study, the relative risk of premature death in overweight (> 110% of standard weight) nonsmoking men was about four times higher than that of nonsmoking men who were at normal weight (100% to 109%) at 30-year follow-up (165). Surprisingly, however, weight loss also was strongly associated with excess overall mortality at this follow-up.

More recently, marked weight fluctuations and high variability in body weight measurements have been reported to be associated with excess total mortality and morbidity, and with mortality from CAD, in both men and women in the Framingham Study cohort (166). The relative risk of these end points in subjects with marked weight fluctuations, as compared with those whose weight was relatively stable, ranged from about 1.3 to 1.9. The negative health consequences of weight fluctuations, including an increased risk of CAD, also has been observed in other cohort studies in which it has been investigated (157).

The Framingham Study and several other large cohort studies have also recently demonstrated significant associations between regional body fat distribution patterns and atherosclerotic CVD and related mortality (156). A high proportion of trunk or abdominal body fat (variously called trunk-abdominal, upper-body, android, male-type, or "apple-shaped" obesity) is reported to be associated with increased risks of developing CVD and premature mortality in both men and women as compared with generalized obesity or typical female fat topography (hip-gluteal, lower-body, gynoid, or "pear-shaped" obesity). Upper-body obesity may be identified by using skinfold measurements (subscapular versus triceps) or by a ratio of waist to hip circumferences of greater than 1.0 in men or 0.8 in women. Computerized tomography has been touted as a much more precise quantitative measurement of regional fat distribution; it can also delineate the amount of deep intra-abdominal or visceral fat stores. Excess visceral fat also appears to be strongly related to an increased risk of CVD, hypertension, and diabetes mellitus (156).

Possible reasons for inconsistencies in the association of overweight and CAD, even by univariate (unadjusted) analysis, has been a topic of much discussion and debate. Proposed contributing factors include a misclassification bias, including fail-ure to distinguish between different fat distribution phenotypes; confounding factors (including the inverse association of obesity with cigarette smoking); or the possibility of protective factors associated with overweight, which counteract other risk factor effects (e.g., associated hormonal changes such as increased circulating estrogen levels) (155).

Postmortem Studies

Autopsy studies, including the International Atherosclerosis Project, failed to find any association between several measures of obesity or remote or recent body weight levels and events of atherosclerosis (37). The few autopsy studies of men with chronic morbid obesity (45.4 kg above a desirable weight or 100% excess weight) surprisingly found no association with significant coronary atherosclerosis, although such men had excess overall age-adjusted mortality rates and were prone to cardiac hypertrophy and CHF (155,167). On the other hand, it is well documented that atherosclerosis is substantially reduced or absent at autopsy in grossly malnourished or cachectic individuals.

Experimental Data

No experimental animal data supporting a relationship between obesity and atherosclerosis are available. Similarly, no controlled trials involving humans to determine the effects of intervention on obesity on either CAD rates or angiographically defined coronary atherosclerosis have been performed.

Secular Trends

Secular trend data also fail to support the hypothesis that obesity is an important independent contributor to atherosclerotic CVD. As previously indicated, NHANES data on a representative sample of the U.S. population have shown that there was a consistent increase in the proportion of the adult population in the United States who were overweight between 1962 and 1980 (154). During the same period, the CVD and CAD mortality rates and stroke progressively and substantially declined, trends attributed to a combination of factors, including a decline in dietary cholesterol and saturated fat intake, associated with a reduced population mean of serum total cholesterol; better detection and more vigorous treatment of hypertension; a marked reduction of cigarette smoking, particularly in men; increased exercise levels; and improved medical management of patients with coronary disease (168).

Biological Relationship of Mechanisms

The relationships between obesity and several metabolic and physiological atherogenic risk factors have been well documented, making it difficult to explain the lack of any clear association between overweight and CAD risk (in observational studies) and the absence of an association between obesity and severity of atherosclerosis based on postmortem findings. For example, hypertension and obesity are clearly related: The prevalence of hypertension is 50% higher in overweight than in underweight adults, and up to one third of hypertensive patients are overweight (169). In addition, changes in body weight in prospective studies in both normotensive and hypertensive patients are associated with changes in the same direction in systolic and diastolic BP levels (169). Furthermore, the two disorders synergistically burden the heart, increase left ventricular stroke work, and produce LVH by different mechanisms (102,109). Weight-reduction programs in obese individuals have consistently noted reduction in systolic and diastolic BP levels in both normotensive and hypertensive patients. Schotte and Stunkard (170) recently reported that a mean weight loss of 10.4 kg in 301 obese patients was accompanied by mean decrease of 10 mm Hg in systolic and 8 mm Hg in diastolic BP. In patients who were hypertensive, every kilogram of weight loss over the first 8 to 10 weeks of treatment was associated with a mean reduction of over 4 mm Hg in systolic pressure and 2 mm Hg to 3 mm Hg in diastolic BP.

Obesity is also commonly associated with alterations in lipoprotein metabolism, which would be expected to enhance atherogenesis (29). Obese individuals generally have increased total body cholesterol production and stores, increased production of very low-density lipoprotein (VLDL) triglycerides by the liver, increased plasma LDL cholesterol levels, and reduced plasma HDL cholesterol levels. Conversely, a reduction of excess weight generally has a favorable impact on the blood lipid profile. For example, in the Framingham Study a 10% reduction in weight was associated with an 11 mg/dL decrease in serum total cholesterol level (171). The beneficial effects of weight loss on reducing elevated blood triglyceride levels are also well documented; however, the contribution of weight reduction to raising low HDL cholesterol levels is quite variable (172).

A variety of epidemiological data indicate that obesity is a major risk factor for non–insulin-dependent (Type II) diabetes mellitus, along with heredity, aging, and reduced physical activity (173). About 80% of individuals with Type II diabetes are obese. The chances for becoming diabetic more than doubles with every 20% excess in body weight. In addition, experimentally induced weight gain in both animals and humans causes cell insulin resistance, the usual underlying principal pathophysiological basis for Type II diabetes (29,173). Diabetes, in turn, by a combination of different mechanisms, markedly increases the risk of CAD, stroke, and occlusive PVD, as well as renal disease, visual impairment, and premature mortality (173). Epidemiological evidence also exists that hyperinsulinemia, common in obese people with or without Type II diabetes, is an independent risk factor for CAD (174). It is postulated that elevated blood insulin levels, due to cell insulin resistance, increase BP levels, contribute to blood lipid-lipoprotein abnormalities, and accelerate the severity of atherosclerosis even in nondiabetic persons (175-177). As previously mentioned, recent data strongly suggest that upper-body obesity (or the presence of large amounts of visceral fat) is more likely than other types of obesity to be associated with hyperinsulinemia, as well as with other risk factors for CVD (156).

Comment

We conclude that despite the contradictory epidemiological data, there is substantial evidence that obesity, particularly the type associated with a predominance of fat in the abdominal region, indirectly increases the risk of CAD by its influence on atherogenic risk factors. In addition, preliminary evidence suggests that large weight fluctuations, so common in dieters, may also adversely affect the risk of CAD. Therefore, preventing obesity or *the loss of excess weight with subsequent maintenance of the attained lower weight*, particularly in those with a tendency for abdominal accumulation of fat, should be important aspects of a program for preventing CVD as well as Type II diabetes mellitus.

Summary

Coronary heart disease is a multifactorial disease. In this chapter the evidence was reviewed on the important contributions of major nonmodifiable and modifiable risk factors, particularly dietary factors, hypertension, cigarette smoking, and obesity. The evidence of the contributing roles of physical activity and fitness and of diabetes mellitus are discussed in other chapters.

References

1. American Heart Association. 1990 heart and stroke facts. Dallas: The American Heart Association; 1989:1-43.
2. Ross, R. The pathogenesis of atherosclerosis—An update. N. Engl. J. Med. 314:488-500; 1986.
3. Hopkins, P.N.; Williams, R.S. Identification and relative weight of cardiovascular risk factors. Cardiol. Clin. 4(1):3-31; 1986.
4. MacMahon, B.; Pugh, T.F. Epidemiology. Principles and methods. Boston: Little, Brown; 1970:17-46.
5. Blackburn, H.; Leon, A.S. Preventive cardiology in practice: Minnesota studies on risk factor reduction. In: Pollock, M.L.; Schmidt, D.H., eds. Heart disease and rehabilitation. 2nd ed. Boston: Houghton Mifflin; 1985:170-192.
6. Leon, A.S. Age and other predictors of coronary heart disease. Med. Sci. Sports Exerc. 19:159-167; 1987.
7. Stokes, J. Cardiovascular risk factors. In: Frohlich, E.D.; Brest, A.N., eds. Preventive aspects of coronary heart disease. Cardiovascular clinics. Philadelphia: Davis; 1990:3-20.
8. Arenson, F.W.; Strong, W.B.; Watkins, L.O.; Balfour, I.C. Pediatric aspects of atherosclerosis and hypertension: The physician's responsibility. In: Hutchinson, R.G., ed. Coronary prevention. A clinical guide. Chicago: Year Book Medical; 1985:9-46.
9. Kannel, W.B. An overview of the risk factors for cardiovascular disease. In: Kaplan, N.H.; Stamler, J., eds. Prevention of coronary heart disease. Philadelphia: Saunders; 1983:20-32.
10. Johansson, W.; Vedin, A.; Wilhelmsen, C. Myocardial infarction in women. Epidemiol. Rev. 5:67-95; 1983.
11. Ayanian, J.Z.; Epstein, A.M. Differences in the use of procedures between women and men hospitalized for coronary heart disease. N. Engl. J. Med. 325:221-225; 1991.
12. Healy, B. The Yentl syndrome (editorial). N. Engl. J. Med. 325:274-276; 1991.
13. Palmer, J.R.; Rosenberg, L.; Shapiro, S. "Low yield" cigarettes and the risk of nonfatal myocardial infarction in women. N. Engl. J. Med. 320:1569-1573; 1989.
14. LaRosa, J.C. Oral contraceptives, lipoproteins, and coronary disease. Perspectives in Lipid Disorders. 6(2):13-19; 1989.
15. Bush, T.L.; Barrett-Connor, E. Noncontraceptive estrogen use and cardiovascular disease. Epidemiol. Rev. 7:80-104; 1985.
16. Henderson, B.E.; Paganini-Hill, A.; Ross, R.K. Decreased mortality in users of estrogen replacement therapy. Arch. Intern. Med. 151:75-78; 1991.
17. Moon, T.E. Estrogen and disease prevention (editorial). Arch. Intern. Med. 151:17-18; 1991.
18. Rosenberg, L.; Hennekens, C.H.; Rosner, B.; Belanger, C.; Rothman, K.J.; Speizer, F.E. Early menopause and risk of myocardial infarction. Am. J. Obstet. Gynecol. 139:47-51; 1981.
19. Gordon, T.; Kannel, W.B.; Hjortland, M.C.; McNamara, M. Menopause and coronary heart disease: The Framingham study. Ann. Intern. Med. 89:157-161; 1978.
20. Wing, R.R.; Matthews, K.A.; Kuller, L.H.; Meilahn, E.N.; Plantinga, P.L. Weight gain at the time of the menopause. Arch. Intern. Med. 151:97-102; 1991.
21. Muller, J.E.; Stone, P.H.; Turi, Z.G.; Rutherford, J.D.; Czeisler, C.A.; Parker, C.; Poole, W.K.; Passamani, E.; Roberts, R.; Robertson, T.; Sobel, B.E.; Willerson, J.T.; Braunwald, E.; the MILS Study Group. Circadian variation in the frequency of acute myocardial infarction. N. Engl. J. Med. 313:1315-1322; 1985.
22. Mitler, M.M.; Kripke, D.F.; Schwab, E.M.; Burke, H.B.; Miller, J.E. Circadian rhythms in myocardial infarction. N. Engl. J. Med. 314:1187-1189; 1986.
23. Quyyumi, A.A.; Mockus, L.; Wright, C.; Fox, K.M. Morphology of ambulatory ST segment change in patients with varying severity of coronary artery disease. Investigation of the frequency of nocturnal ischemia and coronary spasm. Br. Heart J. 33:186-193; 1985.
24. Verdecchia, P.; Schillaci, G.; Guerrieni, M.; Gatteschi, C.; Benemio, G.; Boldrini, F.; Porcellati, C. Circadian blood pressure changes and left ventricular hypertrophy in essential hypertension. Circulation. 81:528-536; 1990.
25. Fletcher, G.F.; Blair, S.N.; Blumenthal, J. Position statement on exercise. Benefits and recommendations for physical activity programs for all Americans, from the American Heart Association. Circulation. 86:340-344; 1992.
26. Leon, A.S. Physical activity and risk of ischemic heart disease—an update 1990. In: Oja, P.; Telema, R., eds. Sport for all. Amsterdam: Elsevier Science; 1991:251-264.
27. NIH consensus conference: Lowering blood cholesterol to prevent heart disease. JAMA. 253:2080-2095; 1985.
28. Anonymous. Report of the national cholesterol education program expert panel on detection, evaluation and treatment of high blood cholesterol in adults. Arch. Intern. Med. 148:36-69; 1988.
29. National Research Council. Diet and health. Implications for reducing chronic disease risk. Washington, DC: National Academy Press; 1989:1-749.
30. The Pooling Project Research Group. Relationship of blood pressure, serum cholesterol, smoking habit, relative weight, and ECG abnormalities to incidence of major coronary events: Final report of the pooling project. J. Chronic Dis. 31:201-306; 1978.

31. Keys, A., editor. Coronary heart disease in seven countries. Circulation. 41[Suppl I]:1-211; 1970.

32. Keys, A. Seven countries. A multivariate analysis of death and coronary heart disease. Cambridge, MA: Harvard University Press; 1980:1-381.

33. Stamler J.; Wentworth, D.; Neaton, J.D. Is the relationship between serum cholesterol and risk of premature death from coronary heart disease continuous or graded? Findings in 356,222 primary screenees of the multiple risk factor intervention trial (MRFIT). JAMA. 256:2823-2828; 1986.

34. Pekkanen, J.; Linn, S.; Heiss, G.; Suchindran, C.M.; Leon, A.S.; Rifkind, B.M.; Tyroler, H.A. Ten-year mortality from cardiovascular disease among men with and without pre-existing cardiovascular disease. N. Engl. J. Med. 322:1700-1707; 1990.

35. Stampfer, M.J.; Sacks, F.M.; Salvini, S.; Willett, W.; Hennekens, C.H. A prospective study of cholesterol, apolipoproteins, and the risk of myocardial infarction. N. Engl. J. Med. 323:373-381; 1991.

36. Robertson, T.L.; Kato, H.; Rhodes, G.G.; Kagan, M.; Marmot, S.L.; Syme, T.; Gordon, R.M.; Worth, J.L.; Belsky, J.S.; Miyanishi, M.; Kawamoto, S. Epidemiologic studies of coronary heart disease and stroke in Japanese men living in Japan, Hawaii, and California: Incidence of myocardial infarction and death from coronary heart disease. Am. J. Cardiol. 39:239-243; 1977.

37. McGill, H.C., Jr., editor. The geographic pathology of atherosclerosis. Baltimore: Williams & Wilkins; 1968, and Lab. Invest. 18(5):463-633; 1968.

38. Reed D,M,; Strong, J.P.; Resch, J.; Hayashi, T. Serum lipids and lipoproteins as predictors of atherosclerosis. An autopsy study. Arteriosclerosis. 9:560-564; 1989.

39. Schettler, G. Atherosclerosis during periods of food deprivation following World War I and II. Prev. Med. 12:75-83; 1983.

40. Goldstein, J.L.; Brown, M.S. Familial hypercholesterolemia. In: Stanbury, J.B.; Wyngaarden, J.B.; Fredrickson, D.S., eds. The metabolic basis of inherited diseases. 5th Ed. New York: McGraw-Hill; 1983:672-712.

41. Scamu, A.M.; Khalil, A.; Neven, L.; Tidore, M.; Dawson, G.; Pfaffinger, D.; Jackson, E.; Carey, K.D.; McGill, H.C.; Fless, G.M. Genetically-determined hypercholesterolemia in a rhesus monkey family due to a deficiency of the LDL receptor. J. Lipid Res. 29:1671-1681; 1988.

42. Wissler, R.W.; Vesselmovitch, D. The development and use of animal models in atherosclerosis research. In: Cardiovascular disease: Molecular and cellular mechanisms, prevention and treatment. New York: Plenum Press; 1987:337-357.

43. Keys, A.; Anderson, J.R.; Grande, F. Prediction of serum-cholesterol responses in man to changes in the diet. Lancet 2:959-966; 1957.

44. Keys, A. Serum cholesterol response to dietary cholesterol. Am. J. Clin. Nutr. 40:351-359; 1984.

45. Hegsted, D.M. Serum cholesterol response to dietary cholesterol: A re-evaluation. Am. J. Clin. Nutr. 44:299-305; 1986.

46. Connor, W.E.; Stone, D.B.; Hodges, R.E. The interrelated effects of dietary cholesterol and fat upon serum lipid levels. J. Clin. Invest. 43:1691-1696; 1964.

47. Grundy, M.S. Monounsaturated fatty acids, plasma cholesterol, and coronary heart disease. Am. J. Clin. Nutr. 45:1237-1242; 1987.

48. Leon, A.S. Physiological interactions between diet and exercise in the etiology and prevention of ischemic heart disease. Ann. Clin. Res. 20:114-120; 1988.

49. Miettinen, T.A. Dietary fiber and lipids. Am. J. Clin. Nutr. 45:1237-1242; 1987.

50. Kinsella, J.E.; Lokesch, B.; Stone, R.A. Dietary n-3 polyunsaturated fatty acids and amelioration of cardiovascular disease: Possible mechanisms. Am. J. Clin. Nutr. 52:1-28; 1990.

51. Kromhout, D. N-3 fatty acids and coronary heart disease: Epidemiology from Eskimos to Western populations. J. Invest. Med. 225:47-52; 1989.

52. Zock, P.L.; Katan, M.B.; Merkus, M.P.; Dusseldorf, M.V.; Harryvan, J.L. Effect of a lipid-rich fraction from boiled coffee on serum cholesterol. Lancet. 335:1235-1237; 1990.

53. Aro, A.; Teirila, J.; Gref, C-G. Dose-dependent effect on serum cholesterol and apoprotein B by consumption of boiled, non-filtered coffee. Atherosclerosis. 83:257-261; 1990.

54. James, J.E. Caffeine and health. London: Academic Press; 1991:139-181.

55. National Diet-Heart Study Research Group. The national diet-heart study final report. Circulation. 37[Suppl. I]:1-248; 1968.

56. Hermann, I.; Holme, I.; Byre, K.V.; Laren, P. Effect of diet and smoking intervention on the incidence of coronary heart disease. Report of the Oslo study group of a randomized trial in healthy men. Lancet. 2:1303-1310; 1981.

57. Multiple Risk Factor Research Group. Multiple risk factor intervention trial: Risk factor changes and mortality results. JAMA. 248:1465-1477; 1982.

58. Multiple Risk Factor Intervention Trial Research Group. Mortality rates after 10.5 years for participants in the multiple risk factor intervention trial. Findings related to a prior hypothesis of the trial. JAMA. 263:1795-1801; 1990.

59. Lipid Research Clinics Program. The lipid research clinics coronary primary prevention trial results. I. Reduction in incidence of coronary heart disease. JAMA. 251:351-364; 1984.

60. Lipid Research Clinics Program. The lipid research clinics coronary primary prevention trial results. II. The relationship of reduction in incidence of coronary heart disease to cholesterol lowering. JAMA. 25:365-374; 1984.

61. Frick, M.H.J.; Elo, O.; Happa, K.; Heinonen, O.P.; Heinsalmi, P.; Helo, P.; Huttenen, J.K.; Kaitaniemi,

P.; Koskinen, P.; Mannien, V.; Maenpaa, H.; Makonen, M.; Mantaari, M.; Norola, S.; Pasternack, A.; Pikkarainen, J.; Romo, M.; Sjoblom, T.; Nikkila, A. Helsinki heart study: Primary prevention trial with gemfibrozil in middle-aged men with dyslipidemia. Safety of treatment changes in risk factors, and incidence of coronary heart disease. N. Engl. J. Med. 317:1237-1245; 1987.

62. Wysowski, D.K.; Gross, T.P. Deaths due to accidents and violence in two recent trials of cholesterol-lowering drugs. Arch. Intern. Med. 150:2169-2172; 1990.

63. Committee of Principal Investigators. WHO cooperative trial on primary prevention of ischaemic heart disease using clofibrate to lower serum cholesterol: Mortality follow-up. Lancet. 2:379-385; 1980.

64. The Coronary Drug Research Project Research Group. Clofibrate and niacin in coronary heart disease. JAMA. 231:360-381; 1975.

65. Canner, P.L.; Berge, K.G.; Wenger, N.K.; Stamler, J.; Friedman, L.; Prineas, R.J.; Friedewald, W. Fifteen year mortality in coronary drug project patients: Long term benefit with niacin. J. Am. Coll. Cardiol. 8:1245-1255; 1986.

66. Buchwald, H.; Varco, R.L.; Matts, J.P.; Long, J.M.; Fitch, L.L.; Campbell, G.S.; Pearce, M.B.; Yellin, A.E.; Edmiston, W.A.; Smink, R.D.; Sawin, H.S., Jr.; Campos, C.T.; Hansen, B.J.; Tuna, N.; Karnegis, J.N.; Sanmarco, M.E.; Amplatz, K.; Castasneda-Zuniga, W.R.; Hunter, D.W.; Bissett, J.K.; Weber, F.J.; Stevenson, J.W.; Leon, A.S.; Chalmers, T.C.; the Posch Group. Effect of partial ileal bypass surgery on mortality and morbidity from coronary heart disease in patients with hypercholesterolemia. N. Eng. J. Med. 323:946-955; 1990.

67. Superko, H.R. Drug therapy and the prevention of atherosclerosis in humans. Am. J. Cardiol. 64:316-386; 1989.

68. Bradford, R.H.; Shear, C.L.; Chremos, A.N.; Dujovne, C.; Downton, M.; Franklin, F.A.; Gould, A.L.; Hesney, M.; Higgins, J.; Hurley, D.P.; Langendorfer, A.; Nash, D.T.; Pool, J.L.; Schnaper, H. Expanded clinical evaluation of lovastatin (EXCEL) study results. I. Efficacy in modifying plasma lipoproteins and adverse event profile in 8,245 patients with moderate hypercholesterolemia. Arch. Intern. Med. 151:43-49; 1990.

69. Gould, K.L. Coronary artery stenosis. New York: Elsevier Science; 1991:121-135.

70. Blankenhorn, D.H.; Nessim, S.A.; Johnston, R.L.; Sanmarco, M.E.; Azen, S.P.; Capshen-Hemphill, L. Beneficial effects of combined colestipolniacin therapy on coronary atherosclerosis and coronary venous bypass grafts. JAMA. 257:3233-3240; 1987.

71. Ornish, D.; Brown, S.E.; Scherwitz, L.W.; Billings, J,H,; Armstrong, W.T.; Ports, T.A.; McLanahan, S.M.; Kirkeeide, R.L.; Brand, R.J.; Gould, K.L. Can lifestyle changes reverse coronary heart disease? The lifestyle heart trial. Lancet. 336:129-133; 1990.

72. Tell, G.S.; Crouse, J.R.; Furberg, C.D. Relation between blood lipids, lipoproteins, and cerebrovascular atherosclerosis. A review. Stroke. 19:423-430; 1988.

73. Kannel, W.B.; Wolf, P.A. Epidemiology of cerebrovascular disease. In: Russell, R.W.R., ed. Vascular disease of the central nervous system. 2nd ed. Edinburgh: Churchill Livingstone; 1983:1-24.

74. Iso, H.; Jacobs, D.R., Jr.; Wentworth, D.; Neaton, J.D.; Cohen, J. Relationship of serum cholesterol to risk of different types of strokes. N. Engl. J. Med. 320:904-910; 1990.

75. Homer, D.; Ingall, T.J.; Baker, H.L., Jr.; O'Fallon, W.M.; Kottke, B.A.; Whisant, J.P. Serum lipids and lipoprotein and cigarette smoking and hypertension. Mayo Clin. Proc. 66:259-267; 1991.

76. Tell, G.T. Cigarette smoking, lipids, lipoproteins, and extracranial carotid artery atherosclerosis. Mayo Clin. Proc. 66:327-331; 1991.

77. Gwynne, J.T. High-density lipoprotein cholesterol as a marker of reverse cholesterol-transport. Am. J. Cardiol. 64: 186-226; 1989.

78. Tyroler, H.A.; Levy, R.I.; Thorn, M.D.; Davis, C.E.; Deev, A.D.; Shestov, D.B. High density lipoprotein cholesterol and coronary heart disease mortality: Experience of white men aged 40 to 59 years in the U.S. lipid research clinics mortality follow-up study. Atherosclerosis Rev. 17:277-286; 1988.

79. Gordon, D.J.; Probstfield, J.L.; Garrison, R.J.; Neaton, J.D.; Castelli, W.P.; Knobe, J.D.; Jacobs, D.R., Jr.; Bangdiwala, S.; Tyroler, H.A. High-density lipoprotein cholesterol and cardiovascular disease. Four prospective American studies. Circulation. 79:8-15; 1989.

80. Castelli, W.P.; Garrison, R.J.; Wilson, P.W.; Abbott, R.D.; Kalousdian, S.; Kannel, W.B. Incidence of coronary heart disease and lipoprotein cholesterol levels. JAMA. 256:2835-2838; 1986.

81. Keys, A.; Karvonen, M.J.; Punsar, S.; Menotti, A.; Fidanza, F.; Farchi, G. HDL serum cholesterol and 24 year mortality of men in Finland. Int. J. Epidemiol. 13:428-435; 1984.

82. Miller, M.E. Associations of high-density lipoprotein cholesterol subclasses and apolipoproteins with ischemic heart disease and coronary atherosclerosis. Am. Heart J. 113:589-897; 1987.

83. Gordon, D.J.; Knoke, J.; Probstfield, J.L.; Superko, R.; Tyroler, H.A. High-density lipoproteins cholesterol and coronary heart disease in hypercholesterolemic men: The lipid research clinics coronary primary prevention trial. Circulation. 74:1217-1229; 1980.

84. Grundy, S.M.; Goodman, D.S.; Rifkind, B.M.; Cleeman, J.I. The place of HDL in cholesterol management. Arch. Intern. Med. 149:505-510; 1989.

85. Miles, L.A.; Fless, G.M.; Levin, E.G.; Scanu, A.M.; Plow, E.F. A potential basis for the thrombotic risks associated with lipoproteins (a). Nature. 339:303-305; 1989.

86. Uterman, G. Lipoprotein (a): A genetic risk factor for premature coronary heart disease. Nutri. Metab. Cardiovasc. Dis. 1:7-9; 1991.

87. Miller, M. Lp(a) and lipoproteins. Nontraditional coronary risk factors. Prev. Cardiol. Rep. 4(3):1-7; 1990.

88. Rhoades, G.G.; Dahlen, G.; Berg, K.; Morton, N.E.; Dannenberg, A.L. Lp(a) lipoprotein as a risk factor for myocardial infarction. JAMA. 256:2540-2544; 1986.

89. Armstrong, V.W.; Cremer, P.; Eberele, E.; Manke, A.; Schulze, F.; Wieland, H.; Kreuzer, H.; Seidel, D. The association between serum Lp(a) concentrations and angiographically assessed coronary atherosclerosis dependence on serum LPL levels. Atherosclerosis. 62:2149-2157; 1986.

90. Grundy, S.M.; Vega, G.L. Role of apolipoprotein levels in clinical practice. Arch. Intern. Med. 150:1579-1581; 1990.

91. Reinhart, R.A.; Gani, K.; Arndt, M.R,.;Broste, S.K. Apolipoproteins A-I and B as predictors of angiographically defined coronary artery disease. Arch. Intern. Med. 150:1629-1633; 1990.

92. Hulley, S.B.; Rosenman, R.H.; Bawol, R.D.; Brand, R.J. Epidemiology as a guide to clinical decisions. The association between triglycerides and coronary heart disease. N. Engl. J. Med. 302:1383-1389; 1980.

93. Cowan, L.D.; Wilcosky, T.; Criqui, M.H.; Barrett-Connor, E.; Suchindran, C.M.; Wallace, R.; Laskarzewski, P.; Walden, C. Demographic, behavioral, biochemical, and dietary correlates and plasma triglycerides. Lipid research clinic program prevalence study. Atherosclerosis. 5:466-480; 1985.

94. Austin, M. Plasma triglycerides a risk factor for coronary heart disease. The epidemiologic evidence and beyond. Am. J. Epidemiol. 129:249-259; 1989.

95. Brunzell, J.D.; Austin, M.A. Plasma triglyceride levels and coronary heart disease. N. Engl. J. Med. 320:1273-1275; 1989.

96. Leon, A.S. Recent advances in management of hypertension. J. Cardiopulmon. Rehab. 11:182-191; 1991.

97. Schnieder, R.E.; Masseri, F.H.; Ruddel, H. Risks for arterial hypertension. Clin. Cardiol. 4:57-66; 1986.

98. Manager, W.M.; Page, I.H. An overview of current concepts regarding the pathogenesis and pathophysiology of hypertension. In: Rosenthal, J., ed. Arterial hypertension: Pathogenesis, diagnosis and therapy. New York: Springer-Verlag; 1986:1-52.

99. Frohlich, E.D. Left ventricular hypertrophy: An independent factor of risk. In: Frohlich, E.D.; Brest, A.N., eds. Preventive aspects of coronary heart disease. Cardiovascular Clinics. Philadelphia: Davis; 1990:85-94.

100. Manolio, T.A.; Levy, D.; Garrison, R.J.; Castelli, W.P.; Kannel, W.B. Relation of alcohol intake to left ventricular mass: The Framingham study. J. Am. Coll. Cardiol. 17:717-721; 1991.

101. Massie, B.M. Myocardial hypertrophy and cardiac failure. A complex interrelationship. Am. J. Med. 66:67-74; 1983.

102. Messerli, F.H. Clinical determinants and consequences of left ventricular hypertrophy. Am. J. Med. 66:51-56; 1983.

103. Marcus, M.L.; Koyangi, S.; Harrison, D.G.; Doty, D.B.; Hiratzka, L.F.; Eastham, C.L. Abnormalities in the coronary circulation that occur as a consequence of cardiac hypertrophy. Am. J. Med. 66:62-66; 1983.

104. Dreslinski, G.R. Identification of left ventricular hypertrophy: Chest roentgenography, echocardiography, and electrocardiography. Am. J. Med. 66:47-50; 1983.

105. Levy, D. Left ventricular hypertrophy. Epidemiologic insights from the Framingham heart study. Drugs. 35[Suppl. 5]:1-5; 1988.

106. Kannel, W.B. Prevalence and natural history of electrocardiographic left ventricular hypertrophy. Am. J. Med. [Suppl.] 66:4-11; 1983.

107. Roccella, E.J.; Bowler, A.E. Hypertension as a risk factor. In: Frohlich, E.D.; Brest, A.M., eds. Preventive aspects of coronary heart disease. Cardiovascular clinics. Philadelphia: Davis; 1990:49-63.

108. MacMahon, S.; Peto, R.; Cutler, J.; Collins, R.; Sorie, P.; Neaton, J.; Abbott, R.; Godwin, J.; Dyer, A.; Stamler, J. Blood pressure, stroke and coronary heart disease. Part I. Prolonged differences in blood pressure: Prospective observational studies corrected for regression dilution bias. Lancet. 335:765-774; 1990.

109. Fraser, G.E. Preventive cardiology. New York: Oxford University Press; 1986:117-147.

110. Morgan, A.D. The pathogenesis of coronary occlusion. Oxford: Blackwell Scientific; 1956:44.

111. Robertson, W.B.; Strong, J.P. Atherosclerosis in persons with hypertension and diabetes mellitus. Lab. Invest. 18:538-551; 1968.

112. Master, A.M.; Dack, S.; Jaffe, H.L. Age, sex and hypertension in myocardial infarction. Arch. Intern. Med. 64:767-780; 1939.

113. Solberg, L.A.; McGarrig, P.A. Cerebral atherosclerosis in selected cases. Lab. Invest. 19:613-619; 1968.

114. Bianchi, G.; Ferrari, P. Animal models for arterial hypertension. In: Genest, J.; Kuchel, O.; Hamet, P.; Cantin, M., eds. Hypertension. 2nd ed. New York: McGraw-Hill; 1983:534-555.

115. Yamaori, Y. Pathophysiology of the various strains of spontaneous hypertensive rats. In: Genest, J.; Kuchel, O.; Hamet, P.; Cantin, M., eds. Hypertension. 2nd ed. New York: McGraw-Hill; 1983:556-581.

116. Dunn, F.G. Prevention of sudden cardiac death. In: Frohlich, E.D.; Brest, A.M., eds. Preventive aspects of coronary heart diseases. Cardiovascular clinics. Philadelphia: Davis; 1990:95-109.

117. Versailles, J.T.; Verscheure, Y.; Lekim, A.; Powrrias, B. Comparison between the ventricular fibrillation

thresholds of spontaneous hypertensive and normotensive rats—investigations of antidysrhythmic drugs. J. Cardiovasc. Pharmacol. 4:430-435; 1982.

118. Collins, R.; Peto, R.; MacMahon, S.; Herbert, P.; Frebach, N.H.; Eberlein, K.A.; Godwin, J.; Qizilbash, N.; Taylor, J.O.; Hennekens, C.H. Blood pressure, stroke and coronary heart disease. Part 2, short-term reductions in blood pressure: Overview of randomized drug trials in their epidemiological context. Lancet. 335:827-838; 1990.

119. MacMahon, S,; Cutler, J.A.; Neaton, J.D.; Furberg, C.D.; Cohen, J.D.; Kuller, L.H.; Stamler, J.; the MRFIT Group. Relationship of blood pressure to coronary and stroke morbidity and mortality in clinical trials and epidemiological studies. J. Hypertens. 4[Suppl. 6]:S14-S17; 1986.

120. Veterans Administration Cooperative Study on Antihypertensive Agents. Effects of treatment on morbidity in hypertension II. Results of patients with diastolic blood pressure averaging 90 through 114 mm Hg. JAMA. 213:1143-1152; 1970.

121. Hypertension Detection and Follow-up Program Cooperative Group. Five-year findings of the hypertension and follow-up program. I. Reduction in mortality of persons with high blood pressure, including mild hypertension. II. Mortality by race, sex and age. JAMA. 242:2562-2576; 1979.

122. Smith, M.W.; the U.S. Public Health Service Hospitals Cooperative Study Group. Treatment of mild hypertension results of a ten-year intervention trial. Circ. Res. 40[Suppl. 1]:95-105; 1977.

123. Medical Research Council Working Party. MRC trial of treatment of mild hypertension: Principal results. Br. Med. J. 291:97-104; 1985.

124. Australian National Blood Pressure Management Committee. The Australian therapeutic trial in mild hypertension. Lancet. 1:1261-1263; 1980.

125. Helgeland, A. Treatment of mild hypertension: A five-year controlled drug trial. The Oslo study. Am. J. Med. 69:725-732; 1980.

126. Stamler, J.; Fainaro, E.; Mojonnier, L.M.; Halls, Y.; Moss, D.; Stamler, R. Prevention and control of hypertension by nutritional means. JAMA. 243:1819-1823; 1980.

127. Stamler, R.; Stamler, J.; Grimm, R., Jr.; Gosch, F.C.; Elmer, P.; Dyer, A.; Berman, R.; Fishman, J.; Van Hell, N.; Civinell, J. Final report of a four-year randomized control trial. The hypertension control program. JAMA. 257:1484-1491; 1987.

128. Winkler, M.A.; Murphy, M.B. Isolated systolic hypertension in the elderly. JAMA. 265:3301-3302; 1991.

129. SHEP Cooperative Research Group. Prevention of stroke by antihypertensive drug treatment in older persons with isolated systolic hypertension. Final results of the systolic hypertension in the elderly program (SHEP). JAMA. 265:3255-3264; 1991.

130. Hansson, L. Reversal of cardiac and vascular hypertrophy by antihypertensive therapy. Am. Heart. J. 121:995-998; 1991.

131. Pegram, B.L.; Froehlich, E.D. Cardiovascular adjustment to antiadrenergic agents. Am. J. Med. 66:94-99; 1983.

132. Sen, S. Regression of cardiac hypertrophy. Experimental animal model. Am. J. Med. 66:87-93; 1983.

133. A Report of the Surgeon General. Reducing the health consequences of smoking: 25 years of progress. DHHS publication no.(CDC) 89-8411, 1989. Washington, DC: U.S. Government Printing Office; 1989:1-687.

134. A Report of the Surgeon General. The health consequences of involuntary smoking. DHHS (CDC) 87-8398. Washington, DC: U.S. Government Printing Office; 1986:1-359.

135. Kuller, L.; Meilahn, E.; Ockene, J. Smoking and coronary heart disease. In: Connor, W.E.; Bristow, J.D., eds. Coronary heart disease. Prevention, complications and treatment. Philadelphia: Lippincott; 1985:65-84.

136. Strong, J.P.; Oalmann, M.C. Effects of smoking in the cardiovascular system. In: Frohlich, E.D.; Brest, A.N., eds. Preventive aspects of coronary heart disease. Cardiovascular clinics. Philadelphia: Davis; 1990:205-221.

137. Svendsen, K.; Kuller, L.H.; Martin, M.J.; Ockene, J.K. Effects of passive smoking in the multiple risk factor intervention trial. Am. J. Epidemiol. 126:783-795; 1987.

138. Garland, C.; Barrett-Connor, E.; Suarez, L.; Criqui, M.H.; Wingard, D.L. Effect of passive smoking on ischemic heart disease mortality of nonsmokers. A prospective study. Am. J. Epidemiol. 121:645-650; 1985.

139. Kannel, W.B. Update on the role of cigarette smoking in coronary artery disease. Am. Heart J. 101:319-328; 1981.

140. Gillis, C.R.; Hole, D.J.; Hawthorne, W.M.; Boyle, P. The effect of environmental tobacco smoke in two urban communities in the west of Scotland. Eur. J. Respir. Dis. 65[Suppl. 133]:121-126; 1984.

141. Hirayama, T. Passive smoking: A new target of epidemiology. J. Exper. Clin. Med. 10:287-293; 1985.

142. Aronrow, W.S. Effect of passive smoking on angina pectoris. N. Engl. J. Med. 299:21-24; 1978.

143. Lee, P.N.; Chamberlain, J.; Anderson, M.R. Relationship of passive smoking to risk of lung cancer and other smoking-associated diseases. Br. J. Cancer. 54:97-105; 1986.

144. Solberg, L.A.; Strong, J.P. Risk factors and atherosclerotic lesions. A review of autopsy data. Arteriosclerosis. 3:187-198; 1983.

145. Strong, J.P.; Richards, M.L. Cigarette smoking and atherosclerosis in autopsied men. Arteriosclerosis. 23:451-459; 1976.

146. Auerbach, O.; Hammond, E.C.; Garfinkel, L. Smoking in relationship to atherosclerosis of the coronary arteries. N. Engl. J. Med. 273:775-779; 1965.

147. Rhoads, G.G.; Blackwelder, W.C.; Stemmerma, G.H.; Hayashi, T.; Kagan, A. Coronary risk factors

and autopsy findings in Japanese-American men. Lab. Invest. 38:304-311; 1978.

148. Anonymous. WHO collaborative trials of coronary heart disease prevention. Lancet. 2:803-804; 1982.

149. Kallio, V.; Hamalainen, H.; Hakkila, J.; Liuurila, O.J. Reduction in sudden death by a multifactorial intervention programme after acute myocardial infarction. Lancet. 2:1091-1094; 1979.

150. Gilman, A.G.; Goodman, L.S.; Rall, T.W.; Muradad, F., editors. Goodman and Gillman's the pharmacological basis of therapeutics. 7th ed. New York: Macmillan; 1985:215-221.

151. Bellet, S,; DeGuzman, M.R.; Kostis, J.B.; Roman, L.; Fleishmann, D. The effect of inhalation of cigarette smoke on ventricular fibrillation threshold in normal dogs and dogs with acute myocardial infarction. Am. Heart J. 83:67-76; 1972.

152. Seltzer, C.C. Effect of smoking on blood pressure. Am. Heart J. 87:558-564; 1974.

153. Aronow, W.S.; Kaplan ,N.M. Smoking. In: Kaplan, N.M.; Stamler, J., eds. Prevention of coronary heart disease. Practical management of the risk factors. Philadelphia: Saunders; 1983:51-60.

154. Van Italie, T.B. Health implications of overweight in the United States. Ann. Intern. Med. 103[Suppl. Part 2]:983-998; 1985.

155. Barrett-Connor, E.L. Obesity, atherosclerosis, and coronary heart disease. Ann. Intern. Med. 103(6) [Suppl. Part 2]:1010-1018; 1985.

156. Despres, J-P.; Moorjani, S.; Lupien, P.J.; Tremblay, A.; Nadeau, A.; Bouchard, C. Regional distribution of body fat, plasma lipoproteins and cardiovascular disease. Arteriosclerosis. 10:497-511; 1990.

157. Bouchard, C. Is weight fluctuation a risk factor? N. Engl. J. Med. 324:1887-1889; 1991.

158. Build and blood pressure study. Vol. 1. Chicago: Society of Actuaries; 1959.

159. 1983 Metropolitan height and weight tables. Stat. Bull. Metrop. Insur. Co. 64:2-9; 1984.

160. National Institutes of Health. Consensus development conference statement: Health implications of obesity. Ann. Intern. Med. 103(6) [Suppl. Part 2]: 1073-1077; 1985.

161. Keys, A.; Fidanza, F.; Karvonen, M.J.; Kimura, M.; Taylor, H.L. Indices of relative weight and obesity. J. Chronic Dis. 25:329-343; 1972.

162. Lew, E.A. Insured lives at the American Cancer Society. Ann. Intern. Med. 103(6) [Suppl. Part 2]: 1024-1029; 1985.

163. Larsson, B.; Bjorntorp, P.; Tibblin, G. The health consequences of moderate obesity. Int. J. Obes. 5:97-116; 1981.

164. Hubert, H.B. The nature of the relationship between obesity and cardiovascular disease. Int. J. Cardiol. 6:268-274; 1984.

165. Garrison, R.J.; Castelli, W.P. Weight and thirty-year mortality of men in the Framingham study. Ann. Intern. Med. 103(6) [Suppl. Part 2]:1006-1009; 1985.

166. Lissner, L.; Odell, P.M.; D'Agostino, R.B.; Stokes, J., III; Kreger, B.E.; Belanger, A.J.; Brownell, K.D. Variability of body weight and health outcomes in the Framingham study. N. Engl. J. Med. 324:1339-1344; 1991.

167. Kral, J.G. Morbid obesity and related health risks. Ann. Intern. Med. 103(6) [Suppl. Part 2]:1043-1047; 1985.

168. Goldman, L.; Cook, E.F. Reasons for the decline in coronary heart disease; medical interventions versus life-style change. In: Higgins, M.W.; Luepker, R.V., eds. Trends in coronary heart disease mortality. The influence of medical care. Oxford: Oxford University Press; 1988:67-75.

169. Dustan, H.P. Obesity and hypertension. Ann. Intern. Med. 103(6) [Suppl. Part 2]:1047-1049; 1985.

170. Schotte, D.E.; Stunkard, A.J. The effects of weight reduction on blood pressure in 301 obese patients. Arch. Intern. Med. 150:1701-1704; 1990.

171. Gordon, T.; Kannel, W.B. Effects of overweight on cardiovascular disease. Geriatrics. 28:80-88; 1973.

172. Alexander, J.K. Obesity and coronary heart disease. In: Connor, W.E.; Bristow, J.D., eds. Coronary heart disease prevention, complications, and treatment. Philadelphia: Lippincott; 1985:111-123.

173. Leon, A.S. Patients with diabetes mellitus. In: Franklin, B.A.; Gordon, S.; Timmis, G.T., eds. Exercise in modern medicine. Baltimore: Williams & Wilkins; 1989:118-145.

174. Pyorala, K. Relationship of glucose tolerance and plasma insulin to the incidence of coronary heart disease: Results from two population studies in Finland. Diabetes Care. 2:131-141; 1979.

175. Zavaroni, M.D.; Bonora, E.; Pagliara, M.D.; Dall'aglio, E.; Luchetti, L.; Buonanno, M.D.; Bonati, P.A.; Bergonazani, M.; Grudis, L.; Passeri, M.; Reavan, G. Risk factors for coronary artery disease with hypersinulinemia and normal glucose tolerance. N. Engl. J. Med. 320:702-706; 1989.

176. Wing, R.R.; Bunker, C.H.; Kuller, L.B.; Matthews, K.A. Insulin, body mass index and cardiovascular risk factors in premenopausal women. Arteriosclerosis. 9:479-484; 1987.

177. Kannel, W.B.; Ross, S.A. (Chairman). Proceedings of a symposium. States of insulin resistance: The interaction between hypertension, glucose intolerance and coronary heart disease. Am. Heart J. 121(4) [Suppl.]:1267-1318; 1991.

Chapter 9

Mechanisms by Which Exercise Training May Improve the Clinical Status of Cardiac Patients

Ray W. Squires

Coronary artery disease (CAD) is a progressive, chronic disorder that is the leading cause of premature death and disability in industrialized nations. Comprehensive cardiac rehabilitation—including education, counseling, adequate medical and surgical treatment, proper nutrition, avoiding tobacco, optimal control of blood lipids and BP and exercise training—has become an accepted component of patient care after myocardial infarction (MI) or coronary revascularization procedures. Exercise training has been the most visible component of cardiac rehabilitation programs over the past 3 decades and has been a popular subject for clinical investigators. Guidelines are widely available for exercise programs for patients with CAD and are generally applied throughout North America (1-4). The concept that exercise may benefit CAD patients is not new. Heberden in 1802 understood at least one way in which habitual physical activity could improve the clinical condition of cardiac patients: He reported an angina pectoris patient "who set himself a task of sawing wood for half an hour every day and was nearly cured" (5). In the latter part of the 19th century Oertel advocated a low-fat diet and walking in the mountains for the treatment of coronary insufficiency (6).

The clinical status of patients with CAD involves several factors:

- Symptoms of exertional intolerance, such as angina pectoris, inappropriate fatigue, exercise-related dyspnea, and claudication
- Exercise capacity as defined by maximal oxygen uptake ($\dot{V}O_2$max), anaerobic threshold, submaximal exercise endurance, muscular strength, and the ability to perform combined dynamic and static activity (for example, carrying an object while walking)

- Survival prognostic factors, such as left ventricular systolic function, residual exertional myocardial ischemia, adequacy of exercise capacity, systolic BP response to exercise, and ventricular arrhythmia
- Classic coronary risk factors, such as tobacco use, an adverse blood lipid profile, hypertension, glucose intolerance, and coronary-prone personality
- Prospects for future morbidity (reinfarction, worsening of symptoms or exercise capacity, reocclusion of catheter-treated coronary arteries, stenosis or occlusion of bypass grafts) or cardiac mortality
- Progression of CAD
- Psychosocial factors and quality of life

Coronary patients are a heterogenous group that we cannot expect to demonstrate consistent and predictable responses to exercise training. Patients differ in many respects:

- The extent of coronary atherosclerotic disease
- Clinical presentation, including acute MI, old silent MI, large versus small infarction, multiple infarctions, whether early thrombolytic therapy was successful or unsuccessful, coronary artery bypass graft (CABG) surgery or catheter-based revascularization, angina pectoris, congestive heart failure (CHF), arrhythmia, and combined coronary and valvular disease
- Left ventricular systolic function (well preserved versus varying degrees of left ventricular impairment)
- Diastolic function
- Ischemia (no residual ischemia versus varying severity and extent of ischemia)
- Age (young adult versus frail elderly)
- Gender

- Risk status for a recurrent event
- Medications
- Classic coronary risk factors, namely, genetic influence, tobacco use, hypercholesterolemia, hypertension, and glucose intolerance
- Revascularization status and restenosis risk (no revascularization, successful versus unsuccessful percutaneous transluminal coronary angioplasty [PTCA], CABG surgery, coronary atherectomy, laser angioplasty, coronary stent placement)
- Coronary anatomy and myocardial perfusion
- Coexisting medical conditions, including metabolic, musculoskeletal, and emotional conditions; nonatherosclerotic cardiac disease, vasospasm, valvular disease, congenital heart disease, primary arrhythmia, subvalvular hypertrophy, left ventricular hypertrophy (LVH), myocardial disease, presence of pacemaker or automatic implantable cardioverter/defibrillator; and other atherosclerotic disease, such as cerebrovascular disease, peripheral vascular disease (PVD), and renovascular disease.

The purpose of this chapter is to describe the mechanisms whereby exercise training may enhance the clinical status of the typical cardiac patient. The topics covered are improvement in aerobic exercise capacity; patients with poor left ventricular systolic function; the benefits of strengthening exercises for cardiac patients; improvement in symptoms of exertional intolerance; exercise training, myocardial ischemia, and blood flow; exercise and secondary prevention of coronary events, mortality, and progression of coronary disease; and improvement in emotional factors with exercise training.

Improvement in Aerobic Exercise Capacity

The ability to perform physical work, including the activities of daily living, occupational and avocational pursuits, formal exercise training, and response to unexpected requirements for physical effort, is an important component of quality of life for cardiac patients. After an uncomplicated MI, exercise capacity may be reduced, probably as a result of inactivity as well as myocardial damage. Spontaneous improvement in aerobic exercise capacity within the first 3 months after MI without exercise training has been reported (7). A further

enhancement of the oxygen transport system of most patients with CAD occurs with habitual exercise training and can be verified by the directly measured $\dot{V}O_2max$. As a result of exercise training, $\dot{V}O_2max$ may increase 10% to 30% or more (8,9). In general, the magnitude of the improvement in $\dot{V}O_2max$ is inversely proportional to the exercise capacity before training (10). The rate of improvement is greatest during the first 3 months of exercise training, but the increase in aerobic capacity may continue for 6 or more months (11).

In one study, exercise training at an intensity of 70% to 85% of maximal heart rate (HRmax) three times weekly for 20 to 40 min, for a duration of 3 to 6 months, resulted in similar increases in $\dot{V}O_2max$ in groups of patients with previous MI ($+6$ ml $\cdot$ kg^{-1} $\cdot$ min^{-1}), CABG surgery ($+8$ ml $\cdot$ kg^{-1} $\cdot$ min^{-1}), and angiographic CAD without MI or revascularization ($+7$ ml $\cdot$ kg^{-1} $\cdot$ min^{-1}) (Figure 9.1) (12). Thus, the ability of some cardiac patients who have suffered an MI or undergone CABG surgery to exhibit a training effect appears to be equivalent to cardiac patients without MI or intervention. Furthermore, patients who receive beta-blocker medications and patients 65 years of age or older experience the same relative magnitude of improvement in exercise capacity as other patients (13).

During the past several years researchers have given attention to relatively low-intensity exercise training for cardiac patients with the thought that compliance with the program might be enhanced and the risks of training (i.e., cardiovascular and musculoskeletal complications) reduced relative to traditional moderate- and high-intensity training. One study randomly assigned patients to either traditional-intensity (65% to 75% of $\dot{V}O_2max$) or low-intensity (< 45% of $\dot{V}O_2max$) exercise training with a duration of 30 to 45 min and a frequency of three sessions/week for 3 months (14). After training, $\dot{V}O_2max$ increased by 11% in the traditional-intensity group ($+3$ ml $\cdot$ kg^{-1} $\cdot$ min^{-1}) and by 14% in the low-intensity group ($+3$ ml $\cdot$ kg^{-1} $\cdot$ min^{-1}). A second study enrolled men with MI and began 3 weeks after the event (15). All patients were encouraged to gradually increase walking to 30 min daily at a comfortable pace. Patients were randomly allocated to either of two 8-week formal exercise programs: a high-intensity program (three times weekly, 30 min/session, at 75% to 85% of HRmax) or a low-intensity program (twice weekly, 30 min/session, with a maximum intensity of resting heart rate 20 beats/min above resting heart rate). Peak exercise capacity in METs (metabolic equivalents), estimated from treadmill test performance, increased by 4 METs in the high-intensity

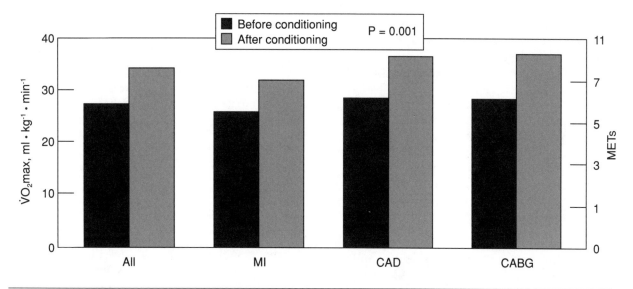

Figure 9.1   Increase in maximal oxygen uptake ($\dot{V}O_2$max) resulting from exercise training in patients with myo-cardial infarction (MI), coronary artery bypass graft (CABG) surgery, and angiographically documented coronary artery disease (CAD). (All = all coronary patients; MET = metabolic equivalent.)
From Hartung, G.H.; Rangel, R. Exercise Training in Post-Myocardial Infarction Patients: Comparison of Results With High Risk Coronary and Post-Bypass Patients. *Arch. Phys. Med. Rehab.*, **62**:147-150, 1981. Reprinted by permission.

patients and by 3 METs in the low-intensity patients. Exercise capacity at 1 year post-MI was similar for both groups.

Coronary patients who exhibit residual exercise-induced ischemia after MI often have below-average $\dot{V}O_2$max and develop evidence of early dependence on anaerobic metabolism for the performance of moderate-intensity physical activity (16). Unfortunately, these patients are less likely to demonstrate an adequate exercise training effect. In a group of 106 coronary patients, 31 of whom developed definite evidence of myocardial ischemia during exercise testing, a 3-month program of exercise training, three times/week at an intensity of 70% to 85% of the HRmax was undertaken (17). Patients with ischemia were allowed to exercise at intensities above their ischemic thresholds during approximately half of the exercise sessions. Exercise capacity, directly measured as $\dot{V}O_2$max, increased a mean of 4.9 METs for the patients without ischemia and 3.5 METs for the ischemic subjects.

The $\dot{V}O_2$max of some patients with CAD does not improve as a result of exercise training, but their physical work efficiency does. For example, 8 patients who participated in a 16-week walking program did not show any increase in aerobic capacity, but did demonstrate a lower oxygen uptake ($\dot{V}O_2$) and heart rate (HR) at a given walking pace on a treadmill after the training program (18).

The improvement in aerobic capacity usually seen after exercise training is a result of adaptation of the oxygen transport system, as defined by the Fick equation: $\dot{V}O_2$ = cardiac output ($\dot{Q}$) × arterial-mixed venous oxygen difference. An increase in the arterial-mixed venous oxygen difference, which is an adaptation of the peripheral circulation that results from an increase in blood volume, capillary density, and oxygen extraction from capillary blood when skeletal muscle performs exercise, is assumed to be the primary training response in cardiac patients (10). Mitochondrial enzymes of oxidative metabolism have been shown to possess increased activity after an exercise training program in coronary patients (19). Whether exercise $\dot{Q}$ increases as a result of training has been controversial. Some relatively early studies (8,20) demonstrated an increase in $\dot{Q}$ after training; an increase in HRmax and in stroke volume (SV) was also observed.

A.A. Ehsani and his colleagues at Washington University (St. Louis, Missouri) has studied extensively the responses of cardiac patients to a much higher intensity and total amount of exercise than what is customarily recommended. They did so to maximize the training stimulus and to redefine the upper limits of the physiological responses, as well as to address the issue of central circulatory adaptation to habitual exercise (21). After a 3-month period of traditional aerobic training (three times weekly, 30 to 40 min/session, 50% to 70% of $\dot{V}O_2$max), patients were gradually brought up to 60 min of exercise, 5 days/week, at an intensity of 70% to 90% of $\dot{V}O_2$max; this level was maintained for the final 3 to 4 months of the year-long training program. Clinicians provided close medical supervision for all exercise sessions. The subjects' mean $\dot{V}O_2$max increased by approximately 40%, about twice the aerobic training effect of more traditional rehabilitation exercise programs. Nine patients continued the high-intensity training for 7 years and demonstrated that the sizable benefits to aerobic capacity can be maintained for the long-term in selected, highly motivated persons (22).

Evidence of improved cardiac output during exercise in the work of Ehsani's group is indicated by the following findings:

- Echocardiographic evidence of improved left ventricular fractional shortening and improved mean velocity of circumferential shortening (23)
- Average 18% increase in SV measured during submaximal exercise i.e., 35% to 65% of $\dot{V}O_2$max (Figure 9.2) (24)
- Improvement in systolic time intervals after training (25)
- Increased exercise left ventricular ejection fraction (LVEF) (rest LVEF unchanged) (26)
- Reversal of exercise-induced and ischemia-related drop in systolic BP (27)

These data are consistent with an improvement in left ventricular function in patients who undertook aggressive exercise training. The impressive physiological adaptations are probably not attainable by patients who exercise at more conservative intensities. Ehsani and colleagues do not recommend high-intensity exercise programs as the norm for cardiac patients, but selected individuals may be candidates for such an aggressive exercise regime.

Exercise Training in Patients With Poor Left Ventricular Systolic Function

Patients with CAD may be classified as high risk for death by a variety of clinical variables, the most important being severe left ventricular dysfunction (28). Traditionally, some patients with low LVEFs were excluded from rehabilitation exercise programs because it was feared that the exertion would precipitate heart failure or dangerous arrhythmias. However, the $\dot{V}O_2$max of ambulatory patients with chronic heart failure has been shown to improve 23% after 4 to 6 months of moderate exercise training (29). Although measures of central cardiac function were unchanged, the systemic arterial-mixed venous oxygen difference, as well as leg blood flow, was improved by the training program. These patients also exhibited reduced

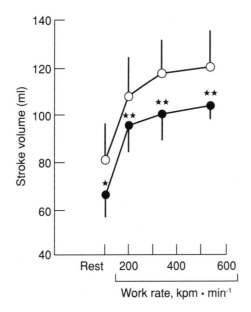
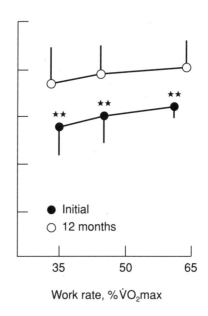

Figure 9.2 Stroke volume at the same absolute work rate (*left*) and the same relative work rate (*right*) before and after 12 months of exercise training. (*p* for each before-after pair < 0.01, except *p < 0.5. kpm · min^{-1} = kilopond meter per minute; $\dot{V}O_2$max = maximum oxygen uptake.)
From Hagberg, J.M.; Ehsani, A.A.; Holloszy, J.O. Effect of 12 Months of Intense Exercise Training on Stroke Volume in Patients With Coronary Artery Disease. *Circulation*, **67**:1194-1199, 1983. Reprinted with permission.

blood lactate levels and better endurance during submaximal exercise following training (30). In England, a 2-month home stationary-cycling program for 11 patients with CAD and LVEFs averaging 19% (55% to 65% being the normal range) resulted an improvement in $\dot{V}O_2$max from 14 to 17 ml · kg^{-1} · min^{-1}. No exercise-related complications were reported (31).

In patients with ischemic left ventricular dysfunction, directly measured aerobic capacity is an important prognostic factor with the subgroup of patients exhibiting exercise capacities of less than 4 METs having a 2-year survival rate of a mere 32% (32,33). It is not known whether increasing $\dot{V}O_2$max by exercise training will improve their survival. In patients with ischemic left ventricular dysfunction, the ability to participate in rehabilitation exercise was associated with a lower-than-expected cardiac mortality based on LVEF alone (34). Selected patients with left ventricular aneurysm after MI have been shown to have better exercise tolerance after training (35).

One study has urged caution in recommending exercise training for patients with moderate-sized anterior Q-wave MIs who exhibit left ventricular asynergy (akinesia or dyskinesia) of 18% or more (36). After a very mild 3-month exercise program that began 15 weeks after MI, these patients demonstrated more cardiac shape distortion, expansion, and wall thinning. LVEF and functional capacity also worsened. Other investigators who have rapidly mobilized similar patients after MI have not observed such deterioration, although patients were not closely matched in all clinical characteristics (37). In a randomized, controlled trial, Giannuzzi et al. (38) evaluated the effects of 6 months of cycle ergometry on left ventricular function and ventricular shape in 49 men who had a first Q-wave anterior wall MI. The subjects had LVEFs of more than 25% and started the study approximately 6 weeks after MI. Graded exercise tests (GXTs) and echocardiography were performed at the beginning of the study and at 6 months. Cycling was done at 80% of HRmax at least three times weekly, for 30 min/session. Exercise capacity improved after training in the exercise group but not in the control group. Subjects in both groups with LVEFs of less than 40% exhibited left ventricular enlargement, regional dilation, and shape distortion. Patients with poor left ventricular function after a Q-wave anterior MI experience adverse ventricular remodeling over time, and standard exercise training does not appear to influence the process. Further investigation is needed before such patients are excluded from exercise training.

Benefits of Strengthening Exercises for Cardiac Patients

Many activities of daily living and some occupational tasks require upper- or lower-extremity static or dynamic muscle strength. Investigators have demonstrated that circuit weight training of moderate intensity is safe and results in improved muscular strength in selected cardiac patients (39). Circuit weight training is thought to be appropriate for patients generally during the later stages of supervised exercise programs (at least 4 months after MI or CABG surgery), although with the trend toward earlier discharge from the hospital and rapid return to work (some patients return to work within 2 weeks of MI), these guidelines need review. For example, Squires et al. (40) introduced mild strength training using standard commercial machines for 13 selected patients during early outpatient (Phase II) cardiac rehabilitation exercise classes. Weight training with machines began an average of 50 days after the cardiac event. Patients progressed within 4 weeks to lifting approximately 40 lb with the arms and 130 lb with the legs. The HR and systolic BP responses were modest, and no clinical problems were observed. Weight training results in improved muscular strength, and it may also improve the ability to perform aerobic exercise especially among patients with weak skeletal musculature (41). Increasing the muscular strength of cardiac patients results in use of a lower percentage of the maximal contractile force during routine tasks and enables patients to accomplish activities at a lower HR and systolic BP, and thus at a lower myocardial oxygen demand. Strength training programs for cardiac patients have improved the patients' perception of their ability to perform strength-requiring activities (42).

Improvement in Symptoms of Exertional Intolerance

Many patients with CAD report that their ability to perform physical tasks is limited by bothersome symptoms. An important outcome from exercise training for many patients is a reduction in the symptoms of effort-related angina pectoris, dyspnea, fatigue, and claudication (43-45). With an increase in $\dot{V}O_2$max after exercise training, a smaller percentage of the exercise capacity is required during routine activities (Figure 9.3). As a result, tasks are performed with less fatigue, dyspnea, and perceived exertion. The productivity and quality of life of the patient may be considerably enhanced. For a specific exercise intensity, the myocardial oxygen requirement, as evidenced by a reduction in the HR and systolic BP (rate-pressure product [RPP]), is reduced by approximately 18% (Figure 9.4) (46). Thus, patients are able to exercise to a higher intensity before the potential achievement of an ischemic or anginal threshold (Figure 9.5).

Exercise Training, Myocardial Ischemia, and Blood Flow

The pathophysiological problem of CAD is an imbalance between the needs of the myocardium for nutritive blood flow and the capacity of the coronary circulation to provide adequate flow. The myocardium extracts essentially all of the available oxygen from the myocardial capillaries and is dependent upon increasing blood flow in order to meet increased metabolic demands for oxygen. The observation that in some cardiac patients the RPP at the ischemic threshold is increased by exercise training, independent of changes in anti-ischemic drug therapy, suggests that myocardial perfusion may be favorably altered (47,48). Thallium perfusion scanning performed before and after a period of exercise training has, in some selected coronary patients, demonstrated improved myocardial blood flow (49). One investigation combined aerobic exercise training, the elimination of cigarette smoking, and a low-fat, low-cholesterol diet for 1 year in 18 cardiac patients. Total cholesterol fell from a mean of 242 mg/dl to 202 mg/dl; the final low-density lipoprotein (LDL) cholesterol was 130 mg/dl. Exercise-induced myocardial ischemia assessed by thallium decreased 54% (50). A total of 105 coronary lesions (2.9 per patient) were identified on baseline quantitative coronary angiography (51). Improvement of myocardial perfusion by thallium exercise testing was independent of changes in coronary atherosclerotic lesions and may have been related to changes in blood lipids, decreased blood viscosity, or the development of collateral vessels.

In animal experiments, exercise training has resulted in increased coronary artery diameter (52), enlarged overall coronary tree size (53), and increased myocardial capillary density (54). Human studies have used the techniques of myocardial perfusion scanning, as reviewed in the previous paragraph, and coronary angiography before and after exercise training. Having recently reviewed the results of five investigations utilizing angiography, Franklin (55) points out the difficulty in visualizing smaller collateral vessels or vessels tunneled into the myocardium. One such study involved 8 men with stable angina who participated in a 1-year supervised exercise program (43). Exercise capacity was improved, and 2 patients with pretraining ischemic electrocardiographic (ECG) changes during treadmill testing reverted to normal. No changes were found in the angiographic appearance of the coronary vessels, the atherosclerotic lesions, or the collateral vasculature. There is no direct evidence that exercise training stimulates coronary collateralization in patients with CAD.

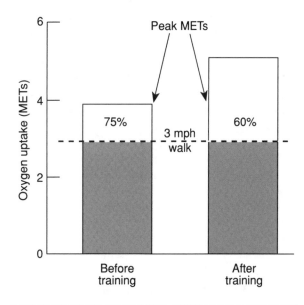

Figure 9.3 Effect of exercise training on peak oxygen uptake in metabolic equivalents (METs) and relative oxygen expenditure (as percent of peak oxygen uptake) for walking 3 mph on a level surface. After exercise training, peak oxygen uptake increases; thus, the relative oxygen cost for the activity decreases.
From Franklin, B.A.; Rubenfire, M. Exercise Training in Coronary Heart Disease: Mechanisms of Improvement. *Pract. Cardiol.*, 6:84-89, 1980. Reprinted with permission.

Exercise and Secondary Prevention of Coronary Events, Mortality, and Progression of Coronary Disease

Although many beneficial effects of exercise training for coronary patients have been appreciated,

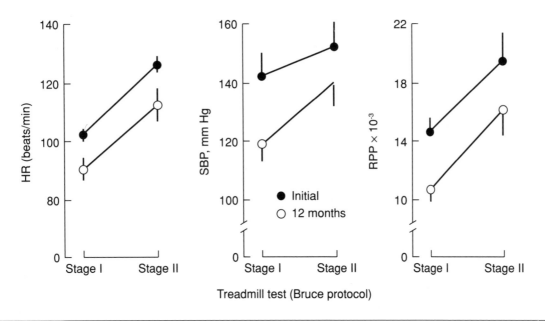

Figure 9.4   Effects of exercise training on heart rate (HR), systolic blood pressure (SBP), and rate-pressure product (RPP) at Stages I and II of the Bruce treadmill protocol. All variables after 12 months of training were significantly ($p < 0.01$) lower than before training.

From Ehsani, A.A.; Martin, W.H.; Heath, G.W.; Coyle, E.F. Cardiac Effects of Prolonged and Intense Exercise Training in Patients With Coronary Artery Disease. *Am. J. Cardiol.*, **50**:246-254, 1982. Reprinted with permission.

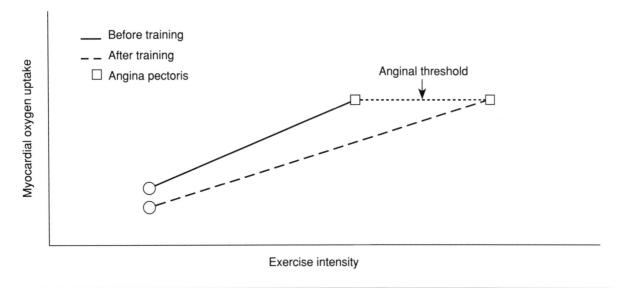

Figure 9.5   Effect of exercise training on exertional angina pectoris.

Modified from Franklin, B.A.; Rubenfire, M. Exercise Training in Coronary Heart Disease: Mechanisms of Improvement. *Pract. Cardiol.*, **6**:84-89, 1980. Used with permission.

the effects of habitual physical activity on survival or prevention of subsequent cardiac events have been difficult to demonstrate. The randomized trials performed thus far have experienced many problems that have limited their findings: insufficient numbers of subjects to achieve adequate statistical power, subject dropouts and crossovers, the inclusion of primarily low-risk patients, and short

durations of observation. The trials generally included an adequate exercise stimulus and some included modification of risk factors and counseling. None of the individual exercise trials demonstrated a significant effect of exercise on subsequent mortality, but trends were favorable in all investigations. Some investigators have pooled data from the trials (meta-analysis) and have reported favorable results (56,57). A 20% to 25% reduction in cardiac events (total mortality, cardiac mortality, and fatal reinfarction) after cardiac rehabilitation, including exercise training, is similar to that demonstrated with other, more expensive, therapies, including revascularization and drug therapy (beta-blockers, lipid-improving agents, and antihypertensives). One randomized trial of cardiac rehabilitation, including exercise training, smoking cessation and dietary advice, and psychosocial counseling, resulted in a reduced 10-year cumulative cardiac mortality (Figure 9.6) (58).

In nonhuman primates, Kramsch et al. (59) demonstrated that regular aerobic exercise training (1 hour of jogging three times/week for about 3 years) reduced the amount of coronary atherosclerosis in the setting of diet-induced hypercholesterolemia and resulted in increased coronary artery diameter. In humans with CAD who underwent two sessions of coronary angiography approximately 2 years apart, a low amount of habitual leisure time physical activity assessed by questionnaire was shown to predict progression of disease (60). Additional risk factors identified for CAD progression in this study were systolic and diastolic hypertension, cigarette smoking, and diabetes mellitus.

Exercise training, in sufficient amounts, appears to retard or even reverse coronary atherosclerosis. A recent investigation studied the effects of 1 year of supervised, moderate intensity exercise on the progression of coronary artery disease (60a). Approximately 60 cardiac patients were randomized into experimental and control groups. All subjects were instructed in a low-fat, low-cholesterol diet and received information regarding the benefits of regular aerobic exercise. The experimental subjects embarked on a supervised and home exercise program, and the control subjects were left to the usual care of their primary physicians. No medications to lower serum cholesterol concentrations were given. Coronary angiography using quantitative techniques was performed before and after the 1-year study. Angiographic progression of disease occurred in 45% of controls and 10% of experimental subjects. No change in the appearance of lesions was observed in 62% of experimental subjects compared with 49% of controls. Regression of atherosclerosis was observed in 28% of experimental subjects versus 6% of controls. Regression of coronary artery disease was observed only in patients who expended an average of 2,200 kilocalories per week in physical activity (approximately 5 to 6 hours of moderate intensity exercise per week).

Exercise training may retard the progression of coronary atherosclerosis by its salutary effects on some of the classic coronary risk factors. Low serum concentration of high-density lipoprotein (HDL) cholesterol is a particularly prevalent risk factor in cardiac patients. Physical training for 3 months has been shown to increase HDL-cholesterol by 15% to 23% in male patients with previous MI, CABG surgery, and angiographically determined disease (61,62). Total LDL cholesterol levels were reduced by 12% and 13% as a result of exercise training (62).

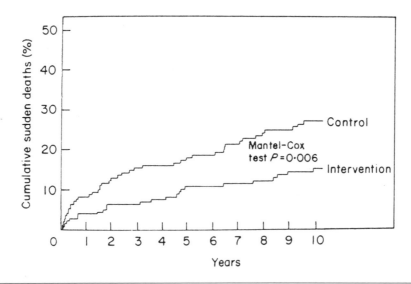

Figure 9.6 Cumulative percentage of sudden cardiac deaths during 10 years of follow-up of multifactorial cardiac rehabilitation intervention and control groups.
From Hamalainen, H.; Luurila, O.J.; Kallio, V.; et al. Long-Term Reduction in Sudden Deaths After a Multifactorial Intervention Programme in Patients With Myocardial Infarction: 10-Year Results of a Controlled Investigation. *Eur. Heart J.*, **10**:55-62, 1989. Reprinted by permission.

Physical activity on a regular basis, especially when used in concert with a modest caloric restriction, is effective in weight loss and maintaining proper body composition. Although a reduction in BP in hypertensive patients after they begin an aerobic-exercise program is not a universal finding, approximately two-thirds of studies have reported a reduction in resting systolic and diastolic BPs (63).

A decrease in insulin sensitivity, leading to hyperinsulinemia and glucose intolerance, has been implicated as an important factor in the development of atherosclerosis in some patients (64). Exercise training results in an increase in insulin sensitivity, a reduction in insulin secretion, and a lower serum insulin concentration (65-67). These alterations in glucose-insulin are presumed to lower the risk of CAD progression.

A high incidence of hyperestrogenemia has been found in young men who have sustained an MI (68). After 1 month of exercise training, estrogen levels decreased markedly and continued to decrease over the 3 months in a study involving 17 men with MI and hyperestrogenemia (62). The reductions in estrogen could not be attributed to change in diet, alteration in smoking behavior, or in changes in medications. Estrogen reduction in these patients as a result of habitual exercise may be beneficial.

Malignant ventricular arrhythmia is a common cause of death in patients with CAD. The threshold for ventricular fibrillation is altered in patients with CAD, due in part to myocardial damage resulting in nonhomogeneity of myocardial excitability (69). Myocardial ischemia, either clinically apparent or silent, is also a major pathogenetic mechanism of sudden cardiac death. The ischemia may be due to increased myocardial oxygen demand in fixed-lesion CAD, coronary artery spasm, or platelet aggregation leading to microthrombi of the coronary arteries. Many patients with CAD who experience sudden cardiac death have severe obstructive disease and often multivessel disease. Habitual physical activity appears to reduce the susceptibility to arrhythmia (70). In the isolated rate heart model, exercise training increases the ventricular fibrillation threshold after experimental MI (71). This benefit may be a result of a decrease of myocardial sympathetic tone, an increase in parasympathetic tone, or both.

Blood platelets and the clotting mechanism have been implicated in the pathogenesis of atherosclerosis and acute arterial occlusion. It is hypothesized that platelet adhesion to the intima and the subsequent release of platelet-derived growth factor initiate intimal plaque formation after vascular injury (72). Acute ischemic syndromes, unstable angina pectoris and acute MI, are believed to follow plaque rupture and subsequent platelet aggregation and thrombus formation (72,73). Partially occlusive thrombi result in unstable angina; complete vessel occlusion leads to acute MI. Patients with CAD often receive antiplatelet therapy to alter the natural history of vessel occlusion. Regular exercise training reduces platelet aggregation in cardiac patients (74) and probably increases fibrinolytic activity (75). Endogenous tissue-plasminogen activator, a potent thrombolytic compound released from endothelial cells, may increase in the blood after exercise (76).

These observations are consistent with an important alteration in the pathophysiology of coronary atherosclerosis and may partially explain the improvement in mortality in the meta-analyses of cardiac rehabilitation exercise training. In healthy subjects, exercise training results in a progressive fall in blood viscosity and improved red cell deformability, which could improve blood flow in atherosclerotic arteries (77). Plasma volume expands and hematocrit decreases slightly as a result of training (76). However, intense physical exercise with a large anaerobic metabolic component may result in a hypercoagulable state in some coronary patients without necessarily resulting in exertional ischemia (78). The change toward a hypercoagulable state after high-intensity exercise is probably less in magnitude than the antithrombotic effects just discussed (76).

Excessive activation of the sympathetic nervous system in response to emotional stress has been postulated as a coronary risk factor (79). Modern life is replete with opportunities for stressful situations that may provoke excessive catecholamine release, elevated HR and increased BP. In individuals without documented CAD and who possess some facets of the coronary-prone personality, exercise training has been shown to reduce the cardiovascular and epinephrine response to mental stress (in the form of mental arithmetic in one study) (80). It is hoped that patients with CAD will experience similar benefits from exercise in terms of their response to stressors. One cross-sectional study evaluated the responses of 39 men to cold-pressor stimulation (81). Fifteen men were very sedentary, 10 performed a moderate amount of exercise on a habitual basis (expending 1,652 kcal/week), 7 were marathon runners (4,257 kcal/week), and 7 were post-CABG patients who exercised moderately in a cardiac rehabilitation program (876 kcal/week). Compared with the sedentary subjects, all exercise groups demonstrated a reduced mean BP response to the cold-pressor test. Reduced BP response to nonexercise stress appears to be a benefit of exercise training in cardiac patients.

Improvement in Emotional Factors With Exercise Training

A cardiac event usually elicits intense emotional responses from patients (82,83). Panic and anxiety surface during the first hours after MI as a result of unfamiliar surroundings, the threat of death, discomfort, and so on. Depression, probably related to a feeling of loss of physical ability or potential as an individual, may occur as early as 3 days after the event or during the early outpatient phase of recovery. The depression is usually transient and may be characterized by typical complaints of fatigue or nonspecific discomfort. Denial is common and may constitute a beneficial response (complete acceptance of the illness but denial of its seriousness) or may be manifest by complete rejection of the reality of the illness. Beneficial denial is associated with a high potential for favorable rehabilitation. Patient quality of life after a cardiac event is not only dependent upon an adequate exercise capacity and freedom from symptoms with usual activities but also on emotional resolution of anxiety and depression.

Psychosocial improvement as a result of cardiac rehabilitation, including exercise training, has been demonstrated for selected cardiac patients. In a controlled, but not randomized, trial of traditional cardiac rehabilitation practices, the following benefits were documented: improved understanding of heart disease, better compliance with treatment recommendations, more positive self-perception, decreased employment-related stress, more enjoyment of leisure time, and more physical and sexual activity (84). In another investigation, which did involve randomization and a control group, exercise training resulted in significant improvement in all measures of depression and anxiety relative to the control group (85). Patients who spent 3 months in a comprehensive rehabilitation program were less distressed psychologically and less dependent upon family support than control subjects, who did not receive rehabilitation (80). In a study of patients who had shown evidence of depression or anxiety, an 8-week exercise program

and behavioral counseling was compared with conventional care (87). Patients in the treatment group experienced an accelerated recovery in anxiety and depression at 8 weeks compared with controls. After 1 year, similar improvements in both groups were observed.

Summary

Although patients with CAD comprise a heterogenous population, most show improved clinical status upon engaging in a program of exercise training. *Clinical status* is defined as both quality and quantity of life and is influenced by symptoms of exertional intolerance, exercise capacity, morbidity and mortality prospects, progression of atherosclerosis, and psychosocial factors. Potential exercise benefits include the following (not all patients will experience all benefits):

- Improvement in aerobic exercise capacity
- Potential improvement in submaximal exercise efficiency
- Increased muscular strength
- Improvement in the symptoms of angina pectoris, effort-related dyspnea, early fatigue, and claudication
- Reduction in myocardial ischemia, potential increase in myocardial perfusion, no evidence for augmented coronary collateralization
- Improvement in morbidity and mortality
- Reduction in classic coronary risk factors (hypertension, hypercholesteralemia, glucose intolerance)
- Potential decreased progression or actual regression of coronary atherosclerosis
- Potential reduction in ventricular arrhythmia
- Improved blood platelet function
- Reduced sympathetic nervous system response to mental and physical stress
- Decreased anxiety and depression and a faster emotional resolution following the cardiac event

References

1. American College of Sports Medicine. Guidelines for exercise testing and prescription. 4th ed. Philadelphia: Lea & Febiger; 1991:93-183.
2. American Heart Association. Exercise standards: A statement for health professionals from the American Heart Association. Circulation. 82:2286-2322; 1990.

3. Pollock, M.L.; Wilmore, J.H. Exercise in health and disease: Evaluation and prescription for prevention and rehabilitation. 2nd ed. Philadelphia: Saunders; 1990:485-642.

4. American Association of Cardiovascular and Pulmonary Rehabilitation. Guidelines for cardiac rehabilitation programs. Champaign, IL: Human Kinetics; 1991:9-15.

5. Heberden, W. Commentary on the history and cure of diseases. In: Willius, F.A.; Keys, T.E., eds. Cardiac classics. St. Louis: Mosby; 1941:224.

6. Wilson, P.K. Cardiac rehabilitation: Then and now. Physician and Sportsmedicine. 16:75-84; 1988.

7. DeBusk, R.F.; Houston, N.; Haskell, W.; Fry, G.; Parker, M. Exercise training soon after myocardial infarction. Am. J. Cardiol. 44:1223-1229; 1979.

8. Clausen, J.P.; Trap-Jensen, J. Effects of training on the distribution of cardiac output in patients with coronary artery disease. Circulation. 42:611-624; 1970.

9. Redwood, D.R.; Rosing, D.R.; Epstein, S.E. Circulatory and symptomatic effects of physical training in patients with coronary-artery disease and angina pectoris. N. Engl. J. Med. 286:959-965; 1972.

10. Detry, J.-M.R.; Rousseau, M.; Vandenbroucke, G.; Kusumi, F.; Brasseur, L.A.; Bruce, R.A. Increased arteriovenous oxygen difference after physical training in coronary heart disease. Circulation. 44:109-118; 1971.

11. Foster, C.; Pollock, M.L.; Anholm, J.D.; Squires, R.W.; Ward, A.; Dymond, D.S.; Rod, J.L.; Saichek, R.P.; Schmidt, D.H. Work capacity and left ventricular function during rehabilitation after myocardial revascularization surgery. Circulation. 69:748-755; 1984.

12. Hartung, G.H.; Rangel, R. Exercise training in postmyocardial infarction patients: Comparison of results with high risk coronary and post-bypass patients. Arch. Phys. Med. Rehabil. 62:147-150; 1981.

13. Williams, M.A.; Maresh, C.M.; Esterbrooks, D.J.; Harbrecht, J.J.; Sketch, M.H. Early exercise training in patients older than 65 years compared with that in younger patients after acute myocardial infarction or coronary artery bypass grafting. Am. J. Cardiol. 55:263-266; 1985.

14. Blumenthal, J.A.; Rejeski, W.J.; Walsh-Riddle, M.; Emery, C.F.; Miller, H.; Roark, S.; Ribisl, P.M.; Morris, P.B.; Brubaker, P.; Williams, R.S. Comparison of high- and low-intensity exercise training after acute myocardial infarction. Am. J. Cardiol. 61:26-30; 1988.

15. Gobel, A.J.; Hare, D.L.; Macdonald, P.S.; Oliver, R.G.; Reid, M.A.; Worcester, M.C. Effects of early programmes of high and low intensity exercise on physical performance after transmural acute myocardial infarction. Br. Heart J. 65:126-131; 1991.

16. Fortini, A.; Bonechi, F.; Taddei, T.; Gensini, G.F.; Malfanti, P.L.; Neri Serneri, G.G. Anaerobic threshold in patients with exercise-induced myocardial ischemia. Circulation. 83 [Suppl. III]:III50-III53; 1991.

17. Ades, P.A.; Grunvald, M.H.; Weiss, R.M.; Hanson, J.S. Usefulness of myocardial ischemia as predictor of training effect in cardiac rehabilitation after acute myocardial infarction or coronary artery bypass grafting. Am. J. Cardiol. 63:1032-1036; 1989.

18. Dressendorfer, R.H.; Smith, J.L.; Amsterdam, E.A.; Mason, D.T. Reduction of submaximal exercise myocardial oxygen demand post-walk training program in coronary patients due to improved physical work efficiency. Am. Heart J. 103:358-362; 1982.

19. Ferguson, R.J.; Taylor, A.W.; Cote, P.; Charlebois, J.; Dinelle, Y.; Peronnet, F.; DeChamplain, J.; Bourassa, M.G. Skeletal muscle and cardiac changes with training in patients with angina pectoris. Am. J. Physiol. 243(Heart Circ. Physiol. 12):H830-H836; 1982.

20. Paterson, D.H.; Shephard, R.J.; Cunningham, D.; Jones, N.L.; Andrew, G. Effects of physical training on cardiovascular function following myocardial infarction. J. Appl. Physiol. Respirat. Environ. Exercise Physiol. 47:482-489; 1979.

21. Hagberg, J.M. Physiologic adaptations to prolonged high-intensity exercise training in patients with coronary artery disease. Med. Sci. Sports Exerc. 23:661-667; 1991.

22. Rogers, M.A.; Yamamoto, C.; Hagberg, J.M.; Holloszy, J.O.; Ehsani, A.A. The effect of 7 years of intense exercise training on patients with coronary artery disease. J. Am. Coll. Cardiol. 10:321-326; 1987.

23. Ehsani, A.A.; Martin, W.H.; Heath, G.W.; Coyle, E.F. Cardiac effects of prolonged and intense exercise training in patients with coronary artery disease. Am. J. Cardiol. 50:246-254; 1982.

24. Hagberg, J.M.; Ehsani, A.A.; Holloszy, J.O. Effect of 12 months of intense exercise training on stroke volume in patients with coronary artery disease. Circulation. 67:1194-1199; 1983.

25. Martin, W.H.; Heath, G.; Coyle, E.F.; Bloomfield, S.A.; Holloszy, J.O.; Ehsani, A.A. Effect of prolonged intense endurance training on systolic time intervals in patients with coronary artery disease. Am. Heart J. 107:75-81; 1984.

26. Ehsani, A.A.; Biello, D.R.; Schultz, J.; Sobel, B.E.; Holloszy, J.O. Improvement of left ventricular contractile function by exercise training in patients with coronary artery disease. Circulation. 74:350-358; 1986.

27. Martin, W.H.; Ehsani, A.A. Reversal of exertional hypotension by prolonged exercise training in selected patients with ischemic heart disease. Circulation. 76:548-555; 1987.

28. Multicenter Postinfarction Research Group. Risk stratification and survival after myocardial infarction. N. Engl. J. Med. 309:331-336; 1983.

29. Sullivan, M.J.; Higginbotham, M.B.; Cobb, F.R. Exercise training in patients with severe left ventricular dysfunction: Hemodynamic and metabolic effects. Circulation. 78:506-515; 1988.

30. Sullivan, M.J.; Higginbotham, M.B.; Cobb, F.R. Exercise training in patients with chronic heart failure

delays ventilatory anaerobic threshold and improves submaximal exercise performance. Circulation. 79:324-329; 1989.

31. Coats, A.J.S.; Adamopoulos, S.; Meyer, T.E.; Conway, J.; Sleight, P. Effects of physical training in chronic heart failure. Lancet. 335:63-66; 1990.

32. Pilote, L.; Silberg, J.; Lisbona, R.; Sniderman, A. Prognosis in patients with low left ventricular ejection fraction after myocardial infarction: Importance of exercise capacity. Circulation. 80:1636-1641; 1989.

33. Mancini, D.M.; Eisen, H.; Kussmaul, W.; Mull, R.; Edmunds, L.H.; Wilson, J.R. Value of peak oxygen consumption for optimal timing of cardiac transplantation in ambulatory patients with heart failure. Circulation. 83:778-786; 1991.

34. Squires, R.W.; Lavie, C.J.; Brandt, T.R.; Gau, G.T.; Bailey, K.R. Cardiac rehabilitation in patients with severe left ventricular dysfunction. Mayo Clin. Proc. 62:997-1002; 1987.

35. Giordano, A.; Giannuzzi, P.; Tavazzi, L. Feasibility of physical training in post-infarct patients with left ventricular aneurysm: A hemodynamic study. Eur. Heart J. 9[Suppl. F]:11-15; 1988.

36. Jugdutt, B.I.; Michorowski, B.L.; Kappagoda, C.T. Exercise training after anterior Q wave myocardial infarction: Importance of regional left ventricular function and topography. J. Am. Coll. Cardiol. 12:362-372; 1988.

37. Rowe, M.H.; Jelinek, M.V.; Liddell, N.; Hugens, M. Effect of rapid mobilization on ejection fractions and ventricular volumes after acute myocardial infarction. Am. J. Cardiol. 63:1037-1041; 1989.

38. Giannuzzi, P.; Temporelli, P.L.; Tavassi, L.; Corra, A.; Gattone, M.; Imparato, A.; Giordano, A.; Schweiger, C.; Sala, L.; Maliverni, C. EAMI—exercise in anterior myocardial infarction: An ongoing multicenter randomized study: Preliminary results on left ventricular function and remodeling. Chest. 101[Suppl.]:315S-321S; 1992.

39. Kelemen, M.H.; Stewart, K.J.; Gillian, R.E.; Ewart, C.K.; Valenti, S.A.; Manley, J.D.; Kelemen, M.D. Circuit weight training in cardiac patients. J. Am. Coll. Cardiol. 7:38-42; 1986.

40. Squires, R.W.; Muri, A.J.; Anderson, L.J.; Allison, T.G.; Miller, T.D.; Gau, G.T. Weight training during phase II (early outpatient) cardiac rehabilitation: Heart rate and blood pressure responses. J. Cardiopul. Rehabil. 11:360-364; 1991.

41. McCartney, N.; McKelvie, R.S.; Haslam, D.R.S.; Jones, N.L. Usefulness of weightlifting training in improving strength and maximal power output in coronary artery disease. Am. J. Cardiol. 67:939-945; 1991.

42. Stewart, K.J.; Mason, M.; Kelemen, M.H. Three-year participation in circuit weight training improves muscular strength and self-efficacy in cardiac patients. J. Cardiopul. Rehabil. 8:292-296; 1988.

43. Kennedy, C.C.; Spiekerman, R.E.; Lindsay, M.I.; Mankin, H.T.; Frye, R.L.; McCallister, B.D. One-year graduated exercise program for men with angina pectoris: Evaluation by physiologic studies and coronary angiography. Mayo Clin. Proc. 51:231-236; 1976.

44. Franklin, B.A.; Wrisley, D.; Johnson, S.; Mitchell, M.; Rubenfire, M. Chronic adaptations to physical conditioning in cardiac patients. Clin. Sports Med. 3:471-512; 1984.

45. Thompson, P.D. The benefits and risks of exercise training in patients with chronic coronary artery disease. JAMA. 259:1537-1540; 1988.

46. Clausen, J.P. Circulatory adjustments to dynamic exercise and effect of physical training in normal subjects and in patients with coronary disease. Prog. Cardiovasc. Dis. 18:459-495; 1976.

47. Raffo, J.A.; Luksic, I.Y.; Kappagoda, C.T.; Mary, D.A.S.G.; Whitaker, W.; Linden, R.J. Effects of physical training on myocardial ischemia in patients with coronary artery disease. Br. Heart J. 43:262-269; 1980.

48. Laslett, L.J.; Paumer, L.; Amsterdam, E.A. Increase in myocardial oxygen consumption index by exercise training at the onset of ischemia in patients with coronary artery disease. Circulation. 71:958-962; 1985.

49. Froelicher, V.; Jensen, D.; Genter, F.; Sullivan, M.; Mckirnan, M.D.; Witztum, K.; Scharf, J.; Strong, M.L.; Ashburn, W. A randomized trial of exercise training in patients with coronary heart disease. JAMA. 252:1291-1297; 1984.

50. Schuler, G.; Schlief, G.; Wirth, A.; Mautner, H.P.; Scheurlen, H.; Thumm, M.; Roth, H.; Scharz, F.; Kohlmeier, M.; Mehmel, H.C.; Kubler, W. Low-fat diet and regular, supervised physical exercise in patients with symptomatic coronary artery disease: Reduction of stress-induced myocardial ischemia. Circulation. 77:172-181; 1988.

51. Schuler, G.; Hambrecht, R.; Schlief, G.; Grunze, M.; Methfessel, S.; Hanet, K.; Kubler, W. Myocardial perfusion and regression of coronary artery disease in patients on a regimen of intensive physical exercise and low fat diet. J. Am. Coll. Cardiol. 19:34-42; 1992.

52. Haslam, R.W.; Cobb, R.B. Frequency of intensive, prolonged exercise as a determinant of relative coronary circumference index. Int. J. Sports Med. 3:118-121; 1982.

53. Wyatt, H.L., Mitchell, J. Influences of physical conditioning and deconditioning on coronary vasculature of dogs. J. Appl. Physiol. 45:619-625; 1978.

54. Rakusan, K.; Wicker, P. Morphometry of the small arteries and arterioles in the rate heart: Effects of chronic hypertension and exercise. Cardiovasc. Res. 24:278-284; 1990.

55. Franklin, B.A. Exercise training and coronary collateral circulation. Med. Sci. Sports Exerc. 23:648-653; 1991.

56. Olridge, N.B.; Guyatt, G.H.; Fischer, M.E.; Rimm, A.A. Cardiac rehabilitation after myocardial infarction: Combined experience of randomized clinical trials. JAMA. 260:945-950; 1988.

57. O'Connor, G.T.; Buring, J.E.; Yusuf, S.; Goldhaber, S.Z.; Olmstead, E.M.; Paffenbarger, R.S.; Hennekens,

C.H. An overview of randomized trials of rehabilitation with exercise after myocardial infarction. Circulation. 80:234-244; 1989.

58. Hamalainen, H.; Luurila, O.J.; Kallio, V.; Knuts, L.R.; Arstila, M.; Hakkila, J. Long-term reduction in sudden deaths after a multifactorial intervention programme in patients with myocardial infarction: 10-year results of a controlled investigation. Eur. Heart J. 10:55-62; 1989.

59. Kramsch, D.M.; Aspen, A.J.; Abramowitz, B.M.; Kreimendahl, T.; Hood, W.B. Reduction of coronary atherosclerosis by moderate conditioning exercise in monkeys on an atherogenic diet. N. Engl. J. Med. 304:1483-1489; 1981.

60. Raichlen, J.S.; Healy, B.; Achuff, S.C.; Pearson, T.A. Importance of risk factors in the angiographic progression of coronary artery disease. Am. J. Cardiol. 57:66-70; 1986.

60a. Hambrecht, R.; Niebauer, J.; Marburger, C.; Grunze, M.; Kalborer, B.; Haner, K.; Schlorf, G.; Kubler, W.; Schulor, G. Various intensities of leisure time physical activity in patients with coronary artery disease: Effects on cardiorespiratory fitness and progression of coronary atherosclerotic lesions. J. Am. Coll. Cardiol. 22:468-477; 1993.

61. Hartung, G.H.; Squires, W.G.; Gotto, A.M. Effect of exercise on plasma high-density lipoprotein cholesterol in coronary disease patients. Am. Heart J. 101:181-184; 1981.

62. Mendoza, S.G.; Carrasco, H.; Zerpa, A., Briceno, Y.; Rodriguez, F.; Glueck, C.J. Effect of physical training on lipids, lipoproteins, apolipoproteins, lipases, and endogenous sex hormones in men with premature myocardial infarction. Metabolism. 40:368-377; 1991.

63. Leon, A.S. Effects of exercise conditioning on physiologic precursors of coronary heart disease. J. Cardiopul. Rehabil. 11:46-57; 1991.

64. Simonson, D.C.; Dzau, V.J. Workshop IX: Lipids, insulin, and diabetes. In: Schoenberger, J.A., ed. Hypertension, lipids and cardiovascular disease: Is insulin the missing link? Am. J. Med. 90(2A):855-865; 1991.

65. Leon, A.S.; Conrad, J.; Hunninghake, D.B.; Serfass, R. Effects of a vigorous walking program on body composition and carbohydrate and lipid metabolism in obese young men. Am. J. Clin. Nutr. 33:1176-1187; 1979.

66. Heath, G.W.; Gavin, J.R.; Hinderliter, J.M.; Hagberg, J.M.; Holloszy, J.O. Effects of exercise and lack of exercise on glucose tolerance and insulin sensitivity. J. Appl. Physiol. 55:512-517; 1983.

67. Donahue, R.P.; Orchard, T.J.; Becker, D.J.; Kuller, H.; Drash, A.I. Physical activity, insulin sensitivity, and the lipoprotein profile in young adults: The Beaver County study. Am. J. Epidemiol. 127:95-103; 1988.

68. Entrican, J.H.; Beach, C.; Carroll, D.; Klopper, A.; Mackie, M.; Douglas, A.S. Raised plasma estradiol and estrogen levels in young survivors of myocardial infarction. Lancet. 2:487-489; 1978.

69. Osborn, M.J. Sudden cardiac death. A. Mechanism, incidence and prevention of sudden cardiac death. In: Giuliani, E.R.; Fuster, V.; Gersh, B.J.; McGoon, M.D.; McGoon, D.C., eds. Cardiology: Fundamentals and practice, 2nd ed. Chicago: Mosby; 1991: 975-1004.

70. Blackburn, H.; Taylor, H.L.; Hamrell, B.; Buskirk, E.; Nicholas, W.C.; Thorsen, R.D. Premature ventricular complexes induced by stress testing: Their frequency and response to physical conditioning. Am. J. Cardiol. 31:441-449; 1973.

71. Posel, D.; Noakes, T.; Kantor, P.; Lambert, M.; Opie, L.H. Exercise training after experimental myocardial infarction increases the ventricular fibrillation threshold before and after the onset of reinfarction in the isolated rate heart. Circulation. 80:138-145; 1989.

72. Fuster, V. Atherosclerosis: Pathogenesis, pathology, and presentation of atherosclerosis. In: Giuliani, E.R.; Fuster, V.; Gersh, B.J.; McGoon, M.D.; McGoon, D.C., eds. Cardiology: Fundamentals and practice, 2nd ed. Chicago: Mosby; 1991:1172-1210.

73. Forrester, J.S.; Litak, F.; Grundfest, W. Initiating events of acute coronary arterial occlusion. Annu. Rev. Med. 42:35-45; 1991.

74. Lehman, M.; Keul, J. Physical activity and coronary heart disease: Sympathetic drive and adrenaline-induced platelet aggregation. Int. J. Sports Med. 7[Suppl. 1]:34-37; 1986.

75. Ferguson, E.W.; Bernier, L.L.; Banta, G.R; Yu-Yahiro, J.; Schoomaker, E.B. Effects of exercise and conditioning on clotting and fibrinolytic activity in men. J. Appl. Physiol. 62:1416-1421; 1987.

76. Eichner, E.R. Coagulability and rheology: Hematologic benefits from exercise, fish, and aspirin. Implications for athletes and nonathletes. Phys. Sports. Med. 14:102-110; 1986.

77. Ernst, E. Influence of regular physical activity on blood rheology. Eur. Heart J. 8[Suppl. G]:59-62; 1987.

78. McGill, D.; McGuiness, J.; Lloyd, J.; Ardle, N. Platelet function and exercise-induced myocardial ischemia in coronary heart disease patients. Thromb. Res. 56:147-158; 1989.

79. Krantz, D.S.; Manuck, S.B. Acute psychophysiologic reactivity and risk of cardiovascular disease: A review and methodologic critique. Psychol. Bull. 96: 435-464; 1984.

80. Blumenthal, J.A.; Fredrikson, M.; Kuhn, C.M.; Ulmer, R.L.; Walsh-Riddle, M.; Appelbaum, M. Aerobic exercise reduces levels of cardiovascular and sympathoadrenal responses to mental stress in subjects without prior evidence of myocardial ischemia. Am. J. Cardiol. 65:93-98; 1990.

81. Rogers, P.J.; Bove, A.A.; Squires, R.W.; Bailey, K.R. Cardiovascular responses to the cold pressor test in exercise-trained and untrained men. J. Cardiopul. Rehabil. 12:518-524; 1988.

82. Cassem, N.H.; Hackett, T.P. Psychological rehabilitation of myocardial infarction patients in the acute phase. Heart Lung. 2:382-388; 1973.

83. Eliot, R.S.; Long, D.R.; Boone, J.L. Rehabilitation. In: Eliot, R.S., ed. Stress and the heart: Mechanisms, measurements, and management. Mount Kisco, NY: Futura Publishing Company; 1988:185-200.

84. Roviaro, S.; Holmes, D.S.; Holmsten, R.D. Influence of a cardiac rehabilitation program on the cardiovascular, psychological, and social functioning of cardiac patients. J. Behav. Med. 7:61-81; 1984.

85. Taylor, C.B.; Houston-Miller, N.; Ahn, D.K.; Haskell, W.; DeBusk, R.F. The effects of exercise training programs on psychosocial improvement in uncomplicated postmyocardial infarction patients. J. Psychosom. Res. 30:581-587; 1986.

86. Burgess, A.W.; Lerner, D.J.; D'Agostino, R.B.; Vokonas, P.S.; Hartman, C.R.; Gaccione, P. A radomized control trial of cardiac rehabilitation. Soc. Sci. Med. 24:359-370; 1987.

87. Oldridge, N.; Guyatt, G.; Jones, N.; Crowe, J.; Singer, J.; Feeny, D.; McKelvie, R.; Runions, J.; Streiner, D.; Torrance, G. Effects on quality of life with comprehensive rehabilitation after acute myocardial infarction. Am. J. Cardiol. 67:1084-4089.

Chapter 10

Behavior Modification for Cardiovascular Risk Factor Reduction

Nancy Houston Miller

C. Barr Taylor

Over the past 20 years much has been learned about how to institute and develop behavioral programs that can help patients with heart disease adopt a healthy lifestyle (1,2). The purpose of this chapter is to review the basic principles of behavior modification that lead toward a more healthy lifestyle. Patients suffering from coronary artery disease (CAD) are faced with many changes, which may include adopting a low-fat, low-cholesterol diet; beginning an exercise program; adhering to long-term medications for management of their disease; losing weight; and quitting smoking. In this chapter we will discuss the general behavioral approaches to these areas and provide an example of how these principles are applied in one program. Among the many models of change that have been developed to explain and guide risk factor modification, those fitting into the general domain of behavior therapy will be the main focus.

Models of Behavioral Change

In its early phases, behavior therapy principles and practice were largely guided by operant (Skinnerian) and classical (Pavlovian) conditioning (3). These models focused on behavior and paid little attention to cognition. More recently, models of behavior change applied to health problems have been developed that include social and cognitive factors. Social learning theory is the most widely cited and applied model; it demonstrates human functioning related to behavioral, cognitive, and environmental factors (4,5). The interventions for the Multiple Risk Factor Intervention Trial, the Lipid Research Clinics Coronary Primary Prevention Trial, and the Stanford Five-City Project, which each encouraged people to make sustained behavior changes over a number of years, were guided by social learning theory.

Self-Efficacy

Social learning theory also emphasizes the importance of self-efficacy as a mediator of behavior change. Self-efficacy is defined as a "person's judgment to organize and execute a course of action to attain a designated type of performance." A person's self-efficacy, or confidence, strongly relates to his or her performance. People are unlikely to undertake tasks when they have little confidence that they will succeed. Self-efficacy is influenced by four main factors:

- **Information and persuasion.** Patients with CAD now receive a bewildering amount of information, often from the mass media, that guides their behavior. The impact of this information is evident on a national level, as seen in such important changes in risk factor modification as smoking rates and in lower levels of cholesterol related to dietary consumption. Despite the importance of the mass media, however, health professionals remain the most credible source of information and are often seminal in encouraging patients to begin the health change process.

  Persuasion from an authority refers to the information and instructions that health care providers impart to their patients, that is, how they educate patients. In addition to imparting information, health care professionals play a critical role in creating positive, and presumably realistic, expectations about the rate, magnitude, and effect of change. Such expectations have been shown to strongly influence behavior (5).

- **Observation of others.** Many important lifestyle changes are undoubtedly influenced by watching others. Some have argued that the value of group cardiac rehabilitation programs may derive from the enhanced opportunity for patients to observe how others are doing.

- **Successful performance of the behavior.** Past and current experience guide the actions of many patients. Unfortunately, patients are more likely to focus on past failures than successes. For instance, smokers may conclude from past failures at quitting that they may have trouble quitting following coronary artery bypass graft (CABG) surgery or a heart attack. In fact, most smokers are able to quit following such an event. Many behavior modification programs request that patients review their previous attempts at changing behavior in an attempt to decide what they can do better or differently the next time.

- **Physiological feedback.** Physiological feedback also guides experience, as evidenced by the fact that the treadmill graded exercise test (GXT) can have a strong effect on a patient's self-efficacy and subsequent behavior (2,6). Post-GXT counseling and feedback on functional capacity, any abnormalities, prognosis, and exercise prescription guidelines amplifies the impact on efficacy in helping patients return to routine activities (2).

Other Models of Behavior Change

A number of other theories have been proposed to help us understand health behavior change. Many years ago, Becker and his colleagues (7) developed the Health Belief Model, which assumes that individuals are likely to change when they believe that they are at risk to develop a problem, that the recommended changes will improve their condition or reduce their risk, and that the changes are within their ability and resources to accomplish. Behavioral interventions often begin after the person has decided to make changes. The Health Belief Model provides insight into factors that need to be considered in helping to motivate patients to change.

Ajzen and Fishbein (8) have emphasized the importance of expectations and activities as precursors of behavior change. The stages of change model posits that change occurs through stages that progress from precontemplation to contemplation, action, and maintenance (9). In this model, different strategies may be needed to move a patient from one stage to another. For instance, individuals still only contemplating behavior change

may need interventions designed to change their beliefs, to clarify the advantages of change, or to improve their efficacy.

Elements of a Successful Behavioral Program

The theories just described, in conjunction with social learning theory, are useful in helping us understand why people change, and they have led to several intervention strategies. However, it is the *practice* of behavior therapy that is the source of most of the interventions that effect and maintain behavior change. (3,10-12). Furthermore, despite innumerable studies, the basic elements of a successful behavioral program derive more from clinical experience than from published research. The 11 basic components that characterize most successful behavioral programs are delineated here (2).

1. *Positive, Accurate Expectations About Results*

The outcome that patients expect from adopting or changing a behavior and their confidence of making that change both influence how likely they are to make and sustain the change. Patients who wish to reduce their serum cholesterol through dietary change are more likely to adopt a low-fat diet if they think that doing so will have some benefit.

Consistent with the Health Belief Model, the behavior change needs to be linked to its physiological effect and its potential long-term benefit.

Creating positive yet accurate patient expectations can be difficult in secondary prevention. For instance, a patient with elevated cholesterol should be encouraged to adopt a low-fat, low-cholesterol diet yet cautioned that such changes may not, in his or her case, have an immediate or large impact on reducing serum cholesterol.

Patients will rapidly abandon programs if their expectations exceed the perceived benefit. For instance, patients may expect sudden and major changes from beginning an exercise program, so when they do not notice immediate changes, they stop exercising.

Patients with positive expectations must also have the requisite skills and tools to make changes and the confidence that they can make the changes. Expectation and confidence are both affected by the principles of social learning theory.

2. *Precisely Defined Behavior Changes*

Specifying the behavior changes that need to be made is the hallmark of behavior therapy. Many questionnaires and surveys have been developed to help individuals define the behavior to be changed. In the area of diet, food frequency forms are used to identify customary dietary patterns and thus possible areas of change. These forms provide a rather global view of dietary behavior, such as the number of servings of meat or complex carbohydrates per day or week. Other interventions are based on analysis of individual food items. Computer technology has made the acquisition of detailed information about individual food selection relatively easy. Most smoking cessation programs include at least some self-monitoring to help patients identify their smoking patterns and high-risk situations that could lead to relapse.

Whereas changes in diet or smoking involve alterations in existing behavior, many other secondary prevention activities involve the adoption of new behaviors, as in the case of beginning an exercise program. The exercise behaviors need to be precisely defined.

3. *Realistic Goals*

Goals for behavior change should be realistic in terms of both the time required to achieve them and the magnitude of change expected. A given program for change should have distal and proximal goals. Distal goals are the desired long-term effects of behavior change, such as an agreed-upon weight loss or a lowering of serum cholesterol. Proximal goals involve the behaviors likely to bring about the distal goals and are the immediate focus of behavior therapy. A realistic proximal goal for weight loss, for example, would be a loss of 0.5 to 1 kg/week.

4. *Contracting*

In our progressively legalistic society, we have come to expect contracts in many of our transactions. Perhaps for this reason, contracts are a useful way of ensuring that a patient is committed to a particular behavior change; they also serve as a reminder in helping the patient achieve that change. Contracts should be written with the patient, they should be realistic, and the goals should be specified in concrete terms that define both the positive and negative consequences of achieving or not achieving a goal. An example of a contract is seen in Figure 10.1.

An alternative to a formal contract is a written agreement, in which a patient agrees to perform certain behaviors. Different from a contract, a written agreement fully describes the expectations of the patient in participating in changing a health behavior or joining a program and indicates actions of the health care professional in supporting the patient. Although this may not be as effective as a contract, it helps to formalize the commitment between the patient and the health care professional that certain changes are to be made. An example of a written agreement is shown in Figure 10.2.

5. *Prevention of Lapse and Relapse*

Relapse prevention theory is derived from studies of alcoholics and drug dependent patients. In studies of alcoholics, Marlatt and colleagues (13) observed that abstinent patients who relapsed justified continued drinking by telling themselves that, since they had already failed in the attempt

Exercise Contract

I, _____, agree to initiate my exercise program tomorrow and to do the following over the next month:

1. Walk 20 to 30 minutes 5 days a week
2. Record my exercise sessions on my daily activity log every evening

If I miss more than three exercise sessions per week I agree to call my support person for help. My support person will send me one postcard reminder in 2 weeks.

This contract will be reevaluated in 1 month.

_____   _____
Your signature   Date

_____   _____
Health Care Provider   Date

Figure 10.1 Exercise contract.

MULTIFIT
Written Agreement

Congratulations! You have joined the MULTIFIT program. Through this program a nurse will counsel you about coronary risk factors such as exercise, diet, and smoking before you leave the hospital and will continue to work with you for the next 12 months to lower your coronary risk.

The more you put into the program the more you will get out of it. We hope that after discussing our mutual expectations, you will formalize your participation by signing the contract below.

We expect you to do the following:

- Be willing to modify your risk factors by exercising regularly; lowering your cholesterol by changing your eating patterns and, if necessary, taking lipid lowering drugs; and stopping smoking
- Complete activity logs, food frequency forms, and questionnaires used to evaluate your progress
- Have your blood drawn for cholesterol levels at 2, 3, 6, and 12 months after your hospitalization and have additional samples drawn if your cholesterol is still elevated after 3 months of dietary therapy
- Discuss your progress with the program nurse at various intervals by telephone

You can expect us to do the following:

- Be committed to giving you support and education for the coming year
- Help you produce a much healthier and happier lifestyle for you and your family

I understand these expectations and agree to participate in the MULTIFIT program as described above.

_____   _____
Your signature   Date signed

_____   _____
Health Care Provider   Date signed

Figure 10.2   Written agreement.

---

to remain dry, they might as well keep on drinking. Researchers then began to focus on what caused the relapse and how it could be avoided the next time. The strategies that developed out of these studies found their most useful application in patients with addictive behaviors. However, many of these techniques are useful for all changes in health behaviors.

In practice, relapse prevention involves preparing people to cope with a lapse (from a new good habit) or relapse (back to an old habit) in behavior that may lead to total relapse or discontinuation of a program. Through relapse prevention training, individuals are taught to identify the situations or feelings that may cause a relapse, to learn skills to cope with these situations, and to practice these skills on a continuing basis.

6. *Modeling*

As mentioned previously, watching others is a powerful source of behavior change. Observing someone else perform behaviors may help the patient feel more efficacious and alleviate questions or concerns about how to go about a change. Group programs provide modeling for many behavior changes, as do videotapes.

7. *Prompting*

Prompts are very useful in helping patients sustain behavior change. Prompts can be as simple as a note on the calendar or a reminder on the refrigerator door. Home-based exercise programs use telephone calls to prompt exercise behavior (14,15). Attendance at a group exercise program can be seen as a type of prompt for exercising.

8. *Feedback*

Feedback, whether provided by a health care professional or a support person, influences behavior change. In home-based exercise programs, feedback from the nurse who monitors the patient's exercise log may be an important component for improving adherence. For a patient engaged in an exercise program following a myocardial infarction (MI), a 6-month GXT can provide extremely gratifying results that may help sustain exercise for the next 6 months.

9. *Problem Solving*

Problem solving is important in overcoming barriers and difficulties with health behavior change. Problem solving involves first specifying the problem in concrete terms, identifying possible solutions, and then developing a plan to implement the solutions. Once this has been completed it is important for the patient to try out the solution and evaluate the effectiveness of the results. The process is repeated if initial solutions have not been successful.

10. *Rewards*

Many programs use monetary or other rewards to influence behavior. Rewards can be as simple as enjoying a television program for exercising or purchasing a new piece of clothing with the money saved from 3 months of nonsmoking. While at the outset many patients develop a plan for rewarding themselves, many do not carry through with their rewards unless encouraged to do so. For many, praise from co-workers, a family member, or health care professional may be an important component of a reward system.

11. *Social Support*

Social support refers to the help that patients receive from family, friends, and society. The absence of social support (social isolation) has been associated with increased mortality from CAD (16). Individuals with greater social support exhibit better compliance than those with less social support. Although many people think of spousal or family support as most beneficial in health behavior change, the use of the "buddy system" to ensure compliance can be highly effective. When support is active and ongoing it can be extremely beneficial, but one needs to be cautious about nagging or inviting guilt for someone's failure to do something.

Stages of Intervention

The principles stated thus far need to be organized into a program to support the basic changes required for modifying a person's behavior. Health behavior change can be conceptualized as occurring in three basic stages:

1. The *antecedent stage*, in which a person is contemplating change
2. The *adoption stage* (corresponding to the action stage in the Stages of Change Model), when a person begins to initiate change

3. The *maintenance stage*, in which the behavior is sustained over months or years.

Different behavioral interventions may be relatively more important during one of these stages then during others.

In the remainder of this section, a general sequence of interventions for typical patients is provided. Health behavior change is a long-term dynamic process, and programs or patients are rarely able to follow this idealized model. Nevertheless, carefully thinking about how to put a program together to maximize and sustain behavior change is important. Most rehabilitation programs put most of the effort in the period immediately following an MI, CABG surgery, or angioplasty, whereas a much longer sustained effort may be needed to achieve significant secondary prevention benefits. In fact, the benefits of secondary risk reduction interventions may not be evident until 3 years or longer after such an event.

Antecedent Stage

Antecedents refer to all the factors that help initiate, hinder, or support change. A person's motivation, expectation, intention, and level of confidence are all important antecedents to change. Most patients in cardiac rehabilitation have been frightened by their surgery or heart disease and are very motivated to make changes to avoid or postpone further problems. As noted previously, a patient's belief about the importance of change, perception of the benefits that change might bring about, and confidence that the extent of changes are within his or her control all need to be addressed in programs.

Providing Information for Change

Since information and instructions are important antecedents to change, programs need to consider how best to provide them. Usually this is done with some face-to-face counseling, often in the hospital or at least soon after discharge. Videotapes, audiotapes, written materials, and even multimedia computer programs can be useful and save labor in this early stage.

It is also important to assess how adequate the program has been in providing the prerequisite material to the patient. A simple test assessing the patient's knowledge about items key to health behavior change can help evaluate the program's success and identify areas where the patient remains confused.

In the antecedent stage, it is important that health care professionals involved in the patient's care provide uniform and consistent messages and instructions. Some programs provide patients with handouts that summarize the features and expectations of the program. In the Stanford Cardiac Rehabilitation Program, we provide a standard form to physicians that requests them to go to the bedside to provide a clear, firm recommendation about the importance of not smoking or remaining a non-smoker. Videotapes and booklets can also help the patient achieve this goal.

Ensuring Patients' Intentions

After patients have sufficient knowledge about what and how to change and the confidence that they can undertake the change, it is important to ask them about their level of intention to change a particular behavior. An easy way to ask this question is to use a simple scale, in which 0 is "very unlikely" and 7 is "very likely." If patients have little or no intention of changing, then some attention should be given to determining if they understand the positive benefits of change and the potential long-term results.

Defining Needed Change

Once a patient is favorable to change, the behaviors that need to be changed must be clearly defined. Self-monitoring or similar evaluation tools are useful for defining these behaviors. New technological interventions can also facilitate this process (17). For instance, DietCoach, developed by the Stanford Cardiac Rehabilitation Program, is a state-of-the-art nutrition education and behavioral change program. This multimedia computer program allows patients to identify their food patterns with a food frequency questionnaire shown on a computer terminal and then to set goals with the help of the instantaneous, color-graphics feedback that delineates what the effects of possible changes in their diet might achieve. A laser disc stores segments in which a dietitian discusses aspects of the program or in which several individuals undergoing dietary change model shopping behavior, food preparation, and other skills. The patient may view these segments as desired. Other color graphics illustrate the fat and other nutrient content of food.

Adoption Stage

Adoption is the early initiation of behavior change. Certain environmental and physical prerequisites are necessary for the adoption of health behavior change, such as purchasing equipment and scheduling time to exercise. Prompting is important during this stage. Also in the adoption stage, the patient tries out new behaviors, which if unsatisfactory or too difficult will require seeking solutions.

Patients frequently have questions and need help in finding ways to cope with the addition or deletion of a behavior. In this regard the telephone is perhaps the most underutilized tool of behavior change. Spending a little time, health care professionals can solve problems and provide positive feedback by telephone. Several studies using the telephone to provide feedback to help MI patients adhere to exercise regimens, for example, have reported adherence rates of 70% to 80% in the first 6 months post-MI (14,15). In a smoking study in which nurses engaged in problem solving by telephone during the adoption stage of smoking cessation, post-MI patients achieved a 71% abstinence rate (confirmed biochemically) at 1 year compared to 45% in a usual-care group (18).

Maintenance Stage

Although there is some overlap between the adoption and maintenance stages of the behavior change process, there are certain elements that play a larger role in ensuring that a health behavior is maintained. For example, one of the most important elements in the maintenance stage is preventing relapses, training for which should begin even prior to the adoption stage. If patients are prepared for lapses and have mastered the skills to cope when faced with these situations, they are much more likely to reinstitute the behavior appropriately.

Although contracting should be initiated in the adoption stage, it also becomes important during maintenance. The patient feels a sense of responsibility to maintain the behavior if a formal agreement has been developed with a co-worker, health care professional, or family member. Additional contracts during maintenance may reinforce the commitment. Finally, social support and rewards are important during maintenance. These help ensure that risk factor changes are sustained for a lifetime.

Unfortunately, relatively little is known about how to provide relatively inexpensive long-term maintenance. Many of the clinical trials involving long-term multifactorial risk reduction have relied heavily on expensive multidisciplinary, clinic-based programs. Commercial group programs obviously provide one avenue for maintenance. Lay programs offer another. The potentially powerful effect of lay-led groups was demonstrated in a study in Norway that enrolled 80,000 persons (out of a national population of 4 million) into lay-led weight-control groups. The dropout rate was less than 10%, with weight losses averaging 14 lb with the aid of follow-up sessions (19). In the more culturally diverse and heterogeneous population of the United States, such successes are not likely, but the Norwegian experience points to the potential of lay-led groups to sustain behavior change.

Telephone follow-up and self-monitoring forms provide other relatively inexpensive tools to help sustain behavior change (15,20).

The MULTIFIT Program

An example of an integrated, behavioral program for cardiovascular risk factor reduction that includes many of the elements described thus far provides an overview of the behavior change process. MULTIFIT is a multiple risk factor intervention program developed at the Standford Cardiac Rehabilitation Program and designed to help patients change their behavior in the year following an MI. The interventions include exercise training, smoking cessation, and diet and drug management of hyperlipidemia, all of which are undertaken at home (21,22). Based on social learning theory and behavior therapy, the program is initiated during hospitalization about 3 days post-MI, and patients are followed for 1 year in the outpatient phase by specially trained nurses who help them manage their risk factors. The following describes the behavior change elements that are incorporated into the MULTIFIT program.

- **Written agreement.** The patient and nurse formalize the patient's participation in the MULTIFIT program with a written agreement.
- **Self-observation forms.** Such forms as a food frequency questionnaire, smoking history form, and self-efficacy form are used to identify areas of needed change.
- **Goal-setting.** Patients are asked to make small incremental changes in their eating behaviors; they receive suggested proximal and distal goals through computer-generated progress reports. Patient and nurse discuss recommended goals by telephone.

- **Contracting.** Contracts are used to commit patients to smoking cessation and exercise training and to define the positive and negative consequences of not achieving a goal.
- **Relapse prevention training.** High-risk situations that may trigger relapse are identified through self-efficacy scales for smoking, and in-hospital counseling by nurses is provided. Patients also identify relapse situations for diet and exercise training, which are monitored on single-item forms. These high-risk situations are monitored using calendars placed on the patient's refrigerator.
- **Modeling.** Patients are introduced to MULTI-FIT through a videotape that incorporates patient testimonials and modeling of behaviors to be changed. Additional videotapes specific to each risk factor are viewed as the behaviors are introduced to the patient.
- **Prompting.** Telephone calls by nurses in the outpatient phase of recovery prompt patients. Telephone calls occur monthly for 5 months and then every 2 months for 6 more months during the maintenance phase. Refrigerator calendars also serve as prompts. Patients are asked to identify their own specific prompts for taking medication once hyperlipidemic medications are prescribed.
- **Feedback.** Positive reinforcement is provided by the nurses through telephone calls. Spousal support is encouraged. Physiological feedback is provided through exercise logs and tests, laboratory cholesterol measurements, and measurement of weight.
- **Problem solving.** Barriers to compliance and getting back on track and difficulties in initiating behavioral changes are discussed and solved by regularly scheduled telephone calls.

Although the methods used to effect behavior change in the MULTIFIT program may seem numerous, compliance rates at 6 and 12 months post-MI remain high. The amount of nursing time spent per patient throughout the 12-month intervention is approximately 9 hours; the majority of contact time occurs by telephone and through the mail.

Summary

The use of behavioral interventions to reduce cardiovascular risk factors has been shown to facilitate a healthy lifestyle in patients with CAD. A systematic approach to incorporating the elements of a successful program of risk factor modification is necessary to achieve change. In addition, organized intervention during the antecedent, adoption, and maintenance stages will help to improve the likelihood of success with the behavior change process.

References

1. Miller, N.H.; Taylor, C.B.; Davidson, D.M.; Hill, M.N.; Krantz, D.S. The efficacy of risk factor intervention and psychological aspects of rehabilitation. Journal of Cardiopulmonary Rehabilitation. 10:198-209; 1990.
2. Taylor, C.B.; Miller, N.H. Education of the coronary patient and family: The behavioral approach. In: Wenger, N.K.; Hellerstein, H.K.; eds. Rehabilitation of the coronary patient, 3rd ed. New York: Churchill Livingstone; 1991.
3. Agras, W.S.; Kazdin, A.E.; Wilson, G.T. Behavior therapy: Toward an applied clinical science. San Francisco: WH Freeman; 1979.
4. Bandura, A. Social learning theory. Englewood Cliffs, NJ: Prentice Hall; 1977.
5. Bandura, A. Social foundations of thought and action: A social cognitive theory, Englewood Cliffs, NJ: Prentice Hall; 1986.
6. Ewart, C.K.; Taylor, C.B.; Reese, L.B.; DeBusk, R.F. Effects of early postmyocardial infarction exercise testing on self-perception and subsequent physical activity. Am. J. Cardiol. 51:1076-1080; 1983.
7. Becker, M.H. The health belief model and personal health behavior. Health Education Monographs. 2:236-508; 1974.
8. Ajzen, I; Fishbein, M. Understanding attitudes and predicting social behavior. Englewood Cliffs, NJ: Prentice Hall; 1980.
9. Prochaska, J.O.; DiClemente, C.C. Stage process of self-change of smoking: Toward an integrative model of change. J. Consult. Clin. Psychol. 51:390-395; 1983.
10. Taylor, C.B.; Miller, N.H.; Flora, J. Principles of health behavior change. In Blair, S.N.; et al.; eds. Resource manual for guidelines for exercise testing and prescription, American College of Sports Medicine. Philadelphia: Lea & Febiger; 1988:323-328.
11. Watson, D.L.; Tharp, R.G. Self-directed behavior change. Monterey, CA: Brooks/Cole; 1981.
12. Goldfried, M.; Davison, C.C. Clinical behavior therapy. New York: Holt, Rinehart & Winston; 1976.
13. Marlatt, G.A.; Gordon, J.R.; eds. Relapse prevention: Maintenance strategies in the treatment of addiction. New York: Guilford Press; 1985.
14. DeBusk, R.F.; Haskell, W.L.; Miller, N.H.; Berra, K.; Taylor, C.B. Medically directed at-home rehabilitation soon after clinically uncomplicated myocardial infarction: A new model for patient care. Am. J. Cardiol. 55:251-257; 1985.
15. King, A.C.; Haskell, W.L.; Taylor, C.B.; Kraemer, H.C.; DeBusk, R.F. Group- versus home-based exercise training in healthy older men and women. JAMA. 266(11):1535-1542; 1991.
16. Ruberman, W.; Weinblatt, E.; Goldberg, J.D.; Chaudhary, B.S. Psychosocial influences on mortality after myocardial infarction. N. Engl. J. Med. 311:552-556; 1984.
17. Wenger, N.K.; Cleeman, J.I.; Herd, J.A.; McIntosh, H.D. Education of the patient with cardiac disease in the twenty-first century: An overview. Am. J. Cardiol. 57:1187-1189; 1986.
18. Taylor, C.B.; Miller, N.H.; Killen, J.; DeBusk, R.F. Smoking cessation after acute myocardial infarction: Effects of a nurse-managed intervention. Ann. Int. Med. 113:118-123; 1990.
19. Grimsmo, A.; Helgesen, G.; Borchgrevink, C.F. Short-term and long-term effects of lay groups in weight reduction. Br. Med. J. 283:1093-1095; 1981.
20. King, A.; Taylor, C.B.; Haskell, W.I.; DeBusk, R.F. Strategies for increasing early adherence and long-term maintenance of home-based physical activity in middle-aged men and women. Am. J. Cardiol. 61:628-632; 1988.
21. DeBusk, R.F.; Miller, N.H.; Superko, H.R.; Dennis, C.A.; Thomas, R.J.; Lew, H.T.; Berger, W.E.; Heller, R.S.; Rompf, J.; Gee, D.; Kraemer, H.C.; Bandura, A.; Ghandour, G.; Shah, R.; Clark, M.; Fisher, L.; Taylor, C.B. A case management system for coronary risk factor modification after acute myocardial infarction. Annals Int. Med. 120:721-729, 1994.
22. Miller, N.H.; Thomas, R.J.; Superko, R.H.; Ghandour, G.; DeBusk, R.F. Lipid-lowering therapy in post-MI patients: Efficacy of a nurse-managed intervention. Anaheim, CA: American Heart Association; November 1991.

Chapter 11

Exercise in the Primary Prevention of Coronary Artery Disease

Ralph S. Paffenbarger, Jr.
Steven N. Blair

The past decade has seen wide acceptance of epidemiological evidence that adequate physical activity promotes physical fitness and counters risks for developing coronary artery disease (CAD), a prime cause of debilitation and premature death. Because exercise is a natural function of the body, its health benefits are thought to come from its effects on all body systems, although the cardiovascular system has received the most attention in recent studies. Recent clinical and epidemiological studies have sought to identify characteristics of physical activity that may have prescriptive value for remedial and intervention purposes. These studies have attempted to define various mechanisms by which exercise appears to exert its salutary influences. This literature is now extensive and highly pertinent, but we intend only to offer an overview of salient epidemiological observations.

The physical activity or exercise we will discuss involves the skeletal muscles' energy expenditure during movement. Physical fitness is a set of characteristics essential to performing physical activity that involves the metabolic, hemostatic, cardiovascular, pulmonary, neurohormonal, and gastrointestinal systems as well as the musculoskeletal structure. Levels of physical activity and fitness influence health, quality of life, and longevity. Precisely what the requirements are for promoting health and longevity, in a clinical or individual sense and on a sociomedical or community scale, have not yet been defined.

The relations among physical activity and fitness, health, quality of life, morbidity, and mortality can be depicted in a pair of flowcharts. The first flowchart shows what ultimately results when physical activity is adequate: Physical activity → Physical fitness → Good-quality life → Low CAD risk → Long life. The second flowchart shows the consequences of physical inactivity: Physical inactivity → Physical unfitness → Poor-quality life

→ High CAD risk → Shortened life. The important relations between these two flowcharts, or the courses they represent, is that correction or avoidance of the problems inherent in the downward path of the second one can result in an adherence or return to the beneficial status represented by the first. In other words, inactive individuals may become physically active, unfit persons become physically fit, and so forth.

Similar flowcharts could be drawn up for the community situation, where programs for maintenance or intervention would be seen to influence rates of CAD incidence and mortality, not to mention expenditures for recreation and treatment facilities.

Physical Activity and Coronary Artery Disease

There used to be ample opportunity for physical activity on the job, and epidemiological studies were designed to assess occupational demands for muscle power. Today, most jobs are mechanized or computerized so extensively that they deny most workers much physical exercise at work. Studies of leisure-time physical activities have now become essential and have shown clearly that leisure-time exertions, such as playing recreational sports, have themselves become essential to the preservation of good health wherever modern "high-tech" work patterns have become the norm.

Table 11.1 shows the findings of three epidemiological studies of the influences of leisure-time physical activity on the relative risks of CAD among populations in England and the United States. The British men in the top panel of the table were middle-aged, middle-class, executive-grade civil servants who were largely confined to desk

Table 11.1   Relative Risk of Coronary Artery Disease (CAD), by Level of Physical Activity in Selected Populations

British civil servants			Sessions of vigorous sports in past 4 weeks	% of men	CAD rate per 100 men[a]	Relative risk of CAD
n	Age at entry	Follow-up period				
7,820 men	45-59 years	1976-1985 (9 years)	0	83	6.3	1.00
			1-3	8	5.1	0.81
			4-7	5	3.6	0.57
			8+	4	2.0	0.32

Multiple risk factor intervention trial			Tertile of physical activity (based on kcal/day)		CAD rate per 100 men[b]	Relative risk of CAD
n	Age at entry	Follow-up period				
12,138 men	35-57 years	1973-1981 (8 years)	low		7.2	1.00
			moderate		6.4	0.88
			high		5.8	0.81

Harvard alumni			Physical activity index (kcal/week)	% of man-years	CAD rate per 1,000 man-years[c]	Relative risk of CAD
n	Age at entry	Follow-up period				
16,936 men	35-74 years	1962-1972 (10 years)	< 2000	62	5.8	1.00
			2000+	38	3.5	0.61

[a]Adjusted for age differences; $p = 0.03$.

[b]Adjusted for age differences; $p < 0.01$.

[c]Adjusted for differences in age, cigarette habit, and blood pressure status; $p < 0.01$.

jobs and were variously inclined to devote some of their leisure hours to physically vigorous recreational sports and hobbies (1-3). After being queried about how many episodes of vigorous exercise they had indulged in during the previous month, such as recreational sports requiring an expenditure of at least 7.5 kcal/min, they were followed for 9 years to evaluate their incidence of CAD. Only 4% reported eight or more sessions of vigorous exercise per month, but their risk of CAD during the follow-up interval was barely one-third that of men who reported no such exercise. A consistent gradient of benefit is seen between these extremes.

The second panel of the table shows a similar but less striking trend of risk associated with three levels of a daily physical activity index derived from interviewing middle-aged American men (Multiple Risk Factor Intervention Trial study subjects) who were in the upper 10% to 15% of risk for developing CAD because of their serum cholesterol and blood pressure (BP) levels and cigarette smoking habits (4). Although their exercise patterns were at best moderate by most standards,

the most active third was twice as energetic as the middle third, which in turn was twice as active as the lowest third, in terms of kilocalories expended per day. During the follow-up interval the CAD rates per 100 men ranged between values close to the one noted for the least active British civil servants. Nevertheless, the most active third in the U.S. group had a relative risk of CAD that was 20% below that of the least active cohort. The influence of physical activity in countering CAD was independent of other recognized predictors, such as cigarette smoking, mostly known to promote CAD. The significance of this study is the finding that the protective effect of physical activity extends to men at the highest levels of CAD risk.

The bottom panel of the table gives similar findings on middle-aged male Harvard alumni followed for CAD incidence for 10 years (5,6). The men were assessed as to their physical activity at entry—including habitual walking and stair climbing and leisure-time sports activities. About 40% of the alumni had a physical activity index of at least 2,000 kcal/week of leisure-time energy expenditure. In this group, 89% included some recreational sports in their habitual patterns, and 67% played vigorous sports, contrasted to a respective 30% and 20% of men with a lower index who played such sports. The relative risk of CAD for the more active alumni was about 40% below that for the less active men.

Although the three studies cited in Table 11.1 differed considerably in their methodologies and populations, they show close parallels in their historical timing and their implications as to the inverse association of physical activity level and CAD risk. Both the British civil servant and the Harvard alumni studies demonstrated that vigorous playing of sports conferred additional benefits against CAD risk over and above the protective influence attributed to moderate or nonvigorous physical activity. When the Harvard alumni follow-up was extended to 16 years, playing sports of any sort was more beneficial than walking or stair climbing without sports. The alumni study also had implications supporting remedial and interventional hypotheses, because college athletes lost CAD protection if they became inactive, but graduates who had been less active as students could acquire a lowered risk if they took up vigorous physical activity as alumni. These experiences exemplify the interrelation of activity, fitness, and health depicted in the flowcharts shown previously.

Epidemiological studies thus far have not resolved questions concerning the relative influences of quantity versus intensity of exercise required for optimum effect, which indeed are thought to become modified with aging. More study will be needed to understand why the British civil servants achieved a significant reduction of CAD risk only if their activity patterns included vigorous sports, while the American men acquired some benefit from ample amounts of light or moderate activity, which was further enhanced by the addition of vigorous sports. From a prescriptive viewpoint, especially for older people, moderate exercise would be preferable to vigorous exertion because it avoids hazards of injury or overstress. Also, it is likely that individuals and community groups may be persuaded more easily to increase nonstrenuous activity than to take up more demanding skills and exertions, though the latter may appeal to many contemporary young people in search of satisfying leisure-time recreation. In the technical sense, the definition of vigorous exercise is linked closely to the concept of physical fitness, and especially to cardiovascular fitness assessed in terms of rate of energy expenditure or percentage of maximal oxygen uptake ($\dot{V}O_2max$), that is, functional capacity.

Physical Fitness and Coronary Artery Disease

Studies of physical fitness, measured primarily as cardiovascular or endurance fitness, have revealed important relations to coronary artery health, and they point in the same direction as the findings on physical activity just discussed. Fitness data from the Multiple Risk Factor Intervention Trial (4) indicate that both treadmill time and the percentage of subjects achieving their target heart rate (THR) were significantly higher among subjects with increased levels of leisure-time physical activity, while their resting and intermediate exercise heart rates (HRs) were lower. The upper third of subjects (based on activity ratings) had a normal estimated mean functional capacity, while the least active group was below average in this measure of fitness. Accordingly, level of CAD risk was inversely related to fitness status (as well as to their physical activity status). It has thus been postulated that the CAD benefits of exercise may be mediated, in part, by its influence on cardiovascular fitness.

Table 11.2 shows the findings of four epidemiological studies of physical fitness as related to CAD and all-cause mortality rates in Norwegian and American populations. The top panel presents data on middle-aged male industrial and government workers in Oslo whose fitness was classified by submaximal ergometer tests and who were followed for CAD mortality for 7 years (7). When distributed into quartiles by increasing levels of fitness, the more fit men had lower BPs, lower HRs, lower serum lipids, and higher maximal heart rates (HRmax), and maximal BPs during exercise and more favorable spirometry findings than those who were less fit. Physical fitness so assessed was a strong inverse predictor of fatal CAD in this population, with the risk in the most fit group reaching but one-fifth that of the least fit group.

The second panel of the table shows the relation of all-cause mortality rates to treadmill fitness test results in the U.S. Railway Study (8). Exercise HRs at various stages of testing of the male railway workers were directly predictive of CAD death rates during the 20-year follow-up interval, with the highest death rate corresponding to the fastest HR. The rates are age-adjusted, but the broad range of ages in this study population, together with its long follow-up period, would seem to add an

Table 11.2   Relative Risk of Coronary Artery Disease (CAD) and All-Cause Death, by Level of Physical Fitness in Selected Populations

Norwegian industry and government workers			Quartile of fitness by submaximal ergometry		CAD death rate per 100 men[a]	Relative risk of CAD death
n	Age at entry	Follow-up period				
2,014 men	40-59 years	1972-1982 (7 years)	1 (low)		5.7	1.00
			2		2.4	0.42
			3		2.2	0.39
			4 (high)		1.1	0.19

U.S. Railway Study			Exercise test heart rate (beats/min)	% of men	CAD death rate per 100 men[a]	Relative risk of CAD death
n	Age at entry	Follow-up period				
2,431 men	22-79 years	1957-1977 (20 years)	128+	22	13.2	1.00
			116-127	28	11.6	0.88
			106-115	27	8.7	0.66
			< 106	23	9.1	0.69

Lipid Research Clinics subjects			Quartile of fitness by submaximal ergometry	CAD death rate per 100 men[b]	Ratio of CAD death rate, quartile 1:4
n	Age at entry	Follow-up period			
4,276 men	30-69 years	1972-1984 (8.5 years)	1 (low)	1.69	(95% CI)
			2	0.91	
			3	0.91	6.5
			4 (high)	0.26	(1.5, 28.7)

Aerobics Center Longitudinal Study			Fitness groups by maximal ergometry	Cardiovascular disease death rate per 10,000 man-years[b]	Test for linear trend slope (95% CI)
n	Age at entry	Follow-up period			
10,244 men	Middle age	1972-1986 (8 years)	low	24.6	−6.0
			moderate	7.8	(−8.8, −3.3)
			high	3.1	

Note. CI = confidence interval.

[a]Adjusted for age differences; $p < 0.01$.

[b]Adjusted for age differences.

impressive experience value to these observations. As in the Multiple Risk Factor Intervention Trial, a high correlation was found between physical activity levels (both work and leisure-time) and ergometric fitness results (9). This pattern matches the sequence of influences depicted in the schematic flowcharts shown earlier.

The third panel of the table shows the levels of fitness among middle-aged men in a Lipid Research Clinics study who were assessed according to HR achieved at Stage 2 of the Bruce protocol to time on the treadmill (10). During an average 8.5-year follow-up the cumulative CAD mortality among men in the least-fit quartile was 6.5 times that of the most-fit quartile. Adjustment for quartile differences in cigarette smoking, BP level, and blood lipoprotein profile did not alter relative risks significantly. In fact, each of these adverse influences contributed independently to CAD mortality rates, as did physical fitness in its countering relationship.

The last panel of the table summarizes some of the results of the Aerobics Center Longitudinal Study, conducted among middle-aged male executive and managerial clients of the Cooper Clinic in Dallas, Texas. The subjects were followed for 8 years for their cardiovascular disease (CVD) death rates, as distributed by fitness groups determined by maximal treadmill performance (11). Low-fit men were those in the first quintile of the fitness distribution; the second and third quintiles were the moderate-fitness group; and the fourth and fifth quintiles were the high-fitness group. The mortality rate for the high-fit group was 88% lower than for the least-fit group. Trends persisted after accounting for differences in cigarette smoking, BP, blood cholesterol, and blood glucose levels; and parental history of CAD. Similar results were seen in 3,120 women in the study with CVD death rates of 7.2, 2.9, and 0.8 per 10,000 woman-years of follow-up for the low-, moderate- and high-fitness groups, respectively.

Physical Activity Versus Physical Fitness

The inverse gradient of death rates by physical fitness categories is steeper, with the exception of the U.S. Railroad Study, than the gradient by physical activity strata. The largest difference in CAD rates between divergent activity groups in Table 11.1 is approximately threefold, among British civil servants (1). In the Norwegian study on physical fitness, the death rates for both CAD and all CVD are five times higher in the most-fit group compared with the least-fit group and are eight times higher in the unfit Cooper Clinic men when compared with their fit counterparts. The reason for the steeper gradient in the fitness studies may be the result of the objective measurement and the relatively more accurate classification of participants as to their fitness status. The assessment of physical activity in the best studies is still somewhat imprecise due to inherent difficulties in measuring this complex and repetitive behavior. This difficulty leads to more misclassification on the primary independent variable and to an underestimate of the true impact of sedentary habits on mortality rates. In contrast, physical fitness is an excellent overall marker for the total amount of habitual activity in which an individual participates, and may provide a better estimate of the true relations between sedentary habits and health.

Lifestyle and Longevity

Exercise, fitness, quality of living, and other elements of lifestyle have been considered for their relations to all-cause mortality and longevity. All-cause death rates among the British civil servants of the previously described study during a 9-year follow-up were lower in men with an exercise-related reduction of CAD risk (1). Accordingly, their survival through middle-age into old age was greater than among men who played no vigorous sports. Table 11.3 shows the relations between physical activity and all-cause mortality in three groups: healthy middle-aged Finnish men (12), Harvard male alumni (13), and men and women aged 70 years and older in Alameda County, California (14). These populations also were studied for their estimated years of added life to age 80 years ascribed to favorable lifestyle characteristics. Of the 636 Finnish men, 287 died during the 20-year follow-up, 106 from CAD. However, men who were habitually vigorous during their daily activities lived an average of 2.1 years longer than those who were less active, the difference due mainly to their contrasting CAD mortality rates. The longer survival in the active group was due largely to avoidance of premature death; in fact, the survival curves for high- and low-activity subjects converged in the last 5 years of follow up to age 80. This convergence of survival rate may have represented a disappearance of differences in physical activity levels, altered influences of activity with aging, or the effect of some other unassessed attribute.

Of the 16,936 Harvard alumni, 1,413 died during the 16-year follow-up, 441 from CAD. The more active men had a 28% lower risk of death from any cause during the follow-up interval than the less active men, as indicated by their relative risks listed in the second panel of the table. A gradient effect (not shown) indicated a steady decline in death rates as exercise levels increased from below 500 kcal/week to an optimum of 3,500 kcal/week. Actuarial models provided estimates of added years of life to be gained by having the benefit of an active lifestyle, as well as other favorable lifestyle elements. After adjusting for age and each of the other habits listed, the data suggest that the largest gain (2.7 years) would be achieved by avoiding hypertension, the second largest (2.3 years) by not smoking cigarettes, and the third largest (1.3 years) by being physically active enough to expend at least 2,000 kcal/week in leisure-time activities. A

Table 11.3 Relative Risk of All-Cause Death, by Level of Physical Activity in Selected Populations

Finnish subjects			Physical activity at baseline	Number of men at baseline	Mean age at baseline (years)	Mean age at death (years)
n	Age at entry	Follow-up period				
636 men	45-64 years	1964-1984 (20 years)	Low	386	54.9	67.4
			High	250	55.2	69.1

Average added years of life from high activity[a] = 2.1.

Harvard alumni			Physical activity index (kcal/week)	Prevalence in man-years (%)	All-cause death rate per 1,000 man-years	Relative risk of all-cause death
n	Age at entry	Follow-up period				
16,936 men	35-74 years	1962-1978 (16 years)	< 2000	62	7.5	1.00
			2000+	38	5.4	0.72

Average added years of life to age 80[b] from high activity = 1.3; cigarette abstention = 2.3; normotension = 2.7.

Alameda County Study			Physical activity at baseline	Adjusted[c] relative risk
n	Age at entry	Follow-up period		
564 men	Over 70 years	1965-1982 (17 years)	Low	(95% CI) 1.37
			High	(1.09, 1.72) 1.0

Added years of life from high activity = 2.0.

Note. CI = confidence interval.

[a]Adjusted for differences in age, blood pressure, serum cholesterol, and cigarette smoking; $p < 0.01$.

[b]Adjusted for differences in age and each of the other characteristics listed; $p < 0.01$ for each characteristic.

[c]Adjusted for differences in age, baseline health status, cigarette smoking, body weight, alcohol intake, sleep habits, whether breakfast eaten, and snacking.

lifestyle combining all of these beneficial characteristics might be expected to gain further added life, because their influences are partly independent. Cross-tabulations of alumni data have shown that the influence of physical activity is not confounded by cigarette smoking nor by a history of hypertension (13). Adequate exercise can be seen as promoting longevity by preventing premature CAD and by decreasing the incidence of hypertension (15) and non–insulin-dependent diabetes mellitus (16, 17), which themselves predispose to CAD. Eschewing cigarette smoking may reduce the risk of death from CAD, stroke, respiratory disease, or lung and other cancers, thus explaining its larger benefit. An active and fit lifestyle may counter the adverse influence of such unwise habits as overeating, alcohol abuse, and cigarette smoking and unfortunate inbred or acquired characteristics, including obesity, unfavorable lipoprotein profile, and hypertension.

The subjects of the Alameda County (California) Study, data for whom appears in the last panel of the table, were a representative sample of the county population who completed an extensive mail-back questionnaire at baseline on behavioral, psychological, social, and health factors (14). Early reports from the study identified seven behavioral risk factors associated with mortality in younger individuals (18). The following were factors related to an improved chance of survival: not smoking cigarettes, maintaining moderate weight, sleeping 7–8 h/night, being physically active, drinking only moderate amounts of alcohol, not snacking between meals, and eating breakfast regularly. As seen in the table, there was a 37% higher risk for all-cause mortality in the low-active men and women as compared with the active subjects. This value is adjusted for the other six behavioral risk factors just listed, as well as for age and baseline health status. Survival analysis indicated a separation of survival curves for the low- and high-active subjects early in the follow-up period (not shown in the table), with an overall difference in longevity of approximately 2 years by the end of 17 years of follow-up. The importance of this study is that the data suggest a considerable survival benefit even in elderly men and women who are physically active.*

Summary

Future studies (epidemiological, clinical, and laboratory) must seek to sort out the mechanisms by which physical activity promotes both short-term and long-range health, reduces CAD incidence, and extends high-quality life. These mechanisms may function via cardiovascular fitness, hemostatic action, metabolic processes, neuroendocrine changes, combinations of these, or other physiological adaptations. The rationale for our interest in physical activity and physical fitness arises from many considerations:

- Engagement in exercise is a natural body procedure and requirement.
- Physical fitness is a continuum that describes the physiological state of the body's systems and determines its capacity to exercise.
- Sedentary lifestyles are a recent development, not previously a characteristic of humankind, yet technological developments, which are partly responsible for contemporary adverse health trends, are here to stay.
- Nearly two thirds of industrialized populations are habitually sedentary and at excessive risk for CAD and its consequences.
- Exercise and total body fitness can counter adverse lifestyles, which tend to promote not only CAD and hypertension but also osteoporosis, non–insulin-dependent diabetes mellitus, and syndromes of anxiety and depression.
- Together with health maintenance, an extension of longevity to its optimum level and an enhancement of the quality of living are likely to accompany a physically active and physically fit way of life.

Acknowledgments

This work was supported by U.S. Public Health Service Research Grants HL 34174 from the National Heart, Lung, and Blood Institute and AG 06945 from the National Institute on Aging.

References

1. Morris, J.N.; Everitt, M.G.; Semmence, A.M. Exercise and coronary heart disease. In: Macleod, D.; Maughn, R.; Nimmo, M.; Reilly, T.; Williams, C., eds. Exercise: Benefits, limits and adaptations. London: E & FN Spon; 1987:4-19.
2. Morris, J.N. Physical activity in the prevention of cardiovascular disease. In: van Erp-Baart, A.M.J.; Katan, M.B.; Kemper, H.C.G.; van der Laan, J.A.M.; Morris, J.N.; de Nobel, E.; Saris, W.H.M.; Weeds, H.W.H., eds. Inspanning en voeding. Alphen aan den Rihn/Brussels: Samsom/Stafleu; 1985:54-63.
3. Morris, J.N. Exercise and the incidence of coronary heart disease. In: Exercise-heart-health. London: The Coronary Prevention Group; 1987:21-34.
4. Leon, A.S.; Connett, J.; Jacobs, D.R., Jr.; Rauramaa, R. Leisure-time physical activity levels and risk of coronary heart disease and death. The multiple risk factor intervention trial. JAMA. 258:2388-2395; 1987.
5. Paffenbarger, R.S., Jr.; Wing, A.L.; Hyde, R.T. Physical activity as an index of heart attack risk in college alumni. Am. J. Epidemiol. 108:161-175; 1978.
6. Paffenbarger, R.S., Jr.; Hyde, R.T.; Wing, A.L.; Steinmetz, C.H. A natural history of athleticism and cardiovascular health. JAMA. 252:491-495; 1984.
7. Lie, H.; Mundal, R.; Erikssen, J. Coronary risk factors and incidence of coronary death in relation to physical fitness. Seven-year follow-up study of middle-aged and elderly men. Eur. Heart J. 6:147-157; 1985.
8. Slattery, M.L.; Jacobs, D.R. Physical fitness and cardiovascular disease mortality: The U.S. railroad study. Am. J. Epidemiol. 127:571-580; 1988.
9. Slattery, M.L.; Jacobs, D.R., Jr.; Nichaman, M.Z. Leisure time physical activity and coronary heart disease death. The U.S. railroad study. Circulation. 79:304-311; 1989.
10. Ekelund, L-G.; Haskell, W.L.; Johnson, J.L.; Whaley, F.S.; Criqui, M.H.; Sheps, D.S. Physical fitness as a predictor of cardiovascular mortality in asymptomatic North American men. The lipid research clinics mortality follow-up study. N. Engl. J. Med. 319:1379-1384; 1988.
11. Blair, S.N.; Kohl, H.W., III; Paffenbarger, R.S., Jr.; Clark, D.G.; Cooper, K.H.; Gibbons, L.W. Physical

*It should be noted that because of the scientific evidence linking physical inactivity to premature death from CAD, the American Heart Association in July 1992 officially elevated physical inactivity to the status of a major risk factor (19).

fitness and all-cause mortality: A prospective study of healthy men and women. JAMA. 262:2395-2401; 1989.

12. Pekkanen, J.; Marti, B.; Nissinen, A.; Tuomilehto, J. Reduction of premature mortality by high physical activity: A 20-year follow-up of middle-aged Finnish men. Lancet. 1:1473-1477; 1987.

13. Paffenbarger, R.S., Jr.; Hyde R.T.; Wing, A.L.; Hsieh, C-c. Physical activity, all cause mortality, and longevity of college alumni. N. Engl. J. Med. 314:605-613; 315:399-401; 1986.

14. Kaplan, G.A.; Seeman, T.E.; Cohen, R.D.; Knudsen, L.P.; Guralnik, J. Mortality among the elderly in the Alameda County study: Behavioral and demographic factors. Am. J. Public Health. 77:307-312; 1987.

15. Paffenbarger, R.S., Jr.; Jung, D.L.; Leung, R.W.; Hyde, R.T. Physical activity and hypertension: An epidemiological view. Ann Med. 23:319-327; 1991.

16. Helmrich, S.; Ragland, D.R.; Leung, R.W.; Paffenbarger, R.S., Jr. Physical activity and reduced occurrence of non-insulin-dependent diabetes mellitus. N. Engl. J. Med. 325:147-152; 1991.

17. Manson, J.E.; Rimm, E.B.; Stampfer, M.J.; Colditz, G.A.; Willett, W.C.; Krolewski, A.S.; Rosner, B.; Hennekens, C.H.; Speizer, F.E. Physical activity and incidence of non-insulin-dependent diabetes mellitus in women. Lancet. 338:774-778; 1991.

18. Berkman, L.F.; Breslow, L. Health and ways of living: The Alameda County study. New York: Oxford University Press; 1983.

19. Fletcher, G.F.; Blair, S.N.; Blumenthal, J.; Caspersen, C.; Chaitman, B.; Epstein, S.; Falls, H.; Froelicher, E.S.; Froelicher, V.F.; Pina, J.L. Position statement on exercise. Benefits and recommendation for physical activity programs for all Americans, from the American Heart Association Circulation. 86:340-344; 1992.

Chapter 12

The Value of Cardiac Rehabilitation: Secondary Prevention

Carl Foster

Matthew Schrager

Jason Cohen

For at least 200 years, exercise has been recognized as a useful means of therapy for patients with cardiovascular disease. Heberden (1) noted in 1772 that one of his patients (presumably with stable angina) was "nearly cured" after half an hour of daily exercise in the form of sawing wood. Although the medical community has frequently forgotten the need for exercise, it is rediscovered periodically and currently enjoys considerable popularity as a central component of heart disease prevention and rehabilitation programs. Even without the possibility of "curing" coronary artery disease (CAD) by reversing the primary pathophysiology of atherosclerotic disease (2), exercise and risk factor modification programs have earned a role in the treatment of patients with CAD because they accelerate the recovery of both objective (3) and subjective (4) effort tolerance, and because they can assist physicians in surveillance (5), thus contributing to improved patient management.

Studies from the early era of cardiac rehabilitation indicate that the mechanism for Heberden's cure had to do with the reduced myocardial oxygen demands for given tasks in physically well-trained persons. Indeed, the genesis for the current popularity of exercise as a therapeutic modality can be traced to this training effect identified in the 1960s (6,7). In 1957 Ekstein described improved cardiac collateralization in dogs with experimentally occluded coronary arteries after the dogs were subjected to vigorous exercise training (8). This finding generated the hope that exercise training might contribute to improved myocardial blood supply and may, accordingly, contribute to a "cure" of the primary pathophysiology of CAD. Significant research has taken place within the rehabilitation community to more clearly define the site of improvement in exercise tolerance with systematic exercise training, peripheral facilitation vs.

myocardial/central circulatory (9,10). Beyond this, as the process of atherogenesis has become more fully understood, the possibility of reversing atherosclerotic disease by changing the milieu that led to its development has emerged as a serious hypothesis. In this chapter we examine data regarding the potential for exercise training (with or without other risk factor interventions) to contribute to the prevention of subsequent cardiac events in patients with known CAD. We will explore the possibility of inducing collateralization and reversing atherosclerosis by means of lifestyle changes as a basis for future research within the cardiac rehabilitation community.

Effects on Morbidity/Mortality

Several randomized clinical trials on the effects of exercise and risk factor modification programs on the survival of patients following myocardial infarction (MI) have been conducted. No single trial has demonstrated unequivocal evidence of improved survival, although there has been a consistently favorable trend in the survival statistics. All the trials have been limited by sample size, drop outs, subject crossover, or other statistical problems. These findings have been disappointing to cardiac rehabilitation professionals, and somewhat surprising in that exercise and risk factor control have an established role in the primary prevention of CAD (see chapter 11). Why should behaviors known to retard the development of atherosclerotic disease not contribute to preventing the progression of the disease? In the late 1980s two studies were published that used the statistical technique of meta-analysis to allow pooling of results from different randomized clinical trials

(11,12). Both analyses demonstrated that significant reductions in mortality could be realized by participation in a rehabilitation program (exercise ± risk factor modification). The magnitude of reduction in mortality, about 20%, was of the same order as that realized from using other forms of medical therapy such as beta blockers, lipid reducing drugs, anticoagulants and smoking cessation programs (11). Neither of these analyses demonstrated a statistically significant effect of program participation on subsequent nonfatal reinfarction, although there was a trend toward more nonfatal reinfarctions in program participants (11). This trend may have relevance to the safety of rehabilitation programs and may influence how exercise and risk factor modification programs interface with conventional medical and surgical management of CAD.

No randomized clinical trials on the effect of rehabilitation programs on morbidity/mortality or other evidence of progression of atherosclerotic disease have been performed in patients following coronary artery bypass graft surgery (CABG surgery), percutaneous transluminal angioplasty (PTCA), or other direct methods of myocardial revascularization. The available evidence suggests that the continuing presence of risk factors for the development of atherosclerotic disease may lead to unfavorable outcomes in CABG surgery and PTCA patients (13). Accordingly, the operating expectation is that participation in exercise and risk factor modification programs should have a favorable effect on subsequent morbidity/mortality in these patients.

Effects on Myocardial Blood Supply

The presence of coronary collateral vessels has been known for three centuries. They are usually associated with significant myocardial ischemia in the absence of acute MI in that area of the myocardium. Since the report by Ekstein (8) of enhanced coronary collateralization in dogs with experimentally occluded coronary arteries, after the dogs were subjected to vigorous exercise training, researchers have attempted to demonstrate that exercise might promote coronary collateralization in patients with CAD. Although there are data favoring the hypothesis that collaterals develop as a normal response to chronic ischemia, the results are far from unequivocal. Collateral development has not been demonstrated in humans as a direct result of either exercise or risk factor modification

(14). This topic has recently been reviewed by Franklin (9).

The presence of unusually large epicardial coronary vessels was noted a generation ago in the autopsy of the well-known marathon runner, Clarence DeMar (15). This observation led to the hypothesis that habitual heavy exertion might promote the development of larger coronary arteries that would not be compromised even with luminal narrowing secondary to atherosclerotic disease. This hypothesis has gained recent support by cross-sectional observations of enhanced vasodilation following nitroglycerin in marathon runners (16), and by longitudinal observations of enhanced coronary flow reserve to dipryidamole following exercise training (17).

The product of heart rate (HR) and systolic blood pressure (SBP), the rate pressure product (RPP) is well accepted as an index of myocardial oxygen consumption. The RPP has traditionally been used as an indirect indication of relative changes in potential myocardial blood flow. The exercise testing literature has suggested that angina and significant ST-segment changes occur at reproducible levels of exertion and of RPP which has fostered the concept of an ischemic threshold. Early studies of the responses to exercise training in patients with CAD suggested that myocardial oxygen demands were reduced during submaximal exercise, leading to a reduction in relative ischemia during ordinary activities (7). Other literature suggested, however, that the maximal RPP did not change in response to exercise training, which led to the widely held belief that exercise training (± other lifestyle changes) would not affect myocardial perfusion. More recently, Ehsani et al. (18) have demonstrated a significantly increased RPP at maximal exercise and reductions in the magnitude of ST segment depression in patients participating in an exercise program of significantly greater intensity, frequency, and duration than usually recommended for patients with CAD. This finding has been replicated in other studies, and is most often observed in patients who have evidence of significant exercise induced ischemia prior to exercise training and who are participants in programs that are somewhat more demanding than the conventional exercise recommendations for CAD patients of 3 days weekly, for 30 to 40 minutes per day, at 60% to 75% of maximal oxygen uptake ($\dot{V}O_2$max)(19-21). This topic has recently been reviewed by Hagberg (10). A 7-year follow-up of the Ehsani high intensity training group has indicated that the increased RPP observed after the first year of training was maintained (22). Only one member of the original group available for follow-up had a subsequent cardiovascular event, CABG surgery. None died from CAD.

Early studies of myocardial perfusion, using radionuclide techniques indicated that there was no systematic change in myocardial perfusion with exercise training despite significant improvement in exercise tolerance (23). Froelicher et al. (21) and Tubau et al. (24) have presented data suggesting that myocardial perfusion seems to improve with exercise training primarily in patients with evidence of significant ischemia prior to training. More recently, a combined dietary and exercise trial by Schuler et al. (25) in patients with CAD, stable angina, and hypercholesterolemia demonstrated a significantly increased exercise tolerance, maximal RPP, and improved myocardial perfusion by thallium scintigraphy following intervention. In a follow-up study from the same laboratory, Neibauer et al. (14) has demonstrated that the same intervention of exercise + low fat diet leads to angiographic evidence of regression of atherosclerotic lesions rather than to collateral formation. Indeed, the only patients who demonstrated collateral formation were those with evidence of significant progression of their atherosclerotic lesions.

Recently, Ornish et al. (26) have demonstrated using quantitative cineangiography that the severity of lesions within the coronary arteries could be reduced following an aggressive program of exercise and risk factor modification (very low-fat vegetarian diet + meditation + exercise + social support). Most of the patients in this trail had significant CAD and evidence of exertional ischemia. Many had either failed conventional medical or surgical therapy or were not considered to be candidates for surgical revascularization. Significantly, the focus of this intervention trial was on the patients total lifestyle with exercise training occupying only a modest role. Beyond the evidence of regression of coronary lesion, the data of Ornish et al. suggest a quantitative relationship between compliance with the intervention program and the magnitude of regression of the atherosclerotic lesions. In a subsequent report from the same study Gould et al. (27) have demonstrated, in addition to a net reduction in luminal narrowing, remodeling of atherosclerotic lesions in a way thought to be consistent with a reduced risk of plaque rupture. In a 4-year follow-up of their original study, Ornish et al. (28) demonstrated evidence for continued regression of coronary lesions in patients participating in their lifestyle modification program of exercise + very low-fat vegetarian diet + meditation + social support.

These findings support the hypothesis that atherosclerotic lesions are dynamic and responsive to changes in the milieu that lead to their development. These findings also suggest that selected patients may be both willing and able to comply with the large scale lifestyle changes that are apparently necessary to provoke regression of atherosclerotic lesions.

Data from the Leiden Intervention Trial, which used a low-fat vegetarian diet as the intervention mode, has further suggested the possibility of regression of coronary lesions with normalization of the lipoprotein profile in patients with known CAD (29). Formal exercise training was not a part of either evaluation or therapy in this trail, although it is fair to point out the Dutch are already rather physically active by North American standards. Other risk factors were not systematically in this trail (e.g.; the same number of patients smoked at baseline and after 2 years of intervention). The mean change in coronary artery diameter, based on computer assisted scoring of angiograms, was moderately related to the ratio of total cholesterol to high density lipoprotein cholesterol. Patients with ratios of less than 5:1 were most likely to demonstrate regression of lesions versus progression or no change.

Negative Effects

The value of any therapy must be judged against the potential for harm from that therapy. Because of the central role of the increase in HR and SBP on the increased myocardial oxygen demands during exercise, exercise is often viewed as a less-than-controllable factor relative to the dynamic balance between myocardial oxygen supply and demand. The somewhat increased risk of acute cardiovascular events during exercise in the population at large (30) and the association between acute ischemia and emergencies during exercise based cardiac rehabilitation programs (31) has engendered a cautious attitude toward exercising the patient with evidence of exercise induced ischemia.

Hossack and Hartwig (31) demonstrated that the combination of electrocardiographic (ECG) evidence of ischemia during exercise, persisting into the recovery period following exercise testing (suggesting fairly profound ischemia), and exercise training beyond one's target heart rate (suggesting prolonged exercise with myocardial ischemia), could account for many of the emergency situations that occur during a community-based cardiac rehabilitation program. The declining rate of complications within the early cardiac rehabilitation experience nationally has been attributed to better monitoring (32). Presumably, one feature of better monitoring is the minimization of the time spent above the ischemic threshold during exercise training.

The trend toward a greater risk of nonfatal reinfarction in patients participating in cardiac rehabilitation programs noted in the meta-analysis of Oldridge et al. (11) is consistent with the increased risk that would be expected from exercising with myocardial ischemia. Further, the association of exercise under ischemic conditions with sustained myocardial dysfunction after exercise (myocardial stunning) in both animal (33) and human (34) models suggests that exercise during ischemia may present a significant risk to the patient. Ornish et al. (26) reported one death within their exercise and lifestyle intervention group. This death was attributed to the patient's exercising in a nonmonitored situation at an intensity significantly beyond that recommended by the staff (i.e., exercise with significant ischemia).

Although there are demonstrable risks associated with more aggressive exercise in patients with CAD, the overall safety statistics for exercise are very encouraging (30). In monitored settings even emergency situations are usually satisfactorily resolved (31,32). Despite the occurrence of one death in the Lifestyle Heart Trial of Ornish et al. (26), there were no reported cardiovascular deaths in other more intensive trails (18,22,25). Preliminary studies of prolonged exercise in CAD patients have failed to demonstrate either catastrophic events or evidence of left ventricular dysfunction during or following sustained submaximal exercise at intensities compatible with those used for exercise training (35-37).

The value of any intervention program is largely related to compliance with the therapeutic regime. Exercise and risk factor modification programs suffer from the same decline in compliance common to all behavioral interventions (38). At the end of 1 year, it is unreasonable to expect more than about 75% of patients will be compliant with a program (39). Unfortunately, patients in most need of the program (e.g., continuing smokers) are even more likely to drop out. As a general principle, it may be assumed that the more complex the behavior change required of the individual, the lower the overall long-term compliance. Certainly, exercise programs with greater intensity, frequency, and duration than normally recommended for healthy adults have higher drop-out rates and a greater

frequency of injuries than conventional programs (40). Although the more aggressive intervention studies by Ehsani et al. (18), Schuler et al. (25), and Ornish et al. (26,28) have documented excellent adherence with fairly significant behavior change, in some cases for periods of several years (22,28), it is still too early in our experience to determine whether less well-selected patients would comply with lifestyle alterations well enough to obviate the need for established therapeutic approaches to chronic ischemia, such as CABG surgery and PTCA.

An Integrative Hypothesis

Clearly exercise and risk factor modification programs have a role in the management of patients with known CAD. There is evidence that such interventions may have a favorable effect on subsequent morbidity and mortality following a patient's first MI. The magnitude of this favorable effect is of the same order as such well-accepted recommendations as the use of beta-blockers or quitting smoking. Reasonable extrapolation of available data suggests that the role of exercise and risk factor modification may also be significant in the management of patients following myocardial revascularization with either CABG surgery or PTCA.

Under any circumstances, significant increases in effort tolerance are to be expected following exercise training. Following conventional clinical exercise programs, it is to be expected that the mechanism of the improved exercise tolerance is mainly via peripheral adaptations. However, following more intense exercise intervention, evidence of improved myocardial blood supply and ventricular function may be present, particularly if the exercise training is coupled with comparatively aggressive treatment of other risk factors. A growing body of evidence suggests that this effect is mediated by angiographically demonstrable regression of atherosclerotic lesions. On the basis of the studies by Ornish et al. (26-28), Schuler et al. (25), and the Leiden Intervention Trial (29), it may be that intervention sufficient to substantially change blood lipids may be necessary to reverse the atherosclerotic process. Given the rather high apparent threshold of exercise needed to significantly change plasma lipoproteins (41), nearly at the level of the high intensity training group of Ehsani et al. (18), it may be argued that either low-fat vegetarian diets or pharmacologic intervention will be needed to allow any possibility for regression of atherosclerotic lesions.

Participation in exercise and risk factor modification programs does, however, carry some risk. Among post-MI patients there is a trend for an increased risk of subsequent nonfatal MI with exercise training. Cardiac emergencies arising during exercise training are most often linked to exercise with an ischemic myocardium or to plaque rupture. These data would suggest that although vigorous exercise may contribute to the long-term improvement of myocardial blood flow, there is an appreciable short-term risk associated with exercise training.

These findings can be understood within the context of the nature of the dose-response curve. With most medical conditions the favorable effects of an applied intervention follow a saturation curve. Unfavorable side effects tend to follow a geometric growth curve. The window between these curves represents the usual therapeutic range for the applied intervention. In the case of cardiac rehabilitation programs, the dose of intervention relates to the intensity, frequency, and duration of the exercise program; the magnitude of effort directed toward dietary and other behavioral changes; and the magnitude of effort directed toward the pharmacological control of ischemia, hyperlipidemia, and hypertension. Favorable effects are related to improved effort tolerance and sense of well-being, the improved medical management attributable to surveillance, and, potentially, to secondary prevention through halting or even reversing the atherosclerotic process. Although there is experimental evidence for this last effect, the results of various studies suggest that it is only likely to occur at relatively high doses of intervention. The side effects of participation in secondary prevention programs may include the usual orthopedic and time constraint problems experienced by healthy adults in fitness programs. These factors may cause patients to drop out from the program, thus negating the favorable effects of even low-dose participation. However, given the comparatively good safety record in contemporary cardiac rehabilitation programs, the relative effectiveness of monitoring to minimize emergencies, and the effectiveness of resuscitation in the setting of a witnessed emergency, the risks of aggressive intervention by the rehabilitation program would appear to be low and acceptable. In the context where the management of the patients already includes steps to minimize ischemia via pharmacological protection, it is to be expected that any real risk related to aggressive lifestyle intervention would

be further minimized. Accordingly, aggressive lifestyle intervention including exercise, diet, and behavior change with the intent of improving myocardial blood flow may represent a valid alternative to direct myocardial revascularization via CABG surgery or PTCA. Certainly in an era when the cost effectiveness of technology dependent medical and surgical therapy is being questioned, secondary prevention of future clinical sequale of CAD via lifestyle change should be encouraged at every opportunity.

Summary

Data collected at a number of levels from epidemiologic to randomized clinical trial to noninvasive evaluation of myocardial perfusion/function to quantitative angiography demonstrate that the clinical sequale of atherosclerotic disease in patients with already established CAD can be minimized by modifications of lifestyle including exercise, diet, and behavior change. Recent data have demonstrated that the atherosclerotic process can even be reversed when the magnitude of lifestyle change is large. These data provide a new context in which to use the term "secondary prevention." Rather than implying merely the slowing of an inevitably progressive disease process, it may now be possible to view cardiac rehabilitation programs, if applied at their greatest level, to be as effective as invasive therapy (CABG surgery/PTCA) relative to "curing" CAD. This provides patients, and their physicians, with a very attractive alternative to conventional therapy for CAD.

References

1. Heberden, W. Commentaries on the history and cure of disease. In: Willins, F.A.; Keys, T.W.; eds. Classics in cardiology, New York: Dover Publishing Inc.; 1961.

2. Ornish, D. Reversing heart disease, New York: Ballantine Books, 1990.

3. Foster, C.; Pollock, M.L.; Anholm, J.D.; Squires, R.W.; Ward, A.; Dymond, D.S.; Rod, J.L.; Saichek, R.; Schmidt, D.H. Work capacity and left ventricular function during rehabilitation from myocardial revascularization surgery. Circulation. 69:748-755; 1984.

4. Foster, C.; Oldridge, N.B.; Hansen, M.A.; Laughlin, J.; Pajak, J.; Plichta, C.R.; Sharkey, R.E.; Schmidt, D.H. Time course of recovery during cardiac rehabilitation. J. Cardiopulm. Rehab. 11:305 (abstract); 1991.

5. Sennett, S.M.; Pollock, M.L.; Pels, A.E.; Foster, C.; Dolatowski, R.; Patel, S. Medical problems of cardiac patients in an outpatient cardiac rehabilitation program. J. Cardiopulm. Rehabil. 7:458-465; 1987.

6. Hellerstein, H.K.; Hirsch, E.Z.; Cumber, W. Reconditioning of the coronary patient. In: Likoff, W.; Moyer, J.H.; eds. Coronary heart disease, New York: Grune & Stratton, 1963: 448-454.

7. Detry, J.M.R.; Gousseau, M.; Vandenbroucke, G. Increased arteriovenous oxygen difference after physical training in coronary heart disease. Circulation. 44:109-119; 1971.

8. Ekstein, R.W. Effect of exercise and coronary artery narrowing on coronary collateral circulation. Circ. Res. 5:230-235, 1957.

9. Franklin, B.A. Exercise training and coronary collateral circulation. Med. Sci. Sports Exerc. 23:648-653, 1991.

10. Hagberg, J.M. Physiologic adaptations to prolonged high intensity training in patients with coronary artery disease. Med. Sci. Sports Exerc. 23:661-667; 1991.

11. Oldridge, N.B.; Guyatt, G.H.; Fischer, M.S.; Rimm, A.A. Cardiac rehabilitation after myocardial infarction: Combined experience of randomized clinical trials. JAMA 260:945-950; 1988.

12. O'Connor, G.T.; Buring, J.E.; Yusuf, S.; Goldhaber S.Z.; Olmstead, E.M.; Paffenbarger. R.S.; Hennekens, C.H. An overview of randomized trials of rehabilitation with exercise after myocardial infarction. Circulation. 80:234-244; 1989.

13. Foster, C.; Tamboli, H.P. Exercise prescription in the rehabilitation of patients following coronary artery bypass graft surgery and percutaneous transluminal coronary angioplasty. In: Miller, H.S.; Shepard, R.; eds. Exercise and the heart in health and cardiac disease. New York: Marcel Dekker Inc.; 1992.

14. Niebauer, J.; Hambrecht, R.; Schlierf, G.; Marburger, C.; Schuler, G. Intensive physical exercise and its impact on collateral circulation in patients with coronary artery disease. Circulation. 88: I-50 (abstract); 1993.

15. Currens, J.H.; White, P.D. Half century of running: Clinical, physiologic and autopsy findings in the case of Clarence De Mar, "Mr Marathoner." N. Engl. J. Med. 265: 988-993; 1961.

16. Haskell, W.L.; Sims, C.; Myll, J.; Bortz, W.M.; St Goar, F.G.; Alderman E.L. Coronary artery size and dilating capacity in ultradistance runners. Circulation. 87: 1076-1082,;1993.

17. Czernin, J.; Barnard, R.J.; Sun, K.; Krivokapich, J.; Brunken, R.; Porenta, G.; Phelps, M.E.; Schelbert, H.R. Beneficial effect of cardiovascular conditioning on myocardial blood flow and coronary vasodilator capacity. Circulation. 88: I-51 (abstract); 1993.

18. Ehsani, A.A.; Heath, G.W.; Hagberg, J.M.; Sobel B.E.; Holloszy, J.O. Effects of 12 months of intense exercise training on ischemic ST segment depression in patients with coronary artery disease. Circulation. 6: 1116-1124; 1981.

19. Raffo, J.A.; Luksic, I.Y.; Kappagoda, C.T.; Mary, D.A.S.G.; Whitaker, W.; Linden, R.J. Effects of physical training on myocardial ischemia in patients with coronary artery disease. Br. Heart J. 43: 262-269,1980.

20. Laslett, L.J.; Paumer, L.; Amsterdam, E.A. Increase in myocardial oxygen consumption indexes by exercise training at onset of ischemia in patients with coronary artery disease. Circulation .71: 958-962; 1985.

21. Froelicher, V.F.; Jensen, D.; Genter, R.; Sullivan, M.; McKirnan, M.D.; Witztum, K.; Scharf, J.; Strong, M.L.; Ashburn, W. A randomized trial of exercise training in patients with coronary heart disease. JAMA. 252:1291-1297; 1984.

22. Rogers, M.A.; Yamamoto, C.; Hagberg, J.M. The effect of 7 years of intense exercise training in patients with coronary heart disease. J. Am. Coll. Cardiol. 10: 321-326; 1987.

23. Verani, M.S.; Hartung, G.H.; Hoepful-Harris, J.; Welton, D.E.; Pratt, C.M.; Miller, R.R. Effects of exercise training on left ventricular performance and myocardial perfusion in patients with coronary artery disease. Am. J. Cardiol. 47: 797-803; 1981.

24. Tubau, J.; Wiztum, K. Froelicher, V.F. Noninvasive assessment of changes in myocardial perfusion and ventricular performance following exercise training. Am. Heart J. 104: 238-248; 1982.

25. Schuler, G.; Schillert, G.; Wirth, A.; Mautner, H-P.; Scheurlen, H.; Thumm, M.; Roth H.; Schwarz, F.; Kohlmeier, M.; Mehmel, H.C.; Kubler, W. Low fat diet and regular supervised physical exercise in patients with symptomatic coronary artery disease: Reduction of stress induced myocardial ischemia. Circulation. 77: 172-181; 1988.

26. Ornish, D.; Brown, S.E.; Scherwitz, L.W.; Billings, J.D.; Armstrong, W.T.; Ports, T.A.; McLanahan, S.M.; Kirdeeide, R.L.; Brand, R.J.; Gould, K.L. Can lifestyle changes reverse coronary heart disease. Lancet 336: 129-133; 1990.

27. Gould, K.L.; Ornish, D.; Kirkeeide, R.; Brown, S.; Stuart, Y.; Buchi, M.; Billings, J.; Armstrong, W.; Ports, T.; Scherwitz, L. Improved stenosis geometry by quantitative coronary arteriography after vigorous risk factor modification. Am. J. Cardiol. 69: 845-853; 1992.

28. Ornish, D.; Brown S.W.; Billings, J.H.; Armstrong, W.T.; Ports, T.A.; Merritt, T.; Sparler, S.; Spann, L.; McLanahan, S.; Scherwitz, L.W.; Kirkeeide, R.L.; Brand, F.K.; Gould, K.L. Can exercise reverse coronary atherosclerosis? Four year results of the lifestyle heart trial. Circulation. 88:I-385 (abstract); 1993.

29. Arntzenius, A.C.; Kromhout, D.; Barth, J.D. Diet, lipoproteins and the progression of coronary atherosclerosis: The Leiden intervention trial. N. Engl. J. Med. 312: 805-811; 1985.

30. Thompson, P.D.; Funk, E.J.; Carleton, R.A. Incidence of death during jogging in Rhode Island from 1975-1980. JAMA 247:2535-2538; 1982.

31. Hossack, K.; Hartwig, R. Cardiac arrest associated with supervised cardiac rehabilitation. J. Cardiopulm. Rehabil. 2: 402-408; 1982.

32. Haskell, W.L. Cardiovascular complications during exercise training of cardiac patients. Circulation. 57: 920-924; 1978.

33. Houmans, D.C.; Sub lett, E.; Dai, X.Y. Persistence of regional left ventricular dysfunction after exercise induced myocardial ischemia. J. Clin. Invest. 77: 66-73; 1986.

34. Kloner, R.A.; Allen, J.; Cox, T.A. Stunned left ventricular myocardium after exercise treadmill testing in coronary artery disease. Am. J. Cardiol. 68: 329-334; 1991.

35. Foster, C.; Gal, R.; Port, S.C.; Schmidt, D.H. Ventricular function during exercise testing and training. Med. Sci. Sports Exerc. 24: S125-747 (abstract); 1992.

36. Lehmann, M.; Durr, H.; Huonker, M.; Keul, J. Mountain hiking with CHD patients: Results of an experimental study. Int. J. Sports Med. 14: 173 (abstract); 1993.

37. Huonker, M.; Durr, H.; Lehmann, M.; Keul, J. Mountain hiking with CHD patients: Doppler echocardiographic analysis of the effects on cardiac dimensions and function. Int. J. Sports Med. 14:173 (abstract); 1993.

38. Oldridge, N.B. Compliance with intervention and rehabilitation exercise programs: A review. Prev. Med. 11:56-62; 1982.

39. Oldridge, N.D.; Donner, A.P.; Buck, C.W.; Jones, N.L.; Andrew, G.M.; Parker, J.O.; Cunningham, D.A.; Kavanagh, T.; Rechnizer, P.A.; Sutton, J.R. Predictors of dropout from cardiac exercise rehabilitation: Ontario Exercise-Heart Collaborative Study. Am. J. Cardiol. 51: 70-74; 1983.

40. Pollock, M.L.; Gettman, L.R.; Mileses, L.R. Effects of frequency and duration of training on attrition and incidence of injury. Med. Sci. Sports Exerc. 9: 31-36; 1977.

41. Superko, H.R. Exercise training, serum lipids, and lipoprotein particles: Is there a change threshold? Med. Sci. Sports Exerc. 23:677-685; 1991.

PART IV

Rehabilitation
of the Cardiac Patient

Chapter 13

Administration of Cardiac Rehabilitation Outpatient Programs

Kathy Berra
Linda K. Hall

The administration of cardiac rehabilitation programs has changed significantly as the size of programs and their sophistication have increased. In previous years programs were often loosely organized and poorly funded and were administered as addenda to nursing on cardiac care units, as physical therapy, or under a broad heading such as noninvasive cardiovascular services. During the 1980s the clinical importance and scientific efficacy of cardiac rehabilitation programs were established (1). As a result, the administration of such programs required a knowledge of clinical practice guidelines, personnel management, budget, policy and procedure formation and implementation, productivity, and quality assurance.

The purpose of this chapter is to outline the administrative components of hospital-based and free-standing cardiac rehabilitation programs. We address such specific issues as budgeting, marketing, staff recruitment and training, record keeping, quality assurance, productivity, public relations, and marketing. Successful administration depends on expertise that is equally strong in business and management (both knowledge and experience) on the one hand, and clinical knowledge and experience on the other. A blending of these skills into daily operation of the program and management of the staff are necessary for providing a high-quality program.

This chapter also provides information to improve current administrative policies, as well as an outline for potential delegation of administrative responsibilities to all staff members. This knowledge should improve the administration and implementation of programs and increase staff participation in the design and delivery of clinical practice.

Successful Administrative Design

In order to operate successfully as a referral service, cardiac rehabilitation programs must (understand and) work within the organizational structure of their hospital, clinic, or community facility. A specific concern would be where and under whom the cardiac rehabilitation program resides in the administrative organization. Typically, cardiac rehabilitation programs are administered under the following leadership areas: nursing, cardiology, cardiovascular surgery, or rehabilitative services. Any of these administrative possibilities have strengths and weaknesses in the management of the program. However, to clarify insurance reimbursement issues, it is preferable for the cardiac rehabilitation program to stand as an autonomous department with its own personnel, policies and procedures, billing codes, and cost center. When evaluated against the "continuity of care" standard of the Joint Commission on Accreditation of Healthcare Organizations (JCAHO), it is difficult to defend a fragmented cardiac rehabilitation program that features education in the nursing department, exercise in the physical therapy department, and nutrition in the dietary area, with no central administration providing teamwork and continuity.

Organizational Schematics and Leadership

Once its place in the administrative framework is established, management of the cardiac rehabilitation department becomes the next critical issue. This section will describe administrative needs and responsibilities that are important to the overall management of a cardiac rehabilitation program. Figure 13.1 depicts several administrative organizational grids that are used in various outpatient cardiac rehabilitation programs. The favored organizational scheme for most programs is Example 1. This scheme allows each person to work within his or her area of expertise and uses an appropriate decision-making chain of command. The program director and the medical director (a physician) work together to manage all the department's clinical and business decisions.

The *program* director (department head, manager, coordinator) is responsible for the overall development, planning, and administration of the program. This requires significant experience with budget, personnel, staff recruitment and training, problem solving, and integration within the hospital's or clinic's many other departments. Quite often, program directors are expected to participate in clinical application and interaction with patients as well as management of all business aspects of the program. It is important to recognize

that limiting the director to primarily providing direct clinical supervision is often the reason why new, innovative, and state-of-the-art programs are not developed.

The *medical* director is responsible for all medical decisions in the clinical application of the department's business. This includes management of emergencies and development of standing orders, guidelines and approval for all exercise prescriptions, decisions with regard to patient disposition when inappropriate responses to therapy arise, and other questions involving medical supervision.

The American Association of Cardiovascular and Pulmonary Rehabilitation (AACVPR) has established required and preferred standards for program and medical directors, which are outlined here. (2)

I. Program director

    A. *Required qualifications*

        1. Bachelor's degree in an allied health field, such as exercise physiology, or licensure in the jurisdiction as a registered nurse

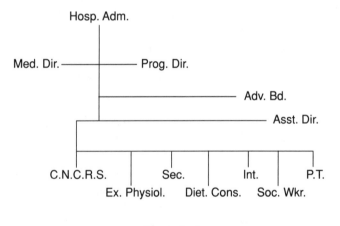

Example 1

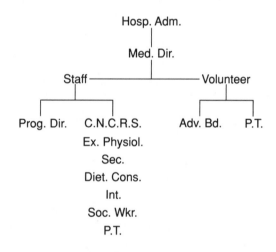

Example 2

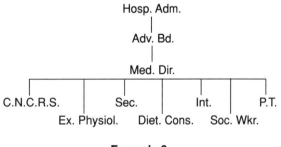

Example 3

Hosp. Adm = Hospital administration
Med. Dir. = Medical director
Prog. Dir. = Program director
Adv. Bd. = Advisory board
Asst. Dir. = Assistant director
C.N.C.R.S. = Clinical nurse cardiac rehabilitation specialist
Ex. Physiol. = Exercise physiologist
Sec. = Secretary
Diet. Cons. = Dietary consultant
Int. = Intern
Soc. Wkr. = Social worker
P.T. = Physical therapist

Figure 13.1 Organizational grids used for management of cardiopulmonary rehabilitation programs.

2. Advanced knowledge of exercise physiology, nutrition, risk factor modification strategies, counseling techniques, and uses of education programs and technologies as applied to cardiovascular rehabilitative services

3. Certification, experience, and training equivalent to those specified for an exercise specialist by the American College of Sports Medicine (ACSM) or the advanced specialty in cardiopulmonary rehabilitation of the American Physical Therapy Association

4. Experience in staff coordination and delivery of cardiovascular rehabilitation services to patients

5. Certification in basic life support (BLS) or advanced cardiac life support (ACLS) (if registered nurse)

B. *Preferred qualifications*

1. Certification, experience, and training equivalent to those specified for program director by the ACSM (3)

2. Certified in ACLS

II. Medical director

A. *Required qualifications*

1. Cardiologist, internist, or other physician with interest and experience in cardiac rehabilitation; licensed to practice in the jurisdiction, and with special competence in rehabilitative care

2. Experienced in exercise testing, prescription, and counseling

3. Certified in ACLS or experienced and knowledgeable in emergency procedures

B. *Preferred qualifications*

1. Board-certified cardiologist

2. Experienced in medical supervision of cardiovascular rehabilitation services

These standards are the only guidelines to date that delineate the necessary educational and knowledge requirements for the administrative positions in managing cardiac rehabilitation programs. The ACSM does have a program director's certification process that can be obtained through written and practical examination (3).

Mission Statements, Goals, and Long-Range Plans

As a management officer of the organization, the program director is responsible for developing immediate, annual, and long-range goals that are consistent with the mission statement of the parent organization. These goals should be specific, with all components of the department's mission addressed: clinical application, marketing, public relations, finances, and new-program development. Maintaining the current programs and planning future new programs should be addressed in this document. Annual goals are necessary in order to carry on and evaluate the daily functions of the department. Such factors as number of projected therapeutic visits, revenues, costs, staffing needs, full-time equivalents (FTEs), equipment, and maintenance expenditures are part of annual goals and objectives. Long-range goals are usually established as part of a business plan encompassing the coming 5 years. This plan is a detailed look at what has occurred during the previous 3 years, what is currently happening, and what should develop in the next 5 years with regard to new patient populations, new therapeutic intervention, reimbursement strategies, marketing and public relations strategies, and prudent fiscal management. The ultimate outcome of annual and future goals is to assure the program's fiscal stability and to maintain state-of-the-art clinical practice.

Most cardiac rehabilitation programs are integrated with other departments within the organization. Consequently the program director is wise to develop interdepartmental goals based on meetings with other departments that share patient- and program-related duties. This helps assure cooperation among departments and commitments, which in turn enhances patient care.

What follows is an example of yearly departmental performance goals, along with a five-year program plan developed by program directors.

Performance Objectives, 1991-1992

1. To continue to review and rework the application of state-of-the-art cardiac and pulmonary rehabilitation on an inpatient and outpatient basis. Because AGH has become a model program that is visited and examined by other practitioners throughout the United States, we need to

continuously examine and measure what we do,

2. To continue with management by team and consensus:
   a. Committee structure
      (1) Goals and objectives
      (2) Led by department members
      (3) Accountability—timelines for completion
   b. Participatory decision making
   c. Department ownership
3. To continue to maintain written job descriptions and the policy and procedure manual in a current state to meet JCAHO guidelines
4. To organize and develop a workshop on managing and developing a complete Phase I-III Cardiac Rehab program:
   a. Development of an educational resource manual
   b. Development of a daily schedule for participants
5. To continue to increase the number of referrals for the pulmonary rehabilitation program
6. To investigate the efficacy of developing additional programs within the department:
   a. Risk Factor Reversal program for CAD (no insult) and PTCA, CABG, and MI patients
   b. Utilization of staff and exercise area for "Shape Down" program
   c. Interrelationship with Dr. Tucker in sports medicine center
7. To continue the annual symposium in the April/May time period
8. To continue speaking locally and in hospitals on stress management and wellness:
   a. Listed in the Staff Development handbook—one 4-hour stress workshop twice each year, two 2-hour time management workshops twice each year
   b. Six workshops yearly on stress, anger, and self-esteem for Lifestages
   c. Interdepartmentally as requested
9. To strengthen the employee fitness program to include more offerings in wellness programs:
   a. Continue smoking cessation
   b. Try to reimplement Lite Life dietary program

10. To lead and assist the staff in completion of two to four research problems:
    a. Iron supplementation study
    b. NIH personality study
    c. Use of nuclear probe in assessing ventricular wall motion study
    d. Others as interested

(Courtesy of Allegheny General Hospital & Linda K. Hall)

Five-Year Goals: 1990-1995

Cardiac Rehabilitation

By 1995 YMCArdiac Therapy (YCT) will continue to serve all cardiovascular patients referred for rehabilitation through individualized programs designed to meet their physical and emotional needs. The YCT Department will provide access to specific cardiovascular risk reduction programs by maintaining high visibility in the medical community. The Cardiac Rehabilitation Program will continue to meet the guidelines of the American Association of Cardiovascular and Pulmonary Rehabilitation (AACVPR) and the American Heart Association (AHA). YCT will pursue cooperative research projects with appropriate physicians and health care professionals in the community. YCT will continue to serve as the national model for YMCAs offering cardiovascular rehabilitation programs. The YCT program directors will continue to participate in the activities of the California Society for Cardiac Rehabilitation, the AACVPR, and the AHA.

Quality Objectives
1991

1. Maintain full capacity of 175 to 190 participants.
2. Recruit 5 new medical supervisors from community hospitals to enhance visibility.
3. Encourage spousal and family memberships with new and existing YCT participants.
4. Enhance medical community involvement and awareness of YCT by having new–referring physician orientation quarterly.
5. Plan and execute a celebration of the 20th anniversary of the program in February. Recruit volunteers for the planning and implementation of this event.

1992-1995

1. Maintain scientific studies as a growing service of the department.
2. Recruit and maintain adequate numbers of highly qualified medical supervisors.
3. Develop new resources for scholarship subsidy.

Easy Going Aerobics

Program Goals

Between 1991 and 1995, YCT will continue to develop and expand the Easy Going Aerobics program. This program will continue to relate specifically to patients referred with low functional capacity due to complex medical conditions. The efficacy of this program will be evaluated through a cooperative research project between Stanford University Department of Cardiology and the YCT Department. This program may expand its scope and direction based on the outcome evaluation of this research.

Quality Objectives
1991

1. Develop a written evaluation of Easy Going participants focused on outcome measure.
2. Consider the group therapy approach as modeled by the Stanford Arthritis Self Care program.
3. Develop active participation in Easy Going efficacy measures with Dr. Randy Thomas, Cardiac Fellow at Stanford.
4. Determine the need for outpatient exercise programs for children and young adults with cystic fibrosis.

1992-1995

1. Implement new program procedures based on the studies of 1991.
2. Evaluate and develop Easy Going services, continuing this as a primary objective of the program.
3. Pursue increased physician awareness and involvement through conferences and written materials.
4. By 1995, the Easy Going Aerobics program will test its protocols and offer them as a training manual to other YMCAs with similar programs.

5. By 1995, the YMCA of the Midpeninsula will be known for its ability to offer medically prescribed and supervised exercise rehabilitation for special populations.

YCT Health Enhancement Programs

Program Goals

Between 1991 and 1995, YCT will pursue the expansion of its health enhancement programs, specifically, the Community Cholesterol Screening Program and the Health Enhancement Program for the Fire Fighters in the city of Palo Alto. The Fire Fighters Program will be offered to the Palo Alto Police Department for integration into its annual budget as an employee benefit. Alternatives to the comprehensive assessment will be offered also. YCT will continue to be available to industry for Cholesterol Screening and Cardiovascular Health lectures and Risk Reduction programs.

Quality Objectives
1991

1. Notification of local industry will be made regarding lipid management programs.
2. Negotiations with the Palo Alto Police Department will be initiated regarding a cardiovascular health program.
3. Enhanced attention will be placed on the older members of the Palo Alto Fire Department and their fitness needs.
4. Members of the Palo Alto Fire Department will be encouraged to utilize fitness facilities as a method of enhancing compliance with programs.

1992-1995

1. The cardiovascular program designed for the Palo Alto Police Department will be instituted.
2. Additional corporate sites will be identified as possible participants in the cardiovascular health enhancement program.
3. Additional industrial sites will be identified and offered cholesterol screening and educational services.

(Courtesy YMCArdiac Therapy,
Palo Alto, California, & Kathy Berra)

Daily Program Operation and Processes

The program director is responsible for the day-to-day management and functioning of the program. She or he manages the staff and their work loads, training, and new-skill acquisition and conducts performance appraisals and evaluations. The staff in larger programs and institutions may include a business manager, public relations consultant, exercise specialists, clinical nurse specialists, physical therapists, dietitians, social workers, and other consultants. In smaller programs the staff may include a half-time clinical nurse specialist and 1 or 2 other part-time staff members. A number of programs operate with 1 or 2 full-time equivalents comprised of 5 to 10 part-time workers. While this latter staffing plan affords program delivery with lower cost (part-time workers receive no benefits), it can interfere with program continuity. In cases in which small programs operate with minimal staff, communications with the parent organization is critical and should be frequent. This is often found in small hospitals, free standing programs, and such community facilities as a YMCA or Jewish Community Center. Just because a program is small and therefore less complex does not imply that communications planning is not important. Annual and long-range goals are even more critical in smaller programs and will aid in bringing in referrals and ensuring financial stability.

Budgetary Considerations and Administration

Large programs, especially those with a great deal of research-grant funding involved in their operations, may have full- or part-time business administrators. In most programs the program director is responsible for the budget. This is one of the most important aspects of program management.

Financial forecasting relative to projected patient volumes and revenues, expenses, reimbursement issues, and unforeseen costs will vary widely between institutions. However, all programs must assess the situation daily relative to projected and actual financial position.

Generally, the central administration starts the budget process 6 months prior to the beginning of a fiscal year. Directors are asked to forecast changes in patient volumes; reimbursement policies that may affect revenues, staff salaries, and

full-time equivalent expectations; and new equipment and programs to be developed with their resultant costs. In an outpatient cardiac rehabilitation program the driving forces behind the budget are the numbers of new patient admissions per year, of reimbursable sessions, and of exercise and laboratory tests, as well as functional evaluations to be provided. These are all revenue producers. On the expense side of the budget in most programs the driving force is staff salaries, which will use from 75% to 85% of the budget allocation.

The budgetary challenge is to provide high-quality care for the greatest number of participants without excessive staffing. This requires that the program director develop accurate job descriptions for all program positions and place the right person with a specific job qualification in the described position. For example: Data entry may be better performed by an employee paid $7.00 to $8.50 per hour than an administrative secretary paid $10.50 to $14.50 per hour.

Salaries are the biggest item in the budget (Table 13.1). One full-time equivalent is figured at 2,080 work hours per year. If the average salary of a clinical specialist is $15.50 per hour, the annual salary is $32,240. Multiplying the salary times the number of full-time equivalents will give the figure for the "Salary, wages, and fees" line item.

Table 13.2 illustrates one means of projecting revenues. The program director usually does this by looking at the records for past years and discussing with the surgery manager, cardiology manager, and all other personnel who will refer to the cardiac rehabilitation department what they

Table 13.1   Sample Expense Budget Items for a Large Cardiac Rehabilitation Program

Item	Expense
Salary, wages, fees	$450,370
Fringe benefits (FICA)	33,559
Consulting services	18,045
Contract maintenance	2,000
Property rental	92,796
Printing and office supplies	4,398
Teaching supplies	9,847
Pubs and subs	260
Travel	4,000
Nondepreciable fixed assets	860
Miscellaneous	1,000
Medical and surgical	5,100
Total	$622,235

Table 13.2 How to Calculate Income Budget Items for a Large Cardiac Rehabilitation Program

Item	Income
Therapeutic exercise	No. of patients × no. of sessions
	Projected attendance × fee per session
Treadmill exercise test	No. of patients projected to be tested per year × fee per test
Cardiovascular consultation	Projected no. of consults × fee per consult.
Laboratory testing	No. of patients × no. of lab tests × fee per test
Community cholesterol screen	No. of screenings × projected no. of participants × fee per test
Risk factor reduction clinics	No. of participants per clinic × projected no. of clinics × fee per participant

expect their numbers to be for the coming year. Once their projected volumes are known, *capture rates* (the number or percentage of these volumes that the cardiac rehabilitation department has had referred in the past) may be applied and revenues projected.

Staff Recruitment and Training

Program success is usually related to two major, significantly interrelated factors: the quality of the rehabilitation staff and the financial health of the program.

Staffing the Program

Recruitment of staff requires careful consideration of administrative and clinical experiences. Before the program recruits new personnel to fill vacant full-time equivalents, a careful audit of abilities, knowledge, and experiences should be made of the existing staff. Deficits should be looked for and noted, and these deficits should be emphasized in recruiting new staff. Along with their ability to fill the job description for the position, new staff

should be sought who will bring new clinical skills to the program. For example, experience in work-hardening, weight-training, and resistance exercise programs; knowledge in patient education and behavior change; and marketing and public relations skills will add strength to the program and enhance its success.

Rehabilitation staff should possess an interest in and an ability to understand the financial as well as the clinical functions of the program. They should have a thorough understanding of the importance of budget projections for future viability as well as the need to comply with existing budget constraints when administering clinical programs. Involving staff in the planning of the annual budget is appropriate and will likely promote staff morale and their sense of being an important part of the program. In addition, it will improve their ability to provide input into future programming needs and development.

Staff Orientation

Staff orientation and training are the critical links to participant safety and satisfaction. The training of staff is the cornerstone of a safe and effective program. Staff members' abilities to convey knowledge about the medical components of cardiac rehabilitation, skill in identifying medical situations of concern, compassion for participants and their families, and enthusiasm for the rehabilitative process are of major importance to the success of the program. Marketing surveys and studies have shown that dissatisfied people tell more people about their unhappiness than happy people their satisfaction (4). Thus it is important from a referral and marketing point of view to keep people happy. This requirement is attained by hiring excellent staff and training them well.

Training may take several months and should ensure that the trainee understand the following factors:

1. The organizational structure and the relationship among programs within this structure
2. The mission statements of the overall organization and of each program
3. Financial overview, with detail on staff responsibilities in the budget process
4. Details concerning program organization and job description
5. Specific outcome measures of the job description

6. Detailed discussion of program components, especially as they relate to the safety of staff and participants

7. Training in medical responsibility, including exercise therapy, counseling, risk factor interventions, exercise testing, prescribing, and other medical components of the programs

8. Training in joint organizational programs, such as smoking cessation and weight control (Many programs find that such programs are more successful when offered to the general public as well as the participant population. In addition, they allow the program to participate in the overall programming of the parent organization.)

The program director provides the model for excellence in staff performance and knowledge acquisition. These are enhanced through the offering of in-service training, continuing education programs, attendance at symposia, and certification of staff in nationally recognized courses (such as ACSM [3]). Additional ongoing training is necessary from the point of view of the AACVPR's guidelines (2) and surveys for accreditation. The JCAHO and the AACVPR recommend continuing education as standards of staffing preparedness. These requirements may be met through staff conferences; attendance at local, regional, state, or national meetings; and other appropriate certification within the aegis of the job description. National certification is available through the American Heart Association (AHA)—for BLS and ACLS—the ACSM, the YMCA, the American Physical Therapy Association, and the American Association of Respiratory Care.

Department Philosophy

Finally, philosophical approaches to applying the program to patients need to be considered. This philosophical ambience is set by the program director and usually encompasses professionalism and expectations, community service by the staff, expectations of participant outcomes, and "extra programming efforts," such as golf and bowling tournaments, picnics, staff educational pursuits, and the relationship of the program to the overall philosophy of the parent organization. The difference between the staff and personnel who meet the job description requirements and those who "see things as they might be or should be and say *why not*" is quite often in the quality of the

leadership and her or his ability to foster individual growth and teamwork. By design, cardiac rehabilitation programs need a variety of health care professionals to provide comprehensive services. As a result, individual growth, communication and team effort become essential to the success of the department.

We have not discussed the actual skills to use in managing people, because these would require volumes for an adequate description. Quite often, staff management is a reflection of the personality and qualifications of the director. Current trends in management lead one to the writings of Deming (5), Imai (6), Kreitner (7), Kiefer and Senge (8), and Koska (9). All these writers espouse a quality-in-management theory that builds on teamwork, examining process, and doing "the right thing right the first time" (5). The openness and statistical evaluation involved in these management techniques require training. These theories are currently so popular that courses in the methods of managing staff are available at weekend seminars and in college programs.

Ancillary Support and Advisory Groups to Aid in Management Success

Management guidelines can be divided into three separate but interrelated areas of responsibility: staff, program, and financial management; medical advisory management; and community relations committee management. Staff and financial management have been covered in previous sections. Here we will discuss the role of medical and community volunteer advisory groups and funding agencies and how they relate to a cardiac rehabilitation program.

Communication With Funding Agencies

Communication with groups and agencies that have the ability to assist the program with community visibility and that may have the ability to influence the financial health of the program is the responsibility of the program and medical directors as well as other members of the staff. Regular communication of program statistics and accomplishments to all agencies associated with both the parent organization and the program in particular is vital to achieving long-range goals. If the cardiac rehabilitation program receives funding from the

☐ 5. Patients must be referred to your service by a physician.

☐ 6. There must be a documented policy regarding admission to your service area for treatment, testing, rehabilitation, and care.

☐ 7. Patient care must be documented by each person who provides or directs the provision of care.

    a. Documentation must be goal directed—it must describe clearly the progress toward identified goals.

    b. Documentation must include assessment, a plan of care, appropriate intervention strategies, plans for follow-up, and evaluation of progress and final outcome.

☐ 8. There must be an individualized plan of treatment established for each patient or client who receives treatment in your service area. The plan of treatment must

    a. include information related to the diagnosis;

    b. include information related to procedures and medications;

    c. include information related to precautions and limitations that would affect the plan;

    d. be periodically reviewed; and

    e. be reviewed by the patient's or client's physician as required by condition, outcomes, and response and be documented orally on tape or in writing.

☐ 9. Signed orders for treatment must be obtained from the patient's or client's physician on a timely basis (91% to 100% of the time).

☐ 10. Staff of the department must contact the patient's or client's physician when warranted by his or her condition.

☐ 11. Care must be provided in accordance with accepted standards of practice.

☐ 12. Care must be provided in accordance with existing physician orders.

☐ 13. A current plan of care addresses the identified needs and planned services to meet those needs and improve the patient's or client's clinical status.

☐ 14. Assessments must be conducted by qualified individuals.

☐ 15. Assessments must identify the problems, needs, and strengths of the patient or client and the services that the family is able to provide.

☐ 16. What your department is providing as care must correspond to the patient's or client's needs as identified in the assessment.

☐ 17. The provision of care must consistently demonstrate individualized, goal-directed care. On admission and periodically throughout the course of care, assessments should be conducted on the individual and his or her family, support system, and home environment as it applies to care and needs.

☐ 18. Goals for intervention must be reasonable and measurable.

☐ 19. There must be written policies and procedures relative to resuscitation, emergent situations, and emergencies. The following specific policies must exist:

    a. Policies and procedures relative to the administration of drugs, route of administration, and exceptions

    b. Policies and procedures relative to IV insertion

    c. Policies and procedures relative to adverse drug reactions

    d. A process to ensure that the drug to be administered is the drug ordered

    e. A policy to ensure that the drug is stable

    f. A process to ensure that there is no contraindication for the patient relative to the drug to be administered

☐ 20. Personnel must be designated as responsible for performing tests and directing or supervising the testing.

☐ 21. Staff who perform tests must have adequate, specific training and orientation to perform the tests.

☐ 22. Current, readily available policies and procedures must be in place and address the following:

    a. Specimen collection

    b. Specimen preservation

    c. Instrument calibration

    d. Quality control and remedial action

    e. Equipment performance evaluations

    f. Test performance

These policies and procedures apply to all aspects of patient care and department function.

☐ 23. The policies and procedures must be reviewed and revised annually to reflect the standards in the field. All quality control checks must be done and records of this documented and maintained.

❏ 24. Distinct plans for education and behavior intervention for the patient or client, when the diagnosis calls for this, must exist.

❏ 25. There must be discharge instructions and guidelines for the patient or client.

Checklist for Management and Administration

❏ 1. There must be a manager (or director) for the service area.

❏ 2. The authority of this manager must be commensurate with the responsibility for the overall management of the department or service area.

❏ 3. There must be a coordinator (or director) of patient services.

❏ 4. The coordinator must take reasonable steps to ensure the availability of services.

❏ 5. The coordinator must take reasonable steps to ensure the quality of services.

❏ 6. The coordinator must take reasonable steps to ensure that there is an appropriate number of qualified staff.

❏ 7. The coordinator must be qualified in his or her health field and must
   a. understand the principles of care for the specific area,
   b. have clinical knowledge and experience in one of the major volume services in the area, and
   c. have access to qualified consultation in areas outside his or her expertise.

❏ 8. There must be written personnel policies and procedures.

❏ 9. Lines of responsibility and accountability must exist and be clearly delineated to all staff.

❏ 10. The coordinator must implement the policies and procedures of the department.

❏ 11. All staff must be oriented to their work, work classification, and expectations of what they will be asked to achieve. Orientation programs must be provided to all staff prior to their assuming patient or client care responsibilities.

❏ 12. Periodic performance evaluations based upon the specific job descriptions must take place.

❏ 13. All staff providing patient and client services must participate in orientation, in-service training, and continuing education programs. Such programs must be provided for staff, and they must be appropriate to the maintenance of skills necessary for the care of the patients and clients. The programs should cover
   a. significant clinical developments,
   b. significant administrative developments, and
   c. skills related to the care or service provided.

❏ 14. An evaluator will be looking at the following:
   a. Administrative policies and procedures
   b. Organizational chart, if available
   c. Budget and financial statements
   d. Orientation, in-service, and continuing education materials
   e. Personnel files
   f. The organization's license, certification, or registration
   g. Written agreements, if appropriate
   h. Program evaluation
   i. Organizational goals and objectives
   j. Previous regulatory and certification reports and responses
   k. Job descriptions
   l. Performance evaluations
   m. Staff interviews
   n. Long- and short-term organizational plans

The tedious parts of management are very important, for if the program is not approved by the various surveying agencies, it will not obtain approval for federal funding and a license to practice. Along with all of the regulations cited, a program must demonstrate that it regularly measures aspects of patient care and its outcome; staff training, preparedness, and performance; and patient evaluations and their outcomes. In all instances in which performance is not up to the standard level, investigation, follow-up, and corrections must be made and all processes involved documented.

Summary

Figures 13.2 to 13.4 summarize the aspects of managing a cardiac rehabilitation program we discussed in this chapter. The figures define tasks specific to each of the job-related responsibilities for successful program management. Each task should be accompanied by written job descriptions and policies and procedures relative to performance. These figures (or similar materials that you create) should be reviewed and revised annually.

Administration of cardiac rehabilitation programs requires detailed planning, carefully monitored implementation, and precise forecasting of clinical and administrative future directions. Administration includes the ability to determine staffing needs and hiring appropriately trained staff. In order to measure success, the adminstrator (program director) and staff must provide a safe and clinically relevant program. This requires constant attention to new medical and surgical advances, to the financial implications of existing programs, and to the future needs of the diverse patient populations they serve.

Irrespective of a program's size, communications and teamwork are the cornerstones of its success. These attributes apply equally in the financial and clinical management areas. The patients, parent organization, medical community, and public benefit from sound administrative policies and procedures.

References

1. National Center for Health Services Research and Health Care Technology Assessment. Health technology assessment reports, cardiac rehabilitation services. DHHS publication no. (PHS) 88-3427. Rockville, MD: U.S. Department of Health and Human Services; 1987:1-89.

2. American Association of Cardiovascular and Pulmonary Rehabilitation. Guidelines for cardiac rehabilitation programs (2nd ed.). Champaign, IL: Human Kinetics; 1994.

3. American College of Sports Medicine. Guidelines for exercise testing and prescription. 4th ed. Philadelphia: Lea & Febiger; 1991.

4. Albrecht, C.; Zemke, R. Service in America. Homewood, IL: Jones-Irwin; 1985.

5. Deming, W.E. Quality, productivity and competitive position. Cambridge, MA: Massachusetts Institute of Technology, Center for Advanced Engineering Study; 1982.

6. Imai, M. Kaizen: The key to Japan's competitive success. New York: McGraw-Hill; 1986.

7. Kreitner, R. Management, a problem solving process. Boston: Houghton Mifflin; 1980.

8. Kiefer, C.F.; Senge, P.M. Thinking and the new management style program. Boston: Alfred P. Sloan School of Management: MIT; 1986.

9. Koska, M.T. Adopting Deming's quality improvement ideas: A case study. Hospitals. 64:58-64; 1990.

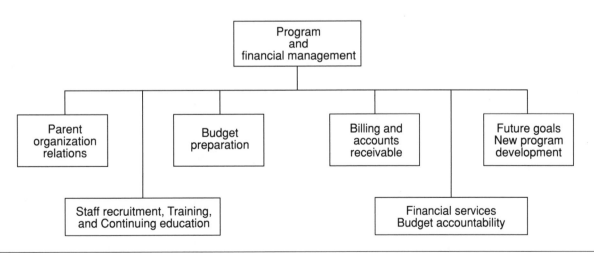

Figure 13.2   Administrative flowchart: program and finance.

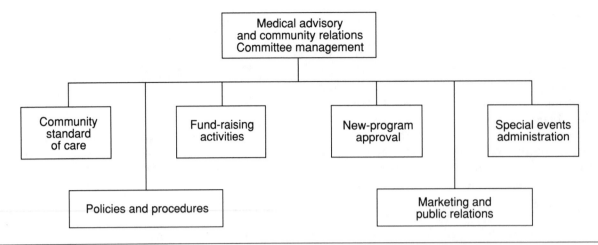

Figure 13.3   Administrative flowchart: medical advisory and community relations.

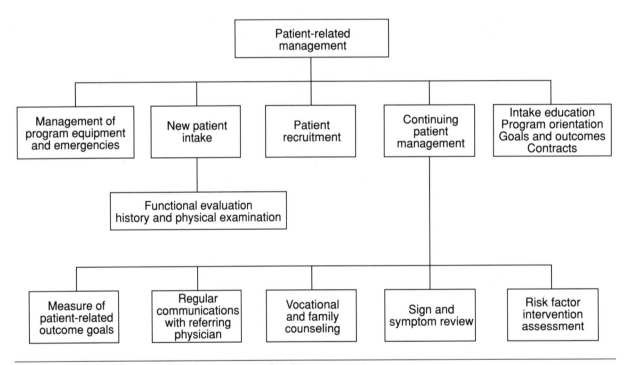

Figure 13.4   Administrative flowchart: patient-related management.

Chapter 14

Rehabilitation of the Cardiac Patient During Hospitalization: Inpatient Programs

Efraim Ben-Ari

The purpose of this chapter is to describe the changes made in the in-hospital rehabilitation program in response to the dramatic decrease in hospital mortality and length of hospital stay post-cardiac event.

The rehabilitation process of patients with cardiac disorders has traditionally been divided into the following four phases:

1. in-hospital,
2. convalescence following discharge,
3. supervised exercise program, and
4. unsupervised maintenance program.

The first phase takes place during the period of hospitalization. During this period many physicians characteristically have been reluctant to permit patients to engage actively in daily activities, wishing to allow time for a firm scar to develop on the myocardium and for cardiac function to recover in a gradual, spontaneous fashion. However, there is increasing acceptance of early hospital discharge: generally, about 3 days after percutaneous transluminal coronary angioplasty (PTCA) and 4 to 14 days after acute myocardial infarction (MI) or coronary artery bypass graft (CABG) surgery (1-3). This trend has resulted in less time being devoted to achieving the following Phase 1 objectives:

- Starting the patient on an in-hospital progressive-activity program
- Providing the patient with a basic understanding of cardiovascular disease (CVD)
- Identifying risk factors relevant to the patient and beginning modification of these for the prevention of coronary artery disease (CAD)
- Using physical activity and educational programs to minimize feelings of invalidism, restore self-confidence, and reduce anxiety

- Promoting early, yet safe, resumption of activity soon after discharge

Changing In-Hospital Care

Based on data compiled by the Professional Activity Survey and the Worcester Heart Attack Study (4), the in-hospital case-fatality rate from acute MI declined from 24.6% in 1970 to 18.8% in 1977 and 15.5% in 1984 (5). Overall, this improving trend may reflect changes in patient care and management or the fact that less severe cases are being admitted to the hospital.

On the other hand, long-term prognosis after an acute MI has not improved. These data reinforce the importance of limiting the extent of acute myocardial damage and preserving jeopardized myocardium early after an MI or CABG surgery. Also, reducing risk factors has been shown to stop the progression or even undo the underlying atherosclerotic process of CAD (6-8). In light of these findings—namely, shorter hospitalization and earlier mobilization following a cardiac event, a decline in in-hospital mortality, and increased public demand for improved health care—Phase 1 rehabilitation directors must constructively reevaluate the goals, means of action, and results of their programs. In fact, because of these trends, some critics raise the question as to the need for a Phase 1 program. In response, it should be noted that several reports, including a recent randomized study, concluded that, compared to controls, patients who participated in Phase 1 cardiac rehabilitation made substantial improvements in self-confidence and in performance of daily activities (9-11).

Designing a Phase 1 Program

Crucial for a successful Phase 1 cardiac rehabilitation program is a design based on the following facts and the plan of action:

- Hospital stay is shorter.
- Compared to previous years, hospitalized patients are older and more acutely ill, making medical care more complex.
- There is increased public pressure to cut hospital costs and at the same time improve the services delivered, including those during the immediate post-hospitalization period.

A plan for developing or upgrading your Phase 1 program should include the following elements:

1. Definition of specific goals and objectives
   - Stratification of patients by diagnosis and demographic makeup
   - Physiological and psychosocial aspects: What do you expect your program to accomplish?
   - Short- and long-term goals: How do you plan for your program to grow?
   - Bedside- and classroom-teaching techniques, means of action, and methods for systematic evaluation of the results
2. Enrollment of other departments and administrators to approve and support the program: staff, budget, space
3. Setting a timetable for every step of your plan

Exercise Testing

In recent years it has become commonplace to perform a submaximal exercise test in uncomplicated patients prior to their hospital discharge. The reasons for performing the test may be summarized as follows:

To evaluate prognosis
- Residual ischemia
- Stratification for possible early discharge or predischarge catheterization
- Indicators of postdischarge angina, MI, death, or restenosis following PTCA

To evaluate functional capacity
- Baseline for follow-up evaluations
- Anginal threshold and medical therapy
- Suitability for return to work

To promote quality of life
- Reassure patient and family
- Promote lifestyle change
- Provide basis for exercise prescription

On the average, the test is performed 7 to 10 days after admission or within 21 days after an MI or CABG surgery (12-14). However, Topol et al. (15) investigated the possibility of performing the test in some uncomplicated post-MI patients 3 days after admission. The study design and results are shown in Figure 14.1. Overall, 136 patients were studied, of which 61 (45%) were identified as low risk, meaning that the following factors were not present:

- Ventricular tachycardia or fibrillation
- Second- or third-degree A-V block
- Pulmonary edema
- Cardiogenic shock
- Infarct extension
- Persistent hypotension
- Sinus tachycardia
- Sustained superventricular tachycardia
- Bundle branch block
- Persistent ST-segment elevation
- Recurrent angina or recent previous MI (6 months)

and had a graded exercise test (GXT). In-hospital follow-up of tested patients revealed that a positive test significantly increased the probability of a short-term adverse cardiac event. Long-term follow-up of the tested patients (8.4 ±1.5 months)

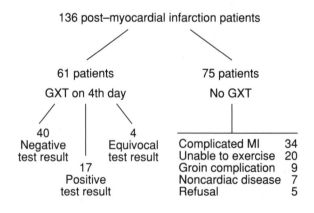

Figure 14.1 Early exercise testing of 136 consecutive patients, 61 of whom underwent graded exercise testing (GXT) on a treadmill on the 4th day of hospitalization (left). On the right are the results of the 75 patients who were not suitable for the test.
From Topol et al. Exercise Testing 3 Days After Acute Myocardial Infarction. *Am. J. Cardiol.*, **60**:960, 1987.

showed no death or deterioration in left ventricular structure or function resulting from taking the GXT. In summary, it is obvious that very early exercise testing is safe and can aid in risk stratification for better patient management and in making decisions about further treatment and early hospital discharge.

Physical Activity

There are numerous excellent reports, such as those presented in Table 14.1, describing step-by-step in-hospital activity protocols. The efficacy of such programs has shown that in low- to moderate-risk patients, early physical activity is safe and has no deleterious effects on left ventricular function (LVF) or volume (16,17). Thus, provided that patients are hemodynamically and electrically stable, mobilization may begin in the intensive care unit. As seen in Table 14.1, patients should first be instructed to sit on the side of their bed. The prime objective here is to prevent orthostatic hypotension and the deleterious effects of prolonged bed rest by first exercising with passive range-of-motion (ROM) movements and sitting at bedside. On day 3 to 5, patients assume self-care activities and slow, supervised walking for up to 5 min two or three times daily. On day 4 to 9, patients are instructed to walk continuously for up to 10 min three times daily and are encouraged to perform some stair climbing (one or two flights). During these low-level activities HR and SBP may increase above resting level by approximately 10 beats/min and 10 mm Hg, respectively (18). More details concerning the exercise prescription in the inpatient program will be found in chapter 17.

A source of great confusion is the ambiguous answers patients and family get at the hospital regarding the question, What am I allowed to do after discharge? The Activity Schedule shown in Table 14.2 and the Postdischarge Walking Program found in Table 14.3 are distributed to patients during a special session, which is devoted to a step-by-step explanation of the material. The information should help bridge the gap between what the patients have accomplished in the inpatient program and what they can do when they arrive at home.

Table 14.1   In-Hospital Progressive Activity Program

| Stage | Days of program | | | Activity schedule |
	6-day plan	9-day plan	12-day plan	
I	1	1	1	Use bedside commode. Begin physical therapy range-of-motion exercises to each extremity. Sit at side of bed 5-10 min.
		2	2	Sit in chair 5-15 min twice daily. Begin education program at bedside. Continue physical therapy as above.
	2	3	3	Sit in chair up to 30 min twice daily. Continue physical therapy as above.
II	3	4	5	Move to step-down area: Bathe above waist, shave, and comb hair. Begin self-exercise program with physical therapy supervision. Sit in chair 60-120 min twice daily.
		5	7	Continue self-exercise program with physical therapy supervision. Begin ambulation with physical therapist. Sit in chair 90-150 min twice daily. Begin attending education classes and discussion groups.
		6	8	Take wheelchair shower and use bathroom as desired. Continue physical activity as above.
III	4	7	9	Move to general cardiovascular ward. Dress in street clothes if desired. Be up and around room as tolerated. Begin climbing stairs with physical therapist.
	5	8	11	Take predismissal graded exercise test. Continue physical activity as above. Take standing shower.
	6	9	12	Receive final going-home instructions.

Note. From Squires, R.W. et al. *Mayo Clinic Proceedings*, May 1990; 5:737-751. Reprinted with permission.

Table 14.2 Activity Schedule Following Discharge After Myocardial Infarction or Coronary Artery Bypass Graft Surgery

Activity	Time after discharge (weeks, unless noted otherwise)	Comment
Outside the home		
Be driven in car	As soon as discharged	For short distance.
Walk dog alone	(*See* Table 14.3)	If dog doesn't pull.
Attend religious services	5-7 days	
Attend nearby movie or play	2	
Visit friends	1-2	Short drives or walks, 1-2 h.
Shopping	2-3	*No* carrying. Short walking distances, 10-1 min, rest 5 min, repeat.
Grocery shopping	3-4	As above, one bag at a time, 15.
Restaurant dinner	2-3	Watch what you eat!
Drive locally	2	
Work 3 hours	6-8	Consult your physician.
Work two-thirds time	6-8	Consult your physician.
Work full time	6-8	Consult your physician.
Drive to work	6-8	
Overnight trips	8-10	
Commercial air trips	10-12	Consult your physician.
Three-day, longer trips	12	
Change auto tire	NO!	
Attend major-league ball game	10	In comfortable weather.
Attend local little league	6-8	In comfortable weather.
Swimming	10	Go in slowly; don't jump in.
Golf, riding cart	6-8	In comfortable weather.
Golf, with pull cart	8-12	Start with putting, chipping, and then nine holes.
Inside/around the home		
Walk inside house	As soon as discharged	3-5 times/day, 5 min each.
Climb one flight	As soon as discharged	One step at a time.
Walk in your yard	As soon as discharged	Leisurely walks 5-10 min.
Walk around the block	(*See* Table 14.3)	
Sit in yard	As soon as discharged	In comfortable weather.
Mowing lawn, rider	3-4	
Mowing lawn, push	10-12	
Water lawn	2	
Pull weeds	4	
Gardening	4-6	Light gardening after ground broken.
Sexual relations	2-6	When able to climb two flights.
Beer, wine, cocktails	As soon as discharged	Small drink every 2-3 days.
Friends to visit	1-2	
Out-of-town guests	6-8	
Help make bed, cook, clean up	1-2	Don't rush; make one side.
Put out trash	2	Regular-size bags, one at a time.
Dust, vacuum	2	Slowly, if cleaner moves easily.
Lifting, 20 lbs	3-4	
Laundry	3-4	One load at a time.

Table 14.3   Postdischarge Walking Program

Weeks after discharge	Distance	Time	Note
1	1/4 mile (2 blocks)	Leisurely pace—take 5 min	Twice daily. Also, do activities learned in the hospital.
2	1/2 mile (5 blocks)	Leisurely pace—take 10 min	Twice daily
3	3/4 mile (8 blocks)	Walk 20 min, rest 5 min, repeat	Once daily
4	1 mile (10 blocks)	20 min	Once daily
5	1-1/2 miles (15 blocks)	30 min	Once daily
6	2 miles (20 blocks)	35-40 min	Once daily

The following are some of the questions many patients ask:

1. Must I walk the distance and time specified above?

   No. These are good references to follow, not specific goals you must achieve.

2. How fast should I walk, and what about my heart rate?

   Always walk at a comfortable pace. Immediately after walking, during the first 2 weeks, your heart rate should not be more than 20 beats/min above the standing resting rate. In subsequent weeks, as you increase your walking, your heart rate will increase but not so that you feel a strong pounding in your chest.

3. How should I feel during walking?

   A good general rule to follow is that you should feel your walking is "somewhat hard." Slow down if you feel walking is too hard (heavy breathing, excessive sweating, fatigue, "heavy legs") for you.

4. Should I resume walking after I've stopped to rest because of chest pains or fatigue?

   No! You should never get to this point. Reduce your program to the above outline so that you can walk continuously without these symptoms.

5. What signs should I look for during walking?

   Good signs are light sweating, faster breathing, slight fatigue, and an overall pleasant feeling.

Educational Program

Acute cardiac events are attended by chaos for both the patient and family. Initially there is panic and anxiety, followed by the threat of death, transient depression, and denial of the seriousness of the disease or rejection of its reality. Therefore, the health professional, who is seen as the person responsible for teaching patients about their post–cardiac event care, needs to be far more than just a provider of information. In my experience, during the first 2 months after hospital discharge only about half of all patients comply with the information given in-hospital, a proportion that decreases to less than 30% by 4 months following discharge.

Cardiac events affect all family members. It is important to recognize sources of stress, such as overprotection of the cardiac patient by family members, and to understand that grief is normal to a certain extent. When such reactions are noted, the cardiac rehabilitation staff or other health professionals should help family members cope with the problem. This counseling may make for a smoother recovery and the resumption of good-quality life. Hence, family members, as well as the patient, should attend as many educational classes as possible while the patient is in the Phase 1 program. Readers are encouraged to refer to material dealing with postcardiac psychosocial concerns (19-22).

In designing an educational program, more attention than traditionally has been given must be paid to the patient's selected needs. For example, Thompson et al. (23) reported that normalization of lifestyle was significantly higher on the priority list of patient and spouse, followed by risk factor modification. And, of those who had smoked at the time of admission, 39% selected smoking cessation as the last of seven priorities. These findings, obviously, call for special programming, emphasizing smoking cessation.

To be effective, then, the educational program must be carefully structured, taking into account patients' needs, the issues included in the plan of action noted previously, and the following criteria for successful lifestyle change:

- The patient must believe that he or she is susceptible to the disease and would be significantly affected by the disease.
- The patient must believe that the action that he or she will take will lessen the severity of the disease.
- The patient must understand that the threat of the disease is greater than taking health-related actions.
- A stable and relaxed preoperative emotional state is very important for early postdischarge resumption of good-quality life.
- All members of the health team should emulate the program's doctrine.
- Information must be up-to-date, consistent, and simple.
- Staff must exhibit to the patient genuine interest, warmth, and friendliness.

Home-Based Program

Unfortunately, many patients are not enrolled in Phase 2 supervised outpatient cardiac rehabilitation programs. Even so, home-based activity and dietary programs serve as a good alternative and form a foundation that can support long-term adherence to a change in lifestyle. The pioneering work of DeBusk et al. (24,25) and Pollock et al. (26) (see chapter 17 for an update) provided home-based programs for low- to moderate-risk patients. They and, more recently, Coats et al. (27), in their work with chronic heart-failure patients, make it clear that medically directed home-based programs are safe, inexpensive, and effective. The important point is that the inpatient cardiac rehabilitation experience and staff involvement can provide patients with the confidence, educational materials, answers to questions, and motivation that will allow them to continue their program after discharge. A follow-up and patient-support program should be developed to ensure adherence.

Thus, due to the changes noted previously in in-hospital care, the cardiac rehabilitation team faces, in addition to changes in the duration of the Phase 1 program, the added challenge of implementing a home-based exercise and risk factor modification program. Special attention should be given to patients who will not, for whatever reason, join a Phase 2 cardiac rehabilitation program. Such attention can be in the form of additional class

time, a written, step-by-step home-based activity program, and/or periodic telephone follow-up.

Methods

A wide variety of teaching methods and tools are available. Choosing the ones that will best work for you should be done in full concert with your plan of action. Written materials, if merely handed out, are ineffective because many patients are not able to read above the fifth-grade level (28) and because the lack of time available for education programs (in-hospital) often makes teaching difficult. Thus, a variety of techniques, including audiovisual aids, booklets, tapes, group sessions, bedside teaching, and follow-up support structure, as well as a sound program and professional staff, should be applied. Information must be prioritized, made clear, repeated and reinforced as frequently as possible (29). Modifiable risk factors, such as cigarette smoking, depressed mood, and obesity have been related to noncompliance (30,31); in one study, involvement of physicians in the educational program increased the 8-week compliance rate from 36% to 96% (31). An example of a postoperative classroom educational program schedule, including class outline and time schedule, is shown in Table 14.4. This program is coordinated with other departments. The plan is to have each patient and/or spouse attend as many of these sessions as possible.

Summary

In recent years in-hospital care has gone through dramatic changes including decline in hospital mortality following an acute MI, shorter hospitalization and earlier mobilization following a cardiac event, and increased public demand for reduced costs and improved health-related services. In response, Phase 1 cardiac rehabilitation objectives, program content, and methods must be constructively reevaluated to fit these changing trends and demands. In addition to changes in current in-hospital programs, this includes detailed information so that postdischarge education and home exercise become an integral part of Phase 1 programming. Special attention should be given to stratification of patients not only by clinical diagnosis but also by level of education, number and level of risk factors for CAD, availability of a Phase 2 program, and the patient's preference.

Table 14.4 Program Schedule for In-Hospital Postsurgery Cardiac Rehabilitation and Education

Event	Action
Family information meeting	While you are in the recovery room, family members are invited to an information meeting. A nurse and a counselor will explain all aspects of the recovery period. The meeting is held Tuesdays and Thursdays at 2:30 p.m.
Physical exercise	Physical activity will start as soon as possible. Daily activities including some exercises and walking.
Dietary instructions	Heart-healthy eating instructions will be given Monday through Friday from 3:30 p.m. to 4:30 p.m.
Medications	The pharmacist will explain medications and their effects, on Mondays and Thursdays at 4:00 p.m.
Stress management	The practice of various stress management techniques with a special counselor is held Monday through Thursday at 5:00 p.m.
Risk factor modification	Making the right modification in lifestyle may prevent worsening of your heart disease. What risk factors there are and how to modify them will be explained in detail on Tuesdays and Thursdays at 3:00 p.m.
Discharge	This is the final meeting to review all instructions, your follow-up schedule, and *dos* and *don'ts*. Meet Mondays, Wednesdays, and Fridays at 12:30 p.m.

References

1. DeBusk, R.F.; Blomquist, C.G.; Kouchoukos, N.T.; Luepker, R.V.; Miller, H.S.; Moss, A.J.; Pollock, M.L.; Reeves, T.J.; Selvester, R.H.; Stason, W.B.; Wanger, G.S.; Willman, V.L. Identification and treatment of low-risk patients after acute myocardial infarction and coronary artery bypass graft surgery. N. Engl. J. Med. 314:161-166; 1986.

2. DeBusk, R.F. American college of physicians position paper. Evaluation of patients after recent acute myocardial infarction. Ann. Intern. Med. 110:485-488; 1989.

3. Topol, E.J.; Burek, K.; O'Neill, W.W.; Kewman, D.G.; Kander, N.H.; Shea, M.J.; Kirscht, J.; Juni, J.E.; Pitt, B. A randomized controlled trial of hospital discharge three days after myocardial infarction. N. Engl. J. Med. 318:1083-1088; 1988.

4. Goldberg, R.J.; Gore, J.M.; Alpert, J.S. Recent changes in attack and survival rates of acute myocardial infarction (1975 through 1981). The Worcester heart attack study. JAMA. 255:2774-2779; 1986.

5. Greeland, P.; Henrietta, R.S.; Goldbourt, U.; Behar, S.; the Israeli SPRINT Investigators. Inhospital and one-year mortality in women after myocardial infarction. Circulation. 82[Suppl. III]:468; 1990.

6. Ornish, D.; Brown, S.E.; Scherwitz, L.W.; Billings, J.H.; Armstrong, W.T.; Ports, T.A.; McLanahan, S.M.; Rirkeeide, R.L.; Brand, R.J.; Gould, K.L. Can lifestyle reverse coronary heart disease? Lancet. 336:129-133; 1990.

7. Brown, G.; Albert, J.J.; Fisher, L.D.; Schaefer, S.M.; Lin, J.T.; Kaplan, C.; Zhao, X.Q.; Bisson, B.D.; Fitzpatrick, V.F.; Dodge, H.T. Regression of coronary artery disease as a result of intensive lipid-lowering therapy in men with high levels of apolipoprotein B. N. Engl. J. Med. 323:1289-1298; 1990.

8. Blankenhorn, F.H.; Nessim, S.A.; Johnson, S.A.; Sanmarco, M.E.; Azen, S.P.; Cashin, H.L. Beneficial effects of combined colestipol niacin therapy on coronary atherosclerosis and coronary venous bypass grafts. JAMA. 257:3233-3240; 1987.

9. Knapp, D.; Gutmann, M.; Regis, S.; Squires, R.; Pollock, M. Follow-up activity level among coronary artery by-pass surgery (CABS) patients (Ab). Med. Sci. Sports Exerc. 14:178; 1982.

10. Gulanick, M. Is phase 2 cardiac rehabilitation necessary for early recovery of patients with cardiac disease? A randomized, controlled study. Heart Lung. 20:9-15; 1991.

11. Opitz, J.L. Physical activity following myocardial infarction. Psychiatr. Ann. 8:80-83; 1978.

12. Markiewicz, W.; Houston, N.; DeBusk, R.F. Exercise testing soon after myocardial infarction. Circulation. 56:26-31; 1977.

13. Theroux, P.; Waters, D.D.; Halphen, C. Prognostic value of exercise testing soon after myocardial infarction. N. Engl. J. Med. 310:341-345; 1979.

14. DeBusk, R.F.; Haskell, W. Symptom-limited versus heart-rate limited exercise testing soon after myocardial infarction. Circulation. 61:738-743; 1980.

15. Topol, E.J.; Juni, J.E.; O'Neill, W.W.; Nicklas, J.M.; Shea, M.J.; Burke, K.; Pitt, B. Exercise testing 3 days after acute myocardial infarction. Am. J. Cardiol. 60:958-962; 1987.

16. Rowe, M.H.; Jelinek, M.V.; Liddell, N.; Hugens, M. Effects of rapid mobilization on ejection fractions and ventricular volumes after acute myocardial infarction. Am. J. Cardiol. 63:1037-1041; 1989.

17. Dion, W.F.; Grevenow, P.; Pollock, M.L.; Squires, R.W.; Foster, C.; Johnson, W.D.; Schmidt, D.H. Medical problems and physiologic responses during supervised inpatient cardiac rehabilitation: The patient after coronary artery bypass grafting. Heart Lung. 11:248-255; 1982.

18. Silvidi, G.E.; Squires, R.W.; Pollock, M.L.; Foster, C. Hemodynamic responses and medical problems associated with early exercise and ambulation in

coronary artery bypass graft surgery patients. J. Cardiac Rehabil. 2:355-362; 1982.

19. Rhoda, L.F. The cardiac family recovery program training manual. Minneapolis: Heartmates Inc.; 1990.

20. Marshall, J.; Hawrysio, A. Inpatient recovery following myocardial infarction and coronary artery bypass graft surgery. J. Cardiovas. Nursing. 2:1-12; 1988.

21. Dobson, M.; Tattersfield, A.E.; Adler, M.W.; McNicol, M.W. Attitudes and long-term adjustment of patients surviving cardiac arrest. Br. Med. J. 3:207-212; 1971.

22. Granger, J.W. Full recovery from myocardial infarction: Psychosocial factors. Heart Lung. 3(4):600-609; 1974.

23. Thompson, D.L.; Fernicola, J.; Langenbach, B.S.; Parker, C. Patient-directed educational priorities in phase 1 cardiac rehabilitation. J. Cardiopul. Rehabil.-Annual Meeting, November 9-11, 1990.

24. DeBusk, R.F.; Haskell, W.L.; Miller, N.H.; Berra, K.; Taylor, C.B.; Berger, W.E., III; Lew, H. Medically directed at-home rehabilitation soon after clinically uncomplicated acute myocardial infarction: A new model for patient care. Am. J. Cardiol. 55:251-257; 1985.

25. DeBusk, R.F.; Blomqvist, C.G.; Kouchoukos, N.T.; Luepker, R.V.; Miller, H.S.; Pollock, M.L.; Selvester, R.H.; Stason, W.B.; Wanger, G.S.; William, V.L. Identification and treatment of low-risk patients after acute myocardial infarction and coronary artery bypass surgery. N. Engl. J. Med. 314:161-166; 1986.

26. Pollock, M.L.; Pels, A.E.; Foster, C. Exercise prescription for rehabilitation of the cardiac patient. In: Pollock, M.L.; Schmidt, D.H., eds. Heart disease and rehabilitation. 2d ed. New York: Wiley; 1986:475-515.

27. Coats, A.J.S.; Adamopoulos, S.; Meyer, T.E.; Conway, J.; Sleight, P. Effects of physical training in chronic heart failure. Lancet. 335:63-66; 1990.

28. Hellerstein, H.K.; Friedman, E.H. Sexual activity and the post-coronary patient. Arch. Intern. Med. 125:987-999; 1970.

29. Tullio, M.R.; Granata, D.; Broccolino, M.; Dossena, M.G.; Pedroni, P.; Zaini, G.; Recalcati, F.; Belli, C. Early predictors of smoking cessation after myocardial infarction. Circulation. 396[Suppl. III]:82; 1990.

30. Tardif, G.S. Sexual activity after a myocardial infarction. Arch. Phys. Med. Rehabil. 70:763-766; 1989.

31. Gonzalez-Fernandez, R.A.; Rivera, M.; Torres, D.; Quiles, J.; Jackson, A. Usefulness of a systematic hypertension inhospital education program. Am. J. Cardiol. 65:1384-1386; 1990.

Chapter 15

Hospital- and Home-Based Cardiac Rehabilitation Outpatient Programs

Barry A. Franklin
Kimberly Bonzheim
Tom Berg
Scott Bonzheim

Cardiac rehabilitation and its progressive incorporation into the mainstream of contemporary medical care are responsible for some impressive gains in the management of patients with cardiovascular disease (CVD) (1). These patients include the traditional patients of past years—myocardial infarction (MI), coronary artery bypass graft (CABG) surgery, and percutaneous transluminal coronary angioplasty (PTCA) patients—in addition to coronary patients with or without residual ischemia, compensated heart failure, cardiomyopathies, and worrisome arrhythmias; a variety of categories of patients with nonischemic heart disease; patients with concomitant pulmonary disease; patients who have undergone new interventions, such as pacemaker implantation, cardioverter-defibrillator implantation, heart valve repair or replacement, and cardiac transplantation; elderly patients; and medically complex patients taking multiple cardiac and other medications (2). The nearly 2,000 North American cardiac rehabilitation programs and thousands of others throughout the world are prized by patients for the interventions they provide to help prevent or retard the progression of the disease process and to restore and maintain optimal physical, psychological, emotional, social, and vocational functioning. These outpatient programs offer special services that are often lacking in the acute-care setting, including exercise therapy; patient and family education; and psychosocial, nutritional, and vocational counseling.

The purpose of this chapter is to review contemporary issues and concerns in hospital- and home-based outpatient cardiac rehabilitation, with specific reference to program models, staffing, facilities and equipment, exercise testing and training, emergency and surveillance procedures, compliance, quality assurance, and reimbursement considerations. Community-based programs are specifically discussed in the next chapter.

Program Models: Group Versus Home

Participation in a supervised, exercise-based group rehabilitation program is not always practical. Home exercise training may be a reasonable alternative for many cardiac patients. Advantages of home-training programs include lesser cost, increased availability, increased convenience, and the promotion of independence and responsibility among recovering coronary patients (3). Such programs can be effective in improving functional capacity, especially for low-risk patients (4). Drawbacks, however, include the limited means of teaching patients necessary principles and proscriptions for exercise, the lack of opportunity to counsel and encourage lifestyle changes for coronary risk reduction, and the lack of medical surveillance, emergency care, and peer support. Several techniques have been proposed to overcome these limitations, including regular telephone contact between patients and rehabilitation staff and transtelephonic exercise electrocardiographic (ECG) monitoring (4).

Although supervised group programs often involve increased cost and extended travel time, considerable data demonstrate the safety, efficacy, and cost effectiveness of this model. In addition, supervised programs can provide emergency support for patients and ongoing surveillance information for referring physicians. Such programs are appropriate for the wide range of medically complex patients eligible for cardiac rehabilitation services, including those at intermediate risk and high risk for future cardiac events. Moreover, supervised exercise training facilitates education about exercise and lifestyle changes for coronary artery disease (CAD) risk reduction, provides variety and recreational opportunities, offers staff reassurance and peer support, and enhances the potential for compliance and safety.

Staffing

The success of a cardiac rehabilitation program is closely tied to the selection of qualified allied health care personnel, acting in conjunction with the referring physician's individual treatment plan. The staff should possess the clinical experience and competencies needed to guide interventions aimed at restoring and maintaining functional capacity and effecting favorable modification of CAD risk factors. The collective knowledge base of the persons assigned to provide rehabilitative services should include a comprehensive and up-to-date understanding of CVD, cardiovascular nursing and emergency procedures, appropriate diagnostic studies, medications, nutrition, exercise physiology, health psychology, vocational issues, and medical and educational strategies for risk factor modification.

The multidisciplinary cardiac rehabilitation staff should include both licensed and nonlicensed health care professionals. The minimum staff required for a program to provide cardiovascular rehabilitation services is a physician or medical director, a program director or coordinator, and a registered nurse (5). When possible, it is recommended that the services of an exercise physiologist, physical therapist, registered dietitian, psychologist, social worker, vocational rehabilitation counselor, occupational therapist, health educator, and pharmacist be recruited to complement the "core" personnel. However, staff selection and utilization must also consider cost-containment and reimbursement issues.

The specific competency guidelines and required and preferred qualifications of cardiac rehabilitation personnel are largely derived from previously published standards (5,6). For example, guidelines for professional education and minimal competencies, outlined as general and specific behavioral objectives for program directors, exercise specialists, and exercise test technologists, have been developed by the American College of Sports

Medicine (ACSM) (6). Involvement of ACSM-certified personnel in preventive and rehabilitative exercise programs is desirable because of the specific knowledge, skills, and competencies associated with each level of certification. It is important that staff participate in professional conferences and continuing-education activities and that certification of personnel be undertaken to ensure that competency standards are maintained.

Facilities and Equipment

Although settings for outpatient cardiac rehabilitation may vary, the success of any program is attributed, at least in part, to its accessibility, hours of operation, and facilities and equipment.

Gymnasium Facilities and Equipment

The following monitoring devices and exercise equipment and facilities are commonly found in many outpatient cardiac rehabilitation programs (5):

1. Multichannel ECG telemetry monitor
2. Emergency equipment (e.g., defibrillator, drugs, O_2, IV apparatus, suction machine)
3. Sphygmomanometer and stethoscope
4. Perceived-exertion scale
5. Pain/discomfort scales
6. Large clock with sweep second hand
7. Anthropometric equipment
   - Skinfold calipers
   - Tape measure
   - Scale
8. Recreational game equipment
   - Mats
   - Balls
   - Volleyball stands
9. Exercise equipment and facilities
   for the lower extremities
   - Stationary-cycle ergometers
   - Treadmills
   - Stair-climbing devices
   - Resistance equipment
   - Walking areas
   for the upper extremities
   - Arm ergometers
   - Dumbbells
   - Resistance equipment
   - Rubber bands
   - Hand weights

for both the lower and upper extremities

- Arm-and-leg ergometers (e.g., the Schwinn Air-Dyne)
- Cross-country ski machines
- Rowing machines
- Warm-up and cool-down area

Aquatic Exercise Programs

The availability of a swimming pool offers additional exercise opportunities for patients with concomitant musculoskeletal and orthopedic problems. Water provides an ideal medium for aerobic exercise and adds therapeutic alternatives and variety to a gymnasium-based cardiac rehabilitation program. Water walking, that is, striding in waist- to chest-deep water at 1.5 to 2.0 mph, requires the same energy expenditure as fast walking or jogging on land (7). The effects of water's resistance and buoyancy make high levels of energy expenditure possible with reduced strain on the musculoskeletal system (8). Water offers approximately 12 times the resistance of air. When walking and pulling with the arms, this resistance causes the use of both the extensor and flexor muscles of a submerged body part. Buoyancy at shoulder depth is equal to the body's experiencing a 90% weight loss. A water level between the midriff and armpits is recommended to allow exercisers better movement control.

Heart rates (HR) during water activities tend to be lower than those observed on land. Consequently, less demand is placed on the myocardium for any given oxygen uptake or work rate. This may be attributed, at least in part, to decreased orthostatic pressure, which facilitates venous return. Moreover, excess metabolic heat from the exercise is more easily dissipated in water, enhancing temperature regulation.

A recent study involving identical aerobic routines performed on land and in water showed that 80% of maximal oxygen uptake ($\dot{V}O_2max$) was required during both, despite a 13% lower HR response in the water (9). The Institute for Aerobics Research suggests that one deduct 17 beats/min from the prescribed target HR on land to adjust for the decreased chronotropic reserve in the water (10). A 6-s pulse count (times 10) is recommended for use in accounting for the rapid decrease in HR that occurs with cessation of activity in water (11). Ratings of perceived exertion (RPE) can also serve as a useful and important adjunct to HR as an intensity guide for exercise training.

Appropriate candidates for water aerobics classes include "low-risk" patients who can accurately monitor their exercise intensity, as demonstrated by their participation in a Phase II program or its equivalent. Equipment that can be added to water routines to provide variety and modulate the exercise intensity includes pull buoys, weights, kickboards, balls, plastic jugs, swim fins, hand paddles, deep-water vests, and styrofoam dumbbells. Aqua shoes can also be used to ensure stable footing and protect the feet from rough pool bottoms.

Swimming, even at slow, comfortable speeds, can result in masked anginal symptoms, and near-maximal values for HR and oxygen uptake ($\dot{V}O_2$) in patients with ischemic heart disease (12). Exercise intensity is extremely variable and highly dependent on skill and mechanical efficiency. Because of these concerns, swim training should be carefully prescribed for some cardiac patients and proscribed for others (13). Upright aquatic exercise is much easier to monitor and regulate for those patients who enjoy water activities.

Contraindications to Exercise Training

Absolute contraindications are those known or suspected medical conditions that may preclude or delay entrance into or continuation of an exercise-based cardiac rehabilitation program. In some instances appropriate medical and surgical interventions may alleviate the problem. The following are common contraindications to participation in inpatient or outpatient cardiac exercise programs (6):

- Unstable angina
- Resting systolic blood pressure (BP) greater than 200 mm Hg or resting diastolic BP greater than 110 mm Hg
- Orthostatic BP drop of 20 mm Hg or more
- Moderate to severe aortic stenosis
- Acute systemic illness or fever
- Uncontrolled atrial or ventricular dysrhythmias
- Uncontrolled sinus tachycardia (> 120 beats/min)
- Uncontrolled congestive heart failure (CHF)
- Third-degree heart block without pacemaker
- Active pericarditis or myocarditis
- Recent embolism
- Thrombophlebitis
- Resting ST displacement (> 3 mm)
- Uncontrolled diabetes
- Orthopedic problems that would prohibit exercise

Recently, concerns have been raised regarding the potential deleterious effects of exercise training for patients with silent myocardial ischemia or those recovering from large anterior wall MIs (i.e., with greater than 18% left ventricular asynergy) (14). Some experienced clinicians have suggested that asymptomatic patients who demonstrate significant ST-segment depression should refrain from vigorous exercise training, citing biopsy studies of ischemic myocardium that show increased fibrosis (15). Moreover, a preliminary report by Jugdutt et al. (16) showed that some patients respond adversely to exercise training soon after anterior wall MI, demonstrating further deterioration in both global and regional left ventricular function (LVF). An accompanying editorial commentary by Iskandrian (17) stated that "until further studies become available it may be advisable not to enroll patients with large anterior Q waves in an exercise training program soon after myocardial infarction." However, other investigations of painless exercise-induced ST-segment depression have allayed concerns regarding risk and have demonstrated better survival, milder disease, and higher exercise-training intensities in such patients compared with those with angina (18,19). In addition, recent radionuclide and echocardiographic studies in patients with CHF, anterior wall MI, or both, indicate that infarct expansion and deterioration in LVF are unlikely outcomes of exercise training (20-22).

Risk Stratification

Identification of patients soon after acute MI who are at increased risk for subsequent cardiac events offers two major benefits: (1) patients at moderate to high risk can be evaluated for more intensive pharmacotherapy, interventional cardiac catheterization, PTCA, or CABG surgery and (2) patients at low risk can be spared immediate cardiac catheterization and unwarranted restriction of their vocational and leisure-time activities. The triaging of patients into ECG-monitored or nonmonitored exercise-based rehabilitation programs can also be facilitated using the level of risk stratification in which the patient has been placed (23).

DeBusk et al. (24) emphasized in their risk stratification algorithm that it is the degree of left ventricular dysfunction (LVD) and residual resting or exercise-induced myocardial ischemia, manifested as significant ST-segment depression, angina pectoris, or both, that determines the risk of future cardiac events. In this algorithm, 50% of the patients were in the low-risk group (< 2% annual mortality rate) because of an absence of resting or exercise-induced myocardial ischemia and of severe LVD, 30% were at moderate risk (10% to 20% first-year mortality rate) because of resting or exercise-induced ischemia in the presence of moderate to good LVF, and 20% were at high risk (> 25% first-year mortality rate) because of clinically evident severe pump failure or severe LVD.

It should be emphasized that risk status can be influenced by numerous interventions and lifestyle habits (Figure 15.1). Accordingly, patients may move on the risk stratification continuum from one subset to another. For example, multicenter trials have confirmed that mortality from acute MI can be decreased by approximately 25% with thrombolysis (25). Patients at moderate risk are those most likely to experience a reduction in mortality from PTCA or CABG surgery (24). The Beta-Blocker Heart Attack Trial showed that a daily dose of 180 to 240 mg of propranolol, initiated 5 or more days after MI, decreased annual mortality by more than 25% as compared with a placebo (26). Major clinical trials of aspirin in post-MI patients have also yielded encouraging results (27). Risk factor interventions aimed at smoking cessation and lipid and lipoprotein modification have demonstrated significant reductions in cardiovascular-related morbidity and mortality (28). Indeed, partial regression of coronary arteriosclerosis has been reported with lipid-lowering drugs and intensive lifestyle changes (29,30). Moreover, pooled data from randomized trials of secondary

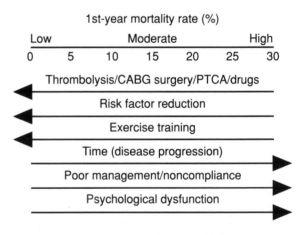

Figure 15.1 Risk stratification continuum (based on myocardial ischemia and left ventricular dysfunction), indicating variables that may potentially influence the patient's risk status. (PTCA = percutaneous transluminal coronary angioplasty)

prevention have shown increased survival with participants in exercise-based cardiac rehabilitation programs (31,32). In contrast, time (disease progression), poor patient management or compliance, and psychological dysfunction (33), manifested as hostility or social isolationism, can lead to increased risk and a poorer prognosis. Although many health insurers inappropriately consider "low-risk" patients ineligible for exercise-based cardiac rehabilitation, education, and counseling services, it is important to maintain their position at the far left of the continuum, obviating the need for even costlier interventions. The cardiac rehabilitation staffs, acting in conjunction with the referring physicians' individual treatment plans, have a unique opportunity to coordinate many of the interventions and lifestyle habits, favorably modifying the patients' risk status.

Exercise Testing: When and How Often?

Although risk stratification has aided in identifying patients who are at moderate to high risk for a future coronary event, the accuracy in predicting patient prognosis remains imperfect. Unfortunately, exercise-based cardiac rehabilitation, regardless of its comprehensive nature, does not necessarily prevent the worsening of CAD (34). Sequelae may include new symptoms, deterioration in ST-segment and T-wave responses, and electrical instability. Since ventricular tachycardia and other worrisome forms of exertion-related ventricular ectopy may be the harbingers of ventricular fibrillation and sudden cardiac death, graded exercise tests (GXTs) should be conducted at regular intervals, and additional diagnostic studies and therapeutic strategies should be considered for patients who demonstrate significant abnormalities.

After an Uncomplicated Myocardial Infarction

Exercise testing of the convalescing patient soon after an uncomplicated MI is used not only to assess functional status, but also as a diagnostic, prognostic, and therapeutic guide (13). The test also serves to promote patient self-confidence, providing reassurance that various physical activities, including lifting or carrying, stair climbing, and physical exertion in general, can be undertaken safely.

Whether the predischarge GXT should be limited by volitional fatigue or signs and symptoms, or stopped when an arbitrary "submaximal" end point is achieved, remains controversial (13). A recent survey showed that the majority of physicians still preferred "low-level" GXTs soon after acute MI (35). For this reason, these tests are generally terminated once a predetermined HR response (usually 70% to 75% of the age-predicted maximal HR [HR max], an HR of 120 to 140 beats/min, or a peak rate of 30 beats/min above rest), workload (usually up to 5 METs [metabolic equivalents]), or RPE (usually "somewhat hard" to "hard") is attained. However, a test may, in the absence of signs or symptoms, safely continue until peak or symptom-limited workloads are reached (36).

After a low-level GXT has been satisfactorily completed, the patient may be given home exercise guidelines and scheduled for a symptom-limited GXT (SL-GXT) within 6 weeks. The results of this later GXT can facilitate individualized prescriptions for exercise-based cardiac rehabilitation (Phase II or III) and identify residual myocardial ischemia and life-threatening forms of ventricular ectopy. Another GXT may be scheduled after an additional 3 to 6 months of physical conditioning to update the exercise prescription and assess improvement in functional capacity. Evidence of a training effect may be verified by a reduction in the HR, double product, or RPE at a given submaximal work load. Thereafter, a GXT once yearly is adequate, although more frequent tests may be necessary if the patient demonstrates signs or symptoms that are suggestive of a deterioration in clinical status (37).

After Coronary Artery Bypass Graft Surgery

Exercise testing should also be performed at regular intervals for patients who have undergone CABG surgery, regardless of the location or type of rehabilitation program. Treadmill or cycle ergometer testing has proved to be valuable in assessing functional capacity and in prescribing levels of physical activity in the posthospital phase after revascularization surgery (usually 3 to 5 weeks). Arm ergometer testing at this time may be uncomfortable because of midsternal incisional pain but is usually well tolerated at 6 to 8 weeks postoperatively (13). Follow-up testing procedures are similar to those recommended after acute MI— that is, following an additional 3 to 6 months of exercise training and yearly thereafter.

After Percutaneous Transluminal Coronary Angioplasty

The frequency of GXTs soon after PTCA may be more intense than that typically recommended after MI or CABG surgery. Although PTCA has a high initial-success rate, restenosis occurs in 25% to 40% of dilated lesions, usually within 6 months. Preliminary signs or symptoms of restenosis, manifested by significant ST-segment depression, the provocation of angina pectoris, or both, may be apparent with GXT as early as 2 to 3 days after PTCA (38). A better time period for initial evaluation of PTCA patients is 2 to 5 weeks, followed by another test to volitional fatigue at 6 months, assuming that no symptoms become apparent before this time (39,40). Thereafter, it appears reasonable to reevaluate these patients on an annual basis.

Drug Therapy: Special Considerations for Exercise Testing and Prescription

Cardiac rehabilitation program guidelines should address the need for GXTs to accommodate changes in medication and dosage adjustments. In some instances, repeat exercise testing may be clinically warranted to assess the efficacy of new-drug therapy, for example, antiarrhythmic agents. However, in other situations, exercise testing may not be necessary to revise the prescribed training intensity. Pharmacological treatment in cardiac exercisers may include the following: diuretics, beta-blockers, vasodilators, angiotensin-converting enzyme (ACE) inhibitors, calcium antagonists (slow channel-blocking agents), digitalis, antiarrhythmic agents, central nervous system–active drugs, and alpha-receptor blockers. Special considerations for exercise testing and prescription are reviewed elsewhere (6,41) and found in chapter 25.

Safety of Outpatient Cardiac Exercise Therapy

The safety and incidence of cardiac events associated with cardiac exercise therapy programs is extensively reviewed in chapter 28 and summarized briefly below, with specific reference to hospital and home-based outpatient programs.

Identifying High-Risk Patients

Although life-threatening events and deaths are rare, the identification of high-risk patients and the use of prudent guidelines for reducing the incidence of cardiovascular complications are important. It is difficult to identify cardiac patients who may be predisposed to cardiovascular complications during exercise training. Certain characteristics, however, have emerged. Patients with previous MI who have LVD, marked exercise induced ST-segment depression with or without angina pectoris, serious ventricular arrhythmias, or a low MET capacity appear to be at increased risk for exercise-related cardiovascular complications. Cardiac arrest victims are also more likely to disregard appropriate warm-up and cool-down procedures or exceed the prescribed training HR range, such as exercise intensity violators. From this type of information, a profile of the "high-risk" patient has emerged (Table 15.1) (42).

Reducing the Incidence of Cardiovascular Complications

Recommendations for reducing the incidence of cardiovascular complications during exercise-based cardiac rehabilitation include the following (42).

Ensure Medical Clearance and Follow-Up, Including Serial Graded Exercise Testing

Exercise testing should be performed before the physical conditioning program begins and at regular intervals during training to assess the patient's response or lack of response to exercise. Periodic GXTs also help identify cardiac patients who are at increased risk for exercise-related cardiovascular complications and allows the exercise prescription to be appropriately modified. Coronary arteriography should be considered for all patients with evidence of exercise-induced myocardial ischemia to exclude severe coronary stenosis that may place an individual at increased risk. Although once-a-year testing is generally considered adequate, more frequent tests may be necessary if the patient's clinical status changes or medication adjustments are made (6,37).

Provide On-Site Medical Supervision

Although low-risk cardiac patients can safely and effectively participate in home exercise programs, with or without transtelephonic ECG monitoring,

Table 15.1 Patient Characteristics Associated With High Risk for Exercise-Related Cardiovascular Complications

Clinical status	Exercise test data
Multiple myocardial infarctions	Low exercise tolerance (≤ 4 METs)
Impaired left ventricular function (ejection fraction < 25%)	Chronotropic impairment off drugs (< 120 beats/min)
Rest or unstable angina pectoris	Inotropic impairment (decrease in systolic blood pressure with increasing workloads)
Serious dysrhythmias at rest	Myocardial ischemia (angina and/or ST-depression ≥ 0.2 mV)
High-grade left anterior descending coronary artery lesions and/or significant (≥ 75% occlusion) multivessel atherosclerosis on angiography	Malignant cardiac dysrhythmias (especially in patients with impaired left ventricular function)
Low serum potassium	
Previous sudden cardiac death	

Personal characteristics during exercise	Other
Disregard for appropriate warm-up and cool-down	Cigarette smoker
Consistently exceeds prescribed training heart rate	Male gender

Note. MET = metabolic equivalent.

moderate- to high-risk patients should receive on-site medical supervision. The utilization of personnel to monitor and supervise exercise training of high-, intermediate-, and low-risk patients is summarized in Table 15.2 (5). It is recommended that the immediate posthospital exercise intervention (Phase II) and maintenance (Phase III or IV) programs have minimum staff-to-patient ratios of 1:5 and 1:15, respectively.

Van Camp and Peterson (43) reported 29 cardiovascular complications (21 cardiac arrests and 8 MIs), including 3 fatal events, during 2,351,916 hours of outpatient cardiac exercise training. Accordingly, the incidence of complications was one cardiac arrest per 111,996 patient-hours, one MI per 293,990 patient-hours, and one fatality per 783,972 patient-hours of exercise. It should be emphasized, however, that this seemingly low mortality rate applies only to medically supervised programs equipped with a defibrillator and appropriate emergency drugs. Recent reports indicate that up to 90% of all cardiac arrests that occur under such conditions are successfully resuscitated without ensuing MI.

Establish an Emergency Plan

The rehabilitation staff should be prepared to handle cardiovascular emergencies, including the performance of cardiopulmonary resuscitation (CPR) and patient stabilization for transport to a hospital or medical center. To this end, "mock" codes and CPR practice sessions should be conducted regularly and documented, along with reviews of crash cart equipment, medications, and supplies. The defibrillator should be charged and checked daily, and outdated drugs should be replaced. A plan of action should be established whereby specific responsibilities are assigned to each staff member.

Use Instantaneous ECG Monitoring

Although the use of costly continuous ECG monitoring as a routine procedure in cardiac exercise programs has been questioned, particularly in low-risk patients, instantaneous ECG (which records ECG rate, rhythm, and repolarization through defibrillator paddles; Figure 15.2) can be used to provide valuable surveillance data to program staff and referring physicians. We have employed this spot-monitoring technique in our cardiac rehabilitation program for several years and have found it to be an effective way to screen for ST-segment depression, serious ventricular arrhythmias, and exercise intensity violators (44). Participants in our program are encouraged to practice frequent self-monitoring of their pulse and to obtain instantaneous ECGs when symptoms occur, when cardiac

Table 15.2 Utilization of Program Personnel in the Supervision of Cardiac Exercise Therapy

Staff member	Patient risk for exercise-related cardiovascular complications		
	High (hospitalized)	High/Intermediate (ambulatory)	Low (maintenance)
Supervising physician	IA	IA or IS	IS
Program director or coordinator	IA	IA	IS
Registered nurse	IA	IR	NA
Exercise specialist or leader	IA	IA	IA

Note. IA = immediately available in the facility if requested by personnel authorized to visually supervise the exercising patient; IR = in room, that is, should be in the exercise room; IS = indirect supervision, that is, individual provides substantial influence for policy and procedure development affecting exercise services delivered to patients; also, substantially involved in planning, review of progress, and discharge assessments for each patient's exercise intervention; NA = not applicable. Material adapted from *AACVPR: Guidelines for Cardiac Rehabilitation Programs.* Champaign, IL: Human Kinetics. 1991. Reproduced with permission.

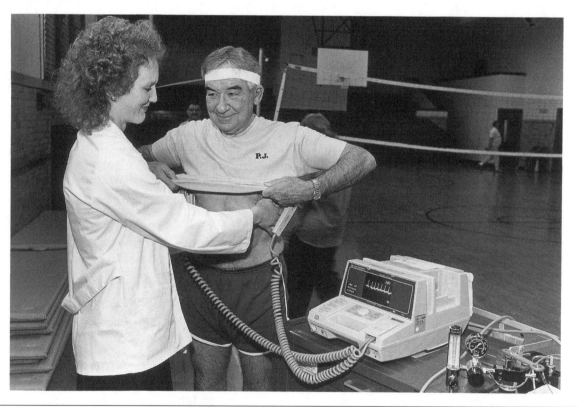

Figure 15.2 Obtaining instantaneous electrocardiographic rhythm strips with defibrillator paddle electrodes during outpatient cardiac exercise programs.

rhythm is irregular, or when HR is accelerated or bradycardic. This monitoring procedure facilitates the recording and classification of dysrhythmias that would otherwise go undetected (Figure 15.3) and is particularly helpful in enhancing patient safety and management.

Mandate Appropriate Warm-Up and Cool-Down Procedures

Cardiovascular complications during exercise-based rehabilitation programs are more likely to occur during the warm-up and cool-down phases. A gradual warm-up, such as brisk walking or mild

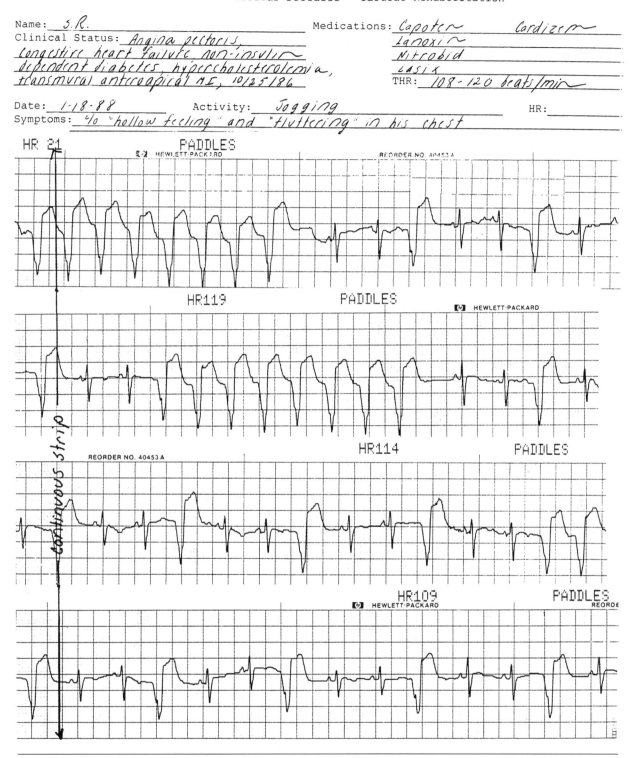

Figure 15.3 Ventricular arrhythmias documented by instantaneous electrocardiography in a symptomatic patient during a Phase III gymnasium exercise session.

resistance cycle ergometry, serves to decrease the occurrence of ECG and wall motion abnormalities, which are suggestive of myocardial ischemia, and ventricular arrhythmias, which may be provoked by sudden strenuous exertion (13). A cool-down enhances venous return during recovery, reducing the possibility of postexercise hypotension and related sequelae. Moreover, it ameliorates the potential, deleterious effects of the postexercise rise in plasma catecholamines (45).

Our experience suggests that the best warm-up for a given aerobic exercise is that activity performed at a lower intensity. Hence, participants who jog during the endurance phase should conclude the warm-up period with moderate to brisk walking. Similarly, for participants who use the stationary-cycle ergometer, "zero" load or mild tension cycling serves as an ideal warm-up or cool-down. Cardiorespiratory warm-up activities can also be modified to incorporate playground balls and individual, partner, or group activities or relays.

Promote Patient Education

Participants should be informed of major premonitory signs and symptoms, including arrhythmias, chest pain or pressure, and dizziness, which may signify a deterioration in clinical status or impending cardiovascular complications. Warnings should also include mention of abdominal discomfort, which many exercisers fail to recognize as possibly being of cardiac origin.

It is imperative that patients know their prescribed HR range for training, what work loads will achieve this range, how to take their pulse accurately, and the effect that medications and environmental factors have on the exercise intensity. There should be a method by which patients report, before each exercise therapy session, changes in signs, symptoms, HR responses, and medications.

Emphasize Strict Adherence to Prescribed Training Heart Rates

The safety of high-intensity exercise training regimens has been challenged in retrospective reports of cardiac patients who developed cardiovascular complications during or shortly after medically supervised rehabilitation. Hossack and Hartwig (46) identified patients at increased risk of untoward events as those having a markedly ischemic exercise ECG, an above-average aerobic capacity, and poor compliance to the prescribed training HR

(THR) range. These and other recent data (47) suggest that patients should be encouraged to exercise at the lower end of their THR range. Patient documentation of exercise HRs at each exercise session is recommended. Moreover, staff should regularly review training records to identify chronic intensity violators, that is, patients who consistently exceed their prescribed THR, and counsel them.

Employ a Mild to Moderate Exercise Intensity and Perceived Exertion Guidelines

The lower the intensity, the less likely it is that an exercise-related cardiovascular complication will occur. Considerable evidence suggests that the threshold (minimal) intensity for exercise training increases in direct proportion to the pretraining $\dot{V}O_2$max (48); for most cardiac patients, the threshold probably lies between 40% and 60% of $\dot{V}O_2$max, which is equivalent to 60% to 70% of HR max (6) (Figure 15.4). Improvement in aerobic capacity with low to moderate training intensities suggests that interrelationships among the training intensity, frequency, and duration may permit a decrease in the intensity to be partially or totally compensated for by increases in the exercise duration or frequency, or both (6).

We have employed Borg's category or category-ratio scales for RPE (see Tables 17.7 & 17.8, p. 258) as a useful and important adjunct to HR as an intensity guide (49). Ratings greater than 13 to 15 (on the 15-grade scale) or 4 to 6 (on the 10-grade scale) usually indicate an exercise intensity that is too high, regardless of the HR response.

Maintain Supervision During the Recovery Period

Since cardiovascular complications often occur after exercise, it is important that staff remain on-site until all exercisers have exited the shower and changing areas (a minimum time of 15 min is recommended). Accordingly, many cardiac rehabilitation programs have extended their emergency alarm systems into the locker room.

Modify Recreational Game Rules and Minimize Competition

Because of the relative consistency of energy expenditure in walking, jogging, and stationary-cycle ergometry, these activities lend themselves particularly well to the regulation of exercise intensity. In contrast, myocardial and aerobic demands during game activities are influenced, to a large extent, by team members and opponent expertise. Also,

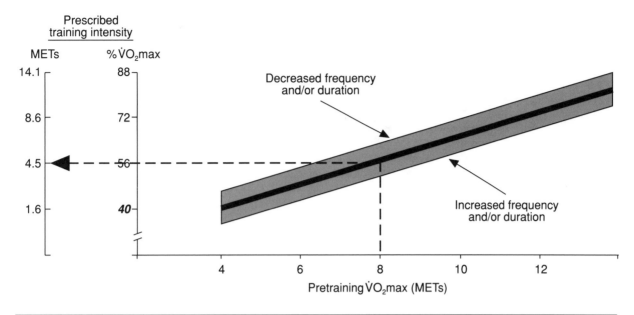

Figure 15.4   Theoretical relation between aerobic capacity in METs (metabolic equivalents) and the threshold (minimal) intensity for exercise training, expressed as a percentage of the maximal oxygen uptake ($\dot{V}O_2$max). The threshold intensity for training increases in direct proportion to the $\dot{V}O_2$max before training; however, it can be modulated by altering the exercise duration or frequency, or both. For example, a patient with a peak capacity of 8 METs would exercise at approximately 56% of his or her $\dot{V}O_2$max, or 4.5 ± 0.5 METs, to further increase his functional capacity.

From Franklin, B. et al. (48), with permission.

the excitement of competition may increase sympathetic activity and catecholamine excretion and lower the threshold to ventricular fibrillation. Exercise leaders should minimize competition and modify game rules to decrease the energy cost and HR response to play.

Adapt the Exercise to the Environment

Cardiac patients can exercise safely in cold weather if they take proper precautions. For patients who suffer from angina pectoris when inhaling cold air, discomfort can be reduced or alleviated if they wear a face mask to warm the inspired air. Additionally, patients should consider the wind-chill factor, change wet clothing, wear several layers of light clothing that they can shed or replace as necessary, stay moving to increase body heat production, and protect body areas that have a large surface area–to–mass ratio (e.g., the hands and feet). Because of a poor vasoconstriction response, an uncovered head may incur a tremendous loss of body heat.

Hyperthermic conditions may constitute an even greater hazard than cold weather for cardiac exercisers. Simultaneous increases in core temperature and metabolism can result in a disproportionate myocardial oxygen demand. Men not acclimated to heat who were exposed to temperatures greater than 24°C experienced added HR increases of 1 beat/min per °C while exercising (Figure 15.5) and 2 to 4 beats/min per °C with concomitant increased humidity (50). Moreover, excessive sweating may alter serum and cellular electrolytes (sodium and potassium), causing dysrhythmias. Patients who exercise in warm weather should maintain hydration by drinking fluids before, during, and after physical activity; decrease exercise intensity at ambient temperatures above 80°F (27°C), 75% relative humidity, or both; exercise during the cooler parts of the day (i.e., early morning or evening); wear minimal amounts of porous, light-colored, loose-fitting clothing to facilitate cooling by evaporation; and progress exercise gradually to allow for acclimatization. (Refer also to chapters 20 and 21.)

Emergency and Surveillance Procedures

Cardiac rehabilitation programs should establish procedures regarding the on-site treatment of complications and medical emergencies. Emergency equipment and first-aid supplies should be readily

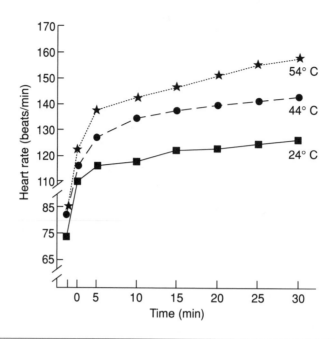

Figure 15.5   Influence of environmental temperature on heart rate responses at a constant exercise work load. Heart rate increases approximately 1 beat/min for each °C increment in ambient temperature above 24°C. Adapted from Pandolf, K.B. et al. (50).

available. Staff should be prepared to attend musculoskeletal injuries and the rare instance of a life-threatening cardiovascular complication. This includes performing CPR and stabilizing the patient for transport to a nearby hospital or emergency center. To this end, staff who have direct or supervisorial contact with patients should participate in regular reviews of emergency cart equipment, medications, and supplies; the reviews should be documented. Emergency drills should be conducted at least every 2 months, and a "plan of action" should be established, by either the medical director of the program or the medical advisory committee, in a policy and procedure manual that follows guidelines of the American Heart Association (AHA) and the Joint Commission on Accreditation of Healthcare Organizations (JCAHO). The manual should include algorithms for code situation responses and instructions in the use of emergency equipment. Specific responsibilities of individual staff members, such as performing CPR, calling emergency medical services, moving participants from the immediate area, and waiting for and directing the emergency medical service to the area, should also be delineated.

Ideally, the exercise-testing and training facilities should be complemented by an alarm system to alert all personnel of an emergency situation. This system should have numerous activation sites distributed in all relevant areas, with information transmitted to a central circuit board that identifies the specific site where the injury or complication has occurred. This would allow for patients or staff to set off the alarm, activating the emergency plan by immediately summoning staff to the area of the untoward event. Locations of special concern include locker and shower rooms, because there is often little supervision in these areas. Finally, telephone numbers for emergency assistance should be clearly posted on all telephones.

Staff Training and Certification

Personnel who relate to patient care should be proficient in Basic Life Support (BLS) as designated by the training and certification programs for emergency cardiac care that are provided by the AHA. It is also recommended that all staff (non-physicians) who are medically responsible for patients during dynamic activities (i.e., personnel who have been assigned by the medical director as having a significant role in the emergency plan) be certified in Advanced Cardiac Life Support (ACLS) (5). Moreover, it is recommended that at least one supervisory staff member who is both certified and licensed to provide ACLS be present during all exercise-training sessions involving intermediate- and high-risk patients. These certifications suggest adequate knowledge and skill to address the needs of the patient in an emergency situation. Timely renewal of BLS and ACLS certifications should be mandatory.

Early Warning Signs and Symptoms of Increasing Risk

Changing patterns of signs or symptoms can alert the rehabilitation staff to early warning signals that may precede exercise-related cardiovascular complications or other medical emergencies. It is difficult to predict which patients may experience cardiac arrest or acute MI during exercise. Neither superior fitness, regular exercise participation, nor the absence of cardiac risk factors guarantees protection against an exercise death. Nevertheless, cardiovascular complications during exercise are often preceded by increased intensity, frequency, or duration of angina in patients with this symptom; anginal drug therapy that is less effective than usual; and new or changing patterns of arrhythmias, especially if the episodes of arrhythmia are associated with light-headedness or syncope (5). Indications of LVD or CHF may be signified by higher RPEs during standard submaximal work loads, worsening symptoms of shortness of breath at rest or during exercise, swelling of the ankles with associated weight gain, and increased fatigue. If patients are appropriately educated to assist in identifying such warning signs and symptoms, their self-monitoring can greatly enhance staff efforts at ongoing surveillance. Such findings should be documented in the participant's chart, reviewed with the participant, and promptly reported to the referring physician.

Interventions

A clinical assessment should be obtained in response to the early warning signs and symptoms just noted. This may include an evaluation of the heart and lungs by auscultation, measures of HR and BP, telemetry ECG monitoring for ST-segment displacement or arrhythmias, and a 12-lead ECG for evidence of new or changing patterns (e.g., MI, ischemia, or heart block) compared to a prior ECG. Interventions may include a phone call to the referring physician to report the findings and receive directives, use of nitroglycerin and oxygen, establishment of an intravenous line as a safety precaution, and rapid transport to the closest emergency room.

Compliance Issues in Cardiac Rehabilitation

In medical practice, *compliance* is defined as "the extent to which a patient's behavior in terms of taking medications, following diets, or executing other lifestyle changes coincides with the clinical prescription" (51). Four factors must be considered for successful patient treatment: (1) recognition of ill health, (2) correct diagnosis of illness, (3) provision of proper treatment, and (4) patient compliance with the therapeutic plan (52). Thus, even the best treatment programs by well-intentioned staff can be nullified by poor patient compliance.

The motivation of an individual to adhere to a prescribed therapeutic regimen is of critical importance when evaluating patient compliance. It is the responsibility of the rehabilitation staff, including the physician, physiologist, nurse, and dietitian, to educate and motivate their patients. Patients who perceive themselves as having close contact with their physician and rehabilitation staff seem to derive more from the program and achieve better compliance. Motivation to comply with a prescribed therapy appears to be highest soon after an acute cardiac event (53,54). With time, however, compliance often decreases. Patients are also influenced by their perceived susceptibility to recurrent cardiac events. If they do not feel that they are vulnerable, they are more likely to be poor compliers.

Long-term compliance to the exercise component of the rehabilitation program appears to be predicated on two major objectives: (1) educating patients as to why and how they should be physically active and (2) motivating them to adhere to a physical conditioning regimen. Unfortunately, exercise testing and exercise prescription are sometimes emphasized more than the education and motivation components of the program. Consequently, negative variables often outweigh the positive ones that contribute to sustained participant interest and enthusiasm (Figure 15.6) (55). Such imbalance leads to a decline in program adherence and effectiveness. To counteract this problem, cardiac rehabilitation staff should incorporate a strong educational component as well as selected motivational strategies.

Educational Component

Several program offerings serve to promote the educational component. Films, booklets, lectures,

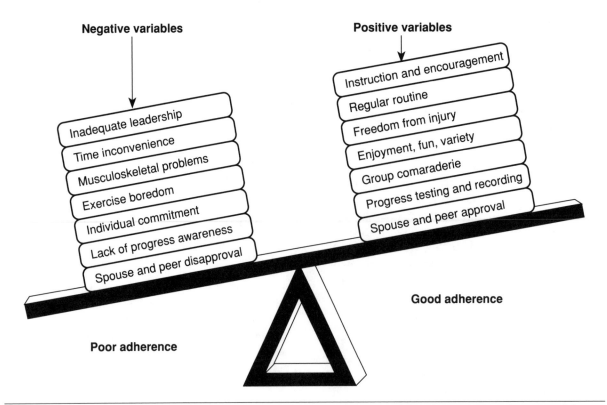

Figure 15.6 Variables that affect compliance to exercise training programs. Negative variables often outweigh positive ones, resulting in poor adherence.

workshops, and group discussions help participants understand the benefits of risk factor modification and regular physical activity. Bulletin boards and educational murals facilitate the dissemination of current literature and human interest stories related to exercise and physical fitness. A program newsletter can provide information on physical activity, heart disease, weight control, stress, and nutrition. Also, periodic group meetings for participants and spouses allow for the discussion of such topics as exercise prescription, medications, diet, and weight control.

Motivational Strategies

Motivation is a major factor in exercise program effectiveness, safety, and long-term compliance. Research and empiric experience suggest that selected exercise program modifications and motivational strategies may enhance participant interest and enthusiasm, as well as long-term compliance (55). Examples of such strategies are listed here:

- Minimize musculoskeletal injuries with a moderate exercise prescription.
- Encourage group participation.

- Emphasize variety and enjoyment in the exercise program.
- Incorporate a personalized, positive approach to participants and realistic goal setting.
- Employ periodic fitness testing, including lipid and lipoprotein profiling and body composition assessment, to evaluate patient progress.
- Recruit spouse support in promoting the exercise program.
- Encourage participant documentation of daily exercise achievements through progress charts or logs.
- Provide music during exercise sessions.
- Recognize individual accomplishments through extrinsic rewards (e.g., T-shirts, trophies, and certificates).
- Provide well-trained, highly motivated, and enthusiastic exercise leaders.

Quality Assessment and Improvement

Quality assessment and improvement, also termed "quality assurance," describes the hospital's efforts to assess and improve the quality of patient care. The process involves a coordinated effort to bring together the various activities in a cardiac program that are designed to detect, control, and hopefully prevent the occurrence of errors. Each hospital-based cardiac rehabilitation program is subject to an audit by the JCAHO. The auditors review documented policies and procedures for the department based on the hospital's mission and goals. These policies and procedures should incorporate the standards of care from national organizations, such as the ACSM (6), the American Association of Cardiovascular and Pulmonary Rehabilitation (AACVPR) (5), and the AHA (37), as well as state guidelines and recommendations for quality assessment and control. The achievement of safe and appropriate patient care should be a program's primary objective. Program policies should be designed under the advisement of medical, legal, and insurance consultants and be systematically reviewed and updated.

The current *Accreditation Manual for Hospitals* details the various standards that the JCAHO uses during its audits (56). The chapters entitled "Quality Assessment and Improvement" and "Hospital-Sponsored Ambulatory Care Services" should be of special interest to health care professionals in cardiac rehabilitation. The JCAHO evaluates how effectively the policies and procedures are coordinated and integrated and how the process can be improved. This emphasis should alleviate the negative image associated with quality assessment, thus allowing staff to pursue self-appraisal and continued professional growth and ultimately facilitating the best possible patient care.

Program Evaluation

Program evaluation is an ongoing process that uses objective and subjective information. All cardiac rehabilitation programs should be evaluated in terms of their contribution to revenues, allocation of resources, cost, productivity, growth, public image, and continued strategic fit within the organization. Services offered to the patient, family, and community should also be reviewed.

It is important to define measurable physiological, psychological, and vocational objectives to evaluate favorable outcomes from the services offered. Suggested efficacy measures for evaluation of exercise programming, lipid and lipoprotein modification, hypertension control, weight reduction, stress management, time to return to work, and psychosocial functioning are published elsewhere (5). The JCAHO provides guidelines for

evaluation of services relative to their effectiveness and appropriateness through collection of data, assessment of information, actions taken to correct problems, evaluation of outcomes, conclusions, and reappraisal of programs and their components. The results of these evaluations should be periodically reviewed and used to improve patient outcomes.

Reimbursement Considerations

Contemporary cardiac rehabilitation services have been increasingly assessed for both appropriateness and effectiveness. When submitting for insurance reimbursement, one must consider diagnosis codes, recognized procedures, the utilization review guidelines published by each insurer, and personnel licensure requirements. Maintaining regular communication with the director of provider relations from each insurer should provide an update on which services are covered, based on the patient's diagnosis.

Sources of outpatient reimbursement for medical services are found in both private industry (Blue Cross and Blue Shield, health maintenance organizations [HMOs], preferred provider organizations [PPOs], and private insurance companies) and the public sector (Medicare, Medicaid, and the Civilian Health and Medical Program for the Uniformed Services [CHAMPUS]). Currently, third-party payers are more likely to reimburse for telemetry ECG–monitored exercise sessions (Phase II) rather than for maintenance exercise classes. This practice may stem in part from an American Medical Association (AMA) survey that overwhelmingly (87% of an expert panel of respondents) endorsed telemetry ECG monitoring as "essential to the safety and efficacy of a prescribed regimen of exercise in coronary rehabilitation" (57). In contrast, Phase III and IV programs are generally offered as a patient pay service.

Over the past decade, cardiac rehabilitation services have been reviewed by several third-party payers and associations. In 1985, Blue Cross and Blue Shield acknowledged that cardiac rehabilitation was indicated for patients recovering from an MI or CABG surgery. However, the insurer suggested that, for the majority of individuals, *three visits* to a physicians office or cardiac rehabilitation program were usually adequate. Three years later, the Blue Cross and Blue Shield perspective changed considerably by triaging patients according to risk stratification: low-risk patients were deemed ineligible for formal cardiac rehabilitation services, intermediate patients were candidates for Phase II cardiac rehabilitation (three times weekly for 8 to 12 weeks), and high-risk patients could receive even more intensive surveillance. Similar recommendations, including for patients with stable angina pectoris, were offered by expert panels of the AMA (57) and the American College of Cardiology (ACC) (23). The Medicare Research Group, however, deferred a specific recommendation on the need for ECG monitoring, citing insufficient data to resolve the issue (58).

Recently, CHAMPUS, a major insurance carrier in the South, reversed a long-standing policy of denying reimbursement for cardiac rehabilitation services, making their coverage retroactive to October 1987. In arriving at this decision, the carrier's Office of Program Development surveyed contemporary scientific literature. The position statements of national associations, including the October 1987 Diagnostic and Therapeutic Technology Assessment (DATTA) report of the AMA (57) and the August 1988 report of the Office of Health Technology and Assessment (OHTA) (58), were also reviewed. It was found that cardiac rehabilitation services are an integral part of the treatment of patients with CAD, including those with previous MI, CABG surgery, or chronic stable angina pectoris. Further, in October 1988 the American College of Physicians (ACP) published a report (59) that endorsed cardiac rehabilitation as appropriate for such patients, as well as those with residual LVD. More recently, a position paper prepared by the Ad Hoc Task Force on Cardiac Rehabilitation of the ACC highlighted the value of cardiac rehabilitation services following PTCA and valvular surgery (60). CHAMPUS concluded that these reports reflect the consensus of national medical organizations that cardiac rehabilitation has become the standard of care within the medical community by which individuals are restored to their optimal physical, medical, and psychosocial status after a cardiac event.

Resistance to covering cardiac rehabilitation services may stem, at least in part, from the perception that few data are available regarding the benefit of these programs. There is also a lack of agreement on reimbursing providers that do not carry state certification or licensure. Cardiac rehabilitation providers must interact with a wider constituency than they have to date—including consumers, physicians, allied health professionals, associations, and health care insurers—to share new information describing the efficacy of exercise-based cardiac rehabilitation (31,32) and its cost-effectiveness (61,62).

In October 1992 the federal government's Agency for Health Care Policy and Research (AHCPR) announced that a $1,137,000 contract had been awarded to the AACVPR to develop clinical practice guidelines for identifying patients who would benefit from cardiac rehabilitation and determine which rehabilitation services provide the most benefit. AACVPR is responsible to coordinate the activities of a multidisciplinary panel of experts, appointed by the AHCPR administrator, who will develop medical review criteria, standards of quality, and performance measures based on a careful search of the scientific literature. These guidelines, which are scheduled for publication in 1994, should enable physicians, other health care practitioners, and patients to make more informed clinical decisions on the appropriateness of cardiac rehabilitation services.

Third-party reimbursement generally provides the major source of income for a hospital. Because cardiac rehabilitation is not a large revenue producer, and insurance coverage is limited, it is important to explore and procure alternative sources of revenue to maintain the financial viability of any program. These may include the sponsorship of cardiovascular health-and-fitness programs for business and industry, police and fire fighter screenings, evaluation and therapy programs for special-patient populations (e.g., diabetics and persons with multiple sclerosis), conferences, and funded research. The ultimate goal is to utilize staff, facilities, and equipment to their fullest potential.

Prospects for the Future

In a provocative editorial, DeBusk (63) recently suggested that the current gymnasium-based cardiac rehabilitation program model suffers from the following shortcomings: (a) difficulty in distinguishing its effects from those of a physician's care, (b) lack of support from physicians, (c) inconvenience of the group format, and (d) relatively low participation rates (< 15% of all eligible patients). He proposed unsupervised (home) exercise training as a viable alternative to promote weight management, enhance psychological status, and improve physical endurance in low-, moderate-, and high-risk patients. However, home exercise training programs also have limitations, including the lack of opportunity to teach and encourage exercise principles and coronary risk reduction and the absence of medical surveillance, emergency cardiac care, and peer support (3). In some cases supervised programs may be best, especially for moderate- to high-risk patients. On the other hand, exercise training can be carried out safely and effectively at home for patients without significant LVD or exercise-induced myocardial ischemia. Contemporary models must be developed to ensure that all patients with CAD can participate in comprehensive programs of secondary prevention (28). The challenge for clinicians developing these models is to incorporate techniques to facilitate optimal compliance and overcome many of the current limitations of supervised and unsupervised programs, while maximizing their benefits.

Although it has been suggested that current thrombolytic and revascularization procedures would likely diminish the impact of adjunctive cardiac exercise programs on survival and that the importance of physical conditioning as a prerequisite for returning to work has decreased (63), exercise training remains a pivotal component of rehabilitative care for patients with MI and following myocardial revascularization procedures. Low- to moderate-intensity exercise training, especially when combined with education and behavior modification, can produce beneficial changes in functional capacity, cardiac function, coronary risk factors, psychosocial well-being and possibly improve survival in patients with CAD (2,48). Incorporating more aggressive efforts at smoking cessation and diet and drug management for hypercholesterolemia should further enhance the efficacy and attractiveness of cardiac rehabilitation programs for physicians, patients, and third-party payers (63).

Summary

Hospital- and home-based cardiac rehabilitation outpatient programs include interventions designed to prevent or retard the progression of the disease process and to restore and maintain optimal physical, psychological, emotional, social, and vocational functioning. Although physical conditioning may enhance these objectives, exercise alone should not be expected to alter global functioning or risk status. A comprehensive approach, including physical activity, patient and family education, and psychosocial, nutritional, and vocational counseling is important. Attention to program models, staffing, facilities and equipment, exercise testing and training, emergency and surveillance procedures, compliance-promoting strategies, and quality assurance measures should serve to optimize the safety, efficacy, and cost-effectiveness of secondary prevention programs.

References

1. Franklin, B.A. Cardiac rehabilitation: It's more than exercise. Phys. Sportsmed. 14:177-180; 1986.
2. Franklin, B.A. Introduction: Physiologic adaptations to exercise training in cardiac patients: Contemporary issues and concerns. Med. Sci. Sports Exerc. 23:645-647; 1991.
3. Wenger, N.K. Supervised versus unsupervised exercise training following myocardial infarction and myocardial revascularization procedures. Annals Academy of Medicine. 21:141-144; 1992.
4. DeBusk, R.F.; Haskell, W.L.; Miller, N.H.; Berra, K.; Taylor, C.B.; Berger, W.E.; Lew, H. Medically directed at-home rehabilitation soon after clinically uncomplicated acute myocardial infarction. A new model for patient care. Am. J. Cardiol. 55:251-257; 1985.
5. American Association of Cardiovascular and Pulmonary Rehabilitation. Guidelines for cardiac rehabilitation programs. Franklin, B.A.; Hall, L. eds. Champaign, IL: Human Kinetics; 1991.
6. American College of Sports Medicine. Guidelines for exercise testing and prescription. 4th ed. Philadelphia: Lea & Febiger; 1991.
7. Vickery, S.R.; Cureton, K.J.; Langstaff, J.L. Heart rate and energy expenditure during aqua dynamics. Phys. Sportsmed. 11:67-72; 1983.
8. Evans, B.; Cureton, K.; Purvis, J. Metabolic and circulatory responses to walking and jogging in water. Research Quarterly for Ex. and Sport. 49:442-449; 1978.
9. Lindle, J. Water exercise research. The AKWA Letter. 3:11, 13; 1989.
10. Windhorst, M.; Chossek, V. Aquatic exercise association manual. Port Washington, WI: Aquatic Exercise Association; 1988.
11. AEA Heart Rate Study. The AKWA Letter. 2:9; 1987.
12. Magder, S.; Linnarsson, D.; Gullstrand, L. The effect of swimming on patients with ischemic heart disease. Circulation. 63:979-986; 1981.
13. Franklin, B.A.; Hellerstein, H.K.; Gordon, S.; Timmis, G.C. Cardiac patients. In: Franklin, B.A.; Gordon, S.; Timmis, G.C., eds. Exercise in modern medicine. Baltimore: Williams & Wilkins; 1989: 44-80.
14. Myers, J.; Froelicher, V.F. Predicting outcome in cardiac rehabilitation. J. Am. Coll. Cardiol. 15:983-985; 1990.

15. Hess, O.M.; Schneider, J.; Nonogi, H.; Carroll, J.D.; Schneider, K.; Turina, M.; Krayenbuehl, H.P. Myocardial structure in patients with exercise-induced ischemia. Circulation. 77:967-977; 1988.

16. Jugdutt, B.I.; Michorowski, B.L.; Kappagoda, C.T. Exercise training after anterior Q wave myocardial infarction: Importance of regional left ventricular function and topography. J. Am. Coll. Cardiol. 12:362-372; 1988.

17. Iskandrian, A.S. Exercise training after anterior Q wave myocardial infarction: Harmful or beneficial. J. Am. Coll. Cardiol. 12:373-374; 1988.

18. Mark, D.B.; Hlatky, M.A.; Califf, R.M.; Morris, J.J., Jr.; Sisson, S.D.; McCants, C.B.; Lee, K.L.; Harrell, F.E., Jr.; Pryor, D.B. Painless exercise ST deviation on the treadmill: Long-term prognosis. J. Am. Coll. Cardiol. 14:885-892; 1989.

19. Schuler, G.; Shlierf, G.; Wirth, A.; Mautner, H.P.; Scheurlen, H.; Thumm, M.; Roth, H.; Schwartz, F.; Kohlmeier, M.; Mehmel, H.C. Low fat diet and regular, supervised physical exercise in patients with symptomatic coronary artery disease: Reduction of stress-induced myocardial ischemia. Circulation. 77:172-181; 1988.

20. Sullivan, M.J.; Higginbotham, M.B.; Cobb, F.R. Exercise training in patients with severe left ventricular dysfunction: Hemodynamic and metabolic effects. Circulation. 78:506-515; 1988.

21. Froelicher, V.F.; Jensen, D.; Genter, F.; Sullivan, M.; McKirnan, M.D.; Witztum, K.; Scharf, J.; Strong, M.L.; Ashburn, W. A randomized trial of exercise training in patients with coronary heart disease. JAMA. 252:1291-1297; 1984.

22. Giannuzzi, P.; Temporelli, P.L.; Tavazzi, L.; Corrá, U.; Gattone, M.; Imparato, A.; Giordano, A.; Schweiger, C.; Sala, L.; Malinverni, C. EAMI-exercise training in anterior myocardial infarction: An ongoing multicenter randomized study; preliminary results of left ventricular function and remodeling. Chest. 101:315S-321S; 1992.

23. American College of Cardiology. Position report on cardiac rehabilitation: Recommendations of the American College of Cardiology. J. Am. Coll. Cardiol. 7:451-453; 1986.

24. DeBusk, R.F.; Blomqvist, C.G.; Kouchoukos, N.T.; Leupker, R.V.; Miller, H.S.; Moss, A.J.; Pollock, M.L.; Reeves, T.J.; Selvester, R.H.; Stason, W.B. Identification and treatment of low-risk patients after acute myocardial infarction and coronary-artery bypass graft surgery. N. Engl. J. Med. 314:161-166; 1986.

25. European Cooperative Study Group for Streptokinase Treatment in Acute Myocardial Infarction. Streptokinase in acute myocardial infarction. N. Engl. J. Med. 301:797-802; 1979.

26. β-Blocker Heart Attack Study Group. The β-blocker heart attack trial. JAMA. 246:2073-2074; 1981.

27. Lewis, H.D., Jr.; Davis, J.W.; Archibald, D.G.; Steinke, W.E.; Smitherman, T.C.; Doherty, J.E., III; Schnaper, H.W.; LeWinter, M.M.; Linares, E.; Pouget, J.M.; Sabharwal, S.C.; Chesler, E.; De Mots, H. Protective effects of aspirin against acute myocardial infarction and death in men with unstable angina. Results of a veterans administration cooperative study. N. Engl. J. Med. 309:396-403; 1983.

28. Gattiker, H.; Goins, P.; Dennis, C. Cardiac rehabilitation: Current status and future directions. West. J. Med. 156:183-188; 1992.

29. Brown, G.; Albers, J.J.; Fisher, L.D.; Schaefer, S.M.; Lin, J.T.; Kaplan, C.; Zhao, X.Q.; Bisson, B.D.; Fitzpatrick, V.F.; Dodge, H.T. Regression of coronary artery disease as a result of intensive lipid-lowering therapy in men with high levels of apolipoprotein B. N. Engl. J. Med. 323:1289-1298; 1990.

30. Ornish, D.; Brown, S.E.; Scherwitz, L.W.; Billings, J.H.; Armstrong, W.T.; Ports, T.A.; McLanahan, S.M.; Kirkeeide, R.L.; Brand, R.J.; Gould, K.L. Can lifestyle changes reverse coronary heart disease? Lancet. 336: 129-133; 1990.

31. Oldridge, N.B.; Guyatt, G.H.; Fischer, M.E.; Rimm, A.A. Cardiac rehabilitation after myocardial infarction–combined experience of randomized clinical trials. JAMA. 260:945-950; 1988.

32. O'Connor, G.T.; Buring, J.E.; Yusuf, S.; Goldhaber, S.Z.; Olmstead, E.M.; Paffenbarger, R.S.J.; Hennekens, C.H. An overview of randomized trials of rehabilitation with exercise after myocardial infarction. Circulation. 80:234-244; 1989.

33. van Dixhoorn, J.; Duivenvoorden, H.J.; Pool, J. Success and failure of exercise training after myocardial infarction: Is the outcome predictable? J. Am. Coll. Cardiol. 15:974-982; 1990.

34. Gamble, P.; Froelicher, V.F. Can an exercise program worsen heart disease? Phys. Sportsmed. 10:69-77; 1982.

35. Hamm, L.F.; Stull, G.A.; Serfass, R.C.; Ainsworth, B. Prognostic endpoint yield of high-level versus low-level graded exercise testing. Arch. Phys. Med. Rehabil. 69:86-89; 1988.

36. Topol, E.J.; Burek, K.; O'Neill, W.W.; Kewman, D.G.; Kander, N.H.; Shea, M.J.; Schork, M.A.; Kirscht, J.; Juni, J.E.; Pitt, B. A randomized controlled trial of hospital discharge three days after myocardial infarction in the era of reperfusion. N. Engl. J. Med. 318:1083-1088; 1988.

37. Fletcher, G.F.; Froelicher, V.F.; Hartley, L.H.; Haskell, W.L.; Pollock, M.L. Exercise standards: A statement for health professionals from the American Heart Association. Circulation. 82:2286-2322; 1990.

38. el Tamini, H.; Davies, G.J.; Hackett, D.; Fragasso, G.; Crea, F.; Maseri, A.; O'Sullivan, C. Very early prediction of restenosis after successful coronary angioplasty: Anatomic and functional assessment. J. Am. Coll. Cardiol. 15:259-264; 1990.

39. Miller, D.D.; Liu, P.; Strauss, H.W.; Block, P.C.; Okada, R.D.; Boucher, C.A. Prognostic value of computer-quantitated exercise thallium imaging early after percutaneous transluminal coronary angioplasty. J. Am. Coll. Cardiol. 10:275-283; 1987.

40. Wijns, W.; Serruys, P.W.; Reiber, J.H.; de Feyter, P.J.; van den Brand, M.; Simoons, M.L.; Hugenholtz, P.G.

Early detection of restenosis after successful percutaneous transluminal coronary angioplasty by exercise redistribution thallium scintigraphy. Am. J. Cardiol. 55:357-361; 1985.

41. Zohman, L.R. Exercise stress test interpretation for cardiac diagnosis and functional evaluation. Arch. Phys. Med. Rehabil. 58:235-240; 1977.

42. Franklin, B.A. Safety of outpatient cardiac exercise therapy: Reducing the incidence of complications. Phys. Sportsmed. 14:235-248; 1986.

43. Van Camp, S.P.; Peterson, R.A. Cardiovascular complications of outpatient cardiac rehabilitation programs. JAMA. 256:1160-1163; 1986.

44. Franklin, B.A.; Reed, P.S.; Gordon, S.; Timmis, G.C. Instantaneous electrocardiography: A simple screening technique for cardiac exercise programs. Chest. 96:174-177; 1989.

45. Dimsdale, J.E.; Hartley, H.; Guiney, T.; Ruskin, J.N.; Greenblat, D. Postexercise peril: Plasma catecholamines and exercise. JAMA. 251:630-632; 1984.

46. Hossack, K.F.; Hartwig, R. Cardiac arrest associated with supervised cardiac rehabilitation. J. Cardiac Rehab. 2:402-408; 1982.

47. Friedwald, V.E., Jr.; Spence, D.W. Sudden cardiac death associated with exercise: The risk-benefit issue. Am. J. Cardiol. 66:183-188; 1990.

48. Franklin, B.A.; Gordon, S.; Timmis, G.C. Amount of exercise necessary for the patient with coronary artery disease. Am. J. Cardiol. 69:1426-1432; 1992.

49. Borg, G. Psychophysical bases of perceived exertion. Med. Sci. Sports Exerc. 14:377-381; 1982.

50. Pandolf, K.B.; Cafarelli, E.; Noble, B.J.; Metz, K.F. Hyperthermia: Effect of exercise prescription. Arch. Phys. Med. Rehabil. 56:524-526; 1975.

51. Sackett, D.L. Introduction. In: Sackett, D.L.; Haynes, R.B., eds. Compliance with therapeutic regimens. Baltimore: Johns Hopkins University Press; 1976:1.

52. Dishman, R.K. Compliance/adherence in health related exercise. Health Psychol. 1:237-276; 1982.

53. McMahon, M.; Miller, P.; Wikoff, R.; Garrett, M.J.; Ringel, K. Life situations, health beliefs, and medical regimen adherence in patients with myocardial infarction. Heart Lung. 15:82-86; 1986.

54. Miller, P.; Wikoff, R.L.; McMahon, M.; Garrett, M.J.; Ringel, K. Indicators of medical regimen adherence for myocardial infarction patients. Nurs. Res. 34:272-286; 1985.

55. Franklin, B.A. Motivating and educating adults to exercise. J Phys Ed Rec. 49:13-17; 1978.

56. The Joint Commission on Accreditation of Healthcare Organizations. Accreditation manual for hospitals. 1992:31-37.

57. Diagnostic and therapeutic technology assessment (DATTA): Coronary rehabilitation services. JAMA. 258:1959-1962; 1987.

58. Cardiac Rehabilitation Services. Health technology assessment reports. Rockville, MD: U.S. Department of Health and Human Services, NCHSR; 1987.

59. Health and Public Policy Committee, American College of Physicians. Cardiac rehabilitation services. Ann. Intern. Med. 109:671-673; 1988.

60. Ad Hoc Task Force on Cardiac Rehabilitation, American College of Cardiology. Position paper on cardiac rehabilitation services following PTCA and valvular surgery: Guidelines for use, May 1990.

61. Levin, L.A.; Perk, J.; Medback, B. Cardiac rehabilitation—a cost analysis. J. Intern. Med. 230:427-434; 1991.

62. Ades, P.A.; Huang, D.; Weaver, S.O. Cardiac rehabilitation participation predicts lower rehospitalization costs. Am. Heart J. 123:916-921; 1992.

63. DeBusk, R.F. Why is cardiac rehabilitation not widely used? West. J. Med. 156:206-208; 1992.

Chapter 16

Community-Based Cardiac Rehabilitation Outpatient Programs

Henry S. Miller, Jr.
Gerald F. Fletcher

Rehabilitation of the cardiac patient should begin shortly after admission to the hospital and continue well beyond the immediate recovery period for maximum safe, functional capacity and lasting lifestyle changes that significantly reduce risk factors to be accomplished. This chapter will give basic guidelines for the development of community-based outpatient cardiac rehabilitation programs and variations that may enhance convenience for the patient.

Although in the past the level of cardiac rehabilitation has been described in terms of Phase I, II, III, and IV, based on continuous electrocardiographic (ECG) monitoring and time after the cardiac event; this system does not always seem appropriate in community-based settings. Due to rapid progress in the diagnosis and therapy areas of cardiovascular disease (CVD), most patients are able to enter outpatient cardiac rehabilitation programs 2 to 3 weeks after their cardiac event or surgery. If carefully screened and stratified according to life-threatening risk, low-risk and many moderate-risk patients do not need to participate in a traditional hospital-based monitored Phase II program. Therefore, it is suggested that the terms *inpatient program* and *outpatient program* are more accurate descriptions of cardiac rehabilitation programs.

Comprehensive Cardiac Rehabilitation

A community outpatient program is designed to focus on the rehabilitative needs of the cardiac patients once they have been discharged from the hospital. Its goals are to develop and foster lifestyle alterations that will allow participants to return to a normal productive life. The multiple intervention therapy should include dietary and psychological modifications in addition to exercise activities to improve functional capacity and aid the patient in returning to work. The task of the program is essential to replace destructive lifestyle habits with disease prevention behavior. This must be a long-range commitment on the part of both the rehabilitation center and the participant. Patient response to rehabilitation efforts is variable and depends on such factors as disease severity, compliance, and social situations. The optimal length of time needed for maximum benefit from a multiple intervention cardiac rehabilitation program is also dependent on these factors. Our experience indicates that it requires 3 to 12 months, usually greater than 6 months, to produce significant lasting gains in risk factor modification in most patients.

A successful rehabilitation program is one that insures that these gains will be maintained. However, only a program that can achieve reasonable compliance by meeting the unique needs of the community participants can enjoy success. Ideally, a cardiac rehabilitation program should begin for patients before they return to work, fit into their daily routines, and convey the message that lifestyle changes have a beneficial impact upon quality of life and progression of disease. Additionally, the program should begin and end at a time that does not significantly conflict with the patient's employment, be easily accessible, have ample space for the multiple intervention therapy, and provide an atmosphere that is conducive to positive health behaviors. Well-trained personnel who understand the unique characteristics of the community participants are extremely helpful in providing a program that is able to attain good compliance and rehabilitative success.

History of Community-Based Outpatient Programs

Hospital cardiac rehabilitation programs were instituted in the United States in the late 1960s and became more refined in the early 1970s. A few community-based outpatient programs were available to selected patients during this time. The enthusiasm of a few physicians and hospitals about the need for patient rehabilitation determined the areas of the nation in which this was practiced. As an example of one method in which a cardiac rehabilitation system was established, the Division of Vocational Rehabilitation Services in North Carolina, through the state's affiliate of the American Heart Association (AHA), provided in 1974 a grant to Wake Forest University to develop community-based outpatient cardiac rehabilitation programs in which patients discharged from the hospital and others with CVD could be evaluated and rehabilitated for return to work. Patient education and risk factor modification, in addition to the dietary interventions and exercise initiated in a hospital program, were expanded progressively. This multidisciplinary approach used in the inpatient programs was continued. Personnel required for these programs consisted of the program director, medical director, dietitian, psychologist, vocational counselor, exercise specialists, physicians, nurses, physical therapists, and others. The number of personnel required was dependent on the size of the program and whether graded exercise tests (GXTs) were performed at the rehabilitation site.

Once or twice each year workshops for team members from other communities who wished to start a program were held, usually at the Wake Forest Rehabilitation Program. This allowed the sharing of good and bad experiences with the beginning programs to help them avoid problems that might result in failure. The original multidisciplinary model has since been modified by programs in other communities to fit their personnel and facilities. However, all programs must provide the essential therapeutic components of exercise and dietary, psychological, and vocational evaluation and therapy.

The Division of Vocational Rehabilitation Services has played an active role in both the initiation and maintenance of cardiac rehabilitation in North Carolina, as have corresponding segments of the bureaucracy in other states. Vocational rehabilitation counselors are involved in all cardiac rehabilitation programs in North Carolina. Counselors facilitate patients' return to work by evaluating their physical and emotional capabilities with regard to work involvement. They can assist in job change or modification and serve as liaisons to alleviate employer-employee differences when the patient returns to work.

As such outpatient programs proliferated around the state, developing a mechanism to assure that the established guidelines and standards are met by all groups engaging in long-term therapy for cardiac patients became essential. To assure this, in 1983 the North Carolina General Assembly ratified rules and certification standards for community-based outpatient cardiac rehabilitation programs. This North Carolina Cardiac Rehabilitation Plan has been officially recognized as the basis for the establishment of programs since March 1, 1984. Similar cooperative arrangements with state licensing and medical agencies have been developed in other states.

In North Carolina and elsewhere, official program guidelines (1) are regularly updated by the existing outpatient programs. The centers now providing rehabilitation therapy for cardiac and other medical patients in the out-of-hospital programs have adopted these guidelines and work together to improve and preserve high-quality, appropriately staffed, safe programs for patients. An annual cardiac rehabilitation symposium for the state and surrounding area promotes an exchange of ideas, discussion of problems, and the development of better programs. More than 50 outpatient programs are certified in North Carolina, and staff from the 30 or so cardiac rehabilitation programs participate in the activities of the North Carolina symposium.

Implementation of Community-Based Outpatient Programs

The development of the community-based outpatient cardiac rehabilitation programs involves careful planning and successful completion of several preparation phases. Attendance at a workshop designed to demonstrate the operation of an outpatient program provides insight into the problems that frequently arise in the course of program development. The following sections will address specific issues that we have found to require special attention before the initiation of a community-based outpatient program.

Rapport With the Medical Community

Early contact with the local and regional medical communities is essential in the development of a sound and successful program. At the outset, the program organizer should emphasize the safety and effectiveness of the program to community physicians and make them aware that the rehabilitation program will complement and not replace their own patient care. Physicians should be invited to visit the program and participate in it. Every effort should be made to allay any fears the private physicians may have of losing their patients to the program physicians. Such fears have arisen in most communities in which an outpatient program is planned, and failure to address the issue properly at the outset can have a negative impact on the development and growth of the program.

Personal Letter and Survey of Potential Patient Availability

A brief letter should be sent to all appropriate physicians in the community to describe the intent to establish a cardiac rehabilitation program. This letter should be the first major contact to the medical community, assuring physicians that they are the first to be consulted and informing them that the program is in the planning and development stage. A description of the proposed program should be enclosed to provide the physician with a clear idea of the program goals and the methods to be employed to achieve them. A questionnaire that evaluates the reaction of the physicians to the concept of the new program should be included on a postage-paid card. An estimate of the number of potential patients each physician might refer can be assessed by the same method. A follow-up planning meeting, phone calls, and office visit may help to better familiarize the physicians more thoroughly with the proposed program.

County Medical Society and Hospital Medical Staff Meetings

In most areas, meetings of the county medical society (or analogous organization) and hospital medical staff are the best forums in which to present the concept and details of a community-based outpatient program. The presentation should include documented evidence of regression of coronary artery lesions and, more importantly, decrease in mortality (2-7); exercise methods and risk factor control methods to be used; and the results you expect. These meetings can be used to dispel any fears that local physicians may have about the safety of the program, and they provide an excellent opportunity for the program's medical director to emphasize to the referring physicians that rehabilitation therapy complements, and does not replace, the patient care that they provide. A description of the ongoing interaction that will be maintained between the medical director and referral physicians in the form of written progress reports, notes, and phone calls about patient medications and medical problems can be emphasized. The referral physicians must know that they control all the medical management of their patients. At the hospital medical staff meetings, the nurses, physical therapists, and dietary staff responsible for cardiovascular patient care should be invited. They frequently have more daily contact with the patients than the physicians and can significantly influence referrals of patients to the community program.

Brochures and Fliers

At the meetings just described, a brochure or flier describing the program and enrollment procedures can be distributed (and later disseminated) to the physicians' offices and areas in the hospital where cardiovascular patients are treated. This greatly simplifies the referral process for the physician and the hospital personnel. The brochure should be attractive, informative, and professional in its wording and appearance, since it may be the only contact that many physicians, nurses, and even patients will have with the program. A poorly prepared brochure may be more detrimental than none at all.

Identification of Patient Potential

Since a program cannot exist without a sufficient number of patients to offset expenses, a careful and critical appraisal of the number of patients required and their availability should be established before starting the program. Several methods of accomplishing this are examined here.

Survey of the Medical Community

In the previously noted questionnaire and letter sent to physicians, respondents should be asked to indicate the number of patients she or he sees each year who would qualify for cardiac rehabilitation and the percentage of these patients that is likely to attend the program. Generally, the results of the survey will substantially overestimate the number of patients who are eventually referred; actual referrals are approximately 30% of the projected number.

Contact With Hospital Staff

Following the introductory meeting, the program's medical director should contact the appropriate members of the hospital staff, that is, cardiologists, internists, family physicians, and coronary care unit (CCU) and other cardiovascular nurses. It is appropriate to ask the hospital rehabilitation staff to promote rehabilitation as a means of recovery once the patient leaves the hospital. Patients are more receptive when the full impact of the myocardial infarction (MI) or surgery is foremost in their thoughts.

Referral Agencies

Though the majority of patients will originate from referring physicians, some agencies can also provide referrals. Vocational Rehabilitation counselors and social service personnel frequently acquire clients for evaluation and rehabilitation to determine physical limitations relative to employment and independent home living. These people should be made aware of the cardiac rehabilitation program and have brochures and other information pertaining to referral procedures available in their offices. (It is also advantageous to have a vocational counselor as a member of the rehabilitative team to assess the employment status of patients.)

Media Coverage

When it appears that there is sufficient support for the program and the starting date has been established, the local media can be contacted to publicize the program. As a new community service, a cardiac rehabilitation program will be of widespread interest to the public, and media coverage is easily obtained. Discuss the nature of the approach thoroughly with the program planning staff or board of directors and a group of referring physicians, and be careful not to overdo the media blitz. Representatives of the local heart association, Vocational Rehabilitation counselors, and others should be contacted early in the development stage of the program, as they can provide valuable assistance in promoting the program in both the medical and lay communities and provide valuable insight from the perspective of their agencies.

Program Development

The nature and scope of a cardiac rehabilitation program should be established early in the development period. The level of disability and the types of patients that are accepted in the program markedly influence the required personnel, equipment, and facilities. In addition, this outpatient program may be the center for conducting and monitoring home-based and workplace rehabilitative exercise and risk factor screening education, which will add to staff and equipment.

Admission Diagnosis

Specific admission criteria should be established. These criteria must be communicated to physicians, nurses, and other medical personnel to ensure that appropriate patients are being referred to the program. Medical insurance or personal financial responsibilities for patient services may be related to the admission diagnosis. Preplanning with the medical care providers to determine which medical problems they will reimburse is very important.

The admission diagnoses that may be considered are outlined here.

1. **Myocardial infarction**
   a. 2 to 3 weeks after the event or at the discretion of the personal physician and medical director.
   b. Adequate control of complications, including angina, congestive heart failure (CHF), and arrhythmias is preferable.

2. **Percutaneous transluminal coronary angioplasty (PTCA)**
   a. 3 to 4 days after procedure.

3. **Postoperative cardiovascular surgery**
   a. 3 weeks after aortocoronary bypass surgery.
   b. 3 to 4 weeks after valvular, congenital, or peripheral vascular surgery. The exact admission date will depend on the condition of the patient and is always at the discretion of the referring physician and medical director.

4. **Stable Angina pectoris**
   a. At any time.
   b. Recent changes in medication for angina control are permissible at the discretion of the patient's personal physician.

5. **Hypertension**
   a. Patients with low functional capacity (< 7 METs [metabolic equivalents]) who need physical conditioning while evaluating blood pressure (BP) control with exercise.

6. Arrhythmias

a. Activity-induced arrhythmias without coronary disease or any arrhythmias with associated heart disease.

7. Pacemakers

a. 3-4 days after implantation for evaluation of rate change with exercise and patient conditioning.

8. Other

Medical conditions that benefit from exercise, dietary therapy, and risk factor control, including the following:

a. Diabetes
b. Cardiomyopathies
c. Peripheral vascular disease (PVD)
d. Valvular heart disease
e. Renal disease
f. Limiting arthritis
g. Obesity

Risk Level Stratification

Risk stratification of patients with CVD has been discussed by a number of authors (8-14). Risk levels are designated as low, intermediate or moderate, and high. Fortunately, 50% to 55% of the patients who have had an MI or coronary artery bypass graft (CABG) surgery are at low risk. The risk level is determined based on the evidence of residual ischemia, left ventricular ejection fraction (LVEF), the presence or absence of CHF, and the complexity of ventricular ectopy. Table 16.1 indicates the authors' assessment of the risk levels based on personal experience and the literature.

In addition to determining acceptable risks, the rehabilitation team should carefully identify contraindications for entry of patients in community-based outpatient cardiac rehabilitation programs. The list of contraindications includes, but is not limited to, the following:

- Untreated hypertension of 200/110 mm Hg or greater at rest
- Uncontrolled or unstable angina
- Uncontrolled atrial or ventricular arrhythmias
- Third-degree heart block without pacemaker therapy
- Acute pericarditis or myocarditis
- Severe aortic or mitral stenosis or insufficiency that has not been appropriately treated
- Symptomatic CHF, inadequately treated
- Uncontrolled diabetes
- Acute systemic illness or fever of unknown origin

Table 16.1 Guidelines for Risk Stratification

Risk level	Signs and symptoms
Low	Functional capacity ≥ 7 METs No myocardial ischemia Normal left ventricular function (ejection fraction ≥ 50%) No significant ventricular ectopy after 3rd day
Intermediate (moderate)	Evidence of myocardial ischemia ST-segment depression ≥ 2 mm Reversible myocardial perfusion abnormalities on exercise thallium imaging Left ventricular ejection fraction = 35%-49% No complex ventricular ectopy (as listed under "High") No decrease in blood pressure with exercise
High	Recurrent angina with ischemic ST-segment changes > 24 hours following admission Congestive heart failure signs and symptoms Left ventricular ejection fraction ≤ 0.35 High-grade ventricular ectopy, i.e., multifocal ventricular beats, nonsustained and sustained ventricular tachycardia, R-on-T phenomenon, ventricular fibrillation Functional capacity ≤ 5 METs on exercise testing that is limited by angina, significant ST-segment depression, or insufficient blood pressure response Decrease or failure to increase systolic blood pressure with exercise Persistent ischemic ST-segment changes and/or angina following exercise

Note. MET = metabolic equivalent.

- Thrombophlebitis or recent embolism
- Orthopedic or arthritic problems that would prohibit significant exercise

Most of these problems can in time be corrected or controlled and will allow the patient with an adequate functional capacity to participate in the rehabilitation program.

Personnel

The organizational structure of a community-based outpatient cardiac rehabilitation program need not be complex but should have the personnel required to provide patient assessment, exercise therapy, supervision, and emergency care. In many community programs, a board of directors may include business professionals, physicians, nurses, and other medical or allied health personnel who can assist in organizational and financial planning and medical support. The medical personnel should include one or two major patient referral physicians. This board's activities are perhaps more important during the initial development of the program, but the board can be valuable in an advisory capacity after the program is operational.

The two key positions in the rehabilitation program are the program director and the medical director. The primary responsibility of the program director is to coordinate personnel and all phases of the program; he or she may also serve as exercise director, nurse, or nutritionist. A bachelor's degree in an allied health field, such as exercise physiology, nursing, physical therapy, or other rehabilitation discipline, should be required, with an advanced degree and certification preferable. A knowledge of exercise physiology and nutrition, the benefits or risk factor modification and patient education, and experience in leadership is very important. Certification by the American College of Sports Medicine (ACSM) as program director or exercise specialist or equivalent certification by another organization is preferable and should be encouraged (14).

The medical director, a physician, works closely with the program director and medical staff to organize all medical aspects of the program and frequently serves as the supervising physician for exercise testing and exercise therapy. It is important that this physician be well qualified, respected in the community, and have good relations with local hospitals' medical staff and medical practice groups. These attributes will allow recruitment of local physicians to serve as exercise-testing and exercise therapy monitors and will minimize the perceived threat of patient loss. All medical aspects of the program, including patient safety, emergency procedures, and the medical aspects of personnel training, are the responsibility of the medical director.

A registered nurse who is licensed in the area and has experience or subspecialty training in cardiac rehabilitation is a vital member of the team. The nurse frequently has contact with hospital nursing personnel and plays a vital role in patient referrals. If not serving as the program director, the nurse's primary role is to assist the medical director in coordinating and supervising the medical aspects of the program and in staff and patient education.

If the program director is not an exercise specialist, it is necessary to have someone trained in exercise physiology or experienced in the exercise training of adults who can work with the medical program directors and other physicians in developing exercise prescriptions and coordinating the exercise program. Physical therapists are utilized in many programs as exercise supervisors and leaders and also are valuable for the design of specific exercise prescriptions for patients with exercise limitations.

A registered dietitian, who can assess nutritional needs and instruct patients in dietary therapy, is vital. Similarly, a psychologist, psychiatrist, or other mental health professional should be part of the staff and be available to evaluate and provide appropriate stress management and other psychotherapy for patients in need. Vocational counselors, occupational therapists, and additional exercise leaders, as needed to provide adequate personnel for patient exercise supervision and comprehensive multiphasic rehabilitation therapy, are essential (13,14).

There is no definite ratio of exercise supervisory personnel to number of patients established. As a rule of thumb, there should be 1 exercise leader to every 10 patients in the first 8 to 12 weeks of the program and perhaps 1 per 15 patients after this time. The number and the level of training and certification of the exercise personnel required depends on the risk level, exercise restrictions, and medical problems of the patient population. Most of the personnel employed by a rehabilitation program (physicians, nurses, physical therapists, psychologists, dietitians, and counselors) are licensed by a state medical licensing agency, have a medical specialty certification, or both; however, exercise physiologists, specialists, and technicians are not. The competency of these persons can be evaluated by their educational degrees, specialty training, and experience in exercise leadership of rehabilitation and adult fitness subjects. It is recommended that they be certified by the ACSM as exercise test technologists, exercise specialists, or program directors (14). This certification attests to their education and experience, knowledge, and qualification to do their respective jobs. All personnel should have basic life support (BLS) training and one or two of the staff involved with patient exercise testing and the training of the high-risk patients should be certified in advanced cardiac life support (ACLS).

Emergency Procedures

The program director, medical director, nurse, and exercise coordinator or leader should establish an emergency system. This should include specific staff assignments for each emergency task. Emergency drills should be held in the testing laboratory, exercise areas, and dressing rooms at least every 3 months after the emergency routine is established and at any time there is a personnel change. Detailed records of the presence of a physician or nurse and of the exact times that all phases of cardiac resuscitation are initiated—identification of heart rhythm, initiation of cardiopulmonary resuscitation (CPR), when defibrillation was accomplished, when oxygen was applied, when IVs were started—are all very important. Records of available drugs should also be kept. Staged practice of emergency procedures minimize the time required to carry out protocols and sharpen the skills of each team member.

Facility

The facility that is selected should be conveniently located, adequate in size, and easily accessible to patients and staff and should have convenient parking. Failure to comply with these requirements could jeopardize the recruitment of patients and staff (especially medical staff) and make compliance poor. The floor area should be large enough to accommodate the expected needs and the anticipated growth of the program. In addition, it is preferable if the available space for patient testing, consultation, and education and staff meetings can be expanded as numbers increase. Areas for screening patient records, emergency procedures, and storage of exercise equipment are essential.

Facilities currently used for cardiac rehabilitation programs in our area are university gymnasiums, community colleges, public-school facilities,

YMCAs, YWCAs, community recreational centers, religious recreational centers, hospital facilities, and independently operated centers of rehabilitation. With good planning, the time of the exercise phase of the rehabilitation program may be worked around a facility's other high-priority usage times, particularly at YMCAs and colleges or universities. Lastly, the cost of the facility should be reasonable, to minimize the program cost to the patient. Whenever possible, unused space within the community should be sought as a community service to keep the program costs within the means of the patient population.

Equipment

As the size, scope, and location of the program and facility vary, so will the equipment required. However, in all programs, a stethoscope, BP cuff, drugs, IV solutions, defibrillator, suction, and oxygen for patient emergency treatment and monitoring are absolutely essential.

The required exercise equipment varies. Exercise mats, nets and balls for games, free weights, resistance equipment, and water exercise supplies depend on the available room, facilities, and finances. It is essential to have a method for recording heart rates (HRs) and obtaining BPs in each exercise area with a 12-lead ECG recorder available in the facility. Defibrillator paddles are an excellent way to identify and record HRs and heart rhythms. If exercise testing and other patient evaluation methods are performed in the outpatient rehabilitation setting, a treadmill, cycle ergometer, and multichannel ECG recorder will be required in addition to the equipment and supplies noted for the exercise area. Equipment for obtaining anthropometric measurements, a spirometer, an instrument for body fat determination, and balance scales are also desirable in that they allow the effect of the program on the respective parameters to be determined.

Medical Records

An outpatient program held in a university gymnasium, church, community center, or other location must provide a secure location for patients' medical files. Policy and procedures should be implemented for their security as well as the availability of essential patient information for the staff. A community-based program should be required to provide the following:

- Complete, accurate, and updated medical records for each patient
- A system that allows easy accessibility of essential patient information in case of emergency
- A file for the informed consent documents that are signed by the patient before exercise testing and participation in the rehabilitation program
- A mechanism for patient record confidentiality with a patient consent form for release of medical information

Types of Exercise: General Considerations

All types of aerobic activity may be beneficial to the cardiac patient. Varying the activity and making the exercise fun for the participant increases compliance. The following sections provide general physiological information about various types of exercise. The mode, intensity, and duration of exercise used in the exercise prescription are discussed in chapter 17.

Dynamic Versus Isometric Exercise

The physiological response to increasing *dynamic (isotonic) exercise* in young to middle-aged persons is an increase in HR with an associated increase in stroke volume (SV). In older patients the increase in HR predominates, with little increase in SV. Systolic BP increases progressively with maintenance of, or slight decrease in, diastolic BP. Improved oxygen extraction, associated with redistribution of blood flow to working muscles, increases the systemic arteriovenous oxygen difference.

With *isometric exercise* the increase in HR is modest and is not related to the intensity of the effort, and the increase in cardiac output ($\dot{Q}$) is slight. High-intensity isometric activity can cause an increase in systolic BP, which can provoke angina, increase left ventricular dysfunction (LVD), and arrhythmias; this is the basis for limiting isometric activity in rehabilitation of patients with recent MI. Because a pressure load causes little improvement in cardiovascular function, isolated isometric training has not been a major component of cardiac rehabilitative physical activity. Combined isotonic and isometric training, however, may produce a substantial training effect in appropriately selected coronary patients (15). The enhanced muscle strength from resistance training often aids in dynamic endurance exercise. However, rehabilitation

professionals should take care, particularly in the home or workplace, since wall motion abnormalities may be aggravated by isometric activity, even in exercise-trained coronary patients (16).

Arm Versus Leg Exercise

Ideally, both arm and leg exercise should be included in a training regimen (17), since their effects are only modestly interchangeable. After leg training, the HR and BP responses to leg work decrease, but there is a lesser improvement in the responses to arm work. After arm training, the predominant decreases in HR and BP response occur with arm work. In one study (18), 50% of the improvement in exercise performance was a result of a generalized training effect and the remainder reflected predominantly improvement in oxygen extraction by trained skeletal muscle. A work load approximately 50% of that used for leg training is appropriate and safe for arm training (17). At a comparable oxygen uptake, arm work results in a higher HR and systolic BP response than does leg exercise. Since most occupational and recreational activities entail both arm and leg work and often involve predominantly arm work, specific arm muscle exercises must be included along with walking, cycling, and other lower-extremity activities in rehabilitative exercise training to improve physical performance.

Upper-Body Exercise

One recent review specifically addressed myocardial and aerobic requirements for upper-body exercising. This has become important in patients with paraplegia, amputations, and neurological, vascular, and certain other orthopedic and musculoskeletal problems of the lower extremities. In this setting, particularly a center where general medical rehabilitation programs are active, upper-extremity activity is very important in patients with associated CVD. In addition, upper-extremity activity is important to consider in patients whose occupational and work activity is predominantly done by arm activity (19).

Weight Training

In addition to the aforementioned, there are data available on weight training for improving strength and maximal power output in coronary artery disease (CAD) (20). In the studies that have been alluded to previously, it has been demonstrated that dynamic weight training in combination with aerobic dynamic exercise is a more effective method of increasing muscle strength and maximal power output in conditioned patients with CAD than aerobic endurance training alone. This is important in the overall care of the patient in community-based programs and certainly adds variety for those who have interest in weight training because of previous athletic interests or current interests in various training modalities.

Home and Workplace Cardiac Rehabilitation Programs

An alternate location for cardiac rehabilitation that may be applicable to many patients is the home-based or workplace (individual) program. Data (21,22) are available from two centers regarding the safety and efficacy of this kind of program, which is convenient for patients who live far from any facility and who may not need personal medical supervision. If the exercise is done at home or at the workplace, HR and rhythm may be monitored by transtelephonic ECG transmission and symptoms reported by voice transmission. If a patient chooses a nearby facility, such as a YMCA or exercise club, there is usually an exercise leader or someone to work closely with him or her within a group. In these individual and home programs, however, the use of an exercise prescription of less intensity than in a supervised setting (perhaps 60% to 70% of maximum) and regular and perhaps more frequent GXTs is of vast importance.

Today, more and more physicians, occupational and rehabilitation nurses, and other health professionals are recommending exercise to their patients, either at home, a shopping mall, or the workplace. Unfortunately, many times these patients have been given no further instruction than to "just walk," even though they are often in need of more supervised cardiac rehabilitation. A specific cardiac rehabilitation exercise prescription must be prescribed for each individual, as it is no longer acceptable to prescribe the same exercise routine for all persons. Certain objective data—including exercise level achieved on a GXT, baseline and peak HRs and BP, and a measured or estimated peak metabolic level (maximal oxygen uptake [$\dot{V}O_2$max])—are needed from the GXT to properly prescribe an exercise routine. Calculations can then be made from these data for a safe,

effective exercise prescription. This specific exercise prescription is particularly important for people exercising on their own at home or the workplace. (The means of developing an exercise prescription are discussed in chapter 17.)

An example of an exercise training program at home or at the workplace is outlined in Figure 16.1. All six levels can be designated initially or, if the patient's exercise program is difficult to determine initially, over two follow-up visits (23). The intensity of exercise can be altered if the individuals are overachieving or underachieving their target heart rate (THR) range. Each exercise level should be performed for approximately six exercise sessions, or 2 weeks, before progressing to the next level. When the individual achieves Level 6, the exercise routine can be maintained if appropriate, or retesting can determine a new exercise level.

Coronary Risk Factor Modification at Home and in the Workplace

Patient and spouse education and risk factor modification are intricate parts of the community rehabilitation program; the mechanisms and content of these are described elsewhere. Workplace cardiac programs can also be effective in gathering and dispensing health information about modification of coronary risk factors. Increased motivation for changing unhealthy behaviors, such as a sedentary lifestyle, may be found in the camaraderie of colleagues working toward common goals of improved health, a benefit of implementing programs in the workplace.

The group of risk factors for heart attack and stroke, some of which are modifiable, have been identified by the AHA and include heredity, male sex, increasing age, smoking, high BP, physical inactivity and elevated blood cholesterol. (It should be noted that the AHA recently elevated physical inactivity to the status of risk factor [24].) Other contributing factors are diabetes mellitus, obesity, and excess emotional stress (25).

Using the AHA's publication, *Heart Facts* (25), to emphasize the need for risk factor control may improve compliance. The following information, for example, might influence patients positively:

The chance of developing heart or blood vessel disease increases significantly as the number of risk factors increases. . . . To the contrary, at-risk individuals who take action to lower

Individual Exercise Training Program

Name: _____

Target heart range: _____   Target MET range: _____

Instructions: This exercise prescription is designed to *gradually* increase your level of exercise over the next 12 weeks. (1) Starting with Level 1, put an X in the small box each day you exercise. When you complete 6 days, move to the next level. (2) Record the date each time you start a new level. (3) At any time, if you have *questions* or experience any *problems*, please notify a staff member.

Level	Calisthenics	Walking/jogging	Cycling	Other
1 Date _____ ☐☐☐ ☐☐☐ 2 weeks or more	12 repetitions each	1.5 miles in _____ minutes	15 minutes _____ Resistance _____ rpm or mph	
2 Date _____ ☐☐☐ ☐☐☐ 2 weeks or more	15-20 repetitions	2.0 miles in _____ minutes	15 minutes _____ Resistance _____ rpm or mph	
3 Date _____ ☐☐☐ ☐☐☐ 2 weeks or more	15-20 repetitions	2.25 miles in _____ minutes	15 minutes _____ Resistance _____ rpm or mph	
4 Date _____ ☐☐☐ ☐☐☐ 2 weeks or more	15-20 repetitions	2.5 miles in _____ minutes	15 minutes _____ Resistance _____ rpm or mph	
5 Date _____ ☐☐☐ ☐☐☐ 2 weeks or more	15-20 repetitions	2.75 miles in _____ minutes	15 minutes _____ Resistance _____ rpm or mph	
6 Date _____ ☐☐☐ ☐☐☐ 2 weeks or more and then maintain	15-20 repetitions	3.0 miles in _____ minutes	15 minutes _____ Resistance _____ rpm or mph	

Figure 16.1   Individual exercise training program. The professional giving the prescription fills in the blanks in the Walking/Jogging, Cycling, and Other columns. (rpm = revolutions per minute; mph = miles per hour.) Reprinted with permission from Fletcher, B.J. Cardiac Rehabilitation in the Work-Place: Current Concepts. *Am. Assoc. Occup. Health Nurses J.* **38**: 443, 1990.

blood cholesterol below 200 mg/dL, stop smoking, and maintain a blood pressure of below 140/90 mm Hg experience a significant drop in risk of coronary artery disease. Control of diabetes, weight reduction, changing a sedentary lifestyle, and implementing stress management strategies are also linked to lowered risk of cardiovascular disease (25).

Such changes may take place in a home or workplace rehabilitation program, as well as a community rehabilitation setting.

Individual nutrition guidelines along with the individual exercise prescription are important first steps in helping implement a program of coronary risk factor modification. Experienced health professionals can personalize recommendations, thus meeting individual needs and increasing the likelihood of adherence to the recommended regimen (26). Group classes taught by health professionals at a convenient location can be very successful in coronary risk factor modification and health education when scheduled at a time and location convenient for employees. Health education classes provided in a program of risk factor modification are more likely to be attended and the information used if the class presentation takes into consideration such participant characteristics as education and socioeconomic background, gender, previous experiences of group members, perceived needs and interests of the group members as determined by survey, and work and travel schedules (27,28).

Motivation to participate in a program of behavior change is very important if the modification of risk factors is to be successful. Health care providers can increase participation by taking a positive approach, focusing more on those risk factors that participants can and are willing to change than on those that may be more difficult to modify (29). In addition, individual goals to be achieved in the rehabilitation programs are more likely to be met if mutually developed by the participant and the health care provider. Sloan and Gruman (30) have described several factors that positively influenced voluntary participation in programs of risk factor modification. Women were more likely than men to enroll in these programs. The perceived support of supervisors that participate resulted in a more positive effect. Also positive, but to a lesser extent, was the intention to change health behaviors that are based on increased perceived risk of illness. With the recent finding of decreased progression and even regression of arterial plaque formation by adherence to a risk factor control program (specific diets, exercise, and BP control), the message of the benefits of multidisciplinary cardiac rehabilitation program to the patient is even more persuasive.

Financial Support for the Program

A major problem that confronts a new program is the establishment of sound financial support. For the most part, financial problems result from poor planning or lack of good financial policies and procedures. The board of directors may be very helpful in establishing the policies and raising start-up funds.

Seed Money or Start-Up Grant

Although some programs are conducted for a short time with volunteer help, it is generally agreed that a program should be self-sustaining. A small grant, start-up "seed" money, or a loan may support the program until the number of patients required to generate adequate revenue can be acquired. Ideally, these funds should maintain the program for 6 months to 1 year to cover the delay in third-party payment.

Adequate financing may be a continuing problem for many programs, since many insurance carriers in the United States do not reimburse for rehabilitation therapy. Increasing the program income rapidly enough to become self-sustaining even in a 6- to 9-month period is at times difficult; a contingency plan and other methods of generating income should be available.

Insurance Carriers and Other Agencies

The greatest proportion of a program's income will come from claims filed with medical insurance carriers. If possible, contact should be made with the major medical insurance carriers in the area to make them aware of the program and to establish a system of filing claims. Blue Cross and Blue Shield, for instance, requires that the billing party have a provider number, which is assigned by the carrier to a program if it meets the requirements as a provider of services. Medicare may require that a provider qualify for certification by that agency. Other carriers may have other requirements, which should be determined early in the planning stages. It is essential that any questions the insurance carrier has regarding the reimbursement for rehabilitation services be answered well before the cardiac rehabilitation program begins. These issues are more difficult to resolve after the program has begun.

Patient's Responsibility

Initial discussion with incoming patients should always include their financial responsibility and the fact that they must assume any unpaid balance not reimbursed by the medical insurance carrier. Patients with group major medical plans typically have the most comprehensive coverage for the various services rendered in a cardiac rehabilitation program; often 80% of the charges are covered, with the patient being responsible for the 20% balance. Other policies may have more limited coverage. Presenting these facts to the patients at the time of entry will allow them to make an early decision and arrangements to assume the responsibility for part or all of the program costs. Some programs require their patients to pay 20% of the estimated cost within the first 2 weeks of participation, which helps provide operating monies while awaiting the insurance payments.

Auxiliary Income

As the testing laboratory and exercise equipment are rarely used full time, it is possible to supplement the program's income by offering risk factor screening tests, physical fitness appraisals, and work evaluations for local industry. In addition, GXTs, preventive exercise programs, and executive fitness programs can be a source of extra revenue if staff, facilities, and equipment are available. Utilization of the staff and facilities to the utmost will make the program financially solvent as it serves additional community needs.

Liability

Premises liability insurance and malpractice insurance are necessary. *Premises liability insurance* covers claims resulting from injury during participation on the premises. *Malpractice insurance* covers members of the staff for malpractice claims. In most programs, the malpractice insurance carried by the medical director and participating physicians and nurses is more than adequate to cover exercise testing and exercise therapy. However, exercise specialists may not be adequately insured. The ACSM has group insurance for professional personnel associated with preventive and rehabilitative exercise programs that can be acquired by the staff members. Information about this plan is available from the national office (American College of Sports Medicine; 401 W. Michigan Street, P.O. Box 1440; Indianapolis, Indiana 46206-1440). Regardless of the approach taken, the financial level of premises and malpractice coverage should be clearly established early in the planning stages by the program administrators after sufficient consultation and be in place before starting operation.

Communication

Problems may arise from many areas within a cardiac rehabilitation program, but the most common underlying cause is a lack of communication. Being sure that all staff are knowledgeable about the initial and subsequent assessment information as it affects the rehabilitation therapy of each patient is vitally important. Daily review of patient exercise and event information alerts everyone to any problems. Patient staffing conferences, in which an open discussion of each patient's medical information, evaluation results, rehabilitation goals, and therapy is held, provides an excellent opportunity for staff communication. In addition, a meeting of the entire staff every 2 to 4 weeks should be required to discuss the monthly activity schedule, special events, problems, and future directions.

Referral Physicians

The staff must maintain continuous communication with the referring physicians regarding the status and progress of their patients. This is accomplished by sending routine progress reports and reports of all tests on all patients during their time in the program, in addition to telephoning about any significant medical events.

Medical Community

Even though individual referring physicians have information concerning their patients, it is important to present the status of the rehabilitation program to the medical community. A presentation in the form of a progress report to the county medical society and, more importantly, to the hospital medical staff is an excellent way to again remind the medical community of the value of the program and its progression. This can also serve to familiarize new physicians with the program and enhance patient referrals.

Patients

A program newsletter is one of the most frequently used methods of keeping patients informed about program events, attendance records, and the rehabilitative accomplishments of the participants. This publication is also an excellent way of providing patients with exercise tips, heart-healthy recipes, and medical information. Special discussions and lectures, weekly educational presentations, and even questionnaires to evaluate patients' perception of the program and staff can be used very successfully to benefit the patients and the program. Most important is the one-on-one staff discussion of test results with each patient, at which time the progress toward rehabilitation goals and therapeutic direction can be presented. Many patient problems are solved early or avoided through an effective communication system.

Evaluation

To assess the effectiveness of the program and its impact upon participants, methods of evaluation to assess outcomes should be established early. The evaluation may include a method to document changes in risk factors, morbidity and mortality, return to work, and improvement in functional capacity. A record of the effect that the program has on changes in the cognitive domains (knowledge and understanding of heart disease and rehabilitation) and affective domains (attitudes and psychosocial traits) can be very helpful in assessment. Input from referring physicians as to the program's effectiveness in their patients is always beneficial to the program's success. Well-designed methods of evaluation that are utilized regularly provide valuable insight into staff and program effectiveness, pinpoint trouble areas that may require immediate attention, and provide statistical data that can be useful to others in the field of rehabilitation and document the therapeutic outcomes of your program.

Summary

This chapter has identified some of the major facets of the development of a community-based cardiac rehabilitation program and has discussed special problems that are often responsible for inhibiting the growth and effectiveness of a program. Most problems that are anticipated can be minimized, if not solved, before the program begins.

Excellent studies in the literature have supported the effectiveness of our rehabilitation methods. Whether one experiences an improvement in lifestyle, regression of arterial occlusive lesions, or a reduction in CVD mortality, most patients experience some improvement (2-7).

In conclusion, the key to making this beneficial, effective, and proven method of therapy successful is careful planning, good financial support, staff dedication, perseverance, and effective communication.

References

1. North Carolina Cardio-Pulmonary Rehabilitation Society. Organizational guidelines for cardiac rehabilitation programs in North Carolina. Winston-Salem, NC: North Carolina Cardio-Pulmonary Rehabilitation Society; 1987.

2. Blankenhorn, D.H.; Nessim, S.A.; Johnson, R.L.; Sanmarco, M.E.; Azen, S.P.; Cashin-Hemphill, L. Beneficial effects of combined colestipol-niacin therapy on coronary atherosclerosis and coronary venous bypass grafts. JAMA. 257:3233-3240; 1987.

3. Brown, G.; Albers, J.J.; Fisher, L.D.; et al. Regression of coronary artery disease as a result of intensive lipid-lowering therapy in men with high levels of apolipoprotein B. N. Engl. J. Med. 323:1289-1298; 1990.

4. Ornish, D.; Brown, S.E.; Scherwitz, L.W.; et al. Can lifestyle changes reverse coronary heart disease? Lancet. 336:129-133; 1990.

5. Schuler, G.; Rainer, H.; Gunter, S.; Gruze, M.; Methfessel, S.; Hauer, K.; Kubler, W. Myocardial perfusion and regression of coronary artery disease in patients on a regimen of intensive physical exercise and low fat diet. J. Am. Coll. Cardiol. 19(1):34-42; 1992.

6. Oldridge, N.B.; Guyatt, G.H.; Fischer, M.E.; Rimm, A.A. Cardiac rehabilitation after myocardial infarction. Combined experience of randomized clinical trials. JAMA. 260:945-950; 1988.

7. O'Connor, G.T.; Buring, J.E.; Yusuf, S.; Goldhaber, S.Z.; Olmstead, E.M.; Paffenbarger, R.S.; Hennekens, C.H. An overview of randomized trials of rehabilitation with exercise after myocardial infarction. Circulation. 80:234-244; 1989.

8. DeBusk, R.T.; Blomqvist, C.G.; Kouchoukos, N.T.; Luepker, R.V.; Miller, H.S.; et al. Identification and treatment of low-risk patients after acute myocardial infarction and coronary artery bypass graft surgery. N. Engl. J. Med. 314:161-166; 1986.

9. Debusk, R.F. American college of physicians position paper. Evaluation of patients after recent acute myocardial infarction. Ann. Intern. Med. 110:485-488; 1989.

10. Balady, G.J.; Weiner, D.A. Risk stratification in cardiac rehabilitation. J. Cardiopul. Rehab. 11:39-45; 1991.

11. Beller, G.A.; Gibson, R.S. Risk stratification after myocardial infarction. Mod. Concepts Cardiovasc. Dis. 55(2):5-10; 1988.

12. The Multicenter Post Infarction Research Group. Risk stratification and survival after myocardial infarction.

13. American Association of Cardiovascular and Pulmonary Rehabilitation. Guidelines for cardiac rehabilitation programs. Champaign, IL: Human Kinetics; 1991.

14. American College of Sports Medicine. Guidelines for exercise testing and prescription. 4th ed. Philadelphia: Lea & Febiger; 1991.

15. Kelemen, M.H.; Stewart, K.J.; Gillilan, R.E.; et al. Circuit weight training in cardiac patients. J. Am. Coll. Cardiol. 7:38; 1986.

16. Sagiv, M.; Hanson, P.; Besozzi, M.; et al. Left ventricular responses to upright isometric handgrip and deadlift in men with coronary artery disease. Am. J. Cardiol. 55:1298; 1985.

17. Franklin, B.A. Exercise testing, training, and arm ergometry. Sports Med. 2:100; 1985.

18. Thompson, P.D.; Cullinane, E.; Lazarus, B.; et al. Effect of exercise training on the untrained limb exercise performance of men with angina pectoris. Am. J. Cardiol. 48:844; 1981.

19. Grais, S.L.; McClintock, S.; Franklin, B.A.; et al. Myocardial and aerobic requirements for an upper body exercise: Implications for cardiac rehabilitation. Arch. Phys. Med. Rehabil. 72:563-566; 1991.

20. McCartney, N.; McKelvie, R.S.; Haslam, D.R.S.; et al. Usefulness of weightlifting training in improving strength and maximal power output in coronary artery disease. Am. J. Cardiol. 67:939-945; 1991.

21. Fletcher, G.F.; Chiaramida, Aj.; LeMay, M.R.; et al. Telephonically-monitored home exercise early after coronary artery bypass surgery. Chest. 86:198-202; 1984.

22. DeBusk, R.F.; Haskell, W.L.; Miller, N.H.; et al. Medically directed at-home rehabilitation soon after clinically uncomplicated acute myocardial infarction: A new model of patient care. Am. J. Cardiol. 55:251-257; 1985.

23. Fletcher, B.J.; Thiel, J.; Fletcher, G.F. Phase II intensive monitored cardiac rehabilitation for coronary artery disease and coronary risk factors—A six session protocol. Am. J. Cardiol. 57:751-756; 1986.

24. Fletcher, G.F.; Blair, S.N.; Blumenthal, J.; et al. Position statement on exercise. Benefits and recommendation for activity programs for all Americans—from the American Heart Association. Circulation. 86:340-344; 1992.

25. American Heart Association. 1993 heart facts. Dallas: American Heart Association Publication No. 550362; 1993.

26. Martin, J.E. Strategies to enhance patient exercise compliance. In: Franklin, B.A.; Gordon, S.; Timmis, G. eds. Exercise in modern medicine. Baltimore: Williams & Wilkins; 1989:73-83.

27. Planning, implementing, and evaluating learning experience for adults. Nurse Educator. November/December 31-36; 1978.

28. O'Donnell, M.P.; Ainsworth, T.H. Health promotion in the workplace. New York: Wiley; 1984:55-65.

29. Mason, J.; Ogden, H.; Barreth, D.; Martin, L.Y. Interpreting risks to the public. J. Prevent. Med. 2(3):133-139; 1986.

30. Sloan, R.P.; Gruman, J.C. Participation in workplace health promotion programs: The contribution of health and organizational factors. Health Educ. Q. 15(3):269-288; 1988.

Chapter 17

Exercise Prescription for Cardiac Rehabilitation

Michael L. Pollock
Michael A. Welsch
James E. Graves

Cardiac rehabilitation is the process of restoring psychological, physical, and social functions in people with manifestations of coronary artery disease (CAD). In the past 40 years there has been a profound shift from a conservative approach that discouraged physical activity by patients with angina pectoris and those who had had a myocardial infarction (MI) to one of encouraging as much activity as a patient's symptoms and medical status permit. Six weeks of bed rest after MI used to be the standard treatment (1). Fortunately, many cardiologists (2-5) questioned this conservative approach. They demonstrated the safety and effectiveness of low- to moderate-intensity physical activity for the anginal patient; the early use of a bedside chair; low-level ambulation, and range-of-motion (ROM) exercises for the stabilized MI patient; and progressive, endurance-stimulating exercises for those whose MIs had healed (2-6).

The benefits of cardiac rehabilitation on morbidity and mortality are not fully proven although they are strongly suggested (7-10). The effect of cardiac rehabilitation on quality of life, however, is not disputed (9-14). Cardiac rehabilitation includes exercise training and a wide spectrum of medical, physical, and psychosocial behavior changes. The multiple intervention approach to risk factor modification (smoking cessation, proper diet, stress management and exercise) in cardiac rehabilitation favors decreased morbidity and mortality (15,16).

Strict bed rest has a significant detrimental effect on physiological function (17-19). After just a few days or weeks, the patient has significantly decreased cardiorespiratory fitness, blood volume, red blood cell count, nitrogen and protein balance, strength, and flexibility and increased problems of orthostatic hypotension and thromboembolism (17-19). In patients who have undergone coronary artery bypass graft (CABG) surgery, physical activity can decrease postsurgical stiffness and prevent complications of postsurgical atelectasis. Other potential benefits of cardiac rehabilitation include a decrease in the incidence and severity of depression and anxiety, improved self-esteem, and a reduction in Type A behavorial characteristics such as hostility and anger (20-22). Part III of this book further discusses some of these benefits.

The purpose of this chapter is to provide the reader with the current accepted guidelines for the prescription of exercise for the cardiac patient. Therefore, a review of the recent guidelines for exercise therapy published by the American Heart Association (AHA) (23), the American College of Sports Medicine (ACSM) (24) and the American Association of Cardiovascular and Pulmonary Rehabilitation (AACVPR) (25) will be presented. Additional reviews of the role of early exercise and other aspects of cardiac rehabilitation on various medical, physiological, psychological, and social factors related to CAD can be found elsewhere (6,13,20,26). Although this chapter will focus primarily on the prescription of exercise for the traditional cardiac patient (uncomplicated MI and/or CABG), specific guidelines for other cardiac populations will also be presented.

General Guidelines and Preliminary Considerations

Before presenting the specific guidelines for exercise prescription for the various phases of cardiac rehabilitation, a brief discussion follows regarding several issues that require some preliminary considerations.

243

Risk Stratification

Participants in cardiac rehabilitation programs have traditionally been patients who were considered at low risk for additional cardiovascular complications. However, due to medical advances in the treatment of cardiovascular disease (CVD), an increasing number of patients are surviving acute cardiovascular events and may benefit from an organized cardiac rehabilitation program. Current cardiac rehabilitation programs, therefore, include the traditional MI and CABG patients as well as patients with severe left ventricular dysfunction (LVD), congestive heart failure (CHF), heart transplantation, exercise-induced ischemia, peripheral vascular disease (PVD), dysrhythmias, pacemakers, coronary angioplasty, valvular repairs, nonischemic CAD, pulmonary disease, diabetes mellitus, and many elderly heart patients (24).

Because of the wide range of patients currently enrolled in cardiac rehabilitation programs, the prescription of exercise and other strategies for risk factor modification have become complex for the cardiac rehabilitation specialist. Only when the cardiac rehabilitation specialist is aware of the patient's complete medical history, prognosis, functional ability, and personal needs, goals, and preferences can an exercise plan that maximizes safety, efficacy and adherence be prescribed (24).

An important addition to the rehabilitation process is the stratification of patients into risk categories based on their medical history and prognosis for future major cardiovascular events and rate of survival during the first year following an MI or CABG. Several guidelines and algorithms exist that may help health professionals in the design of a patient's program in regard to the appropriateness of exercise training (27-29). One such algorithm was proposed by DeBusk et al. (27) and suggests stratifying patients into three main risk categories (low, intermediate, and high) based on the extent of myocardial ischemia, LVD, the patient's hospital course, early entry into cardiac rehabilitation and the results of a symptom-limited graded exercise test (SL-GXT). This stratification usually takes place 3 to 6 weeks following hospital discharge and identifies those patients in need of a more formal and monitored cardiac rehabilitation program (Figure 17.1).

The Health and Public Policy Committee of the American College of Physicians (ACP) has recently established guidelines that help stratify patients based on their risk for developing further significant cardiovascular problems (28). The AHA, ACSM, and AACVPR strongly recommend using this method of risk stratification in the design of each patient's program in regard to the appropriateness of exercise training, the type and the intensity of the exercise prescribed, and the nature of medical monitoring and supervision needed (23-25).

The ACP define low-, intermediate-, and high-risk patients as follows (28):

Low-risk patients

- Uncomplicated clinical course in hospital
- No evidence of myocardial ischemia
- Functional capacity greater then 7 METs (metabolic equivalents)
- Normal left ventricular function (LVF) (left ventricular ejection fraction [LVEF] > 50%)
- Absence of significant ventricular ectopy

Intermediate-risk patients

- ST-segment depression greater than or equal to 2 mm flat or downsloping
- Reversible thallium defects
- Moderate to good LVF (LVEF 35% to 49%)
- Changing pattern or new development of angina pectoris

High-risk patients

- Prior MI or infarct involving 35% or more of the left ventricle
- LVEF less than 35% at rest
- Fall in exercise systolic blood pressure (BP) or failure of systolic BP to rise more than 10 mm Hg on exercise tolerance test
- Persistent or recurrent ischemic pain 24 h or more after hospital admission
- Functional capacity less than 5 METs with hypotensive BP response or ST-segment depression of 1 mm or more
- CHF syndrome in hospital
- ST-segment depression of 2 mm or more at a peak rate of 135 beats/min or less
- High-grade ventricular ectopy

Although every patient entering a cardiac rehabilitation program needs some basic training (usually a minimum of 6-12 sessions as recommended by the AHA [23]), those at low risk (approximately 50%) can be placed in a home exercise program or, once the recovery phase is completed, may be treated like most participants entering an adult fitness program. The intermediate- and high-risk patients, however, usually require a longer, more formal program with extensive monitoring while engaged in physical activity until they have become medically stable.

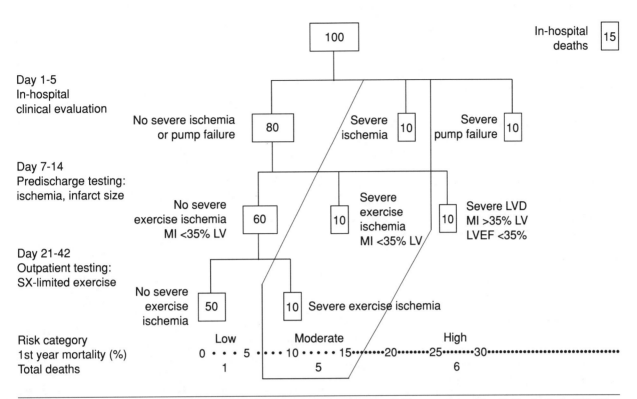

Figure 17.1 Prognostic stratification after acute myocardial infarction (MI) as proposed by DeBusk et al. (27). The size of each patient subset (numbers in boxes) in the algorithm is approximate and varies according to the patient population. Stratification of patients into the three main risk categories (low, moderate, and high) is based on the extent of left ventricular (LV) and left ventricular dysfunction (LVD). A variety of clinical observations and tests may be used to detect these abnormalities at various times after acute MI (LVEF = left ventricular ejection fraction; SX = symptom).

From DeBusk et al.: Identification and Treatment of Low-Risk Patients After Acute Myocardial Infarction and Coronary Bypass Graft Surgery. *N. Engl. J. Med.* 314:161-166, 1986. Reprinted with permission.

The Cardiac Rehabilitation Plan

For the majority of cardiac patients involved in cardiac rehabilitation the optimal period of a comprehensive rehabilitation plan is variable; many recommend up to 1 year (24,25,30). The cardiac rehabilitation plan should be individually tailored and based on the patient's medical history, prognosis, functional capacity, and specific needs. The program should be aimed to maximize safety, efficacy, and adherence. The program plan may be partioned into four distinct phases, recently defined by the ACSM as follows (24).

Phase I: Inpatient Phase   Phase I involves immediate inpatient exercise rehabilitation that emphasizes patient education (i.e., informal discussions with nurses and physicians) and counseling. Exercise therapy should include musculoskeletal ROM activities and activities of daily living (sitting, standing, and walking).

The main purpose of Phase I is to counter the deconditioning effects of prolonged bed rest and to prepare the patient for a return to normal daily activities.

Phase II: Early Outpatient, Clinic or Home-Based Phase   Ideally, Phase II should commence within 3 weeks of hospital discharge. The main purpose of this phase is to progressively improve patient's functional capacity, lower cardiovascular risk factors and prepare the patient for a return to his or her vocation. This phase should include exercise training and generally should last up to 3 months.

Exercise training should include progressive, light to moderate aerobic and strength-training activities. In addition, patients should continue to receive risk factor education as well as psychological support and vocational guidance.

Phase III: Late Outpatient, Community-Based or Home-Based Phase   The main purpose of

Phase III is to allow a patient to continue to improve his or her physical status. There should be a continued emphasis on patient education and risk factor modification.

The transition from Phase II to Phase III should be based on clinical, physiological and psychological information. Patients are moved into this phase when medically stable and desired outcomes from exercise therapy have been achieved (usually 6 to 12 weeks).

Phase IV: Community-Based Maintenance Phase Phase IV is generally used to provide patients with a means to monitor and maintain the results achieved during the earlier phases of rehabilitation.

Exercise Prescription for the Cardiac Patient

A clear understanding of the patient's needs, medical history, and present medical and physiological status is necessary to prescribe exercise safely and adequately. Because patients vary greatly in health status and physical fitness, body composition, age, motivation, and needs, an individual approach to exercise prescription is recommended. To be most effective, each exercise prescription should have specific guidelines concerning the frequency, intensity, duration, mode, and progression of the exercise program. In addition, a well-rounded program should be emphasized. The well-rounded program includes aerobic activities for the development or maintenance of cardiorespiratory fitness and proper weight control, and strength and muscular endurance activities, and flexibility exercises to develop and maintain strength and flexibility.

Many of the principles of exercise prescription outlined by the ACSM for healthy people are appropriate for the cardiac patient. The major differences are related to the application of these principles to the patient and how they affect the regulation of frequency, intensity, and duration; the rate of progression; and the selection of mode of training. Because of the potential medical problems associated with the diseased heart and the time required for cardiac patients to heal properly, program modifications and avoidance of certain activities are necessary.

Basic Components of a Training Session for Cardiac Patients

The basic components of a training session for cardiac patients are shown in Table 17.1. Cardiac patients need longer warm-up and cool-down periods than normal, healthy people and may require

Table 17.1   Components of a Training Session for Cardiac Patients

Component	Phase	Duration (min)
Warm-up	I	15-20
	II-IV	10-15
Muscular conditioning	II-IV	10-20
Aerobic exercise	I	5-20
	II	10-60
	III and IV	30-60
Cool-down	I-IV	15

Note. From Pollock, M.L. and J.H. Wilmore: *Exercise in Health and Disease: Evaluation and prescription for prevention and rehabilitation.* Philadelphia, W.B. Saunders, 1990. Reprinted by permission.

modifications of the endurance phase of the session, depending on their medical condition and phase of training. As a result of the low state of fitness and the adverse effects of bed rest and surgery on the musculoskeletal system of the cardiac patient, there is a need for special stretching and joint readiness exercise during Phase I. Generally, a Phase I patient is weak and cannot tolerate long bouts of physical activity. Thus, the aerobic phase should start with short ambulation periods, which are performed two or three times daily.

Once patients enter Phase II, they are generally ready for low-level muscle-conditioning activities. Emphasis is placed on dynamic and rhythmic exercise that does not impede normal breathing. Activities could include light calisthenics, light weight training (initially 1 to 5 lb), and various other low-resistance apparatus. The exercise time for a cardiac patient during the latter part of Phase II and Phase III and IV is similar to the exercise components recommended for a healthy person (30).

Specific details about exercise prescriptions are discussed in subsequent sections.

Rate of Progression

Figure 17.2 shows the average estimate of progression of training for cardiac and noncardiac groups. Progression is dependent on the participant's age, level of fitness, and health status. The slightly slower rate of progression at the beginning of the program for the MI patient, compared to the CABG patient, is the result of a reluctance on the part of the primary physician and rehabilitation staff to progress these patients rapidly. Generally, by 4 to

Cardiac rehabilitation/ physical therapy	Ward activity[a]	Patient education
Step 2: 1.5 METs Ward TX: Active-assistive ROM to major muscle groups, active ankle exercises, 5 repetitions; deep breathing (supine/sitting) twice daily.	Feed self. Partial morning care (washing hands and face, brushing teeth in bed). Bedside commode.	Answer patient and family questions regarding progress, procedures, reason for activity limitation. Explain RPE scale.
Step 3: 1.5 METs Ward TX: Active ROM to major muscle groups, active ankle exercises, 5 repetitions; deep breathing (sitting) twice daily.	Begin sitting in chair for short periods as tolerated 2 times daily. Bathe self. Bedside commode.	
Step 4: 1.5 METs Ward TX: Active exercises: shoulder flexion and abduction; elbow flexion; hip flexion; knee extension; toe raises; ankle exercises, 5 repetitions; deep breathing (standing) twice daily.	Bathroom privileges. Sit in chair 3 times daily. Up in chair for meals. Bathe self, dress, comb hair (sitting).	
Step 5: 1.5–2 METs Ward TX: Active exercises: shoulder flexion, abduction, and circumduction; elbow flexion; trunk lateral flexion; hip flexion and abduction; knee extension; toe raises; ankle exercises, 5 repetitions each (standing) twice daily. Monitored ambulation of 100-200 ft, twice daily, with physician approval.	Bathroom privileges. Up as tolerated in room. Stand at sink to shave and comb hair. Bathe self and dress. Up in chair as tolerated.	Answer patient and family questions. Orient to ICCU phase of recovery. Present discharge booklet and other printed material (AHA). Encourage patient and family to attend group classes or do 1:1 sessions.
Step 6: 1.5–2 METs Ward TX: Standing: Exercises outlined in step 5, 5-10 repetitions; once daily. Monitored ambulation for 5 min (440 ft). Exercise Center: Transport to IEC for monitored ROM/strengthening exercises from step 5, 5-10 repetitions; leg stretching (posterior thigh muscles, gastrocnemius), 10 repetitions; treadmill and/or bicycle 5 min; and stair climbing (2-4 stairs) with physician approval.	Continue ward activity from step 5. Increase ambulation up to 1 lap (440 ft) with assistance if appropriate, twice daily. Walk short distance in hall (room and quad areas) as tolerated.	Instruction in pulse taking and rationale. Explain value of exercise. Present T-shirt and activity log. Begin discharge instructions with patient and family when appropriate. Encourage group class attendance or offer 1:1 as needed.
Step 7: 1.5–2.5 METs Ward TX: Standing: Exercises from step 5 with 1 lb weight each extremity, 5-10 repetitions, once daily. Monitored ambulation for 5-10 min (440-1,000 ft).	Continue ward activity from step 6. Sit up in chair most of the day. Increase ambulation up to 3 laps (up to 1,100 ft) daily.	

(continued)

Table 17.2 *(continued)*

Cardiac rehabilitation/ physical therapy	Ward activity[a]	Patient education
Step 7 (continued) Exercise Center: Transport to IEC for monitored ROM/strengthening exercises from step 6 with 1 lb weight each extremity, 5-10 repetitions; leg stretching, 10 repetitions; treadmill and/or bicycle 5-10 min; and stair climbing (4-8 stairs).		
Step 8: 1.5–2.5 METs Ward TX: Standing: Exercises from step 5 with 1 lb weight each extremity, 10 repetitions, once daily. Monitored ambulation for 10 min (up to 1,980 ft) if appropriate. Exercise Center: Ambulate to IEC for monitored ROM/strengthening exercises from step 6 with 1 lb weight each extremity, 10 repetitions; leg stretching, 10 repetitions; treadmill and/or bicycle 10-20 min; and stair climbing (10-12 stairs).	Continue ward activity from step 7. Increase ambulation up to 5 laps (up to 1,980 ft) daily.	Give instruction in home exercise program. Initiate referral to Phase II if appropriate. Explain PD-GXT and upper-limit heart rate.
Step 9: 1.5–2.5 METs Ward TX: Standing: Exercises from step 5 with 2 lb weight each extremity, 10 repetitions, once daily. Monitored ambulation if appropriate. Exercise Center: Ambulate to IEC for monitored ROM/strengthening exercises from step 6 with 2 lb weight each extremity, 10 repetitions; leg stretching, 10 repetitions; treadmill and/or bicycle 20-25 min; and stair climbing (12-14 stairs).	Up as tolerated in room and quad area. Increase ambulation to 6 laps (up to 2,640 ft) daily.	
Step 10: 1.5–3 METs Ward TX: Exercises from step 5 with 2 lb weight each extremity, 10 repetitions, once daily. Monitored ambulation if appropriate. Exercise Center: Ambulate to IEC for monitored ROM/strengthening exercises from step 6 with 2 lb weight each extremity, 10 repetitions; leg stretching, 10 repetitions; treadmill and/or bicycle 25-30 min; and stair climbing (14-15 stairs).	Up as tolerated in room and quad area. Increase ambulation up to 8 laps (up to 3,300 ft) daily.	

Note. Heart rates, blood pressures, and comments are recorded on the Inpatient Data Record or Exercise Log. AHA = American Heart Association; CCU = cardiac care unit; ICCU = intensive cardiac care unit; IEC = inpatient exercise center; MET = metabolic equivalent; PD-GXT = predischarge graded exercise test; ROM = range of motion; RPE = rating of perceived exertion; TX = treatment.

[a]Activities performed alone, with family, or with primary nurse. "Laps" refers to the distance around the ICCU at Mount Sinai Medical Center, Milwaukee, WI, approx. 424 ft.

Table 17.3 Inpatient Physical Activity and Education Program Schedule and Guidelines for Open-Heart Surgery Patients

Cardiac rehabilitation/ physical therapy	Ward activity[a]	Patient education
Step 1: 1.5 METs a.m. Ward TX: Sitting with feet supported: Active-assistive to active ROM to major muscle groups, active ankle scapular elevation/depression, retraction/protraction, 3-5 repetitions; deep breathing. Monitored ambulation of 100 ft as tolerated. p.m. Ward TX: Sitting with feet supported: Active ROM to major muscle groups, 5 repetitions; deep breathing. Monitored ambulation of 100-200 ft with assistance as tolerated.	Begin sitting in chair (when stable) several times a day for 10-30 min. May ambulate 100-200 ft with assistance, 1-2 times daily.	Orient to CVICU. Reinforce purpose of physical therapy and deep-breathing exercises. Orient to exercise component of rehabilitation program. Answer patient and family questions regarding progress.
Step 2: 1.5 METs Ward TX: Sitting: Repeat exercises from step 1 and increase repetitions to 5-10; deep breathing twice daily. Monitored ambulation of 200 ft with assistance as tolerated (stress correct posture) twice daily.	Continue activities from step 1.	Continue above.
Step 3: 1.5–2 METs Ward TX: Standing: Begin active upper-extremity and trunk exercise bilaterally without resistance (shoulder flexion, abduction, internal/external rotation, hyperextension, circumduction backward; elbow flexion; trunk lateral flexion and rotation; trunk lateral flexion and rotation; knee extension [if appropriate]); ankle exercises, 5-10 repetitions, twice daily. Monitored ambulation of 300 ft twice daily.	Increase ambulation to 300 ft or approximately 3 corridor lengths at slow pace with assistance twice daily.	Begin pulse-taking instruction when appropriate and explain RPE scale. Answer questions of patient and family. Reorient patient and family to ICCU. Encourage family attendance at group classes.
Step 4: 1.5–2 METs Ward TX: Standing: Active exercises from step 3, 10-15 repetitions, twice daily. Monitored ambulation of 424 ft twice daily.	Increase ambulation to 1 lap at slow pace with assistance twice daily.	
Step 5: 1.2–2.5 METs Ward TX: Standing: Active exercises from step 3, 15 repetitions, once daily. Monitored ambulation for 5-10 min (424-848 ft) as tolerated. Exercise Center: Walk to IEC for monitored ROM/strengthening exercises from step 3, 15 repetitions; leg stretching (posterior thigh muscles, gastrocnemius), 10 repetitions; treadmill or bicycle 5-10 min (refer to treadmill/bicycle protocol) with physician approval.	Increase ambulation up to 3 laps (up to 1,320 ft) daily as tolerated. Begin participating in daily ADL and personal care as tolerated. Encourage chair sitting with legs crossed.	Orient to IEC. Continue instruction in pulse taking and use of RPE scale. Explain value of exercise. Present T-shirt and activity log.

(continued)

Table 17.3 *(continued)*

Cardiac rehabilitation/ physical therapy	Ward activity[a]	Patient education
Step 6: 1.5–2.5 METs Ward TX: Standing: Active exercises from step 3 with 1 lb weight each upper extremity, 15 repetitions, once daily. Monitored ambulation for 10-15 min (up to 1,980 ft) if appropriate. Exercise Center: Walk to IEC for monitored ROM/strengthening exercises from step 5 with 1 lb weight each upper extremity, 15 repetitions; leg stretching, 10 repetitions; treadmill and/or bicycle 15-20 min; and stair climbing (6-12 stairs) with assistance.	Increase ambulation up to 5 laps (up to 1,980 ft) daily. Encourage independence in ADL. Encourage chair sitting with legs elevated.	Give discharge booklet and general discharge instructions to patient and family. Encourage group class attendance. Individual instruction by physical therapist, nutritionist, pharmacist.
Step 7: 2–3 METs Ward TX: Standing: Active exercises from step 3 with 1 lb weight each upper extremity, 15 repetitions, once daily. Monitored ambulation for 15-20 min (up to 3,300 ft) if appropriate. Exercise Center: Walk to IEC for monitored ROM/strengthening exercises from step 5 with 1 lb weight each upper extremity, 15 repetitions; leg stretching, 10 repetitions; treadmill and/or bicycle 20-30 min; and stair climbing (up to 14 stairs) with assistance.	Continue activities from step 6. Increase ambulation up to 8 laps (up to 3,300 ft) daily.	Discuss and initiate referral to Phase II program if appropriate. Reinforce prior teaching. Give instruction in home exercise program. Explain PD-GXT and upper-limit heart rate.
Step 8: 2–3 METs Ward TX: Standing: Exercises from step 3 with 2 lb weight each upper extremity, 15 repetitions, once daily. Monitored ambulation if appropriate. Exercise Center: Walk to IEC for monitored ROM/strengthening exercise from step 5 with 2 lb weight each upper extremity, 15 repetitions; leg stretching, 10 repetitions; treadmill and/or bicycle 20-30 min; and stair climbing (up to 16 stairs).	Continue activities from step 7. Increase ambulation up to 9 laps (up to 3,746 ft) daily.	Reinforce prior teaching.

[a]Activities performed alone, with family, or with primary nurse.

Note. Heart rates, blood pressures, and comments are recorded on the Inpatient Data Record or Exercise Log. ADL = activities of daily living; CVICU = cardiovascular intensive care unit; ICCU = intensive cardiac care unit; IEC = inpatient exercise center; PD-GXT = predischarge graded exercise test; ROM = range of motion; RPE = rating of perceived exertion; TX = treatment. From Pollock, M.L., and J.H. Wilmore: *Exercise in Health and Disease: Evaluation and prescription for prevention and rehabilitation.* Philadelphia, W.B. Saunders, 1990. Reprinted by permission.

when the cardiac rehabilitation staff is supervising the patient, (2) ward activity, when the primary nurse or patient (on his or her own) supervises the program, and (3) patient education. These guidelines were designed so that at step 6 of the MI program and step 5 of the CABG protocol the patient goes to an inpatient exercise center once a day for physical activity (36). In general, the patient may be advanced one step each day, although the rate of progression should be individualized and depend on how successfully the patient is able to adapt to each stage of the program. Patients who appear to be at higher risk or who are symptomatic during exercise should be treated more conservatively.

The ACSM provides the following guidelines to modify or terminate a Phase I exercise session for cardiac patients (24):

- Fatigue
- Failure of monitoring equipment
- Light-headedness, confusion, ataxia, cyanosis, dyspnea, nausea or any peripheral circulatory insufficiency
- Onset of angina with exercise
- Symptomatic supraventricular tachycardia
- ST displacement (3 mm) horizontal or down-sloping from rest
- Ventricular tachycardia (three or more consecutive premature ventricular contractions [PVCs])
- Exercise-induced left bundle branch block
- Onset of second- or third-degree atrioventricular block
- R-on-T PVC
- Frequent multifocal PVCs (30% of the complexes)
- Excessive hypotension (> 20 mm Hg drop in systolic BP during exercise)
- Excessive BP rise (systolic BP ≥ 220 mm Hg or diastolic BP ≥ 110 mm Hg)
- Inappropriate bradycardia (drop in HR greater than 10 beats/min) with an increase or no change in workload

Exercise Prescription for Phase I

Some of the more important aspects of Phase I cardiac rehabilitation include the need to maintain working capacity, strength, and flexibility and to counter the deconditioning effects of prolonged bed rest. In this section the type, intensity, and duration of exercises for the Phase I cardiac patient will be discussed. In addition, some details regarding discharge planning and the physiologicical responses to exercise will be addressed.

Range-of-Motion Exercises

The use of upper-extremity ROM exercises is an important component of the early recovery phase from heart surgery and MI. Due to surgical trauma to the muscles and bones of the upper body, these areas may become atrophied and are vulnerable to the development of adhesions. Upper-extremity ROM exercises may enhance blood flow to the damaged areas and accelerate tissue repair. In addition, ROM may enhance muscular strength and flexibility, thereby preventing the development of undue weakness and poor posture.

ROM exercises used in the cardiovascular intensive care units for surgical patients typically include shoulder flexion, abduction, and internal and external rotation; elbow flexion; hip flexion, abduction, and internal and external rotation; and ankle plantar and dorsal flexion, inversion, and eversion (38). Initially, five repetitions of each activity should be performed one or two times daily, with a gradual progression to 10 to 15 repetitions twice daily. When patients can comfortably execute 10 to 15 repetitions, 1- to 3-lb wrist weights may be added. As discussed previously, patients who experience sternal movement or clicking or who have postsurgical sternal wound complications should refrain from these activities until they are medically stable. A detailed description of upper-body exercise for surgical and MI patients can be found elsewhere (30).

Ambulation

Two commonly encountered medical problems associated with a reduction in blood volume found following bed rest or CABG surgery are orthostatic hypotension and reflex tachycardia (33). Prior to ambulation, orthostatic BP measurements should be taken to avoid possible cardiovascular complications. This may be done by taking a BP measurement on the patient in the sitting position and a second reading after the patient has been standing for 30 s. A patient who is asymptomatic and has a small (< 10 mm Hg) drop in systolic BP between measurements can be cleared for exercise as long as the systolic BP is above 90 mm Hg. Patients who exhibit a 10 mm Hg to 20 mm Hg drop in orthostatic systolic BP may need further evaluation prior to engaging in the ambulatory phase of the program. A drop in orthostatic systolic BP of 20 mm Hg or more is considered a contraindication to exercise (27).

The types and progression of activities are described in Tables 17.2 and 17.3. Ambulatory activities in Phase I should be low in intensity (approximately 1.5 to 3 METs) and initially include self-care activities (eating, sitting), which are gradually progressed to slow walking, ROM exercise, and other activities of daily living. Preferably, these activities are performed a minimum of twice daily under medical supervision.

During the latter steps of the inpatient program, patients may progress more rapidly, and other activities such as stair climbing can be introduced. In addition, the duration of the ambulatory part of the exercise session may be progressively extended to up to 20 min. When patients are physically stronger, they can participate in a more formalized physical activity program that may include stationary cycling, stair climbing, and treadmill walking.

Exercise Intensity

Activities performed in Phase I typically do not exceed 2 to 3 METs. Although there is no set rule in determining the training (target) heart rate (THR) for the inpatient, two methods are generally used (30): 1. the use of a fixed low-level HR and 2. a specified number of beats above the patient's standing resting HR. The first method, a fixed low-level training HR (e.g., a THR of 120 beats/min), may not be appropriate because of the wide range of resting HRs among patients. For example, surgical patients tend to be somewhat tachycardic (110 to 120 beats/min), whereas patients on beta-blockers may be bradycardic, with resting HRs as low as 50 to 60 beats/min (39-41). Consequently, training at a fixed HR of 110 to 120 beats/min for surgery patients probably would not provide a sufficient training stimulus, whereas beta-blocked patients would have to double their HRs to reach the preset level. Thus, the use of standing resting HR plus 10 to 20 beats/min is an appropriate index of intensity for both surgical and medical patients.

In addition, the use of the Borg rating of perceived exertion (RPE) scale is encouraged after the first few days in the hospital (30,42). Patients should aim to achieve levels of 10 to 12 (light) on the 15-point category RPE scale (42-44).

Discharge Planning

During the final days in the hospital, patients should be prepared for the continuation of the rehabilitation program after discharge. If available, an organized outpatient program should be recommended to most patients, but in particular to patients who are considered at moderate to high risk (25,30) or if medical management is in transition; that is, if new medications are being used or medications are being adjusted. Prior to discharge, patients should be encouraged to visit the outpatient facility (if in the same hospital) at which they plan to continue their rehabilitation.

The predischarge plan should include strategies for risk factor modification, dietary counseling, education on medications, an emergency plan, and an exercise prescription for use at home.

The exercise prescription should include a list and description of the ROM exercises, information on walking and stationary cycling, and recommendations for stair climbing and other activities of daily living. Basic guidelines on exercise prescription should be reemphasized: namely, warm-up, cool-down, progression, frequency, intensity, duration, and modes of activity. Table 17.4 provides the basic components of the exercise program following hospital discharge.

In addition, patients should receive basic instructions in HR measurement, the use of the RPE scale and a brief explanation of the normal and abnormal responses to exercise training. If necessary, special instructions for exercising in a hot or cold environment should be included.

The use of exercise testing prior to hospital discharge may provide critical data regarding a patient's risk for subsequent coronary events. Patients who have a poor exercise capacity (< 6 METs), who develop angina pectoris with additional ST-segment depression (> 1 mm from rest) or complex dysrhythmias, or who fail to increase systolic BP during submaximal exercise are at greater risk for reinfarction and sudden death (45,46). Prehospital discharge exercise testing also provides further guidelines for the resumption of normal activities of daily living and may help reassure the patient and spouse by demonstrating that physical activity can be performed without developing significant symptoms.

It is important to note that, because of today's trend toward earlier hospital discharge, fewer predischarge graded exercise tests (GXTs) are done. Most programs administer low-level (approximately 5 METs or HR of 130 beats/min) GXTs within 3 weeks of surgery or an event and wait until 3 to 6 weeks after hospital discharge before an SL-GXT is performed.

Heart Rate, Hemodynamic, and Rating of Perceived Exertion Response to Exercise

As discussed previously, inpatient exercise is usually performed within a 2- to 3-MET range. Typically, HR responses for range-of-motion exercises and ambulatory activities during the first few days of rehabilitation are no more than 5 to 10 beats/min above resting level (33,38). SBP usually does not rise more than 5 mm Hg during ROM activities and 10 to 20 mm Hg during ambulation (33,38). A fall in systolic BP could be the result of exercise-induced LVD and is a criterion for terminating the exercise session. RPEs for both activities are generally between 10 and 12 (light) on the category RPE scale (see Table 17.7). The RPE concept is not presented to the patient until the third or fourth day of hospitalization, due to early comprehension problems resulting from excessive fatigue and medication (33,38).

Phase II: Outpatient Cardiac Rehabilitation

Organized, supervised outpatient cardiac rehabilitation has become an important part of the rehabilitation process and should begin when the patient is discharged from the hospital.

Timing and Location

Most experts believe that the first few weeks after discharge are the most crucial for the patient with regard to the need for medical supervision as well as the initiation of a risk factor intervention program. Because of the many anxieties and apprehensions that exist when the healing process is incomplete and because medication dosages are often altered at this time, it is contradictory not to have a well-planned and well-administered outpatient program.

Ideally, the Phase II program should be organized as a hospital-based program, although a community-based or home program may be implemented if an outpatient program is not available. Patients involved in a home program should be encouraged to periodically attend a hospital-based outpatient facility for further evaluation and to monitor progress.

As defined earlier, the outpatient phase of cardiac rehabilitation is the intermediate stage, during which the patient progresses from a restricted low level of training to a less restricted moderate-level program of physical activity.

The contraindications and guidelines used to modify or terminate exercise in the Phase I program are appropriate for the outpatient program as well (24,25).

Exercise Prescription for Phase II

During Phase II, the purpose of the exercise prescription for the cardiac patient should be the development of functional capacity. This section addresses the principles of exercise prescription (intensity, frequency, duration, mode of training, and the rate of progression) as applied to the cardiac patient.

Determination of Intensity of Training

The intensity of an aerobic activity is the energy required to perform that activity relative to its maximum metabolic cost, that is, the maximum oxygen uptake ($\dot{V}O_2$max). Therefore, to obtain a desired training intensity, $\dot{V}O_2$ or some equivalent index must be measured. In the following paragraphs, four different techniques frequently used to determine an appropriate training intensity for a cardiac patient are discussed.

Heart Rate.   The upper limit for the THR in the outpatient program may vary considerably, depending on medical status, symptomatology, method of calculation, RPE, personal preference, and whether the patient has performed an SL-GXT (24,37,47,48). Table 17.4 describes the standards recommended in the outpatient program. Generally, the THR estimated for hospital discharge can be used for the first 3 to 6 weeks of the outpatient program and for patients with functional capacities of 5 METs or less.

At 3 to 6 weeks following a cardiac event or surgery an SL-GXT is typically performed to evaluate the patient's medical status. The test results are used to modify the exercise prescription and to further define the patient's risk status (e.g., the need for continued ECG monitoring, physical capacity for return to work, changes in medications, etc.).

There are three primary methods of calculating the THR. Method I (percent of the maximal HR [HRmax]): THR = specified percentage of HRmax. Method II (percentage of HRmax reserve): THR = resting HR + specified percentage of the difference between HRmax and resting HR. Method III (percentage of maximal METs): THR = HR at $\dot{V}O_2$ that is a specified percentage of $\dot{V}O_2$max.

All three methods are acceptable, although method I generally yields significantly lower THRs than the others (37). Table 17.5 compares values calculated according to the three methods. The table shows that the THRs for both healthy adults and cardiac patients calculated by methods II and III are in close agreement. The THR of healthy

Table 17.4   Guidelines for Exercise Prescription for Cardiac Patients as Compared With Healthy Adults

Prescription	Phase I (inpatient program)	Phase II (discharge to 3 months)	Phase III (after 3 months)	Healthy adults
Frequency	2-3 times/day	1-2 times/day	3-5 times/week	3-5 times/week
Intensity	MI: RHR +20 CABG: RHR +20	MI: RHR +20: RPE 13 CABG: RHR +20: RPE 13	60-85% of HRmax	60-85% of HRmax
Duration	MI: 5-20 min CABG: 10-20 min	MI: 20-60 min CABG: 20-60 min	30-60 min	20-60 min
Activity	ROM,treadmill, bike, one flight of stairs	ROM, treadmill (walking, walking-jogging), biking, arm ergometer, calisthenics, weight training	Walking, biking, jogging, swimming, calisthenics, weight training, endurance sports	Walking, jogging, running, biking, swimming, calisthenics, weight training, endurance sports

Note. CABG = coronary artery bypass graft surgery patient; HRmax = maximal heart rate; MI = myocardial infarction patient; RHR = resting heart rate (beats/min), ROM = range-of-motion exercise; RPE = rating of perceived exertion. From Pollock, M.L., and J.H. Wilmore: *Exercise in Health and Disease: Evaluation and prescription for prevention and rehabilitation*. Philadelphia, W.B. Saunders, 1990. Reprinted by permission.

Table 17.5   Comparison of Training Heart Rate Calculated by Three Methods

Group	n	Age (years)	$\dot{V}O_2$max (METs)	Standing resting HR (beats/min)	HRmax (beats/min)	Intensity multiplier used to calculate training HR, %	Method I: % of HRmax (beats/min)	Method II: % of HRmax reserve (beats/min)	Method III: HR at % of $\dot{V}O_2$max (beats/min)
Healthy males	10	36.2 ± 3.2	11.9 ± 1.5	78.7 ± 12.6	186.2 ± 11.0	70	130.1 ± 7.5	154.0 ± 8.6	158.9 ± 9.0
						85	158.3 ± 9.1	170.2 ± 9.6	174.3 ± 11.4
Cardiac patients	10[a]	50.8 ± 8.3	9.8 ± 2.4	81.0 ± 17.7	152.7 ± 21.5	70	106.9 ± 14.8	131.2 ± 19.0	126.1 ± 20.5
						85	129.8 ± 18.2	141.8 ± 20.3	139.9 ± 22.8

[a]Seven coronary artery bypass graft and 3 myocardial infarction patients, 9 weeks postevent.

Note. HR = heart rate; HRmax = maximal heart rate; MET = metabolic equivalent; $\dot{V}O_2$max = maximal oxygen capacity.

adults calculated by method I was approximately 25 beats/min and 13 beats/min (10% to 15%) lower than that calculated by the other methods at 70% and 85% of maximum, respectively. For cardiac patients, the difference was approximately 20 beats/min and 11 beats/min, respectively. It seems, therefore, that method I is too conservative (24,37,49). If it is used, several investigators have recommended adding 10% to 15% to the calculated THR in order to achieve an appropriate training response (24,37,47,49).

Method II was first developed by Karvonen et al. (50). Table 17.6 provides a sample calculation for a THR range of 60% to 80% of HRmax reserve. The ACSM and AACVPR recommend a starting intensity of 55% to 70% of HRmax reserve with a gradual increase to 60% to 85% of HRmax reserve as tolerated (24,25). The AHA recommends starting at 50% to 60% of HRmax reserve (23).

A common criticism of method II is the variability of resting HR. Resting HR values vary greatly depending on time of measurement, posture, whether the patient smokes, eating, emotional stress, medications, and environmental conditions. To improve the accuracy of the method it is recommended that the resting HR be determined by multiple readings on different days under standardized conditions (15). On the other hand, even a 10 beat/min error in the resting HR only affects the HRmax reserve value by 2% to 3%. This error becomes even less significant when a training HR range is calculated.

Table 17.6   Method of Calculating Training Heart Rate (Upper and Lower Limits) Using HRmax Reserve

	Lower limit (60% of HRmax reserve)	Upper limit (80% of HRmax reserve)
HRmax	190	190
Resting HR	− 70	− 70
HRmax reserve	120	120
Intensity (multiplier used)	× .60	× .80
	72	96
Resting HR	+ 70	+ 70
THR	142	166

Note. HR = heart rate; HRmax = maximal heart rate; THR = training heart rate. From Karvonen et al.: The Effect of Training Heart Rate: A Longitudinal Study. *Ann. Med. Exp. Biol. Fenn.* 35:307-315; 1957.

Method III plots the relationship between HR and $\dot{V}O_2$ (51). A THR may then be chosen from HRs that correspond to $\dot{V}O_2$ values of 50% to 85% of $\dot{V}O_2$max achieved (24). However, because this method requires both an accurate measure of HRmax and $\dot{V}O_2$max, it may not always be practical.

Although most exercise tests for cardiac patients (approximately 85%) are terminated due to symptoms of fatigue (26), some tests are stopped at submaximal workloads due to abnormal cardiac signs or symptoms. In these cases the THR should be prescribed 5 to 10 beats/min below the point at which the clinical manifestations occurred.

For patients on beta-adrenergic-blocking agents the determination of the THR requires special consideration. When these drugs are administered, the patient's HR and BP are significantly reduced, although the relationship between the percentage of HRmax and the percentage of $\dot{V}O_2$max is not altered. Therefore, the determination of the THR and method of doing so are similar for patients on or off beta-blockade. However, it is important that the THR in patients on beta-blockers is determined from exercise tests that are performed during the time of day when the patient will be exercising (or similar time from which the drug was administered), to assure similar HR and BP responses (30).

No matter what method of calculation is used, the exercise leader must understand that the THR is only one of many physiological responses that can be monitored during exercise training. Understanding the use of RPE, BP responses, ECG changes, and signs and symptoms (fatigue, skin color, breathing pattern, sweat rate) to determine if a patient is responding appropriately to the exercise stimulus is important for safety and efficacy.

Rating of Perceived Exertion. The RPE scale was conceived and introduced by Borg in the early 1960s and is an important adjunct to HR in monitoring the intensity of training in cardiac patients (42,43,44,47). The original scale was a 15-grade category ranging from 6 to 20, with a descriptive marker of subjective physical effort at every odd number. This scale was modified by Dr. Borg in 1985 (see Table 17.7). A more recent 10-grade category scale with ratio properties and similar verbal descriptions has also been developed by Borg (see Table 17.8) and is used with equal success as the original scale. Ratings of perceived exertion and HR are linearly related to each other and to work intensity (42). In addition, RPE correlates highly with a variety of other physiological parameters such as pulmonary ventilation, and lactate (42).

Table 17.7   Rating of Perceived Exertion (RPE) Scale

15-point category RPE scale

6	No exertion at all
7	Extremely light
8	
9	Very light
10	
11	Light
12	
13	Somewhat hard
14	
15	Hard (heavy)
16	
17	Very hard
18	
19	Extremely hard
20	Maximal exertion

Note. From *An Introduction to Borg's RPE-Scale* by G. Borg, 1985, Ithaca, NY: Mouvement. Copyright 1985 by Gunnar Borg. Reprinted by permission.

Table 17.8   Borg Scale With Ratio Properties

10-point category-ratio (CR-10) scale

0	Nothing at all
0.5	Very, very weak (just noticeable)
1	Very weak
2	Weak (light)
3	Moderate
4	Somewhat strong
5	Strong (heavy)
6	
7	Very strong
8	
9	
10	Very, very strong (almost maximal)
•	Maximal

Note. From "A Category Scale With Ratio Properties for Intermodal and Interindividual Comparisons" by G. Borg. In H.G. Geissler and P. Petzoid (Eds.) *Psychophysical Judgment and the Process of Perception*, 1982. VEB Deutscher Verlag der Wissenschaften, Berlin. Reprinted by permission.

Thus the RPE scales provide valuable subjective information related to the amount of strain or fatigue the patient is experiencing during exercise.

The original 15-point scale was validated in a young population and related to actual HR. Adding a zero to each number would reflect the actual HR at a given level of work; that is, a rating of 6 or 7 would reflect a resting HR of 60 or 70 beats/min and a rating of 19 or 20, an HRmax of 190 or 200 beats/min. Because HRmax declines with age, actual HR values and RPE do not match in older adults. However, the linear relationship between HR and work intensity remains for individuals at all ages. When RPE is expressed in terms of relative intensity (percentage of $\dot{V}O_2$max), RPE values are similar for both younger and older individuals. Thus, the use of the RPE scales to establish relative exercise intensity is valid if the HR is expressed relative to a percentage of maximum (30). Table 17.9 shows a classification system for exercise intensity that has been included in the recent statements on exercise from the ACSM (52) and the AHA (23). The classification system is based on 30 to 60 minutes of endurance training and incorporates two methods of calculating the THR (HRmax or HRmax reserve method) and RPE with its descriptive marker.

During the early stages of the Phase II program, the recommended RPE range (11 to 13 on the category RPE scale, or 4 to 6 on the category-ratio scale)

Table 17.9   Classification of Intensity of Exercise Based on 30 to 60 Minutes of Endurance Training

Relative intensity		Rating of perceived exertion	Classification of intensity
HRmax	$\dot{V}O_2$max or HRmax reserve		
< 35%	< 30%	< 10	Very light
35%-59%	30%-49%	10-11	Light
60%-79%	50%-74%	12-12	Moderate (somewhat hard)
80%-89%	75%-84%	14-16	Heavy
≥ 90%	≥ 85%	> 16	Very heavy

Note. HRmax = maximum heart rate; $\dot{V}O_2$max = maximum oxygen uptake. From Pollock, M.L., and Wilmore, J.H. *Exercise in Health and Disease: Evaluation and Prescription for Prevention and Rehabilitation.* Philadelphia, W.B. Saunders, 1990.

is only slightly higher than the range provided upon discharge from the hospital. After the initial 3 to 6 weeks and an SL-GXT, the current ACSM and AACVPR guidelines recommend an RPE range of 12 (somewhat hard) to 16 (hard), which corresponds to an intensity of 50% to 85% of HRmax reserve (24,25).

Since RPE increases with increasing work loads and fatigue and decreases in proportion to HR when adaptation to training occurs, knowledge of a patient's RPE informs the exercise leader of how the participant is adjusting to the exercise program and when further progression in training should occur.

Although the usefulness of the RPE scale has been clearly shown in many different populations, its value must be interpreted in proper context. In addition, the exercise leader should consider that approximately 10% of the population are either underraters or overraters or simply cannot use the scale with any accuracy (53).

Metabolic Equivalents. Knowledge of the metabolic cost of certain activities provides another way of determining the appropriate exercise intensity. The appropriate range for intensity of conditioning activities for cardiac patients as recommended by the ACSM is usually 40% to 85% of the patient's maximal functional capacity (24). Since data on the energy cost of most activities now exists, activities that fall within the prescribed range may provide adequate stimulation for improving cardiorespiratory function. When choosing activities, the exercise leader will have to take into account the variability of the energy cost of the activity due to the patient's skill level and enthusiasm, as well as the climate and geographical location in which the activity will be performed (24,54,55). Any of these factors may complicate a person's attempt to stay within the prescribed exercise range. Difficulties in maintaining the prescribed exercise intensity may be overcome by including additional physiological indicators of intensity (i.e., HR and RPE), which adjust for personal and environmental changes.

Although this method of prescribing exercise has some distinct disadvantages, patients involved in home exercise programs may benefit, since it will provide them with additional guidelines as to what daily activities may be safe and appropriate. The AHA (23) provides a list of energy requirements of various activities (Table 17.10). The ACSM (24), and Pollock and Wilmore (30) provide additional lists of various exercise and leisure-time activities with an estimate of their metabolic cost in kilocalories (kcal) and METs.

Anaerobic Threshold. Cardiopulmonary exercise testing to evaluate the functional capacity of cardiac patients has gained in popularity in recent years. Knowledge of both the cardiac and pulmonary responses to exercise testing have led to more precise and safer exercise prescriptions. In addi-

tion, some programs have begun to use the anaerobic threshold (AT) for the prescription of exercise for CAD patients (56).

The concept of the AT was first proposed by Wasserman et al. (57), who defined AT as "the level of exercise $\dot{V}O_2$, above which aerobic energy production is supplemented by anaerobic mechanisms." A physiological characteristic of the AT is the nonlinear rise in ventilation and carbon dioxide production ($\dot{V}CO_2$), while $\dot{V}O_2$ continues to rise in a linear fashion (58). Although the exact mechanism which causes the AT is presently not well understood, some investigators have found the AT to be highly reproducible (58). Because the AT generally falls within the prescribed range of exercise for HR and METs, training near the AT is an appropriate stimulus for cardiorespiratory training. However, sophisticated equipment is needed to determine the AT. And even with such equipment and an experienced clinician, the AT remains difficult to determine. If the AT can be accurately identified from an exercise test it may have important implications for patients for whom high-intensity exercise is contraindicated. Training intensities should be prescribed slightly below the HR that corresponds to the AT, ensuring that the patient is performing aerobic work (59).

As a result of training adaptation, the AT tends to occur at higher workloads, which should be considered by the exercise specialist when adjusting the exercise prescription. However, given the uncertainties of measuring, defining, or describing the AT, its use in exercise prescription is limited until further research has demonstrated adequate reproducibility or understanding of the phenomenon across a broad spectrum of patients. The use of the AT method to prescribe exercise should be done only in conjunction with the standard and accepted methods of prescription.

Frequency and Duration of Training

The recommended frequency and duration of training during the Phase II program are shown in Table 17.4. A near-daily program is recommended. This typically means three supervised exercise sessions in an organized outpatient program and four additional sessions at home each week. For patients who are not stable, whose medications are still being adjusted, whose risk status has not been determined, or who are at high risk, the home program would not be recommended.

The exercise sessions during the early stages of the Phase II program are of short duration (15 to 20 min each). Depending on medical status and

Table 17.10 Estimated Energy Requirements of Selected Activities

Activity	METs	Activity	METs
Mild		*Moderate* (continued)	
Baking	2.0	Playing drums	3.8
Billiards	2.4	Sailing	3.0
Bookbinding	2.2	Swimming (slowly)	4.5
Canoeing (leisurely)	2.5	Walking (3 mph)	3.3
Conducting an orchestra	2.2	Walking (4 mph)	4.5
Dancing, ballroom (slow)	2.9	*Vigorous*	
Golf (with cart)	2.5	Badminton	5.5
Horseback riding (walking)	2.3	Chopping wood	4.9
Playing a musical instrument:		Climbing hills	
Accordion	1.8	No load	6.9
Cello	2.3	With 5-kg load	7.4
Flute	2.0	Cycling (moderately)	5.7
Horn	1.7	Dancing	
Piano	2.3	Aerobic or ballet	6.0
Trumpet	1.8	Ballroom (fast) or square	5.5
Violin	2.6	Field hockey	7.7
Woodwind	1.8	Ice skating	5.5
Volleyball (noncompetitive)	2.9	Jogging (10-minute mile)	10.2
Walking (2 mph)	2.5	Karate or judo	6.5
Writing	1.7	Roller skating	6.5
Moderate		Rope skipping	12.0
Calisthenics (no weights)	4.0	Skiing (water or downhill)	6.8
Croquet	3.0	Squash	12.1
Cycling (leisurely)	3.5	Surfing	6.0
Gardening (no lifting)	4.4	Swimming (fast)	7.0
Golf (without cart)	4.9	Tennis (doubles)	6.0
Mowing lawn (power mower)	3.0		

Note. These activities can often be done at variable intensities, assuming that the intensity is not excessive and that the courses are flat (no hills) unless so specified. Categories are based on experience of tolerance; if an activity is perceived to be more than indicated, it should be judged accordingly. MET = metabolic equivalent (3.5 ml · kg^{-1} · min^{-1} oxygen uptake). From Fletcher, G.F., Froelicher, V.F., Hartley, L.H., Haskell, W.L., and Pollock, M.L. Exercise Standards: A Statement for Health Professionals From the American Heart Association. *Circulation* 82:2286-2322, 1990. Reprinted by permission.

fitness levels, some patients may require an extra exercise session each day during the early stages of rehabilitation if their caloric expenditure is not sufficient. As the patient progresses, the duration of the exercise session can gradually increase in 5-min increments per week until a 45-min session is attained. Once a 45-min duration of training has been attained, frequency of training can be reduced or maintained between 3 to 5 times/week. For most patients this may take 4 to 6 weeks. The standard formal outpatient program usually consists of three visits/week, and includes both the exercise and educational components of rehabilitation.

Mode of Training

There are many activities that provide adequate stimulation for improving cardiorespiratory func-tion, flexibility/ROM, and strength. When choos-ing an activity, the cardiac rehabilitaton specialist should take into account the patient's medical sta-tus, level of fitness, interests and needs, as well as the available equipment, facilities, climate, and geographical location (24,54,55). At this stage of rehabilitation, highly competitive activities should be avoided, as they may result in inappropriate cardiovascular and hemodynamic responses. Par-ticipation in a variety of activities is recommended to ensure a well-rounded program. The modes of training recommended for the Phase II program are listed in Table 17.4.

Several methods of training have been suggested for use during the Phase II program and they in-clude continuous (single or dual mode), circuit

(circuit training and circuit weight training), and interval.

The continuous training method (usually walking, cycling, or a combination) imposes a submaximal energy requirement that is maintained throughout a training period (24). The advantages of this type of training are the ease of prescribing exercise and the ability to monitor the patient.

Circuit training has been shown to be an excellent method of conditioning to improve both muscular strength and cardiovascular endurance in cardiac patients (30). Circuit training incorporates a combination of lower body (stationary cycling, treadmill walking, and stair climbing) and upper body exercises (rowing, light weights, and wall pulleys). Patients exercise for 5 to 12 min on each modality, alternating arm and leg activities. Circuit weight training (CWT) is a series of resistance-training exercises designed to improve both muscular strength and cardiorespiratory fitness (60,61). Generally, circuit weight training results in significant gains in strength but only modest improvements in $\dot{V}O_2$max in both healthy and patient populations (60,61). As a result of these modest improvements in cardiorespiratory fitness, it is recommended that circuit weight training be utilized only in conjunction with, rather than serve as a substitute for, regularly performed aerobic exercise (30).

Interval training is defined as work followed by properly prescribed relief (rest) periods (24). The advantage of this method of training is that patients with low exercise tolerance may perform a greater amount of physical work during an exercise session.

Regardless of the method of training, the exercise prescription should include exercises that encompass all the major muscle groups of the body (24).

Endurance Activities. The ACSM has classified endurance activities on the basis of the rate of energy expenditure (24). Some activities, such as walking, jogging, and cycling can be easily maintained at a constant rate of energy expenditure, whereas the energy expenditure for other activities (basketball and racquetball) are highly related to a person's skill level. Because precise control of the exercise prescription in the cardiac patient is necessary, the choice of activity should be one that can be easily maintained at a constant intensity and inter-individual variability in energy expenditure is low.

Walking. Walking is safe from the standpoint of both a cardiovascular and orthopedic risk and has been found to be an excellent activity for improving aerobic fitness (62-64). Walking is also simple in nature, which allows most people to participate. The compliance to walking programs is usually high (65) because walking requires no special skills, facilities, or equipment and can be incorporated into most busy lifestyles.

Table 17.11 shows a 12-step walking program that can be used in an outpatient or home program. The patient progresses from step to step as tolerated. A patient should be stable at a step for 1 to 2 weeks before progressing to a higher level. One of the objectives of the program is to have patients progress to the point that they expend a minimum of 250 to 300 kcal/session, or 1,000 kcal/week (24,30,66-68). Because the caloric expenditure per exercise session for cardiac patients in Phase I begins at a much lower level (approximately 50 kcal/session) (38), it typically takes the cardiac patient several weeks or months longer than healthy individuals to reach this minimum (see Figure 17.2) (37). This amount of activity improves a participant's aerobic capacity 15% to 30% over 4 to 6 months. Therefore, at a slow to moderate walking speed, patients must eventually walk 45 to 60 min/session, or increase the training frequency or both, to reach the required caloric expenditure.

The use of hand-held weights during walking increases the energy cost of the exercise (69-73). Walking with 3-lb weights on the wrist or in the hands and using an arm-swing up to shoulder height increases the oxygen cost by 1 MET and the HR by approximately 10 to 12 beats/min (72,73). On the other hand, just holding the weight without any arm movement has little additional benefit (74). BP responses resulting from the use of hand-held weights are usually small; thus, their general use is not contraindicated for most individuals, including patients with hypertension (70,72,73). However, the use of hand-held weights is associated with a significantly greater number of orthopedic problems of the elbow joint (34).

Jogging. Although jogging is generally not recommended for patients in the early stages of the Phase II program, some individuals may progress to a level at which higher-intensity exercise may be tolerated. Cardiac patients entering a jogging program usually begin with short periods of jogging interspersed with equal distances of walking. As they progress, they will walk less and jog more. However, it should be noted that several investigations have shown that high-intensity efforts are associated with a greater risk for developing further cardiovascular complications (75-77). In addition, there is a strong relationship between high-impact activities (such as jogging) and orthopedic

Table 17.11 Twelve-Step Walking Program for Outpatients

Functional capacity (METs)	Step	Speed (mph)	Treadmill grade (%)	Duration (min)	METs	Energy expenditure (kcal/min)	(kcal/session)
5	1	1.5	0	20-30	2.0	2.0	40.0-60.0
	2	2.0	0	20-30	2.0	2.5	50.0-75.0
5-8	3	2.0	0	5	2.0	2.5	
		2.5		40-60	2.5	3.0	132.5-192.5
	4	2.5	0	5	2.5	3.0	
		3.0	0	40-60	3.0	3.7	
8 or more	5	3.0	0	5	3.0	3.7	
		3.5	0	40-60	3.5	4.2	
	6	3.0	0	5	3.0	3.7	
		3.5	0 (1 min)	40-60	3.5	4.2	
		3.5	2.5 (4 min)		4.2	5.9	
	7	3.0	0	5	3.0	3.7	
		3.5	0 (1 min)	40-60	3.5	4.2	
		3.5	2.5 (6 min)		4.2	5.9	
	8	3.0	0	5	3.0	3.7	
		3.5	0 (1 min)	40-60	3.5	4.2	
		3.5	2.5 (10 min)		4.2	5.9	
	9	3.0	0	5	3.0	3.7	
		3.5	0 (1 min)	40-60	3.5	4.2	
		3.5	2.5 (14 min)		4.2	5.9	
	10	3.0	0	5	3.0	3.7	
		3.5	2.5	40-60	4.2	5.9	
	11	3.0	0	5	3.0	3.7	
		3.5	0 (1 min)	40-60	3.5	4.2	
		3.5	5.0 (2 min)		6.9	7.5	
	12	3.0	0	5	3.0	3.7	
		3.5	0 (1 min)	40-60	3.5	4.2	
		3.5	5.0 (2 min)		6.9	7.5	

Note. The first line in steps 3-12 is the warm-up period. When there are three lines (in steps 6-9, 11, 12) the second and third lines denote interval training; for example, in step 6, the patient alternates 1 min at 0% grade with 4 min at 2.5%. If a treadmill is not available, the higher-intensity segment can include a faster walk and/or use of hand weights (see text). MET = metabolic equivalent. Reprinted with permission from Pollock, M.L., Pels, A.E., Foster, C., and Ward, A.: Exercise prescription for rehabilitation of the cardiac patient. In Pollock, M.L., and Schmidt, D.H. (eds.): *Heart Disease and Rehabilitation, 2nd Ed.* New York, Wiley, 1986, pp. 477-515.

injuries, particularly in beginners, long-term exercisers, the elderly, overweight people, and postmenopausal women (30,78). It would therefore be sensible to consider low-impact activities, which are associated with lower injury rates for many participants.

Stationary Cycling. Stationary cycling is probably one of the best activities that can be used at home. As with walking, stationary cycling is an excellent rhythmic, large-muscle-group activity that stimulates the metabolic and cardiovascular systems. The time components and progressive stages used for the walking program may be used by substituting resistance for speed. Usually, stationary cycling can be initially tolerated at 100 to 300 kilopondmeters (kpm)/min (17 to 50 W). If a patient's power output cannot be tolerated for the minimal required duration, some zero-resistance pedaling may be used or an interval training program incorporated. For example, 1 min of zero-resistance pedaling may be followed by 1 to 3 min of a power output equal to 100 to 300 kpm/min. The patient may initially do this for a total of 10 min. As the patient adapts to the power output exercise, intervals should be gradually increased until the desired duration of exercise can be performed.

An important point to remember when using a cycle ergometer is to make sure that the height of the seat is properly adjusted. The seat should be adjusted so that there is a slight bend in the knee joint when the ball of the foot is resting on the pedal in its lowest position (79).

The use of a proper cool-down period following stationary cycling is important, as postexercise hypotension is a commonly experienced symptom associated with an abrupt cessation of cycling exercise. Thus, easy pedaling against light or no resistance should be continued for several minutes during the cool-down period (30).

Arm-Leg Cycle Ergometry. The use of arm-leg cycle ergometers such as the Air Dyne is a popular mode of exercise in cardiac rehabilitation programs. The Air Dyne ergometer is versatile and allows a participant to train with legs only or arms only, or a combination of arms and legs. The arm-shoulder action is a push-pull movement that develops the muscles used in many commonly performed work and recreational activities. Generally, cycling exercise that combines upper- and lower-body movement will result in less specific muscle fatigue and allows the patient to train longer and/or at a higher $\dot{V}O_2$ than when using arms or legs alone (80). Gleim et al. (81) attributes this to a larger exercising muscle mass. However, submaximal upper- and lower-body exercise results in hemodynamic responses similar to those of treadmill walking when at least 40% of the total power output is performed by the legs (82).

Rowing is also a combined upper- and lower-body exercise, although it is not quite analogous to the push-pull movements performed during Air Dyne cycling. Typically, more emphasis is placed on the use of the trunk musculature than on the arms and shoulders alone (81). Nevertheless, Gleim et al. (81) demonstrated that for a given energy expenditure, the rate-pressure product (RPP) during rowing exercise was comparable with treadmill walking in healthy subjects. Because the RPP: HR (beats/min × systolic BP [mm Hg]) is an indirect measure of coronary blood flow, this implies that walking and rowing result in equivalent myocardial oxygen demands.

Arm Cycle Ergometry. Patients with PVD or orthopedic limitations may benefit greatly from the use of the Air Dyne or by arm cranking. In general, the principles of exercise prescription and the physiological benefits for arm training are similar to those of leg training or a combination of arm and leg training (83,84). However, when prescribing arm exercise, calculating a THR based on the HRmax found during the treadmill or cycle ergometer GXT may result in inappropriately high exercise HRs (85). Several studies comparing leg and arm testing have reported lower HRmax values (approx. 93% of HRmax for the leg test) for arm exercise (86). If the patient is tested on an arm ergometer, the HRmax from that test can be used to determine the THR. Otherwise it is recommended that the THR obtained from the treadmill GXT be reduced by approximately 10 beats/min when applied to training on an arm ergometer. The RPE values found with arm ergometry can also be used to delineate the appropriate intensity for arm cranking (85).

When prescribing exercise for arm training, it is important to remember that at any given submaximal power output, the physiological cost (HR, BP, RPP, and $\dot{V}O_2$) of arm exercise is greater than for leg exercise. However, the absolute workload or power output for arm exercise is significantly less than what can be achieved with leg exercise. Power outputs approximating 50% of those used for leg training are generally appropriate and effective for arm training (85).

Swimming. Although swimming can be introduced in the Phase II program, it is not recommended until after an SL-GXT has been administered and approximately 6 weeks of rehabilitation have been completed. This period should allow sufficient time for healing of the sternum and leg incisions in the surgery patient and the heart tissue of the MI patient.

The advantages of a swimming program are many: it is an aerobic activity involving both arms and legs; the water buoyancy helps venous return and HR; swimming causes fewer musculoskeletal injuries; and it can be therapeutic for patients with arthritis, intermittent claudication, limb amputations, or paralysis (87-90).

The wide variations in skill level and energy cost of swimming among patients are major problems in regulating swimming programs (87-90). For nonswimmers and those with poor skills, swimming may be an anaerobic activity. Walking in waist- or chest-deep water while paddling backward with the arms and the use of flotation devices around the waist for swimming on the back are two excellent ways of introducing water activities to patients. They are suitable for the nonswimmer and the swimmer with poor skills. It is recommended that nonswimmers begin their program on the side or back, using the sidestroke or elementary backstroke. Frequent stops at the side of the pool should be made to count the pulse. It is important to have the patient avoid entering cold water or becoming uncomfortable in a pool in which the temperature is too cold.

After patients have had a chance to adjust to their water activities, their exercise may be regulated like other aerobic exercise. The duration should be gradually increased to 30 to 45 min; RPE and HR responses may be used to regulate the intensity. The HR in water, in the prone position, is lower for a given work load than measured on a treadmill or cycle ergometer. Therefore, if the THR for water is estimated from a treadmill or cycle GXT, the calculated prone or supine swimming HR should be reduced 5 to 10 beats/min.

Stairclimbing and Stair Stepping. Because climbing stairs is a component of most people's daily routines, and because the development of new equipment has facilitated the use of stair stepping as an exercise mode, stair-climbing exercise has become quite popular in Phase II programs.

Few studies have evaluated the effects of stair-climbing exercise on cardiac patients (91-93). Holland et al. (92) reported no significant differences in clinical manifestations between conventional treadmill exercise and the revolving-stair ergometer in rehabilitated patients with CAD. In addition, they showed that cardiovascular and hemodynamic responses to submaximal and maximal exercise were similar between the two testing modes. This finding suggests that the use of a THR calculated from a treadmill GXT would be appropriate for stair-stepping exercise. Reddy et al. (93), however, found that in patients with moderate to severe CHF, climbing three flights of stairs was a strenuous and anaerobic exercise, which resulted in significant fatigue and dyspnea.

In general, the newer stair-stepping devices can be regulated to a low level of intensity and would be appropriate for use in the clinically stable CAD patient. However, some precautions should be taken when using these devices. For patients with CHF, weak thigh muscles, orthopedic problems (i.e., arthritis, knee, and ankle problems), stair-climbing devices may be contraindicated. In addition, some of the older model stair-climbing machines cannot be regulated below 30 steps/min and so may present too great an initial exercise intensity for the low-fit or high-risk patient (30).

Resistance Training. Along with the ROM/flexibility exercises previously described for Phase I, resistance (i.e., strength) training should be emphasized during Phase II of cardiac rehabilitation. This training should be integrated as part of a well-rounded program and should address the patient's preparation for return to work or leisure activities.

Since most home- and job-related tasks require upper- and lower-body static and dynamic strength, improvements in muscular strength and endurance may facilitate the patient's return to a fully active lifestyle (30).

Traditionally, cardiac patients were told to avoid resistance training because it was associated with an increased pressure load on the heart and a decreased venous return, thus placing the patient at higher risk for a cardiac event (94-96). The increased pressure load was a direct result of large increases in HR, systolic and diastolic BP, and mean arterial pressure (94-96). The decreased venous return was the result of the absence of an active muscle pump (94-97). However, most recent data have shown that the increase in BP with exercise is directly related to the amount of muscle mass being used and the relative percent of maximum at which it is stimulated (98-101). For example, when comparing static and dynamic exercise performed by handgrip and double-legged knee extension, mean arterial pressure increases were found to be similar for each mode of exercise, but greater for knee extension (100). Thus, in contrast to what some have interpreted about arm exercise, the HR, $\dot{V}O_2$, and BP responses are greater for leg exercise than for arm exercise.

Early studies on subjects with CVD suggested that isometric exercise caused LVD (reduced LVEF, regional wall motion abnormalities and increased cardiac dysrhythmias), with a transient reduction in the SV index, particularly in those patients with already compromised ventricles (95,102). Other studies, however, found that brief periods of isometric resistance training were not dangerous for selected patients with cardiac disease (103).

The majority of investigations focusing specifically on the effects of resistance training in patients with CAD generally report similar cardiovascular and hemodynamic responses to such training in normal subjects (104-107). Haslam et al. (108) have shown that cardiac patients performing light- to moderate-intensity strength training of up to 60% of maximal volitional contraction (MVC) were able to maintain their RPP at or below 85% of the maximum RPP found during an SL-GXT. Other programs have shown the safety of strength training, with no added incidence of ischemia, dysrhythmia, or frequency and intensity of angina pectoris (109-112). It appears that even though diastolic BP increases during resistance training, the greater perfusion of blood through the myocardium may alleviate some of the potential adverse effects of the increase (113). One program observed and followed patients for up to 3 years and found no serious cardiovascular or orthopedic complications (110).

Studies looking at the feasibility and effectiveness of dynamic-resistance training on muscular strength in CAD patients report improvements similar to those found in normal subjects (30,114). Keleman et al. (105) evaluated low-risk CAD patients engaged in circuit weight training (see p. 533a) for a period of 12 weeks. The intensity of training used increased HR and BP to up to 60% of values at maximum effort. Measures of strength increased by an average of 24% in the resistance training group, while control subjects, who participated in a traditional program, showed no changes in strength. Ghilarducci et al. (111) have shown strength gains from 12% to 53% following high-intensity resistance exercise, without complications during training or testing. These large increases may have been partially the result of the low initial levels of strength of these patients (114). In light of this research, resistance training under proper medical guidance is both a safe and effective form of exercise training in selected patients with CAD.

The following criteria for abstaining from participation in resistance training have been established by the ACSM and AACVPR (24,25):

- Abnormal hemodynamic responses with exercise
- Ischemic changes during graded exercise testing on the ECG
- Poor LVF
- Uncontrolled hypertension or dysrhythmias
- Peak exercise capacity less than 6 METs

Exercise Prescription for Resistance Training. Once the patient is properly screened, resistance training should be initiated with careful consideration of the patient's medical status and functional capacity. Although a recent study demonstrated that machine-resistance exercise in early outpatient rehabilitation did not result in abnormal cardiovascular responses (ECG and BP) (112), most patients begin their resistance training following hospital discharge with 10 to 15 repetitions of 3- to 5-lb wrist weights or dumbbells and progress to 5- to 7-lb weights before the 6-week SL-GXT (30). Following an SL-GXT at 4 to 6 weeks, general restrictions on lifting can be eliminated, which will allow patients to progress to heavier weights and the use of barbells or resistance exercise machines as their medical condition permits (30).

Several methods are available for determining an appropriate resistance training load in cardiac patients. One method simply starts the patient at the lightest weight on the weight stack (24,30). At this weight the patient performs 10 to 12 repetitions or exercises up to an RPE of no greater than 13 (somewhat hard). Gradually progress the patient to the next higher weight using increments of 5 to 10 lb (or 3% to 5% of the previous weight) every 1 to 2 weeks. Other methods include starting the training load at 30% to 50% of a one-repetition maximum (1RM) or the maximum weight that can be lifted 2 or 3 times (90% of 1RM) (114). One RM is the maximum amount of weight that can be lifted one time. Studies evaluating cardiovascular responses during 1RM testing generally do not report any significant cardiovascular complications (106,111,112). However, because more research is needed to determine the safe limits of high-intensity strength testing and resistance training of patients with CAD, starting the patient at the lightest weight on the weight stack is recommended.

Guidelines for resistance training for cardiac patients include a minimum of 8 to 10 exercises involving the major muscle groups, performed a minimum of two times per week. Each exercise should consist of one set of 12 to 15 repetitions at an intensity that corresponds to an RPE of 15 to 16. Each exercise should be performed throughout the patient's ROM to maximize the potential benefits (115). Rest periods between exercises should not exceed more than 1 to 2 min. These guidelines differ somewhat from those established by the AACVPR, who recommend two or three sets of exercise. The rationale for these differences is based on two factors. First, the time it takes to complete a well-rounded exercise program is important. Programs that last longer than 60 min/session are associated with higher dropout rates (65). Second, several investigators have noted considerable gains in strength (greater than 25%) following training programs using one set of 10 to 15 repetitions to fatigue (115-117). The strength gains noted by training one set are not much different from those found by using additional sets (115-117). As a result of this research the ACSM's current recommendation for healthy individuals is a minimum of one set of 8 to 12 repetitions to fatigue (52). The authors support these current recommendations for cardiac patients as well, although the number of repetitions should be slightly higher (12 to 15) and the perceived intensity lower (RPE values not to exceed 15 to 16).

Proper form, including lifting the weight slowly and smoothly, should be emphasized (118). If possible, patients should avoid holding the breath or using excessive force when gripping the bars of the machines as this could cause an added increase in BP. Patients should be instructed to lift the weight in 2 s while exhaling and to lower it in 4 s while inhaling. Exhaling while lifting helps to avoid a Valsalva maneuver. Studies that have conducted static contractions with the Valsalva maneuver have shown significant increases in BP (119). In contrast to these studies a recent investigation (120) suggests that increasing intrathoracic pressure by performing a brief Valsalva maneuver during resistance training is not detrimental and may actually help offset the increase in systolic BP, thereby limiting the increase in left ventricular transmural pressure. Therefore, a brief Valsalva maneuver is not necessarily contraindicated. However, patients recovering from surgery should avoid activities that may put undue pressure on the sternum.

Muscular strength and endurance may be developed by means of isometric, isotonic, or isokinetic exercises using the overload principle. However, because isometric exercise may result in left ventricular decompensation in patients with poor LVF, pure isometric contractions should be avoided (95). In addition, because high-intensity resistance training has been associated with significant increases in BP in young healthy individuals (121), dynamic low- to moderate-resistance exercises are recommended (30).

Additional guidelines regarding resistance training for healthy adults and low-risk cardiac patients have been established by the ACSM and AACVPR and include the following (24,28):

- When 12 to 15 repetitions can be lifted comfortably, increase the weight loads gradually (3% to 5%).
- Include exercises for both the upper and lower body (arms/shoulders, trunk, lower back, abdomen, and hips and legs) and exercise large muscle groups before small ones.
- Terminate the exercise session in the event of dizziness, dysrhythmias, unusual shortness of breath, chest pain, or other warning signals.

Monitoring During Resistance Training. Initially, monitoring of the CAD patient during resistance training should include HR and heart rhythm, BP, RPP, and RPE to determine safety. BP and HR responses as well as rhythm strips should be recorded prior to and during the training session.

However, because BP returns to a level within normal limits 10-15 s after a resistance training exercise (121), it may be necessary to measure BP during the activity to provide a more accurate measure of arterial pressure. This may be done by recording pressures at nonmoving sites (e.g., the ankles during arm exercise). Patients should be instructed to stay within their THR. However, it should be noted that HR typically contributes less to the increase in cardiovascular stress during resistance training than does BP (122). The use of the RPP may be a better indicator of myocardial stress than BP or HR alone, and should therefore be periodically monitored to ensure that the patient does not exceed the RPP at which symptoms or ECG changes suggestive of ischemia became apparent during the SL-GXT (24). Initially, the RPE should range from 11 to 13 on the category RPE scale or 2 to 4 on the category-ratio scale and should be monitored at each exercise station. As the patient adapts to and tolerates the training well the RPE range may be progressed to 15 or 16 on the category RPE scale.

Rate of Progression

The rate of progression during the Phase II program should be gradual. However, during the initial 4 to 6 weeks of rehabilitation, patients are still considered in the starting stage of the exercise program. Exercise training should therefore be individualized and continue to be conducted at low intensities. Patients should be progressed first by increasing the frequency and duration of training and later the intensity of exercise. Proper introduction to an exercise regimen may reduce the risk of further cardiac injury, minimize muscle soreness or orthopedic injury and increase the chance for long-term adherence.

After completion of the 6-week SL-GXT, training intensity for the low- to moderate-risk patient can usually increase to 70% of HRmax reserve and continue to progress to a 250 to 300 kcal expenditure per exercise session (24,30). As stated earlier, it may take cardiac patients weeks to months longer than healthy individuals to reach this level of energy expenditure (37).

The progression of caloric expenditure in Figure 17.2 usually stops at 300 to 400 kcal per exercise session. The need for greater energy expenditure and high-intensity exercise is not necessary for patients to achieve adequate health and fitness (25). However, in several studies, high-intensity, high-volume training in selected cardiac patients elicited both central and peripheral adaptations (123-127). In this series of studies, MI patients were exposed to a rigorous training regimen, with training intensities up to 90% of VO_2max and training frequencies of 5 days/week for a period of 9 months. Results clearly showed an improvement in markers of central function: increased SV, maximal RPP, and LVEF (123-127). Markers of ischemia: A reduction in ST-segment depression and significantly less angina at maximal efforts also showed improvement after training (123-127). Although these findings are provocative, they must be interpreted with caution, since it is also known that high-intensity training is associated with a greater risk for major cardiovascular complications (75,76).

Warm-Up and Cool-Down

Each exercise session should incorporate a warm-up and cool-down period of 10 to 15 min each. The warm-up period should be designed to increase the metabolic rate gradually from a resting level to a level of energy expenditure needed for the conditioning phase of the session. Typically, this may be accomplished with low-intensity cardiovascular activities. In addition, light ROM exercises and low-level calisthenics may help prepare the muscles, joints, and ligaments for the added stress of the exercise.

Proper warm-up may prevent potential musculoskeletal injuries as well as cardiovascular complications (128-130). Barnard et al. (128) demonstrated serious ECG abnormalities (ST-segment depression and dysrhythmias) in middle-aged adults when sudden exercise was undertaken without proper warm-up. Foster et al. (129) also reported a significant decrease in LVEF in healthy individuals who started exercise abruptly.

The importance of the cool-down period is equal to that of the warm-up period. The major purpose of cooling down is to keep active the primary muscle groups that were involved in the exercise. Since most cardiovascular exercises involve the musculature of the legs and are performed in the upright position, blood tends to pool in the lower extremities upon cessation. Therefore, patients should be encouraged to continue to exercise at a gradually diminishing rate during the cool-down period. As described before, postexercise hypotension has been found to be particularly evident after stationary cycling.

Continued activity during the cool-down period will also reduce the risk of cardiac dysrhythmias. Plasma catecholamine levels tend to be markedly elevated during the immediate postexercise recovery period. This can cause significant dysrhythmias in high-risk individuals. Many cardiovascular events occur during the first few minutes of

recovery (130). Therefore, close surveillance of the patient during the first 15 min after exercise is highly recommended.

Phases III and IV: Community-Based Cardiac Rehabilitation Program

The Phase III program may be conducted in an organized and supervised community-based setting and Phase IV denotes a long-term maintenance program that can be unsupervised. The Phase III and IV programs should provide the cardiac patient with an opportunity to continue the conditioning programs of Phase I and Phase II. Participants in Phase III and IV have typically been out of the hospital for 6 to 12 weeks. In addition, they should be clinically stable, knowledgeable about cardiac symptoms, and able to self-regulate exercise regimens. They should have a minimum functional capacity of 5 METs (24).

Table 17.4 shows the guidelines for exercise prescription used in Phase III and IV. At this stage of training, the exercise prescription is similar for both MI and CABG patients and becomes closer to that recommended for the healthy adult. The intensity of training is based on the patient's medical and physical status and on the results of an entry SL-GXT. The initial intensity prescribed is usually 60% to 70% of the HRmax reserve. As the patient continues to progress in the program, the intensity may reach 85% of functional capacity (24).

The duration of training should be between 30 and 60 min, depending on available time and the intensity of the exercise (24,30). Note that this time range does not include the time needed for warm-up, muscular conditioning, and cool-down. Normally, the duration of training for cardiac patients is longer than what is recommended for healthy adults because the former are training at lower intensity.

Frequency of training should be a minimum of 3 days/week and, if time is available, up to 5 days/week. As in Phase II, an energy expenditure of 250 to 300 kcal/session and 1,000 kcal/week are important thresholds for developing and maintaining fitness.

Table 17.4 shows the wider variety of activities now available to the participant of the Phase III and IV programs. The activity still depends on medical status, functional capacity, needs and desires, time, and available facilities. Generally, highly competitive games are not recommended for high-risk individuals. Special preparation may be required for those patients who want to resume normal work and leisure activities; for example, the muscles needed to perform specific tasks may need specific training.

If local patients prefer to train at home rather than as part of a supervised program, they should be encouraged to have periodic evaluations of their training routines. These evaluations may occur once every 2 weeks to several months, depending on medical status and level of training. Preferably these sessions are conducted in the Phase II or community-based facility and should simulate exercise conditions at home.

Considerations for Special Populations

The cardiac rehabilitation specialist should be aware of certain specific problems and needs that may be associated with exercise prescriptions for special patient populations (see also Part V). The purpose of this section is to present some patient populations that deserve such additional attention.

Percutaneous Transluminal Coronary Angioplasty Patients

The number of percutaneous transluminal coronary angioplasty (PTCA) procedures has risen dramatically over the past few years. Many patients who undergo a PTCA are discharged within 36 h of the procedure, leaving little time for providing them with a comprehensive inpatient program. In addition, because the angioplasty often results in immediate improvements in clinical status (i.e., in ECG abnormalities, LVF, and angina) and work capacity, many patients deny the need for further medical intervention. It is therefore critical that these patients be made aware of the importance of exercise and risk factor modification, especially since 20% to 30% of PTCA patients will experience restenosis during the first 6 months after the procedure (131,132). Just because the procedure was successful does not mean that the patient should ignore the fact that he or she has significant CAD.

The PTCA patient can typically begin slow ambulation and ROM exercises approximately 24 hours after the procedure. Prior to discharge from the hospital the patient should be encouraged to visit a multidisciplinary Phase II program. Because the restenosis rate may range from 20% to 30%, it is important that patients become knowledgeable concerning the signs and symptoms of restenosis

and be given clear instructions about when to seek medical attention (131,132).

If the patient is given an SL-GXT prior to or shortly after discharge, this information may be used to prescribe exercise. Generally, the rules outlined for the CABG patient apply for the PTCA patient, with the PTCA patient usually progressing a little faster (133). If the patient is also recovering from an MI, however, the guidelines outlined for the MI patient should be used.

Typically, at 2 weeks after discharge, the patient returns to the hospital for a follow-up visit with the cardiologist. If the patient is not enrolled in an outpatient program it is advisable to have him or her meet with a member of the cardiac rehabilitation staff for further instructions regarding exercise and diet. At this time the patient's exercise progress should be evaluated and the prescription modified if necessary. In addition, it is helpful to review the principles of exercise and to provide the patient with instructions on measuring HR, and on using the RPE scale.

Elderly Patients

An increasing number of cardiac patients are above the age of 65 years. These patients are particularly susceptible to the adverse effects of bed rest (13) so early mobilization is especially important to return them to active and independent lifestyles. The elderly patient is often poorly fit and may suffer from significant muscle atrophy, orthostatic intolerance, hypertension, diabetes mellitus, and degenerative bone disease, in addition to CAD which may further complicate the exercise prescription (24).

Individualization of the exercise prescription is essential for elderly patients to minimize the risk of cardiovascular and orthopedic complications; nevertheless the design should follow the principles described earlier in the chapter. Generally, the goal of physical activity is to maintain functional capacity for independent living.

Intensity

Exercise intensity is generally prescribed using the previously described techniques. However, recent data suggests the need to reevaluate the methods used to determine exercise intensity in the elderly. It is generally accepted that the relative HRmax reserve corresponds to relative $\dot{V}O_2$max. However, there may be an exception in the elderly. Panton et al. (134) have shown that the use of the HRmax reserve method in 60- to 80-year-old persons results in an underprediction (5% to 10%) of the true exercise intensity (based on percent $\dot{V}O_2$max). In this study the percent of HRmax method more closely represented the percent $\dot{V}O_2$max and may therefore provide a more precise estimation of exercise intensity.

The elderly coronary patient generally starts with a lower intensity of exercise because of limited functional capacity and additional medical conditions (osteoporosis, hypertension, orthostatic hypotension) that may affect exercise performance (24). Exercise training at intensities as low as 30% to 40% of $\dot{V}O_2$max improves cardiorespiratory fitness in very low-fit individuals (135). In contrast, high-intensity/high-impact exercise in elderly individuals may result in a significant increase in the incidence of musculoskeletal injuries (78), in addition to greater risk of cardiovascular complications.

Duration and Frequency

The duration and frequency of exercise should also be modified for the elderly. Interval training (2 to 6 min, with 1-min to 2-min rests) is often necessary for these individuals in both the inpatient and early outpatient phase. As the patient better tolerates the activity, the exercise time may be gradually lengthened to 30 to 60 min of continuous exercise. The frequency of exercise should be two to three times a day during the initial stages of the program and progressed up to 5 times per week when longer durations of exercise can be sustained (135).

Mode of Training

The types of activities that should be emphasized include those that involve low impact to the feet and legs and a rhythmic use of the large muscle groups. Walking, stationary cycling, and a combination of arm- and leg-work are excellent activities for the elderly patient. Swimming may be particularly beneficial to patients who, in addition to their cardiovascular problems, suffer from arthritis or other degenerative bone diseases (135).

Because muscle atrophy and weakness in the elderly have been linked to recurrent falls (a major cause of morbidity and mortality) (136), the need for specific resistance and flexibility exercises is often indicated. Several investigations have shown the feasibility and efficacy of resistance training in the elderly (137-139). Resistance training includes the same activities as described previously for MI and CABG patients but is typically performed with lighter weights and up to 15 or 20 repetitions. The use of variable-resistance machines may be initiated when the patient is clinically stable. However, because many elderly individuals have a limited ROM, it may be necessary to double-pin machines thereby avoiding excessive stress on muscles and joints (30).

As with younger patients, the progression of exercise depends on the older adult's initial level of fitness, medical condition, and need. However, progression is generally slower for the elderly patient. Warm-up and cool-down periods should be longer to allow the body more time to prepare for and recover from the activity. Exercise in hot environments should be avoided, since elderly patients often have impaired mechanisms of heat dissipation (140). More constant supervision may be needed during ambulation during the early phases of cardiac rehabilitation because of the high incidence of orthostatic hypotension and subsequent falls (30).

Patients With Peripheral Vascular Disease

Patients with PVD are often limited in their ambulation as a result of ischemic pain (claudication) in the legs. Typically, the pain disappears upon cessation of the activity.

Recommendations for exercise include both an interval-training method as well as daily exercise (24,141). Interval training may consist of several 1- to 5-min bouts of low-level aerobic exercise followed by 2 to 10 min of rest. As the patient progresses, longer periods of aerobic activity should be introduced, until the patient can sustain 30 to 60 min of continuous aerobic activity (24). Many PVD patients find the RPE scale a useful tool in rating their peripheral discomfort. Generally, when leg discomfort reaches 13 to 15 on the 15-point category RPE scale, patients should stop exercising and recover (34). Other investigators suggest continuous exercise at a level slightly below the onset of significant pain symptoms (grade II, or moderate on the angina scale) (30,142,143). A subjective rating of pain can be made by using the angina scale developed by the ACSM (24).

Grade I: Definite discomfort or pain, but only of initial or modest levels

Grade II: Moderate discomfort or pain from which the patient's attention can be diverted by a number of common stimuli

Grade III: Intense pain from which the patient's attention cannot be diverted, except by catastrophic events

Grade IV: Excruciating and unbearable pain

Depending on where the lesion is located, some patients may tolerate cycling better than walking. In this case a major portion of the exercise session should be performed on the cycle ergometer. However, because walking remains a significant form of transportation, some walking is also recommended (141-143). Alternative exercises during Phases II and III may include swimming and rowing. The progression and prescription of exercise during the initial stages of the exercise program should be guided by the patient's symptoms.

Patients With Left Ventricular Dysfunction

Historically, patients with LVD or CHF were not referred to cardiac rehabilitation programs. However, as a result of the improved medical management of patients with CHF and recent investigations showing the safety and efficacy of rehabilitation, more CHF patients are now enrolled in exercise programs (144-146).

Although the CHF patient generally has a low functional capacity, investigators have reported a lack of correlation between exercise time and the degree of LVD (147). More recent studies have clearly shown that alterations in peripheral mechanisms (impaired vasodilatory capacity of skeletal muscle, reduced aerobic enzyme activity, and increased pulmonary pressures) play a significant role in these patients' marked exercise intolerance (148-150). Because of these peripheral alterations, exercise has been suggested as a therapeutic modality for the CHF patient. The ACSM provides the following guidelines for exercise prescription for patients with LVD (24). In Phase I and early Phase II, interval training using 2- to 6-min low-level exercise bouts interspersed with 1- to 2-min rests or lower levels of training may be an appropriate method of exercise. An increase in the frequency of exercise may be required because of the patient's low level of fitness. Exercise prescriptions for the Phase II program should begin with moderate intensities of 40% to 60% of $\dot{V}O_2$max or should be adjusted to 10 beats/min below any significant signs or symptoms (e.g., angina, exertional hypotension, or complex dysrhythmias). The duration of training should be gradually increased depending on the patient's medical status and tolerance of the exercise. Because the HR response to exercise in the CHF patient may be impaired, the use of BP and ECG to monitor exercise may become more important. RPE responses during exercise should range from 12 to 14, and the use of a dyspnea scale may be indicated. Although ROM exercise would most often be appropriate with the CHF

patient, resistance training and stair-climbing activities may be contraindicated (24,93).

Many patients with CHF receive diuretic agents and other cardiovascular medications to control their condition. Chronic diuretic therapy results in alterations of electrolyte balance (hypokalemia and hypomagnesemia) which may precipitate complex ventricular dysrhythmias (151). In addition, because of left ventricular impairment, patients with CHF are prone to develop exercise-induced hypotension. Therefore, patients with LVD should be monitored continually and have prolonged warm-up and cool-down periods (30).

Transplant Patients

Transplant patients provide challenges to the cardiac rehabilitation staff because of altered hemodynamic characteristics, acute rejection episodes, and markedly reduced exercise capacities. Their low functional capacity is a result of extended periods of inactivity prior to the surgery, the surgical procedure (denervation and low hemoglobin), and the use of immunosuppressant drugs. Resting and exercise HRs in the denervated heart are elevated after surgery (152,153). The denervated heart adjusts more gradually to an exercise load and stays elevated longer during the recovery period. At the onset of exercise, the increase in cardiac output (Q) is primarily the result of an increase in SV augmented by the Frank-Starling mechanism. Later increases are mediated by greater levels of circulating catecholamines (152,154).

The inpatient exercise program for the transplant patient usually starts 3 to 7 days after surgery (30). The progression of the patient is usually slower, with the speed of ambulation or stationary cycling and repetitions of ROM activities lower than for the CABG patient. The prevalence of rejection in the first 3 months after surgery (155) may require the inpatient to exercise during the low-traffic hours of the day to avoid unnecessary contact with patients, visitors, and medical staff. As a result of the slower HR response, transplant patients require a longer warm-up period, and a more gradual increase in workload is necessary.

It is important to realize the effect of some of the immunosuppressant drugs. Cyclosporine may cause hypertension in many patients (156,157). Thus, careful monitoring of systolic and diastolic BP during the training sessions is needed to determine the safety of exercise (24). The effects of prednisone may have a significant impact on the patient's ability to exercise and adapt to training

(158). Prednisone decreases lean body weight (muscle mass and bone density) and affects electrolyte and fluid balance (24).

Exercise prescriptions in the Phase II and III programs include a frequency and duration of training of 3 to 5 days/week for 30 to 60 min/session. Since the HR response to exercise is altered in the denervated heart, the use of the standard HR methods of exercise prescription may not be appropriate. Therefore, exercise intensity should be based on the patient's $\dot{V}O_2$max (159). Generally, the intensity is set at 60% to 70% of the maximal METs achieved on an SL-GXT performed after the first 4 to 6 weeks of rehabilitation. As for the patients with LVD, the use of the RPE scale for the transplant patient is important. With the help of this scale, the exercise prescription based on the patient's maximal MET capacity can be fine tuned.

Summary

This chapter has described in detail how exercise is prescribed to cardiac patients in an inpatient (Phase I), outpatient (Phase II), and community-based (Phase III) or maintenance (Phase IV) program setting.

Inpatient programs for patients without complications usually begin 3 days after MI or 1 to 2 days after CABG. Programs are conducted at a low intensity and emphasize ROM exercise, ambulation, and normal activities of daily living (such as climbing stairs). Outpatient programs are recommended for at least 6 to 12 weeks after hospital discharge, followed by 3 to 6 months in a community-based program and a long-term maintenance program.

Stratification based on the patient's prognosis for future cardiovascular events and rate of survival during the first year following an MI or CABG is crucial. Patient stratification is a major determinant of the design of each patient's program in regard to the appropriateness of training; the type, duration, and intensity of the exercises prescribed; and the level of medical monitoring and supervision needed.

Standards for exercise prescription for each phase of rehabilitation have been recommended by the AHA, the ACSM and the AACVPR. Because of the physical limitations in cardiac patients, progression of exercise is slower, the intensity lower, the frequency greater, and the duration longer than in programs recommended for healthy individuals.

Training programs should be well rounded. Strength training should be included early in the recovery process (Phase II), so that the patient may be better prepared to carry out work and leisure activities. Additionally, ROM exercises should be implemented at each phase of rehabilitation, particularly in surgery patients.

References

1. Lewis, T. Diseases of the Heart. New York: Macmillan; 1933:41-49.
2. Levine, S.A.; Lown, B. The chair treatment of acute coronary thrombosis. Trans. Assoc. Am. Physicians. 64:316-327; 1951.
3. Cain, H.D.; Frasher, W.G.; Stivelman, R. Graded activity program for safe return to self-care after myocardial infarction. JAMA. 177:111-115; 1961.
4. Hellerstein, H.K.; Ford, A.B. Rehabilitation of the cardiac patient. JAMA. 164:225-231; 1957.
5. Naughton, J.; Bruhn, J.G.; Lategola, M.T. Effects of physical training on physiologic and behavorial characteristics of cardiac patients. Arch. Phys. Med. Rehabil. 49:131-137; 1968.
6. Karvonen, M.J.; Barry, A.J., eds. Physical activity and the heart. Springfield, IL: Charles C. Thomas; 1967.
7. O'Connor, G.T.; Buring, J.E.; Yusuf, S.; Goldhaber, S.Z.; Olmstead, E.M.; Paffenbarger, R.S.; Hennekens, C.H. An overview of randomized trials of rehabilitation with exercise after myocardial infarction. Circulation. 80:234-244; 1989.
8. Oldridge, N.B.; Guyatt, G.H.; Fisher, M.E.; Rimm, A.A. Cardiac rehabilitation after myocardial infarction: Combined experience of randomized clinical trials. JAMA. 260:945-950; 1988.
9. Berlin, J.A.; Colditz, G.A. A meta-analysis of physical activity in the prevention of coronary heart disease. Am. J. Epidemiol. 132:612-628; 1990.
10. Fletcher, G.F.; Blair, S.N.; Blumenthal, J.; Caspersen, C.; Chaitman, B.; Epstein, S.; Falls, H.; Froelicher, E.S.; Froelicher, V.F.; Pina, I.L. Statement on exercise: Benefits and recommendations for physical activity programs for all Americans: A statement for health professionals by the committee on exercise and cardiac rehabilitation of the council on clinical cardiology, American Heart Association. Circulation. 86:340-344; 1992.
11. Fox, S.M.; Naughton, J.P.; Haskell, W.L. Physical activity and the preventions of coronary heart disease. Ann. Clin. Res. 3:404-432; 1971.
12. Amsterdam, E.A.; Wilmore, J.H.; DeMaria, A.N., editors. Exercise in cardiovascular health and disease. New York: Yorke Medical Books; 1977.
13. Wenger, N.K.; Hellerstein, H.K., editors. Rehabilitation of the coronary patient, 3rd ed. New York: Churchill Livingstone; 1992.
14. Leon, A.S.; Blackburn, H. Exercise rehabilitation of the coronary heart disease patient. Geriatrics. 32:66-76; 1977.

15. Pollock, M.L.; Schmidt, D.H., editors. Heart disease and rehabilitation, 2nd ed. New York: Wiley; 1986.

16. Kallio, V.; Hamalainen, H.; Hakkila, J.; Luurila, O.J. Reduction in sudden deaths by a multifactorial intervention programme after acute myocardial infarction. Lancet. 2:1091-1094; 1979.

17. Taylor, H.L.; Henschel, A.; Brozek, J.; Keys, A. Effects of bed rest on cardiovascular function and work performance. J. Appl. Physiol. 2:233-239; 1949.

18. Saltin, B.; Blomqvist, G.; Mitchell, J.; Johnson, R.L.; Widenthal, K.; Chapman, C.B. Response to exercise after bed rest and after training. Circulation. 37, 38[Suppl. 7]:1-78; 1968.

19. Convertino, V.; Hung, J.; Goldwater, D.; DeBusk, R.F. Cardiovascular responses to exercise in middle-aged men after 10 days of bed rest. Circulation. 65:134-140; 1982.

20. Morgan, W.P.; Pollock, M.L. Physical activity and cardiovascular health: psychological aspects. In: Landry, F.; Orban, W.A.R., eds. Physical activity and human wellbeing. Miami,FL: Symposium Specialists; 1978:163-181.

21. Blumenthal, J.A. Psychologic assessment in cardiac rehabilitation. J. Cardiopul. Rehabil. 5:208-215; 1985.

22. Taylor, C.B.; Houston-Miller, N.; Ahn, D.K.; Haskell, W.; Debusk, R.F. The effects of exercise training programs on psychosocial improvement in uncomplicated postmyocardial infarction patients. J. Psychosom. Res. 30:581-587; 1986.

23. Fletcher, G.F.; Froelicher, V.F.; Hartley, L.H.; Haskell. W.L.; Pollock, M.L. Exercise standards: A statement for health professionals from the American heart association. Circulation. 82:2286-2322; 1990.

24. American College of Sports Medicine. Guidelines for graded exercise testing and exercise prescription, 4th ed. Philadelphia: Lea & Febiger; 1991.

25. American Association of Cardiovascular and Pulmonary Rehabilitation. Guidelines for cardiac rehabilitation programs. Champaign, IL: Human Kinetics; 1991.

26. Froelicher, V.F. Exercise and the heart: Clinical concepts, 2nd ed. Chicago: Year Book Medical; 1987.

27. DeBusk, R.F.; Blomqvist, C.G.; Kouchokos, N.T.; Luepker, R.W.; Miller, H.S.; Moss, A.J.; Pollock, M.L.; Reeves, T.J.; Sylvester, R.H.; Stason, W.B.; Wagner, G.S.; William, V.L. Identification and treatment of low-risk patients after acute myocardial infarction and coronary bypass graft surgery. N. Engl. J. Med. 314:161-166; 1986.

28. Greenland, P.; Chu, J. Position paper: Cardiac rehabilitation services. Ann. Intern. Med. 109:671-673; 1988.

29. Cheitlin, M.D. Finding the high risk patient with coronary heart disease. JAMA. 259:2271-2277; 1988.

30. Pollock, M.L.; Wilmore, J. Exercise in health and disease: Evaluation and prescription for prevention and rehabilitation. Philadelphia: Saunders; 1990:485-620.

31. Wenger, N.K. The physiological basis for early ambulation after myocardial infarction. In: Wenger, N.K., ed. Exercise and the heart. Philadelphia: Davis; 1978:107-116.

32. Kavanagh, T.; Shephard, R.J.; Doney, H.; Pandit, V. Intensive exercise in coronary rehabilitation. Med. Sci. Sports Exerc. 5:34-39; 1973.

33. Dion Faraher, W.; Grevenow, P.; Pollock, M.L.; Squires, R.W.; Foster, C.; Johnson, W.D.; Schmidt, D.H. Medical problems and physiologic responses during supervised inpatient cardiac rehabilitation: The patient after coronary bypass grafting. Heart Lung. 11:248-255; 1982.

34. Foster, C.; Pollock, M.L.; Anholm, J.D.; Squires, R.W.; Ward, A.; Dymond, D.S.; Rod, J.L.; Saichek, R.P.; Schmidt, D.H. Work capacity and left ventricular function during rehabilitation after myocardial revascularization surgery. Circulation. 69:748-755; 1984.

35. Erb, B.D.; Fletcher, G.F.; Scheffield, T.L. AHA committee report: Standards for cardiovascular exercise treatment programs. Circulation. 59:1084A-1090A; 1979.

36. Pollock, M.L.; Foster, C.; Knapp, D.; Schmidt, D.H. Cardiac rehabilitation program at Mount Sinai Medical Center, Milwaukee. J. Cardiac Rehabil. 2:458-463; 1982.

37. Pollock, M.L.; Pels, A.E.; Foster, C.; Ward, A. Exercise prescription for rehabilitation of the cardiac patient. In: Pollock, M.L.; Schmidt, D.H., eds. Heart disease and rehabilitation, 2nd ed. New York: Wiley; 1986:477-515.

38. Silvidi, G.E.; Squires, R.W.; Pollock, M.L.; Foster, C. Hemodynamic responses and medical problems associated with early exercise and ambulation in coronary artery bypass graft surgery patients. J. Cardiac Rehabil. 2:355-362; 1982.

39. Epstein, S.E.; Robinson, B.E.; Kahler, R.L.; Braunwald, E. Effects of beta-adrenergic blockade on the cardiac response to maximal and submaximal exercise in man. J. Clin. Invest. 44:1745-1753; 1965.

40. Tesch, P.A.; Kaiser, P. Effects of beta-adrenergic blockade on O_2 uptake during submaximal and maximal exercise. J. Appl. Physiol. 54:901-905; 1983.

41. Squires, R.W.; Rod, J.L.; Pollock, M.L.; Foster, C. Effect of propranolol on perceived exertion soon after myocardial revascularization surgery. Med. Sci. Sports Exerc. 14:276-280; 1982.

42. Borg, G.A.V. Psychophysical bases of perceived exertion. Med. Sci. Sports Exerc. 14:377-381; 1982.

43. Noble, B.J. Clinical applications of perceived exertion. Med. Sci. Sports Exerc. 14:406-411; 1982.

44. Pollock, M.L.; Jackson, A.S.; Foster, C. The use of the perception scale for exercise prescription. In: Borg, G.; Ottoson, D., eds. The perception of exertion in physical work. London: Macmillan; 1986:161-176.

45. Theroux, P.; Waters, D.D.; Halphen, C.; Debaisieux, J.C.; Mizgala, H.F. Prognostic value of exercise testing soon after myocardial infarction. N. Engl. J. Med. 301:342-345; 1979.

46. Fioretti, P.; Brower, R.W.; Simoons, M.L.; Das, S.K.; Bos, R.J.; Wijns, W.; Reiber, J.H.; Lubsen, J.; Hugenholtz, P.G. Prediction of mortality in hospital survivors of myocardial infarction. Comparison of predischarge exercise testing and radionuclide ventriculography at rest. Br. Heart J. 52:292-298; 1984.

47. Pollock, M.L.; Foster, C.; Rod, J.L.; Wible, G. Comparison of methods for determining exercise training intensity for cardiac patients and healthy adults. In: Kellerman, J.J., ed. Comprehensive cardiac rehabilitation. Basel, Switzerland: Karger; 1982:129-133.

48. Franklin, B.A.; Hellerstein, H.K.; Gordon, S.; Timmis, G.C. Exercise prescription for the myocardial infarction patient. J. Cardiac Rehabil. 6:62-79; 1986.

49. Metier, C.P.; Pollock, M.L.; Graves, J.E. Exercise prescription for the coronary artery bypass graft surgery patient. J. Cardiac Rehabil. 6:236-242; 1986.

50. Karvonen, M.; Kentala, K.; Musta, O. The effect of training heart rate: A longitudinal study. Ann. Med. Exp. Biol. Fenn. 35:307-315; 1957.

51. Wilmore, J.H.; Haskell, W. Use of the heart rate energy expenditure relationship in the individualized prescription of exercise. Am. J. Clin. Nutr. 24:1186-1192; 1971.

52. American College of Sports Medicine: The recommended quantity and quality of exercise for developing and maintaining cardiorespiratory and muscle fitness in healthy adults. Med. Sci. Sports Exerc. 22:265-274; 1990.

53. Morgan, W.P. Psychophysiology of self-awareness during vigorous physical activity. Res. Q. Exerc. Sport. 52:385-427; 1981.

54. Pollock, M.L.; Wilmore, J.H.; Fox, S.M. Health and fitness through physical activity. New York: Wiley; 1978.

55. Fox, S.M.; Naughton, J.P.; Gorman, P.A. Physical activity and cardiovascular health II. The exercise prescription: intensity and duration. Mod. Concepts Cardiovasc. Dis. 16:21-24; 1972.

56. Roy, B.A. A model for determining exercise intensity in coronary artery disease patients. Med. Sci. Sports Exerc. 24:s114; 1992.

57. Wasserman, K.; Whipp, B.J.; Koyal, S.N.; Beaver, W.L. Anaerobic threshold and respiratory gas exchange during exercise. J. Appl. Physiol. 35:236-243; 1973.

58. Davis, J.A. Anaerobic threshold: Review of the concept and directions of future research. Med. Sci. Sports Exerc. 17:6-18; 1985.

59. Hamm, L.F.; Leon, A.S. Exercise training for the coronary patient. In: Wenger, N.K.; Hellerstein, H.K., eds. Rehabilitation of the coronary patient. 3rd ed. New York: Churchill Livingstone; 1992: 367-402.

60. Morgan, R.E.; Adamson, G.T. Circuit weight training. London: Bell; 1961.

61. Gettman, L.R.; Pollock, M.L. Circuit weight training: A critical review of its physiological benefits. Phys. Sportsmed. 9:44-60; 1981.

62. Pollock, M.L.; Dimmick, J.; Miller, H.S., Jr.; Kendrick, Z.; Linnerud, A.C. Effect of mode of training on cardiovascular function and body composition of middle-aged men. Med. Sci. Sports Exerc. 7:139-145; 1975.

63. Sharkey, B.J.; Holleman, J.P. Cardiorespiratory adaptations to training at specified intensities. Res. Q. 38:698-704; 1967.

64. Jette, M.; Sidney, K.; Campbell, J. Effects of a twelve-week walking program on maximal and sub-maximal work output indices in sedentary middle-aged men and women. J. Sports Med. 28:59-66; 1988.

65. Pollock, M.L. Prescribing exercise for fitness and adherence. In: Dishman, R.K., ed. Exercise adherence: Its impact on public health. Champaign, IL.: Human Kinetics; 1988.

66. Haskell, W.L.; Montoye, H.J.; Orenstein, D. Physical activity and exercise to achieve health-related physical fitness components. Public Health Rep. 100:202-212; 1985.

67. Cooper, K.H. The new aerobics. New York: Lippincott; 1970.

68. Cureton, T.K. The physiological effects of exercise programs upon adults. Springfield, IL: Charles C Thomas; 1969.

69. Zarandora, J.E.; Nelson, A.G.; Conlee, R.K.; Fisher, A.G. Physiological responses to hand-carried weights. Phys. Sportsmed. 14:113-120; 1986.

70. Graves, J.E.; Pollock, M.L.; Montain, S.J.; Jackson, A.S.; O'Keefe, J.M. The effect of hand-held weights on the physiological responses to walking exercise. Med. Sci. Sports Exerc. 19:260-265; 1987.

71. Auble, T.E.; Schwartz, L.; Robertson, R.J. Aerobic requirements for moving handweights through various range of motion while walking. Phys. Sportsmed. 15:133-140; 1987.

72. Graves, J.E.; Martin, A.D.; Miltenberger, L.A.; Pollock, M.L. Physiological responses to walking with hand weights, wrist weights and ankle weights. Med. Sci. Sports Exerc. 20:265-271; 1988.

73. Graves, J.E.; Sagiv, M.E.; Pollock, M.L.; Miltenberger, L.A. Effect of hand-held weights and wrist weights on the metabolic and hemodynamic responses to submaximal exercise in hypertensive responders. J. Cardiac Rehabil. 8:134-140; 1988.

74. Borysyk, L.M.; Franklin, B.; Gordon, S.; Timmis, G.C. Minimal increases in aerobic requirement while walk training with hand weights. Med. Sci. Sports Exerc. 18:598; 1986.

75. Haskell, W.L. Cardiovascular complications during training of cardiac patients. Circulation. 57:920-924; 1974.

76. Hossack, K.F.; Hartwig, R. Cardiac arrest associated with supervised cardiac rehabilitation. J. Cardiac Rehabil. 2:402-408; 1982.

77. Shephard, R.J.: Cardiac rehabilitation in prospect. In: Pollock, M.L.; Schmidt, D.H., eds. Heart disease and rehabilitation, 2nd ed. New York; Wiley; 1986:713-740.

78. Pollock, M.L.; Carroll, J.F.; Graves, J.E.; Leggett, S.H.; Braith, R.W.; Limacher, M.; Hagberg, J.M. Injuries and adherence to walk/jog and resistance training programs in the elderly. Med. Sci. Sports Exerc. 23:1194-1200; 1991.

79. Faria, I.E.; Cavanagh. P.R. The physiology and biomechanics of cycling. New York: Wiley; 1978.

80. Secher, N.H.; Ruberg-Larsen, N.; Binkhorst, R.A.; Bond-Peterson, F. Maximal oxygen uptake during arm cranking and combined arm plus leg exercise. J. Appl. Physiol. 36:515-516; 1974.

81. Gleim, G.W.; Coplan, N.L.; Scandura, M.; Holly, T.; Nicholas, J.A. Rate pressure product at equivalent oxygen consumption on four different exercise modalities. J. Cardiac Rehabil. 8:270-275; 1988.

82. Toner, M.M.; Sawka, M.N.; Levine, L.; Pandolf, K.B. Cardiorespiratory responses to exercise distributed between the upper and lower body. J. Appl. Physiol. 54:1403-1407; 1983.

83. Sawka, M.N. Physiology of upper body exercise. In: Pandolf, K.B., ed. Exercise and sports science reviews, vol. 14. New York: Macmillan; 1986:175-211.

84. Franklin, B.A. Aerobic exercise training programs for the upper body. Med. Sci. Sports Exerc. 21:s141-s148; 1989.

85. Franklin, B.A.; Vander, L.; Wrisley, D.; Rubenfire, M. Aerobic requirements of arm ergometry: Implications for exercise testing and training. Phys. Sportsmed. 11:81-90; 1983.

86. Fardy, P.S.; Webb, D.; Hellerstein, H.K. Benefits of arm exercise in cardiac rehabilitation. Phys. Sportsmed. 5:30-41; 1977.

87. Magder, S.; Linnarson, D.; Gullstrand, L. The effect of swimming on patients with ischemic heart disease. Circulation. 63:979-986; 1981.

88. Thompson, D.L.; Boone, T.W.; Miller, H.S. Comparison of treadmill exercise and tethered swimming to determine validity of exercise prescription. J. Cardiac Rehabil. 2:363-370; 1982.

89. McMurray, R.G.; Fieselman, C.C.; Avery, K.E.; Shops, D.S. Exercise hemodynamics in water and on land in patients with coronary artery disease. J. Cardiac Rehabil. 8:69-75; 1988.

90. Heigenhauser, G.F.; Boulet, D.; Miller, B.; Faulkner, J.A. Cardiac outputs of post myocardial infarction patients during swimming and cycling. Med. Sci. Sports Exerc. 9:143-147; 1977.

91. Verstraete, R.; Ben-Ezra, V. Submaximal cardiovascular response to positive stair climbing and treadmill walking in cardiac patients, abstracted. Med. Sci. Sports Exerc. 19:s57; 1987.

92. Holland, G.J.; Weber, F.; Heng, M.K.; Reese, S.S.; Marin, J.J.; Vincent, W.J.; Mayers, M.M.; Hoffman, J.J.; Caston, A.L. Maximal steptreadmill exercise and treadmill exercise by patients with coronary heart disease: A comparison. J. Cardiac Rehabil. 8:58-68; 1988.

93. Reddy, H.K.; McElroy, P.A.; Janicki, J.S.; Weber, K.T. Response in oxygen uptake and ventilation during stair climbing in patients with chronic heart failure. Am. J. Cardiol. 63:222-225; 1989.

94. Asmussen, E. Similarities and dissimilarities between static and dynamic exercise. Circ. Res. 48[Suppl I]:3-10; 1981.

95. Painter, P.; Hanson, P. Isometric exercise: Implications for the cardiac patient. Cardiovasc. Rev. Reports. 5:261-279; 1984.

96. Lind, A.R.; McNichol, G.W. Muscular factors which determine the cardiovascular responses to sustained and rhythmic exercise. Can. Med. Assoc. J. 96:706-713; 1967.

97. Mitchell, J.H.; Blomqvist, C.G. Response of patients with heart disease to dynamic and static exercise. In Pollock, M.L.; Schmidt, D.H., eds. Heart disease and rehabilitation, 2nd ed. New York: Wiley; 1986: 85-95.

98. Blomqvist, C.G.; Lewis, S.F.; Taylor, W.F.; Graham, R.M. Similarity of the hemodynamic responses to static and dynamic exercise of small muscle groups. Circ. Res. 48[Suppl I]:87-92; 1981.

99. Lewis, S.F.; Taylor, W.F.; Graham, R.M.; Pettinger, W.A.; Schutte, J.E.; Blomqvist, C.G. Cardiovascular responses to exercise as functions of absolute and relative workload. J. Appl. Physiol. 54:1314-1323; 1983.

100. Lewis, S.F.; Snell, P.G.; Taylor, W.F.; Hamra, M.; Graham, R.M.; Pettinger, W.A.; Blomqvist, C.G. Role of muscle mass and mode of contraction in circulatory responses to exercise. J. Appl. Physiol. 58:146-151; 1985.

101. Bezucha, G.R.; Lenser, M.C.; Hanson, P.G.; Nagle, F.J. Comparison of hemodynamic responses to static and dynamic exercise. J. Appl. Physiol. 53: 1589-1593; 1982.

102. Atkins, J.M.; Matthews, O.A.; Blomqvist, C.G.; Mullins, C.B. Incidence of arrhythmias induced by isometric and dynamic exercise. Br. Heart J. 38:465-471; 1976.

103. Debusk, R.F.; Valdez, R.; Houston, N.; Haskell, W. Cardiovascular responses to dynamic and static effort soon after myocardial infarction. Application to occupational work assessment. Circulation 58: 368-375; 1978.

104. Vander, L.B.; Franklin, B.A.; Wrisley, D.; Rubenfire, M. Acute cardiovascular responses to Nautilus exercise in cardiac patients: Implications for exercise training. Ann. Sports Med. 2:165-169; 1986.

105. Keleman, M.H.; Stewart, K.J.; Gillilan, R.E.; Ewart, C.K.; Valenti, S.A.; Manley, J.D.; Kelemen, M.D. Circuit weight training in cardiac patients. J. Am. Coll. Cardiol. 7:38-42; 1986.

106. Butler, R.M.; Beierwaltes, W.H.; Rodgers, F.J. The cardiovascular response to circuit weight training in patients with cardiac diseases. J. Cardiac Rehabil. 7:402-409; 1987.

107. Harris, K.A.; Holly, R.G. Physiological response to circuit weight training in hypertensive subjects. Med. Sci. Sports Exerc. 19:246-252; 1987.

108. Haslam, D.R.S.; McCartney, N.; McKelvie, R.S.; MacDougall, J.D. Direct measurements of arterial blood pressure during formal weightlifting in cardiac patients. J. Cardiac Rehabil. 8:213-225; 1988.

109. Ferguson, R.J.; Cote, P.; Bourassa, M.G.; Corbara, F. Coronary blood flow during isometric and dynamic exercise in angina pectoris patients. J. Cardiac Rehabil. 1:21-26; 1981.

110. Stewart, K.J.; Mason, M.; Kelemen, M.H. Three year participation in circuit weight training improves muscular strength and self-efficacy in cardiac patients. J. Cardiac Rehabil. 8:292-296; 1988.

111. Ghilarducci, L.E.; Holly, R.G.; Amsterdam, E.A. Effects of high resistance training in coronary artery disease. Am. J. Cardiol. 64:866-870; 1989.

112. Squires, R.W.; Muri, A.J.; Anderson , L.J.; Allison, T.G.; Miller, T.D.; Gau, G.T. Weight training during phase II (early outpatient) cardiac rehabilitation: Heart rate and blood pressure responses. J. Cardiac Rehabil. 11:360-364; 1991.

113. Graves, J.E.; Pollock, M.L. Exercise testing in cardiac rehabilitation: Role in prescribing exercise. Cardiology Clinics. 11(2):253-266; 1993.

114. Verrill, D.; Shoup, E.; McElveen, G.; Witt, K.; Bergey, D. Resistive exercise training in cardiac patients. Sports Med. 13:171-193; 1992.

115. Graves, J.E.; Pollock, M.L.; Jones, A.E.; Colvin, A.B.; Leggett, S.H. Specificity of limited range of motion variable resistance training. Med. Sci. Sports Exerc. 21:84-89; 1989.

116. Braith, R.W.; Graves, J.E.; Pollock, M.L.; Leggett, S.L.; Carpenter, D.M.; Colvin, A.B. Comparison of two versus three days per week of variable resistance training during 10 and 18 week programs. Int. J. Sports Med. 10:450-454; 1989.

117. Graves, J.E.; Pollock, M.L.; Leggett, S.L.; Braith, R.W.; Carpenter, D.M.; Bishop, L.E. Effect of reduced training frequency on muscular strength. Int. J. Sports Med. 9:316-319; 1988.

118. Wescott, W.L. Strength fitness: Physiological principles and training techniques, 2nd ed. Boston: Allyn & Bacon; 1987.

119. Ewing, D.J.; Kerr, F.; Leggett, R. Interaction between cardiovascular responses to sustained handgrip and Valsalva manoeuvre. Br. Heart J. 38:483-490; 1976.

120. Lentini, A.C.; McKelvie, R.S.; McCartney, N.; Tomlinson, C.W.; MacDougall, J.D. Left ventricular response in healthy young men during heavy-intensity weight lifting exercise. J. Appl. Physiol: In press.

121. MacDougall, J.D.; Tuxen, D.; Sale, D.G.; Moroz, J.R.; Sutton, J.R. Arterial blood pressure response to heavy resistance exercise. J. Appl. Physiol. 58:785-790; 1985.

122. Hurley, B.F.; Seals, D.R.; Ehsahni, A.A.; Cartier, L.J.; Dalsky, G.P.; Hagberg, J.M.; Holloszy, J.O. Effects of high-intensity training on cardiovascular function. Med. Sci. Sports Exerc. 16:483-488; 1984.

123. Ehsani, A.A.; Heath, G.H.; Hagberg, J.M.; Sobel, B.E.; Holloszy, J.O. Effects of 12 months of intense exercise training on ischemic ST-segment depression in patients with coronary artery disease. Circulation. 64:1116-1124; 1981.

124. Ehsani, A.A.; Biello, D.R.; Schultz, J.; Sobel, B.E.; Holloszy, J.O. Improvement of left ventricular contractile function by exercise training in patients with coronary artery disease. Circulation. 74:350-358; 1986.

125. Martin, W.H.; Ehsani, A.A. Reversal of exertional hypotension by prolonged exercise training in selected patients with ischemic heart disease. Circulation. 76:548-555; 1987.

126. Rodgers, M.A.; Yamamoto, C.; Hagberg, J.M.; Holloszy, J.O.; Ehsani, A.A. The effects of 7 years of intense exercise training on patients with coronary artery disease. J. Am. Coll. Cardiol. 10:321-326; 1987.

127. Hagberg, J.M.; Ehsani, A.A.; Holloszy, J.O. Effects of 12 months of intense exercise training on stroke volume in patients with coronary artery disease. Circulation. 67:1194-1199; 1983.

128. Barnard, R.J.; Gardner, G.W.; Diaco, N.V.; MacAlpin, R.N.; Kattus, A.A. Cardiovascular responses to sudden strenuous exercise-heart rate, blood pressure, and ECG. J. Appl. Physiol. 34:833-837; 1973.

129. Foster, C.; Anholm, J.D.; Hellman, C.K.; Carpenter, J.; Pollock, M.L.; Schmidt, D.H. Left ventricular function during sudden strenuous exercise. Circulation. 63:592-596; 1981.

130. Dimsdale, J.E.; Hartley, L.H.; Guiney, T.; Ruskin, J.N.; Greenblatt, D. Postexercise peril: Plasma catecholamines and exercise. JAMA. 251:630-632.

131. American College of Cardiology/American Heart Association. Guidelines for percutaneous transluminal coronary angioplasty. Circulation. 78:486-502; 1988.

132. King, S.B. Current status of percutaneous transluminal coronary angioplasty. Cardiovasc. Rev. Reports. 9:27-32; 1988.

133. Maresh, C.M.; Harbrecht, J.J.; Flick, B.L.; Hartzler, G.O. Comparison of rehabilitation benefits after percutaneous transluminal coronary angioplasty. J. Cardiac Rehabil. 5:124-130; 1985.

134. Panton, L.B.; Graves, J.E.; Garzarella, L.; Carroll, J.F.; Pollock, M.L.; Leggett, S.H.; Guillen, G.; Lowenthal, D.T. Relative heart rate, heart rate reserve, and oxygen uptake during exercise in the elderly. Med. Sci. Sports Exerc. 24:s185; 1992.

135. Wolfel, E.E.; Hossack, K.F. Guidelines for the exercise training of elderly healthy individuals and elderly patients with cardiac disease. J. Cardiac Rehabil. 9:40-45; 1990.

136. Baker, S.P.; Harvey, A.H. Fall injuries in the elderly. Clin. Geriatr. Med. 1:501-512; 1985.

137. Fiatarone, M.A.; Marks, E.C.; Ryan, N.D.; Meredith, C.N.; Lipsitz, L.A.; Evans, W.J. High-intensity

strength training in nonagenarians: Effects on skeletal muscle. JAMA. 263:3029-3034; 1990.

138. Frontera, W.R.; Meredith, C.N.; O'Reilly, K.P.; Knuttgen, H.J.; Evans, W.J. Strength conditioning in older men: Skeletal muscle hypertrophy and improved function. J. Appl. Physiol. 64:1038-1044; 1988.

139. Panton, L.B.; Graves, J.E.; Pollock, M.L.; Hagberg, J.M.; Leggett, S.H. Effect of aerobic and variable resistance exercise training on strength and body composition of men and women 70-79 years of age. Int. J. Sports Med. 10(2):147; 1989.

140. Williams, M.A.; Esterbrooks, D.J.; Sketch, M.H. Guidelines for exercise therapy of the elderly after myocardial infarction. Eur. Heart J. 5:121-123; 1984.

141. Hall, J.A.; Barnard, R.J. The effects of an intensive 26-day program of diet and exercise on patients with peripheral vascular disease. J. Cardiac Rehabil. 2:569-574; 1982.

142. Boyd, C.E.; Bird, P.J.; Charles, C.D.; Wellons, H.A.; MacDougall, M.A.; Wolfe, L.A. Pain free physical training in intermittent claudication. J. Sports Med. 24:112-122; 1984.

143. Ernst, E.E.; Matrai, A. Intermittent claudication, exercise and blood rheology. Circulation. 76:1110-1114; 1987.

144. Sullivan, M.J.; Higginbotham, M.B.; Cobb, F.R. Exercise training in patients with severe left ventricular dysfunction. Hemodynamic and metabolic effects. Circulation. 78:506-515; 1988.

145. Sullivan, M.J.; Higginbotham, M.B.; Cobb, F.R. Exercise training in patients with chronic heart failure delays ventilatory anaerobic threshold and improves submaximal exercise performance. Circulation.79:324-329; 1989.

146. Minotti, J.R.; Johnson, E.C.; Hudson, T.L.; Zuroske, G.; Murata, G.; Fukushima, E.; Cagle, T.G.; Chick, T.W.; Massie, B.M.; Icenogle, M.V. Skeletal muscle response to exercise training in congestive heart failure. J. Clin. Invest. 86:751-758; 1990.

147. Franciosa, J.A.; Ziesche, S.; Wilen, M. Functional capacity of patients with chronic left ventricular failure: Relationship of bicycle exercise performance to clinical and hemodynamic characterization. Am. J. Med. 67:460-466; 1979.

148. Massie, B.; Conway, M.; Yonge, R.; Frostick, S.; Ledingham, J.; Sleight, P.; Radda, G.; Rajagopalan, B. Skeletal muscle metabolism in patients with congestive heart failure: Relation to clinical severity and blood flow. Circulation. 76(5):1009-1019; 1987.

149. Lipkin, D.P.; Jones, D.A.; Round, J.M.; Poole-Wilson, P.A. Abnormalities of skeletal muscle in patients with chronic heart failure. Int. J. Cardiol. 18:187-195; 1988.

150. Drexler, H. Reduced exercise tolerance in chronic heart failure and its relationship to neurohumoral factors. Eur. Heart J. 12[Suppl. C]:21-28; 1991.

151. Lowenthal, D.T.; Kendrick, Z.V.; Chase, R.; Paran, E.; Perlmutter, G. Cardiovascular drugs and exercise. Exerc. Sport Sci. Rev. 15:67-94; 1987.

152. Savin, W.; Haskell, W.; Schroeder, J.; Stinson, E. Cardiorespiratory responses of cardiac transplant patients to graded, symptom-limited exercise. Circulation. 62:55-60; 1980.

153. Kavanagh, T.; Yacoub, M.; Mertens, D.; Kennedy, J.; Campbell, R.; Sawyer, P. Cardiorespiratory responses to exercise training after orthotopic cardiac transplantion. Circulation. 77:162-171; 1987.

154. Pope, S.E.; Stinson, E.B.; Daughters, G.T.; Schroeder, J.S.; Ingels, N.B.; Alderman, E.L. Exercise response of the denervated heart in long-term cardiac transplant recipients. Am. J. Cardiol. 46:213-218; 1980.

155. Murdock, D.; Collins, E.; Lawless, C.; Molnar, Z.; Scanlon, P.; Pifarre, R. Rejection of the transplanted heart. Heart Lung. 16:237-245; 1987.

156. Schroeder, J.S.; Hunt, S. Cardiac transplantation update 1987. JAMA. 258:3142-3145; 1987.

157. Greenberg, M.; Uretsky, B.; Reddy, P.; Bernstein, R.; Griffith, B.; Hardesty, R.; Thompson, M.; Bahnson, H. Long-term hemodynamic follow-up of cardiac transplant patients treated with cyclosporine and prednisone. Circulation. 71:487-494; 1985.

158. Ramey, E.R. Corticosteroids and skeletal muscle. In: Blaschko, H.; Soyers, G.; Smith, A.D., eds. Handbook of physiology 6. Washington, DC: American Physiological Society; 1975:245-261.

159. Squires, R.W. Exercise training after cardiac transplantation. Med. Sci. Sports Exerc. 23:686-694; 1991.

Chapter 18

Patient Education: Practical Guidelines

Marian Hansen
Mary M. Streff

Most cardiac rehabilitation professionals would confirm that patient education is an integral part of their programs. The lifestyle changes needed to reduce the risk of coronary artery disease (CAD) can be extremely difficult. Maintaining an exercise program, stopping smoking, changing food patterns to control weight or lipids, and successfully managing stress require complex changes in habits that patients have had since early childhood. The educational focus goes beyond knowledge acquisition to helping patients change attitudes and acquire the behavioral skills needed to alter entrenched habits. The ultimate goal is a heart-healthy lifestyle for each patient.

The excellent *Guidelines for Cardiac Rehabilitation Programs*, published by the American Association of Cardiovascular and Pulmonary Rehabilitation (AACVPR) (1), offers definitive listings of educational topics and services. Rather than repeat those recommendations, we will focus on theory and practical suggestions for the process of teaching patients and for understanding the roles of learner and teacher. Many of the individual points deserve longer discussion, so references are offered for further study.

Understanding the Adult Learner

Knowles (2) asserts that adults learn in different patterns than children. Because of their extensive backgrounds and independence, adults bring more to a learning experience and have different expectations than children. Padberg and Padberg (3) discuss the application of Knowles's four principles of adult learning to patient education settings:

Adult learners need an active and controlling role in deciding what will be learned. They have a deep psychological need to see themselves, and have others see them, as independent or self-reliant. Patients' needs are best served when independence and self-direction in learning are respected and promoted.

Learning improves when the material is relevant to a learner's experience. As an individual matures, an expanding reservoir of experience accumulates and becomes an increasingly rich resource for learning. Adults use the experiences they have accumulated over a lifetime to improve learning by building bridges from the known to the unknown, so that new learning is related to a broad base of previous knowledge. In a patient education setting, therefore, the patient's personal background and history can provide multiple opportunities for drawing upon past experience as a resource for learning. Two challenges arise from this principle. First, patients may have misconceptions because of incorrectly linking information received in the past with new information. Second, they may need help in "unfreezing" unhealthy behaviors that stem from years of acquired fixed habits and thought patterns.

Like children, adults usually have phases of growth with corresponding developmental tasks. The developmental tasks of adult years arise from the evolution of social roles within family, work, and community environments. In the middle adult years, for example, developmental tasks might include maintaining an economic standard of living, relating to a spouse, assisting children to become responsible and happy adults, and developing adult leisure-time activities. Usually, adults want to learn information that will help them perform these roles better. The onset of illness interrupts and changes all these roles; the developmental tasks may be harder to accomplish.

Cardiac events may even push a few patients into new tasks that are developmentally older than their chronological years. A middle-aged patient with severe cardiac disease could face developmental tasks from senior years, such as adjusting to decreasing strength, reduced income, or retirement. Cardiac rehabilitation goals are to facilitate patients' returning to their previous roles and developmental tasks and to help them learn to cope with the new challenges.

Adults are most motivated to learn what is immediately applicable in their life setting. They learn largely in response to pressures they feel from problems in life. Although it would appear that patients in a cardiac rehabilitation program have obvious learning needs in common, patients should be assessed as individuals and information tailored to specific needs. Patients also may need help understanding how certain information is linked to their needs, as they often do not see their behavior as unhealthy and are yet not open to new information.

The Learner's Need for Goal Setting

Most participants motivated enough to start a cardiac rehabilitation program have goals in mind. Unfortunately, the patient who starts out motivated does not always stay motivated. Without structured goal setting between the participant and staff at the beginning of a program, it is difficult to help the patient refocus on preset goals and learning needs when motivation begins to fade.

Learning Needs

Wingate (4) investigated patients' perceptions of their learning needs after a myocardial infarction in the coronary care unit (CCU), post-CCU, and at home, through the use of a Cardiac Patient Learning Needs Inventory that listed eight learning categories. In the CCU, patients identified risk factors, anatomy and physiology, and physical activity as important learning needs; after release from the CCU, they selected anatomy and physiology, risk factors, and medications; at home, patients ranked risk factors first, followed by medications and anatomy and physiology. These findings are similar to three other studies using the same inventory (4).

Patients usually have some expectations of what they need and wish to learn. Assessment of the individual's perceived goals and learning needs is crucial. Educators also expect that patients "should" learn certain information. Helping patients to be open to information on unhealthy behaviors requires skill and sensitivity from the educator. Blending the learner's and educator's goals is essential for a successful educational outcome. One possible method for achieving this individualized goal setting is the Outcome Model.

Outcome Model

Girdano and Dusek (5) developed an Outcome Model to be used with clients in the beginning of a health behavior change program. "Clients have a reason for being there, they want something, and no work can be done until they identify what they want (5)." A fundamental principle of the model is that goal statements should be written in positive terms; it is easier to visualize and find the resources to work toward something positive than it is to eliminate something negative. The Outcome Model has six basic steps, presented in the form of questions to ask the client:

1. What do you want?
2. How will things be different or better in your life?
3. What will you accept as proof that you have what you want?
4. What are your useful resources?
5. What has kept you from doing this before?
6. What is your plan of action?

The educator who uses this type of model will promote and enhance self-direction of the learner and will gain insight as to where to focus learning activities. The patient's answers to these questions can also signal to the educator when the patient's expectations of self or the program are unrealistic. The educator can provide feedback and help to shape the goals realistically. For example, a patient who wants to "lose twenty pounds" during a short program needs help to focus on what changes are achievable and what plan of action will produce a reasonable outcome. Girdano and Dusek offer many additional techniques to use within the Outcome Model process (5).

Personal Factors That Affect the Patient as Learner

Many factors affect an individual's ability to achieve the planned learning outcome. When educating about lifestyle changes, the health professional needs to develop an understanding of the learner's ability to absorb the information and adopt the necessary changes. A few of the theories that can help us better understand this process are readiness to change, self-efficacy, self-esteem, and learning styles.

Readiness

Readiness to learn has been conceptualized as one point in time when the learner is open to hearing new information. Girdano and Dusek conceptualize readiness as a continuum of change behaviors. Their definition of readiness is helpful in the cardiac rehabilitation setting: "Readiness is the possession of behaviors, attitudes, skills, and concomitant resources that make it possible for individuals to incorporate a new health behavior into a permanent lifestyle (5)." Girdano and Dusek have developed a Readiness Scale using 10 observable steps that show a progression from knowledge gathering and understanding to complete adoption of the new behavior into the lifestyle. After succeeding in learning the skills of one step, an individual is ready to move on to the next. The 10 steps are as follows:

1. Understands the concepts
2. Values the change, verbalizes as good or right
3. Believes new behavior is possible
4. Visualizes new behavior with low ambiguity
5. Believes in ability to change behavior
6. Can see proof of attainment
7. Possesses new skills
8. Practices skills on regular basis
9. Practices skills in real-life situation
10. Adopts new behavior as lifestyle—without thinking about it

In assessing a patient's readiness for behavior change, the educator can look for cues as to where the person is on the continuum and use the scale to help the learner increase readiness for change. The learner and educator should consider movement through the readiness stages toward the outcome as criteria for success. For example, some patients who are trying to quit smoking do not succeed on their first try. However, if they can be helped to see in a positive way what they have learned about themselves and their habit, they will have moved up on the Readiness Scale and should be more likely to succeed with the next attempt. They should be able to more accurately anticipate what skills they will need to quit.

Self-Efficacy

The third step of the Readiness Scale, "Believes new behavior is possible," is defined as an "internalization that the behavior is possible to achieve and that the behavior, once learned, will result in a new or different and better lifestyle (5)." This definition is very similar to self-efficacy as defined in Bandura's social learning theory (6). Self-efficacy has two components: (1) an outcome expectancy, a person's estimate that a given behavior will lead to certain outcomes, and (2) an efficacy expectation, the conviction that one can successfully execute the behavior required to produce the outcomes. Self-efficacy has been remarkably predictive of whether the individual will actually carry out a behavior. This theory has been tested in the cardiac rehabilitation setting (7-10), for risk factor modification (11), and for other areas of behavior (6,12). Ratings of perceived self-efficacy can help identify individuals at risk of relapse behavior. Low self-efficacy measures in situation-specific areas can identify high-risk situations, and strategies can be targeted toward those behaviors (12). Four sources of information influence self-efficacy expectations, all of which can be used in the learning process.

Physiological cues and emotional arousal. People evaluate their abilities based on their perceptions of strength, capability, and vulnerability. Anxiety is an indicator of vulnerability and low self-esteem; high anxiety impedes learning and can block the development of coping skills. Strategies directed toward reducing the learner's anxiety are important to improving self-efficacy and learning. Self-efficacy can also be improved by strategies that provide feedback on the patient's physiological state (9).

Verbal persuasion. If the learner has some belief in his or her capabilities, the educator can use verbal persuasion, such as in the form of teaching materials, to help the learner achieve a goal. The sooner the learning is reinforced by true mastery, the more likely it is that the behavior will persist.

Vicarious experience or modeling. Seeing others perform the desired behavior successfully provides the learner with hope and ideas on how to achieve the behavior. This vicarious experience is frequently used in cardiac rehabilitation settings, as patients newly admitted to programs set their expectations based on the behavior of patients ready to be discharged. Modeling is the information source being used when former patients visit new patients to answer questions about the long-term outcome of a cardiac event.

Mastery. The best source of information to improve self-efficacy is actually performing the behavior successfully. Once the learner accomplishes this, the behavior is much more likely to be repeated. Educators can use this source of information by helping the learner break down the behavior into small, achievable steps. Patients may choose to modify an easier risk factor before moving on to one that they feel is more difficult. Once mastery of the smaller steps is accomplished, the learner feels more able to move on to the next step.

Self-Esteem

When patients feel a widespread inability to accomplish behavior change, they are often suffering from low self-esteem. McGlashan (13) defines self-esteem as an individual's self-evaluation, the extent to which an individual feels capable, significant, and worthy. Individuals with low self-esteem feel worthless, helpless, and incapable of controlling their lives. They are less motivated to learn and try a behavior change because they cannot visualize a positive outcome. Indicators for low self-esteem are a sensitivity to criticism, a tendency to blame others, a hypercritical attitude, feelings of persecution, and fear of competing with others (5). High self-esteem is a positive resource state that can be tapped in every learning situation, a general "I can learn, I can change" attitude. Learners with high self-esteem respect themselves, recognize their limitations, and expect to grow and improve. They perceive themselves as worthwhile and equal to others and are generally more self-confident, less anxious, and more effective in meeting environmental demands.

A cardiac event often threatens patients' self-esteem. It challenges their ability to master or at least cope with a situation that may be out of their control. McGlashan lists several strategies to help rebuild cardiac patients' self-esteem (13):

- Establish trust
- Inspire hope
- Promote self-care
- Display nonverbal reassurance
- Enhance knowledge
- Encourage healthy support systems
- Provide encouragement and positive feedback
- Promote laughter and humor

Other resources list additional techniques for improving self-esteem (5). Self-esteem strategies can help patients master their current situations and build a positive resource state for future situations.

Preferred Learning Style

People learn in different ways. Merritt (14) developed a Patient Learning Style Questionnaire, based on Canfield's model of learning style, to identify preferences of 125 patients with CAD in both the inpatient and outpatient settings. The majority of patients preferred structured teaching situations, defined as organized instruction with detailed information about learning requirements. Preferred methods of learning were oral presentations accompanied by pictorial, graphic modalities. The significance of this study is not that all patients should be taught using the method preferred by this sample, but that a variety of methods should be available and the method chosen according to the patient's preferred learning style. In addition, the fact that reading was not often identified as a preferred method should raise a note of caution, since most educators rely heavily on written materials when short of time and staff. When written materials are used, they should be visually appealing and well written to entice people who might prefer to learn another way.

Becoming an Effective Educator

Even when armed with the best of adult learning theory and the finest of teaching plans, a health professional is not yet fully prepared for the role of educator. The following aspects of self-exploration and learning should be a normal part of preparation for an effective teaching experience.

Meeting the Challenges

The longer a health professional is in practice, the more obvious become the obstacles to successful patient teaching. This frustration can sometimes stand in the way of sincere patient teaching efforts, unless educators learn to accept and strive to overcome common challenges.

Barriers to Teaching

A number of well-documented factors can act as barriers to patient education in both inpatient and outpatient settings. Barriers to teaching include lack of priority setting, lack of time, and insufficient knowledge or skill (15). Cardiac rehabilitation staff members must share the responsibility of identifying problem areas within the program and work together to minimize the barriers. Strategies might include developing a philosophy for teaching, reviewing content and resources regularly, practicing communication skills, and incorporating specific assessment and teaching methods into program policy (15,16).

Influencing Motivation

A key factor in learning and maintaining new skills is motivation. The patient must recognize the need for new information and be physically and mentally ready to receive it (17). In cardiac rehabilitation an educator must be continually alert to indications of the patient's attitude toward heart-healthy behavior changes. Attempting to force change upon a patient who is not willing or able to accept it will be counterproductive. It may be necessary to demonstrate more than once why a specific change is needed before any further steps can be taken. Once a change is initiated, an educator can help sustain the patient's motivation through consistent guidance, support, and positive reinforcement.

Frustrations of Short-Term Care

Behavior change is a long-term process. Cardiac rehabilitation professionals are generally outcome-oriented and may become frustrated at not knowing the long-term benefits of their efforts. Even studies that have followed patients for 1 or 2 years have varied results in terms of compliance (18-21). More research is needed, but it may also be beneficial to consider another view of patient teaching—one that is process oriented rather than outcome oriented. Guzzetta et al. (22,23) suggest a theory for treating critical-care patients that is useful in any setting. In this holistic, "body-mind-spirit" theory, the mind and body operate on a continuum, and every professional interaction affects more than one aspect of the patient. Each encounter with the patient, including every teaching interaction, has an impact that may not be measurable immediately but is either positive or negative in the long term. Program evaluation based on outcome is still necessary, but the educator also needs to value teaching for its process and should focus attention on assessment methods and teaching techniques that are most likely to have a long-term positive impact.

Seeing the Patient as Individual and Expert

As discussed earlier, the effective educator helps the patient set his or her own goals, objectives, and standards for success (1). However, how often does the potential exist for the patient's goals to be limited or camouflaged by those of the health professional? Out of concern for the patient and the desire to share expertise, an educator may inadvertently block the free expression of a patient by strongly implying what goals and objectives *should be* planned. The educator must be involved in the planning process, but must draw a fine line between facilitating and dictating.

Each patient has developed a unique set of values, beliefs, and goals; so has each health professional. A cardiac rehabilitation program can illustrate the potential conflict between these two value systems. The mean age of health professionals in a given program is likely to be significantly less than that of its patients. In addition, many professionals drawn to the rehabilitation field lead heart-healthy lives with relative ease and may not face the challenges that confront their patients. The professional may find it difficult to understand a patient's lack of motivation or refusal to change and may expect rather quick acceptance or label the patient as uncooperative, unwilling, or lazy. The approach to education may then become routine, which is more stressful and less constructive than when information is tailored to the individual (24). Even worse, patients may begin to view themselves in the same negative terms and become ineffective at making any behavioral changes.

Although not an easy task, it is crucial that health educators learn to put the patient's goals above their own. The cardiac rehabilitation professional may be an expert on medical facts and advice, but the patient is the only expert on his or her own past experiences, beliefs, and feelings. Storlie (25) suggests a teaching philosophy that defines the patient as colleague rather than student and allows the educator to take on a more personal tone and try to know the patient as an individual. Learning should be seen as a personal experience and not all patients can be treated as if they must or want to learn. The only way an educator can truly accept a patient as an individual and an expert resource is through knowing the patient from the patient's perspective.

Applying Theory to Practice

The first part of this chapter discusses learning theories and behavior change—fundamental information for understanding and working with the patient as learner. Equally essential to the educator is the acquisition of communication skills and educational principles that can be applied directly to the teaching process.

Communication

How the patient perceives and relates to the health professional may determine future success in the teaching-learning process (17,24). The previous discussions of Guzzetta's body-mind-spirit theory and Storlie's patient-as-colleague philosophy lend firm support to this concept. Building trust and rapport is an essential beginning to establishing an effective relationship between patient and educator. Excellent resources exist to help the professional enhance specific communication skills (5,17), which include the following basic yet often underused practices:

- Building rapport through communicating acceptance, understanding, and empathy
- Eliciting patient trust and openness through listening, eye contact, and asking open, not closed, questions such as "What do you see as the benefits to you if you stop smoking?" rather than "Do you agree that you should stop smoking?"
- Choosing appropriate responses to patients' verbal cues, such as probing, clarifying, reflecting, or confronting
- Recognizing and clarifying the patient's nonverbal cues, such as facial expression, eye contact, or body posture

The educator who incorporates communication skills into daily practice is able to clearly focus on patients' verbal or nonverbal messages, even in the midst of the busy cardiac rehabilitation environment.

Principles of Education

A number of principles serve as a theoretical base for patient education. One study of critical-care nurses demonstrated that nurses' knowledge and application of teaching and learning principles had a positive effect on increasing knowledge in their patients (26). Knowles's principles, discussed earlier, apply specifically to understanding the adult learner (2). Other principles are particularly applicable to the educator in cardiac rehabilitation:

The environment can be used to focus the patient's attention on what is to be learned (27). This reminder to be aware of what stimuli surround the patient can be valuable in either inpatient or outpatient settings. Educators can use posters, visual aids, written materials, and equipment to convey specific messages to both patient and family.

Success is more motivating than failure (27). This notion seems obvious, but perhaps is not applied as often as it could be. The educator should help patients set goals that are realistic, rather than insurmountable, and guide patients toward working on skills and behaviors that they are able to master.

Insecurity is transferable (28). Fielding questions and solving problems are more difficult than delivering a canned package of information. Educators must feel assured in communication skills and the best use of available resources. This sense of security can have a direct bearing on building trust and rapport with the patient.

Participation enhances learning (28). What better place to apply this than in cardiac rehabilitation? Physical participation in an exercise session is an obvious help, but mental participation in learning other health behaviors is more difficult to ensure. An effective educator facilitates both, from the early goal-setting stages and throughout all phases of the program.

Implications for Practice in Cardiac Rehabilitation

To complete this chapter, here are some final guidelines for consideration. Each area discussed here offers the educator additional strategies, which can be incorporated into any teaching program to help enhance communication and to increase the likelihood of positive outcomes.

Including Family in the Teaching Process

One vital means of confronting the challenges to patient education and effecting a successful outcome is to draw upon the greatest resource available—the patient's family. The family has been identified as one of the most important influences over a patient's ability and willingness to make lifestyle changes (17). The family's emotional investment in the patient far exceeds that of the health professional (28). Family members may be able to retain information when the patient cannot, and they can offer long-term assistance and support. Involving the family as early and as often as possible in the learning process may be the educator's most important key to success.

Relapse Prevention

Both educator and patient enjoy a sense of accomplishment when a new behavior is successfully adopted. However, the challenge that lies ahead is maintaining the change. A relapse prevention training component should be integrated into every cardiac rehabilitation program. One excellent resource on this topic is Marlatt and Gordon's *Relapse Prevention: Maintenance Strategies in the Treatment of Addictive Behaviors* (29). The authors define the purpose of relapse prevention: ". . . to prevent the occurrence of initial lapses after one has embarked on a program of habit change, and/or to prevent any lapse from escalating into a total relapse." The book thoroughly discusses relapse prevention in theory and practice, with sections devoted to strategies for specific behavior changes such as smoking cessation and weight control.

Integrating Education Into an Exercise Program

Many patients enter cardiac rehabilitation with the expectation that the only purpose is exercise. Third-party payers reinforce this image by reimbursing for exercise therapy but usually not doing so for the education required to make permanent lifestyle changes. To compound these concerns, the quality of education may vary from patient to patient if a variety of staff members are teaching but are not careful to coordinate their activities.

The challenge to professionals is all too clear: help the patient recognize cardiac rehabilitation as an opportunity for multiple lifestyle changes while providing consistent resources in a time-efficient, cost-efficient manner. This is not an impossible task, but it is certainly one that requires planning, problem solving, and evaluation. What works for one program may not work for another. Here are two possible approaches that have met with success in some programs.

A Curriculum

Developing a curriculum of topics that can be covered during the exercise sessions will help ensure consistency of educational components. Individual patient goals can be addressed within the set curriculum or separately as needed. For example, the staff of one cardiac rehabilitation department

prioritized what topics should be covered and planned a main topic for each week of a 12-week program. Each topic was small because the staff knew that they would discuss the material as they monitored the patient during exercise. Topics included "how to choose a healthy breakfast at home or in a restaurant" and "how to make exercise enjoyable." A calendar of the topics was posted for the staff. Each week, a set of written materials that explained the appropriate topic was set out for patients to take home at the end of the session. Videotapes were also coordinated to the topic of the week; patients watched the videotapes (using headphones) while exercising. The curriculum allowed the staff to divide material into parts small enough that each could be managed during an exercise session and to coordinate the parts so that all necessary information was included.

Learning Resource Center

A learning resource center is a place within the cardiac rehabilitation facility that contains a variety of written materials, videotapes, audiotapes, posters, bulletin boards, and self-teaching packages. The learning center should be highly visible with appealing displays to entice participation—one program's center is an alcove adjacent to the exercise room. Strategies to draw patients into the center are vital to its use: classes can be scheduled there with time allotted for independent exploration, or patients can be asked to view a specific videotape or learning package based on their learning needs. Patients and families should be invited to use the center on their own; however, several programs have found that participants require assistance in finding what they need and using the equipment.

Guidelines for Written Teaching Materials

Although this chapter emphasizes that knowledge alone is never enough for effective teaching, there is still no question that patients need knowledge on which to base any decisions for change. Most programs depend upon a variety of written materials to impart facts and to supplement or reinforce oral teaching. When time with a patient is extremely limited, written information may be the only available means of introducing important information. The challenge to educators is to choose or develop materials that will appeal to readers, uphold principles, and follow the rules of clear writing. The following guidelines may help.

Evaluate Each Item

Ask four basic questions, based on the list of "practical recommendations to improve retention, recall, and compliance" of Haynes et al. (30):

- *Is it brief?* The more statements presented, the more the patient will forget.
- *Is the most important information given early?* Recall and retention will be greater for information presented in the first third of the communication.
- *Is it well organized?* This should be answered with the above two principles in mind as well as the educator's experience in teaching the topic.
- *Can it be read and understood easily?* Studies show that many patient education materials, including those for cardiac patients (31,32), are written above the average reading level of their intended audience. Readability formulas can be a starting point in assessing materials, but the information they provide is limited and should not take the place of other steps in producing well-written text (33).

Revise, Revise, and Revise Again

Many educators write and develop their own program materials. The following editing suggestions (34,35) will be useful to them:

- Check for long sentences that may be confusing. Shorter sentences are generally better, with subject and verb close together.
- Eliminate unfamiliar large words when smaller words can be substituted.
- Break up the text wherever possible by using headlines and subheads. A question-and-answer format is an effective method for patient teaching materials.
- Check for long paragraphs containing a number of key points that could be made into a bulleted list, such as this one.
- Check for needless words or phrases and delete them.
- Proofread for typing errors, proper punctuation, and grammar; then have the material proofread again by someone who has never read it.

Communicate With the Printing Department

Request consistent use of design elements that will enhance reading (35,36).

- Choose a typeface and type size that are easy to read.
- Allow plenty of white space (unused space on the page)—ample margins, break in the copy as mentioned above, no crowding of text.
- Use **bold type** or *italics* for emphasis, and use them sparingly. Do not use ALL CAPS or underlining, which are more difficult to read.
- Make sure there is plenty of contrast between type and page. Black on white is best; when other combinations are used, each should be evaluated for ease of reading.
- Use illustrations that are easy to follow and that explain or clarify the text.

Summary

The teaching-learning that leads to behavior change is a complex process. Nowhere is this more evident than in a cardiac rehabilitation setting, where professionals share the common goal of helping patients help themselves toward a heart-healthy lifestyle. This chapter should help educators identify and work with a multitude of factors that can influence outcomes within each main element of the education process—learner, teacher, and individual program. Educators should know and respect each patient as an adult learner and should consistently apply theory and strategies that will improve individual and program practices.

References

1. American Association of Cardiovascular and Pulmonary Rehabilitation. Guidelines for cardiac rehabilitation. Champaign, IL: Human Kinetics; 1991.
2. Knowles, M. The modern practice of adult education. New York: Association Press; 1970.
3. Padberg, R.M.; Padberg, L.F. Strengthening the effectiveness of patient education: Applying principles of adult education. Oncology Nursing Forum. 17:65-69; 1990.
4. Wingate, S. Post-MI patients' perceptions of their learning needs. Dimensions of Critical Care Nursing. 9:112-118; 1990.
5. Girdano, D.A.; Dusek, D.E. Changing health behavior. Scottsdale, AZ: Gorsuch Scarisbrick; 1988.
6. Bandura, A.B. Self-efficacy: Toward a unifying theory of behavioral change. Psychol. Rev. 84:191-215; 1977.

7. Gortner, S.R.; Miller, N.H.; Jenkins, L.S. Self-efficacy: A key to recovery. In: Jillings, C.R., ed. Cardiac rehabilitation nursing. Rockville, MD: Aspen; 1988:89-101.

8. Gortner, S.R.; Jenkins, L.S. Self-efficacy and activity level following cardiac surgery. J. Adv. Nurs. 15: 1132-1138; 1990.

9. Ewart, C.K.; Taylor, C.B.; Reese, L.B.; DeBusk, R.F. Effects of early postmyocardial infarction exercise testing on self-perception and subsequent physical activity. Am. J. Cardiol. 51:1076-1080; 1983.

10. Taylor, C.B.; Bandura, A.B.; Ewart, C.K.; Miller, N.H.; DeBusk, R.F. Exercise testing to enhance wives' confidence in their husbands' cardiac capability soon after clinically uncomplicated acute myocardial infarction. Am. J. Cardiol. 55:635-638; 1985.

11. Allen, J.K. Self-efficacy in health behavior: Research and practice. Cardiovascular Nursing. 24:37-38; 1988.

12. Kaplan, R.M.; Atkins, C.J. Specific efficacy expectations mediate exercise compliance in patients with COPD. Health Psychol. 3:223-242; 1984.

13. McGlashan, R. Strategies for rebuilding self-esteem for the cardiac patient. Dimensions of Critical Care. 7:28-38; 1988.

14. Merritt, S.L. Learning style preferences of coronary artery disease patients. Cardiovascular Nursing. 27:7-12; 1991.

15. Corkadel, L.; McGlashan, R. A practical approach to patient teaching. Journal of Continuing Education in Nursing. 14:9-15; 1983.

16. Bille, D.A., editor. Practical approaches to patient teaching. Boston: Little, Brown; 1981.

17. Falvo, D.R. Effective patient education: A guide to increased compliance. Rockville, MD: Aspen Systems Corporation; 1985.

18. Scalzi, C.C.; Burke, L.E.; Greenland, S. Evaluation of an inpatient educational program for coronary patients and families. Heart Lung. 9:846-853; 1980.

19. Sivarajan, E.S.; Newton, K.M.; Almes, M.J.; Kempf, T.M.; Mansfield, L.W.; Bruce, R.A. Limited effects of outpatient teaching and counseling after myocardial infarction: A controlled study. Heart Lung. 12:65-73; 1983.

20. Eyherabide, A.; Yates, B.C. The effects of cardiac rehabilitation on compliance in the coronary artery bypass surgery patient. Cardiovascular Nursing. 21:31-35; 1985.

21. Conroy, R.M.; Mulcahy, R.; Graham, I.M.; Reid, V.; Cahill, S. Predictors of patient response to risk factor modification advice after admission for unstable angina or myocardial infarction. Journal of Cardiopulmonary Rehabilitation. 6:344-357; 1986.

22. Guzzetta, C.E. Can critically ill patients be taught? In: Bille, D.A., ed. Practical approaches to patient teaching. Boston: Little, Brown; 1981:255-270.

23. Guzzetta, C.; Kenner, C.; Dossey, B. Critical care nursing: Body, mind, spirit. Boston: Little, Brown; 1981.

24. Wolff, I. Understanding the patient with coronary artery disease. In: Storlie F., ed. Patient teaching in critical care. New York: Appleton-Century-Crofts; 1975:117-128.

25. Storlie, F.J. The patient as colleague: A personal philosophy. Rehabilitation Nursing. (July/Aug):16-22; 1981.

26. Murdaugh, C.L. Effects of nurses' knowledge of teaching-learning principles on knowledge of coronary care unit patients. Heart Lung. 9:1073-1078; 1980.

27. Redman, B.K. The process of patient teaching in nursing, 4th ed. St. Louis: Mosby; 1980.

28. Storlie, F. Patient teaching in critical care. New York: Appleton-Century-Crofts; 1975.

29. Marlatt, G.A.; Gordon, J.R. Relapse prevention: Maintenance strategies in the treatment of addictive behaviors. New York: Guilford Press; 1985.

30. Haynes, R.B.; Taylor, D.W.; Sackett, D.L. Compliance in health care. Baltimore: Johns Hopkins University Press; 1979.

31. Boyd, M.D.; Feldman, M.A. Health information seeking and reading and comprehension abilities of cardiac rehabilitation patients. J. Cardiac Rehabil. 4:343-347; 1984.

32. Conroy, R.M.; Mulcahy, R. Readability of literature written for cardiac patients. Clin. Cardiol. 8:104-106; 1985.

33. Pichert, J.W.; Elam, P. Readability formulas may mislead you. Patient Education and Counseling. 7:181-191; 1985.

34. Cox, B.G. The art of writing patient education materials. American Medical Writers Association Journal. 4:11-14; 1989.

35. Pocinki, K.M. Writing for an older audience: Ways to maximize understanding and acceptance. American Medical Writers Association Journal. 5:6-10; 1990.

36. Tilden, S.W. Harnessing desktop publishing: How to let the new technology help you do your job better. Pennington, NJ: Scott Tilden, Inc.; 1987.

Chapter 19

Standards for Cardiac Rehabilitation Programs and Practice

Patricia McCall Comoss

Cardiac rehabilitation has come of age. Since its clinical beginnings as an outgrowth of coronary care in the 1960s (1), this specialty has not only survived being called an experiment in the 1970s and a fad in the 1980s (2), but has evolved as a multifaceted clinical service provided by professionals from a number of health care disciplines. Cardiac rehabilitation has emerged in the 1990s as a well-recognized, well-respected part of comprehensive cardiac care.

Signs of maturing are increasingly evident. The introduction of the *Journal of Cardiac Rehabilitation* (now the *Journal of Cardiopulmonary Rehabilitation*) in 1981 (3) and the formation of the American Association of Cardiovascular and Pulmonary Rehabilitation (AACVPR) in 1985 (4) are benchmarks of the specialty's success and stabilization. In the U.S., the specialty is now focused on improving the quality and consistency of its services. Internationally, the emphasis is on increasing awareness of and access to rehabilitative care for cardiac patients (4a). As in any professional field, such concerns are addressed through the development of standards that programs and practitioners can emulate.

While papers addressing some aspects of cardiac rehabilitation have been available since 1972 (5), the proliferation of such documents in the past 5 years has more than doubled the availability of so-called standards. As a result, today's cardiac rehabilitation professionals are challenged not only to be familiar with existing standards, but also to use them effectively in their programs and practice.

It is the purpose of this chapter to describe the purpose of standards, to emphasize the major sources of standards and their significance, and to discuss how to integrate current standards into the daily operation of cardiac rehabilitation programs. After reading this chapter cardiac rehabilitation professionals will be able to

- define *standards* from a legal, professional, and functional perspective;

- identify three major sources of cardiac rehabilitation standards put forth by professional organizations within the field;
- compare and contrast the standards from these three sources;
- identify three major sources of cardiac rehabilitation standards from outside the field;
- discuss how external standards affect the viability of cardiac rehabilitation programs; and
- outline a strategy for integrating standards into cardiac rehabilitation practice.

Definitions and Descriptions of Standards

Standards is a buzzword in today's health care lexicon. Health care professionals in every field can attest to the anxiety experienced at the mere mention of the word. Misuse and overuse of the term often result in apprehension and confusion. To minimize miscommunication, an overview of general standards-related language is presented to the discussion of standards specific to cardiac rehabilitation.

Types of Standards

According to one dictionary, a *standard* is a model or example commonly accepted, adhered to, and used as a basis for measurement (6). Generally then, standards are collections of information about a specific field that can be used as checkpoints against which comparison can be made. As used in health care, the concept of standards can be specifically described from three different perspectives: legal interpretation, professional aspiration, and functional expectation.

From the legal perspective, *standard of care* is a long-standing legal term that means that a health care professional is expected to use the same reasonable care, skill, and diligence in provision of services as would other prudent professionals in the same line of practice (7). Failure to meet the standard of care is the basis of most lawsuits for professional negligence. In court, proof of the standard of care is provided both by written documents, such as published standards, and by the testimony of expert witnesses. The legal standard of care provides consumer protection.

From the professional perspective, *standards of practice* are benchmark behaviors expected from properly trained and experienced professionals in a given field (8). Documents expressing such standards of practice may be labeled as "standards" or "guidelines." While each outlines professional behavior expectations, the distinction between a standard and a guideline has important legal implications. A *standard* is an authoritative statement; a *guideline* is a recommended course of action (9). Professional guidelines and standards of practice promote professional excellence.

From the functional perspective, *standards for cardiac rehabilitation* include both legal standards and professional guidelines available in the field. All sources of standards and guidelines translate into expectations for staff performance and program operation. To assure that performance is congruent with legal standards and that operation is compatible with professional guidelines, cardiac rehabilitation professionals are compelled to collect and assimilate available standards documents and to integrate their contents into local programs and individual practice. Standards for cardiac rehabilitation improve program quality. Table 19.1 summarizes the types of standards and their respective purposes.

Table 19.1 Types of Standards for Cardiac Rehabilitation

Type	Term	Purpose
Legal	Standards of care	Consumer protection
Professional	Standards of practice	Professional excellence
Functional	Standards for cardiac rehabilitation	Program quality

Note. Data compiled from references 7-9.

Terminology

Identifying standards pertinent to cardiac rehabilitation is not as easy as it may sound. Documents that contain program and practice expectations are found under a variety of labels. Among the current titles of such papers are "standards," "guidelines," "positions statements," "recommendations," "rules and regulations," "criteria," and "policies." The origins of major papers using some of these titles are discussed in the next section of this chapter.

Regardless of the specific label used, the common denominator of these standards documents is that each one expresses expectations for professional performance or program operation. All the documents discussed in this chapter meet the general definition of standards as models for comparison. Therefore, the term *standards* will be used in its generic sense throughout the rest of this chapter to emphasize the functional nature of the various published expectations.

Sources and Rationales for Standards

Expectations for cardiac rehabilitation come from a variety of sources. During the past 20 years, groups as diverse as providers and payers, regulatory agencies, and voluntary associations have published their versions of what cardiac rehabilitation ought to be. For discussion purposes, available standards documents can be classified as either being internally generated or externally imposed.

Internal Influence

Most of the existing cardiac rehabilitation standards were developed under the auspices of a professional association by professionals directly involved in the practice of cardiac rehabilitation. Table 19.2 provides a historical listing of major standards in the field (5,10-38).

One of the inherent purposes of a professional association is self-regulation. It is in any association's own interest to try to influence the quality of care that its practitioners provide. Ultimately such internal quality contributes to external credibility. The development of standards and the implementation of certifications based upon those standards are the usual mechanisms through which the goal of self-regulation is accomplished (39).

Table 19.2 Summary of Professional Standards Affecting Cardiac Rehabilitation

Year	Source	Document
1972	AHA	*Exercise Testing and Training of Apparently Healthy Individuals: A Handbook for Physicians*
1974	North Carolina Heart Association	*Organizational Guidelines for Myocardial Infarction Rehabilitation Program*
1975	AHA	*Exercise Testing and Training of Individuals with Heart Disease or at Risk for Its Development: A Handbook for Physicians*
1975	ACSM	*Guidelines for Graded Exercise Testing and Exercise Prescription*
1978	Greater Los Angeles affiliate of the AHA	*Guidelines for Cardiac Rehabilitation Centers*
1978	ACSM	*Position Statement: Recommended Quantity and Quality of Exercise for Developing and Maintaining Fitness in Healthy Adults*
1979	AHA	*The Exercise Standards Book*
1980	ACSM	*Guidelines,* 2nd ed.
1981	ANA and AHA	*Standards of Cardiovascular Nursing Practice*
1984	Orange County, California, chapter of the AHA	*Guidelines for Cardiac Rehabilitation Centers*
1984	North Carolina DHR	*Rules Governing the Certification of Cardiac Rehabilitation Programs*
1986	AACVPR	*Cardiac Rehabilitation Services: A Scientific Evaluation*
1986	ACC	"Position Report on Cardiac Rehabilitation"
1986	Massachusetts Society for Cardiac Rehabilitation	*Guidelines for Cardiac Rehabilitation*
1986	ACSM	*Guidelines,* 3rd ed.
1986	ACC-AHA Joint Task Force	"Guidelines for Exercise Testing"
1987	AMA	"Diagnostic and Therapeutic Technology Assessment: Coronary Rehabilitation Services"
1988	ACP	"Position Paper: Cardiac Rehabilitation Services"
1988	California Society for Cardiac Rehabilitation	*Standards for Cardiac Rehabilitation in California*
1989	ACP	"Position Paper: Evaluation of Patients After Recent Acute Myocardial Infarction"
1990	AACVPR	"Position Paper: Scientific Evidence of the Value of Cardiac Rehabilitation With Emphasis on Patients Following Myocardial Infarction: Exercise Conditioning Component"
1990	ACSM	"Position Stand: The Recommended Quantity and Quality of Exercise for Developing and Maintaining Cardiorespiratory and Muscular Fitness in Healthy Adults"
1990	AACVPR	"Position Paper: The Efficacy of Risk Factor Intervention and Psychosocial Aspects of Cardiac Rehabilitation"
1990	AHA	"A Position Statement for Health Professionals"
1990	ACC-ACP-AHA Joint Task Force	"Clinical Competence in Exercise Testing: A Statement for Physicians"
1990	North Carolina DHR	*Rules Governing the Certification of Cardiac Rehabilitation Programs*
1990	AHA	"Exercise Standards: A Statement for Health Professionals"
1991	AACVPR	*Guidelines for Cardiac Rehabilitation Programs*
1991	ACSM	*Guidelines,* 4th ed.

(continued)

Table 19.2 *(continued)*

Year	Source	Document
1993	ANA	*The Scope of Cardiac Rehabilitation Nursing Practice*
1994	AHCPR	*Clinical Practice Guidelines for Cardiac Rehabilitation*
1995	AACVPR	*Guidelines for Cardiac Rehabilitation Programs*, 2nd ed.

Note. AACVPR = American Association of Cardiovascular and Pulmonary Rehabilitation; ACC = American College of Cardiology; ACP = American College of Physicians; ACSM = American College of Sports Medicine; AHA = American Heart Association; AMA = American Medical Association; ANA = American Nurses Association; DHR = Department of Human Resources; AHCPR = Agency for Health Care Policy & Research. Data compiled from references 5, 10-38.

Historical Processes

The process of writing standards is complex and lengthy. Typically the process proceeds as follows. A group of experts in the practice area is assembled into a standards committee. The committee begins its work by first clarifying the purpose and outlining the scope of the document to be produced. Three critical decisions need to be made at this early stage:

1. Is the document under development intended to impact individual practitioner competence, or will it address how a program ought to be conducted?
2. Should the document be oriented toward practical application or philosophical aspiration?
3. Is the intent to convey minimal expectations for practice (what must *at least* be accounted for) or optimal recommendations (what ought to be done to be the *best*)?

Once these three areas are defined, the committee can focus its attention on content of the standards document. Content is selected and shaped through a combination of extensive review of research and the expert opinions of committee members. Debate over points of content is common and final decisions are made by committee consensus.

As can be seen from Table 19.2, nearly 20 different groups have used a process similar to the one just outlined to produce standards that affect cardiac rehabilitation. While the total number of standards documents is impressive in itself, the single most significant period of standards development occurred in 1990. In the fall of that year, three independently produced sets of standards related to cardiac rehabilitation were released. The fact that the AACVPR, the American College of Sports Medicine (ACSM), and the American Heart Association (AHA) released their respective standards (35-37) within a few months of each other attests to the fact that professionals in the field were feeling an urgent need to update and upgrade their own practice expectations.

The push to clarify professional expectations grew out of three parallel developments in the late 1980s. First, volumes of research were accumulating on the safety and effectiveness of cardiac rehabilitation. Research findings affirmed the long-standing safety record of exercise-based rehabilitation programs (40-42). Evidence emerged to show that program participants lived longer than non-participating peers (43,44) and that even modest levels of exercise provided measurable health improvements (45). And atherosclerotic plaque regression was demonstrated through aggressive drug, diet, and lifestyle interventions (46-48).

The second impetus was experiential; that is practitioners in the field were noticing a change in their patient population. Instead of the stereotypical 60-year-old male post-myocardial infarction (MI) patient being referred for rehabilitation, the patients they were now seeing in their programs were of two diverging groups. A younger, more vigorous group of participants was characterized by the 40-year-old postangioplasty patient who was in and out of the hospital in 3 days, while the older, sicker group was characterized by the 80-year-old patient with recurrent congestive heart failure complicated by diabetes and severe arthritis. Additionally, an increasing number of women of all ages were being referred to cardiac rehabilitation programs. These new populations were a result of both general population shifts and specific developments in interventional cardiology (49). With the new populations came new challenges and the need to change old routines.

The third force for change at the turn of the decade was economics. An increasing emphasis on cost containment coupled with a decreasing availability of insurance reimbursement encouraged the use of alternative program strategies. Thus, research, experience, and economics converged to provide the motivation needed for groups of cardiac rehabilitation professionals to update expectations of themselves and their programs.

As this text goes to press, we are anticipating a second major wave of standards development. In mid-1994, AACVPR will publish the 2nd edition of its *Guidelines for Cardiac Rehabilitation Programs* (38B). At about the same time, *Clinical Practice Guidelines for Cardiac Rehabilitation* will be released by the U.S. Department of Health & Human Services (38A). The latter document is a collaborative project between AACVPR, the Agency for Health Care Policy and Research (AHCPR), and the National Heart, Lung, & Blood Institute (NHLBI). The two documents are expected to be complementary with the AHCPR guidelines heavily emphasizing research results and the AACVPR guidelines offering practical advice.

Current Documents

As previously mentioned, the AACVPR, ACSM, and AHA each released standards related to cardiac rehabilitation in late 1990 (35-37). These three important documents were independently developed, although the AACVPR invited review of its guidelines by contributors to both the AHA and the ACSM documents (50). Each document reflects the perspective of the source organization and offers related points of emphasis, as outlined in Table 19.3.

Despite differences in orientation, the three documents are in substantial agreement on three major issues of change in cardiac rehabilitation programming:

Issue #1: Cardiac Rehabilitation Candidates.
In the past, the appropriate patient to begin an outpatient cardiac rehabilitation program was the uncomplicated MI patient or the recovering coronary artery bypass graft (CABG) surgery patient who entered an outpatient program 8 to 12 weeks after their event. Today, patients are beginning rehabilitation programs while still in the hospital and progressing to outpatient programs immediately

Table 19.3 Overview of Current Guidelines for Cardiac Rehabilitation

Source	Document	Perspective	Emphases	Special features
AACVPR (36)	*Guidelines for Cardiac Rehabilitation Programs*	Multidisciplinary	• Individualized treatment plans • Patient teaching and behavior change of equal importance to exercise • Outcome measures for patients and programs	Incorporates scientific position papers on exercise and risk factor intervention in appendix.
ACSM (37)	*Guidelines for Exercise Testing and Prescription* (4th ed.)	Exercise professionals	• Physiology and rationale for exercise testing and performance • Detailed exercise prescription methods and calculations for healthy, cardiac, and special populations	Includes learning objectives for six levels of personnel certification through ACSM.
AHA (35)	"Exercise Standards: A Statement for Health Professionals"	Physicians	• Evaluation of exercise responses for diagnostic and prognostic purposes • Recommendations and precautions for patients with various heart conditions	Uses frequent "Key Point" captions to highlight important content.

Note. AACVPR = American Association of Cardiovascular and Pulmonary Rehabilitation; ACSM = American College of Sports Medicine; AHA = American Heart Association. Data compiled from references 35-37.

upon discharge. They often complete their structured program in less than 8 to 12 weeks and continue with a self-managed maintenance program thereafter. The patient population has changed dramatically as well. While some patients are younger and more vigorous, many are more medically complex than their predecessors, and others have combinations of chronic diseases. Some types of patients now being seen in cardiac rehabilitation programs would have been considered contraindicated for participation just 10 years ago (51).

AACVPR Guidelines (36), ACSM Guidelines (37), and AHA Standards (35) concur on the concept of an expanded list of patients, compiled as follows, who are appropriate for cardiac rehabilitation:

Patients with CAD
- Post–MI
- Post–CABG
- Post–coronary angioplasty
- Symptomatic ischemia (angina)
- Silent ischemia (ST-depression on exercise test)

Patients with other heart conditions
- Compensated heart failure
- Controlled dysrhythmias
- Automatic implanted cardiovertor-defibrillator
- Pacemakers
- Post–valve replacement
- Cardiomyopathy
- Heart transplant

Patients with other chronic diseases
- Cancer
- Diabetes mellitus
- Hypertension
- Pulmonary disease
- Peripheral vascular disease (PVD)
- Renal disease

Such concurrence points the way to new hope for patients and new opportunities for programs.

Issue #2: Individual Case Management.   In the past, cardiac patients enrolled in rehabilitation programs followed fixed routines dominated by exercise. Today, all three sources of current standards recommend the individualization of each patient's rehabilitation treatment. It is no longer acceptable to apply the same rehabilitation routine to every patient, to offer only one facet of rehabilitation care such as exercise, or to make group program offerings mandatory for all patients. To facilitate an individual case management approach, programs should have alternative methods and

involve patients in making choices among the appropriate options. Each patient's goals and treatment strategies should be recorded in an individualized cardiac rehabilitation treatment plan.

The move toward individual case management has changed the focus of cardiac rehabilitation from what is done to each patient (the *process* of rehabilitation) to what is accomplished by each patient (the *outcomes* of rehabilitation). This individualized approach and outcome focus is compatible with expectations from external sources discussed in a subsequent section of this chapter.

Issue #3: Risk Stratification Criteria.   In the past, most outpatient cardiac rehabilitation programs used continuous telemetry monitoring with all patients while they were exercising. Today, a new strategy for monitoring based on risk stratification is suggested in concert with the individual case management approach discussed earlier. Risk stratification in rehabilitation follows the lead of current cardiology treatment wherein patients are aggressively evaluated for evidence of poor prognosis, i.e., high risk of a recurrent cardiac event. Those found to be at high risk are then aggressively treated, either medically or surgically, in an effort to improve their prognosis.

DeBusk et al. were among the first to extend the concept of risk stratification to rehabilitation (52,53). Their work helped confirm the safety of unmonitored exercise in properly selected patients and set the stage for later recommendations from the American College of Cardiology (ACC) (21) and the American College of Physicians (ACP) (26) that only the highest-risk cardiac patients need to be monitored by telemetry during exercise.

Each of the 1990 standards outlines the respective organization's plan for how to assess risk and assign extent of patient observation. The combined criteria for high risk suggested by AACVPR, ACSM, and AHA are listed here (35-37).

Angina:
- Changing pattern
- New onset

Abnormal blood pressure (BP) response to exercise:
- Drop of more than 10 mm Hg in SBP
- Failure of BP to rise with exercise

Cardiac arrest survivor

Complex dysrhythmia:
- From history
- At rest
- With exercise

Chronotropic incompetence: Exercise heart rate (HR) less than 120 beats/min when patient is off medications

Ejection fraction less than 35%

Exercise capacity less than 5 METs (metabolic equivalents)

Exercise-induced ischemia:
- Silent (ST depression > 2 mm)
- Symptomatic (angina with exercise)

MI complicated by one or more of the following:
- Cardiogenic shock
- Congestive heart failure
- Persistent chest pain

Multiple MIs or large anterior infarction

Patient's inability to comply with exercise prescription or self-regulate exercise

Severe CAD:
- High left anterior descending disease
- Left main disease
- Triple-vessel disease
- Reversible thallium defects

By now, most cardiac rehabilitation programs have responded to the risk stratification challenge by restructuring their programs to include both telemetry monitored and professionally supervised (but unmonitored) blocks of time in their exercise schedule.

Additional Comparisons. Other similarities among the three documents include the following:

- Importance of substantial physician involvement in a rehabilitation program
- Use of a team approach with a staff comprising at least a physician, a program director, and a registered nurse, as well as active involvement by the patient
- Performance of a symptom-limited graded exercise test (SL-GXT) 3 to 4 weeks following the event as the basis for exercise prescription
- Equal emphasis on patient education for risk factor change as on participation in exercise

Similarities as strong and pervasive as these clearly establish a new state of the art for cardiac rehabilitation in the 1990s. When it comes to issues of appropriateness—who should be in the cardiac rehabilitation program and what services should they receive—the published guidelines from the AACVPR, ACSM, and AHA leave little doubt about current professional expectations.

In contrast to the clarity provided by these similarities, differences in some areas among the three current documents cause concern and confusion. Most notably, there is major discrepancy regarding the recommended length of an outpatient cardiac rehabilitation program. While acknowledging the need for individualization of program length and risk-related intensity of monitoring, both the AACVPR (36) and the ACSM (37) state that outpatient cardiac rehabilitation programs may typically last up to 12 weeks. On the same subject, the AHA recommends that "the fewest possible monitored sessions be used," usually 6 to 12 sessions or more (35, p. 2316). Thus, the AHA supports minimal program involvement while the AACVPR and the ACSM attempt to optimize what cardiac rehabilitation can offer.

Other differences between the ACSM and the AHA include methods of exercise prescription and recommendations regarding who should supervise exercise testing and training sessions (54). The AACVPR supports the ACSM's prescription recommendations and offers its own chart of recommendations on the utilization of program personnel (36, p. 40). Inconsistencies in these important areas of program operation can lead to a greater potential for lawsuit should problems arise (55). Therefore, the policies of each cardiac rehabilitation program need to specify which standards are being followed.

External Expectation

Professionals involved in the practice of cardiac rehabilitation are not the only source of expectations about how the specialty should be organized and operated. Groups external to and indirectly involved with cardiac rehabilitation have promulgated standards of their own. Chief among these external sources are state laws, third-party payer criteria, and requirements of inspection and accreditation agencies. Awareness of and adherence to such expectations is often of paramount importance to program survival. Noncompliance can either result in the closing of a program or indirectly contribute to a program's failure to thrive by affecting professional credibility or financial solvency.

State Law

In all fields of health care, the primary role of state government is consumer protection. Mechanisms by which that broad goal is accomplished include the licensing of health care professionals (56) and the mandating of program certification.

Professional Licensure.   Each state has a Department of Professional and Occupational Affairs (or similarly named bureaucratic division) assigned to oversee the licensing process. This department works with a board of experts from each discipline for which a license is required for practice in that state. Applicants for licensure must first meet the board's specifications for education and experience and then must take an extensive written examination, often referred to as state boards. Upon successful completion of the examination, a license to practice in the specific discipline in that state is granted. Because its purpose is consumer protection and legal recognition, the licensing process is general and basic. It is designed to assure a minimum level of competence for entry level practitioners.

Professionals involved in many of the disciplines within the field of cardiac rehabilitation—including physicians, nurses, physical therapists, and psychologists—must be licensed. Licensure for exercise professionals is now being discussed (57,57a). Once licensed, the professional is legally bound to the terms of the state law, which defines requirements and limitations of the specific discipline.

Program Certification.   As of now, there is no national regulation governing the licensure or other approval of cardiac rehabilitation programs. However, concerns about the need for governmental involvement in the regulation of cardiac rehabilitation have grown with the number and types of programs around the country. Supporters of mandatory program certification favor some level of government intervention. Opponents promote the establishment of a voluntary method of program certification, such as one that checks compliance with the internal standards discussed in the previous section. The debate over mandatory versus voluntary program certification is likely to continue for some time. If and when the government insists upon the certification of cardiac rehabilitation programs, related regulations will probably be generated and controlled at a state level. In fact, two states have already passed legislation relative to certification of cardiac rehabilitation programs. Quality concerns provided the impetus in North Carolina, while reimbursement problems served as the motivating force in Massachusetts.

The North Carolina Precedent.   North Carolina entered the cardiac rehabilitation arena in the mid-1970s with the support of the North Carolina Heart Association for the development of inpatient cardiac rehabilitation programs for recovering MI patients (10). The need for outpatient programs quickly followed, and in 1975, with funding from the North Carolina Division of Vocational Rehabilitation, a pilot outpatient program was initiated at Wake Forest University, in Winston-Salem. Using the Wake Forest example, outpatient programs spread across the state by the end of the decade. With rapid program growth came increased concern about program quality.

In response, professionals in North Carolina began work on a mechanism of peer review that would help assure a certain level of program quality. Program guidelines were drafted in 1978 and were voted into law in 1983 by the North Carolina General Assembly. What began as voluntary peer review (program certification) thus became state controlled. As a point of technical clarification, the North Carolina "Rules Governing the Certification of Cardiac Rehabilitation Programs" (34) do not require that every cardiac rehabilitation program be certified. However, many insurance companies in that state have set certification as a requirement for reimbursement; thus, it becomes indirectly compulsory.

The North Carolina certification process is now administered by that state's Department of Human Resources. Two steps are involved. First, written materials must be completed and submitted to obtain provisional approval. Then, within 6 months, an on-site inspection is conducted by a team of cardiac rehabilitation professionals. If program structure and operation meet expectations, the program is certified for a period of 2 years. To date, nearly 50 programs in North Carolina have been certified.

In addition to the obvious advantage of facilitating reimbursement, the most positive outcome reported from the program certification process in North Carolina has been the unification of programs across the state. The biggest disadvantage has been that due to financial constraints, some smaller programs in the state have been unable to meet the structure and staffing criteria to become certified.

The Massachusetts Mandate.   In 1984 professionals involved in the practice of cardiac rehabilitation in Massachusetts organized the Massachusetts Society for Cardiac Rehabilitation (MSCR), whose purposes included improving the quality of existing programs, providing guidelines for the development of new programs, and promoting research. Almost immediately, the new organization became involved in a major reimbursement dispute with Blue Cross regarding coverage of cardiac rehabilitation under its basic policy.

Over the next year, the MSCR spent its energy working with state lawmakers to draft legislation that would mandate cardiac rehabilitation as a basic health insurance benefit. Thanks to their efforts, a law was passed in 1985 requiring "health insurance plans and health maintenance organizations to provide benefits for the expense of cardiac rehabilitation treatment" (58). Coverage was contingent upon program standards to be established by the Massachusetts Department of Public Health. The MSCR played a key role in drafting the standards, which were finally approved as state regulations in 1988 (59). A companion document to the state standards, *Guidelines for Cardiac Rehabilitation*, was published by the MSCR in 1986 (22).

While the Massachusetts legislation got off to a strong start, its implementation has been slower than expected. There has been some confusion about who is responsible for enforcing the regulations on an ongoing basis. Therefore, in 1988 Blue Cross implemented its own review process "to ensure that the hospital's cardiac rehabilitation program conforms to the regulatory provisions" (60). As might be expected, Blue Cross applies strict criteria and requires extensive documentation of each patient's medical necessity, treatment plan, and monthly case reviews.

Economic problems in recent years have played havoc with the health care system in Massachusetts. In 1991, the state's commissioner of insurance was directed to review all health care benefits for which payment was mandatory, examine cost impact of each, and explore alternatives for those services (61). Thus, despite the fact that nearly 60 programs are already certified in Massachusetts, the promise of mandatory reimbursement may be thwarted by the reality of the state's economics.

Comparison of States' Guidelines. Other states aspiring to legislative action can learn valuable lessons from the experiences of North Carolina and Massachusetts. Most notable in both cases was the influence that an organized state society was able to exert. However, neither model necessarily translates to any other state. The substance of the standards in the two states was similar but the process, both initial and ongoing, was quite different, being subject in large part to the larger political agenda in each location. Table 19.4 provides a comparison of the regulations in the two states

Third-Party Payers

Third-party payers are insurance companies that reimburse health care providers for services rendered to patients (62). The term applies to all insurers: public (Medicare, Medicaid), nonprofit (Blue Cross and Blue Shield), and commercial (Aetna, Prudential, etc.). The term *third-party payer* reflects the legal nature of the patient-provider relationship, the first and second parties, respectively. The insurer is the outside, third, party contracted and paid by the patient (or the patient's employer) to provide specified financial coverage for health care.

Third-party payers have no direct authority over health care professionals. They cannot dictate how services, such as cardiac rehabilitation, are to be provided. However, they exert extensive influence by specifying the terms under which payment for services will be made. While compliance with the terms or criteria is voluntary, it is virtually assured, since noncompliance means nonpayment.

Payment terms or criteria are internally derived by each insurance company. Some criteria are clearly based on recent research, as it is interpreted by the medical and technical experts of the insurance company. Other criteria are ambiguous in origin. Still others are periodically challenged and changed. Three issues of importance to the structure and operation of cardiac rehabilitation programs recently encountered third-party scrutiny. A brief review of the incidents that occurred illustrates the standard-setting tactics of third-party payers.

Safety and Effectiveness Review. In 1985 the Health Care Financing Administration, the administrative arm of Medicare, issued a call in the *Federal Register* for evidence showing "the safety, clinical effectiveness, and use of specific elements involved in providing cardiac rehabilitation services" (63, p. 32, 411). A review and analysis of the data submitted were conducted by the Office of Health Technology and Assessment (OHTA) of the U.S. Public Health Service. The 80-page OHTA report concluded that "Cardiac rehabilitation services are considered safe and efficacious therapy to improve the cardiovascular and psychosocial status of patients with documented coronary heart disease to the extent that it [*sic*] improves exercise tolerance and otherwise enhances functional capacity" (64, p. 80). Based on that report, Medicare continued its usual reimbursement of cardiac rehabilitation services under existing criteria.

Subsequently, similar calls were issued for evidence of the value and use of cardiac rehabilitation in specific patient populations, including patients who have undergone percutaneous transluminal coronary angioplasty (PTCA), aortic valve replacement surgery, and heart transplants. In 1991 the Agency for Health Care Policy & Research

Table 19.4   Comparison of Two States' Regulations Governing Standards for Cardiac Rehabilitation Programs

	North Carolina	Massachusetts
Process		
Initiator	North Carolina Division of Vocational Rehabilitation	Massachusetts Society for Cardiac Rehabilitation
Rationale	Program growth and quality control	Reimbursement under basic coverage
Year passed	1983	1985
Official title	Rules Governing the Certification of Cardiac Rehabilitation Programs	Standards Governing Cardiac Rehabilitation Treatment
Stated purpose	"To ensure safe and adequate treatment of individuals in cardiac rehabilitation programs."	"To prescribe basic program components . . . *not* to set the course of treatment for individual patients."
Body administrating the regulations	Department of Human Resources, Division of Facility Services	(To be determined)
Substance		
Regulatory content	Staffing guidelines, patient care expectations, documentation, facilities and equipment (content similar in the two states)	
Emphasis	Staff roles and team coordination	Treatment planning and patient appropriateness
Party conducting on-site inspection	Multidisciplinary team of peers	(To be determined)
Current status	Successful; over 50 programs certified	Being reviewed; nearly 60 programs certified

Note. Data compiled from references 22, 34, and 59.

(AHCPR) concluded that "Patients who have had heart transplants, percutaneous transluminal coronary angioplasty, or heart valve surgery have no unique characteristics that differentiate them from cardiac patients who have had a myocardial infarction or coronary artery bypass graft or who have stable angina in terms of the necessity for participating in supervised rehabilitation programs. Therefore, patients who have had these surgical procedures might be selected for enrollment in cardiac rehabilitation programs on the basis of their physical and psychological conditions" (64A, p. 8). While this report supports selection and stratification of appropriate patients in these groups, programs continue to have difficulty in obtaining Medicare reimbursement for transplant, valve, and PTCA patients.

Medical Necessity Challenge.   In 1987 the Technology Management Department of the Blue Cross and Blue Shield Association requested that ACP commission a paper to review the medical literature on cardiac rehabilitation. The result was a paper by Greenland and Chu entitled "Efficacy of

Cardiac Rehabilitation Services" (65). Based on that paper, Blue Cross revised its clinical recommendations for cardiac rehabilitation coverage, suggesting more selective use of services overall, limiting continuous telemetry monitoring to patients at high risk, and shortening the routine program time frame from 12 weeks to 6 weeks (66). Subsequently, the efficacy paper was criticized for being incomplete (67) and one of the original authors updated his findings and expanded his conclusions (68). Blue Cross, however, did not alter its revised position.

Physician Presence Reversal.   Also in 1987, Medicare intermediaries in several states revised their interpretation of acceptable physician coverage for cardiac rehabilitation programs. Language stating that cardiac rehabilitation services "must be furnished under the direct supervision of a physician" had always been a part of Medicare criteria (69,70). The revision changed the expectation of the physician's location from being "immediately available and accessible for an emergency" to actually being "physically present in the same exercise area as the patient" (71). Many cardiac rehabilitation programs found themselves instantly out of Medicare compliance. Individual programs and organized professional groups launched a campaign citing that the new expectation was unnecessary and unrealistic. Subsequently, Medicare reversed its decision back to the specification of physician availability and added new verbiage to clarify exactly what it meant:

> Direct supervision means that a physician must be in the exercise program area and immediately available and accessible for an emergency at all times the exercise program is conducted. It does not require that a physician be physically present in the exercise room itself, provided that the contractor [Medicare intermediary] does not determine that the physician is too remote from the patients' exercise area to be considered immediately available and accessible. (72, p.1)

As is evident from these examples, both Medicare and Blue Cross set their criteria at a national level. Table 19.5 provides a comparison of major coverage criteria from the two payers.

Both Medicare and Blue Cross give their regional intermediaries considerable flexibility in interpreting and applying national criteria. While regional decisions sometimes give liberal meaning to national criteria and thus may aid reimbursement, they also add inconsistencies in payments from one geographic region to another, making universal reimbursement predictions impossible. Awareness of national developments as well as contact with local insurance representatives is necessary for maintaining a realistic view of the general reimbursement environment and the specific payer expectations under which cardiac rehabilitation services are provided (73).

Accrediting Agencies

Accreditation is the process by which an institution is inspected and approved by an agency that has preannounced expectations. Various accrediting agencies exist, depending upon the type of institution requesting review. For example, osteopathic hospitals are inspected by the American Osteopathic Association (74), while comprehensive rehabilitation hospitals or outpatient centers are usually accredited by the Commission on Accreditation of Rehabilitation Facilities (CARF) (75). The best known and most utilized accrediting agency is the Joint Commission on Accreditation of Healthcare Organizations (JCAHO).

Created in 1951, the JCAHO is a national, nonprofit, voluntary organization dedicated to improving the quality of care provided in health care facilities (76). It fulfills its quality improvement purpose through a well-defined accreditation process. The process centers around the development and dissemination of standards by advisory committees representing most disciplines and major professional organizations in health care.

Participation in the JCAHO accreditation process is both voluntary and expensive. To become accredited, a health care facility must apply to the JCAHO, meet the commission's requirements, pay its fees, and undergo a rigorous on-site review by a JCAHO survey team. The team, usually comprising a physician, nurse, and hospital administrator, evaluates the applicant facility for extent of compliance with the published JCAHO standards. Despite its cost and challenge, many health care facilities choose to participate in the JCAHO process because of the credibility JCAHO accreditation provides within the health care industry and the visibility it offers to the public.

To keep pace with changes in the health care field, the Joint Commission revised its approach to accreditation in 1986. Its "Agenda for Change" document, published that year, initiated a quality improvement strategy and introduced a new definition of quality care (77). JCAHO now defines "patient care quality" as the degree to which patient care services increase the probability of desired patient outcomes and reduce the probability of undesired outcomes (78). This new definition is outcome driven and as such is compatible with the goals emphasized in current guidelines for cardiac rehabilitation (79).

Historically, three types of criteria have been used to evaluate quality and determine a facility's compliance with JCAHO expectations:

- Structure criteria, which focus on the facility's physical plant (space and equipment) and in-house paperwork that describes the facility's use
- Process criteria, which focus on professional performance, policies and procedures, and documentation of services provided (patient charts, etc.)
- Outcome criteria, which focus individually on patient outcomes and collectively on program effectiveness

While all three classes of criteria are still used in the JCAHO process, the most weight is currently placed on the outcome criteria, relatively less on process criteria, and the least on structure criteria.

Table 19.5　Comparison of Criteria for Third-Party Reimbursement of Outpatient Cardiac Rehabilitation Services

	Medicare	Blue Cross
Patient requirements	Physician referral	Physician referral
	Clear medical need	Clear medical need
	ACCEPTABLE DIAGNOSIS:	ACCEPTABLE DIAGNOSIS:
	Within 12 months	Within 12 weeks
	Post–myocardial infarction	Post–myocardial infarction
	Post–coronary artery bypass graft surgery	Post–coronary artery bypass graft surgery
	Stable angina pectoris	Percutaneous transluminal coronary angioplasty
	RISK STRATIFICATION:	RISK STRATIFICATION:
	(Not addressed)	Required, four categories in effect:
		Low risk = ineligible
		Intermediate risk = supervised
		High risk = monitored
		Very high risk = contraindicated
Program requirements	Hospital outpatient departments	Hospital outpatient departments
	Physician-directed clinics and offices	Physician-directed clinics and offices
	Available emergency equipment	
	Exclusive use of area while program is in session	
	Personnel trained in advanced life support and in exercise therapy	(Not specifically addressed)
	Physician in exercise area and immediately available	
	Personnel employed by hospital or physician	
	DURATION OF PROGRAM:	DURATION OF PROGRAM:
	36 visits in 12 weeks	18-24 visits, 6-8 weeks
Services covered	New-patient comprehensive evaluation	New-patient comprehensive evaluation
	Entry and exit treadmill exercise tests	Entry and exit treadmill exercise tests
	EXERCISE THERAPY SESSIONS:	EXERCISE THERAPY SESSIONS:
	With continuous telemetry monitoring *or*	With evidence of appropriate risk stratification:
	Periodic rhythm strips with physician interpretation *or*	High risk = monitored
	Physician observation with prescription revision	Intermediate risk = supervised sessions
Services not covered	Patient/family education	Patient/family education
	Risk reduction counseling	Risk reduction counseling
	Psychological testing or therapy	Psychological testing or therapy
	Physical and occupational therapy	Physical and occupational therapy

Note. Data compiled from references 66 and 72.

Accreditation Manual for Hospitals contains the complete collection of JCAHO standards applied to hospitals (80). A similar manual is available for nonhospital ambulatory health care settings (81). Both types of facilities can apply for accreditation. JCAHO manuals do not contain a chapter of standards specific to cardiac rehabilitation. As a result, in the early 1990s, different sets of standards have been applied to cardiac rehabilitation programs in different settings; fortunately, most of these variations are predictable. JCAHO typically applies two sets of standards when reviewing cardiac rehabilitation programs, one on program operations and the other on professional expectations.

Program Operations. Standards applied to the organization and operation of a cardiac rehabilitation program are those pertinent to the department of the hospital within which the program exists (82). For example, if cardiac rehabilitation is part of the Physical Therapy Department, then the JCAHO's standards for "Physical Rehabilitation Services" will be applied. Likewise, if outpatient cardiac rehabilitation is under the umbrella of ambulatory care at a given institution, then standards for "Ambulatory Care Services" will be followed. JCAHO standards for "Infection Control," "Plant Technology and Safety Management," "Quality Assessment and Improvement" and "Orientation, Training, and Education of Staff," are considered universal and are applied to all hospital services, including cardiac rehabilitation programs.

Professional Expectations. Standards applied to the staff members of a cardiac rehabilitation program are the same as those expected of their peers in other parts of the hospital. For example, physical therapists, occupational therapists, and vocational counselors who practice in cardiac rehabilitation settings are held to expectations for their respective disciplines, as outlined under "Physical Rehabilitation Services." JCAHO has no standards specifically applicable to the role of exercise specialists. Dietitians involved in cardiac rehabilitation are expected to meet the standards for "Dietetic Services," and nurses must conform to expectations expressed under "Nursing Care." In 1991, the JCAHO released revised nursing standards (83). Compared to the previous edition, the new nursing standards emphasize collaborative relationships with other disciplines, focus on the needs of the patient rather than the structure of the nursing department, and encourage improvement and innovation in nursing practice (84). Table 19.6 provides sample checkpoints useful in preparing for a JCAHO inspection.

As Joint Commission continues to fulfill its "Agenda for Change," less compartmentalized, more global standards are expected to emerge. The years 1994 and 1995 will be transition years during which JCAHO will shift toward performance-focused standards that will be organized around functions most relevant to patient care rather than around departments or disciplines (84a).

Impact and Implications of Standards

Standards for cardiac rehabilitation are not intended to be passive reference documents. To match their definition of being models for comparison, standards need to be actively applied to gauge performance. To fulfill their goal of bringing consistent quality to the field, standards need to be universally utilized. The very existence of the impressive array of standards described in this chapter implies their importance and infers that, at the very least, they will be viewed as markers of the excellence they espouse.

The extent of the impact of published standards on a given cardiac rehabilitation program depends upon a variety of factors, including the nature of the sponsoring organization, the length of time the program has been in operation, staff experience with standards, and compatibility of published standards with general operating procedures of the facility. All programs will undoubtedly be affected by standards in some way. However, program staff committed to achieving excellence—to creating the best program possible and to offering optimal services to their patients—will not wait for outsiders to impose changes, but rather will choose to learn about and use available standards to guide both their program's operations and their patient care services. These centers of excellence will set a new pace in meeting evolving expectations.

Achievement of the expectations expressed in the standards documents discussed herein requires a two-step strategy that begins with awareness of what is expected and is followed by application of those expectations to practice.

Awareness of Existing Standards

Knowing what standards are, where they come from, and what they mean, as discussed in this chapter, is the first step toward meeting the myriad expectations that standards documents contain.

Table 19.6   Sample Checkpoints for Preparing for Accreditation by the Joint Commission on Accreditation of Healthcare Organizations

	Program operations	Professional expectations
Structure	Have ready a written description of • program's purpose and goals, • patients' rights and responsibilities, • staff credentials and job descriptions, and • staffing and scheduling guidelines.	Have ready a written plan for • emergency readiness, • instructions for patient safety, • infection control measures, • provisions for patient privacy, • chart confidentiality, • protection of valuables, and • the informed consent process.
Process	Policies and procedures for patient care must • be readily available, • be consistently implemented, • match the facility's mission, • reflect current standards, and • be reviewed and revised annually.	Systematic and timely charting of patient care must include • admission assessment, • physician orders and exercise prescription, • exercise and education notes, and • discharge evaluation.
Outcomes	Aggregate program results on file must include • patient satisfaction questionnaires, • program census and service statistics, and • continuous quality improvement plan.	Individualized treatment plan on each chart must include • problems identified, • outcomes projected, • interventions selected, • results documented, and • comparisons of variables before and after rehabilitation.

Note. Data compiled from reference 78.

Each facility that provides cardiac rehabilitation services needs to keep copies of all applicable standards in its program management files. Each professional practicing in cardiac rehabilitation needs to know which standards are followed in their program operation and where reference copies of the standards documents are kept. The following checklist provides a summary of the major documents discussed in this chapter that should be part of every cardiac rehabilitation program's professional library (22,27,34-38,66,69,78,85-87). Once standards documents are assembled and reviewed, the process of integrating expectations from the various sources and merging them with each program's policies begins.

Checklist of Standards Documents That Should Be Available in Program's Professional Library

❑ *1994 Accreditation Manual for Hospitals* (JCAHO, Oakbrook Terrace, Illinois)

❑ *Clinical and Coverage Recommendations for Outpatient Cardiac Rehabilitation,* 1988 (from local Blue Cross and Blue Shield office)

❑ *Clinical Practice Guidelines for Cardiac Rehabilitation,* 1994, Agency for Health Care Policy and Research, Department of Health and Human Services, Washington, DC

❑ *Exercise Standards: A Statement for Health Professionals,* 1990 (AHA, Dallas)

❑ *Guidelines for Cardiac Rehabilitation Programs,* AACVPR, 1994 (Human Kinetics Publishers, Champaign, Illinois)

❑ *Guidelines for Exercise Testing and Prescription,* 4th ed., ACSM, 1991 (Lea & Febiger, Philadelphia)

❑ *Medicare Coverage Issues: Cardiac Rehabilitation Programs,* 1989 Health Care Financing Administration (from regional Medicare intermediary)

❑ Practice acts for professionals requiring licensure:

- Nurses
- Physicians
- Psychologists
- Physical therapists
- Other: _____
  (From your state's professional/occupational license department)

❑ *Scope of Cardiac Rehabilitation Nursing Practice*, 1993 (American Nurses Association, Washington, DC)

❑ State or regional cardiac rehabilitation standards if available from state or regional society:

- Mandatory: Massachusetts, North Carolina
- Voluntary: check with your state society

Application to Practice

All the standards documents discussed in this chapter contain content that addresses both program and personnel expectations. Being familiar with the documents in general and knowing their similarities and differences in particular help identify practice areas to be reviewed and updated.

Program Issues

Paperwork that describes and supports a cardiac rehabilitation program includes policies that outline how the program operates and procedures that detail the patient care services that are provided. Ideally, such paperwork is researched and referenced to the latest published standards in the field. Each program is expected to have a complete and current collection of such paperwork, and day-to-day program operations are expected to match written policies (88). Three key questions need to be asked to determine if program policies are compatible with standards discussed herein.

1. When was the last time policies were revised? If the most recent revision predates 1991, current policies do not consider the three significant standards released at the end of 1990.
2. If policies were revised during or after 1991, do they include footnotes or references to verify that AACVPR, ACSM, and AHA standards were reviewed and incorporated into the latest policy edition?

3. Are there specific policies and procedures that address the program changes repeatedly emphasized by these three sources of standards?

Table 19.7 summarizes key patient care issues and offers standards-based recommendations for program policy updates (35-37).

Personnel Issues

Standards affect cardiac rehabilitation professionals not only by setting guidelines for how programs ought to be run but also by specifying expectations of those who run them. Job descriptions are to personnel what policies and procedures are to programs: they provide detailed expectations. Each professional practicing in cardiac rehabilitation is responsible for knowing the relevant job description and for fulfilling its expectations. Just as program policies need to be updated periodically, so do job descriptions. Professionals should check when their job descriptions were last revised and whether they included current performance expectations. Most standards documents include expectations about the competence, currency, and credentials of cardiac rehabilitation professionals. Table 19.8 lists recommendations for the development of personnel policies related to published personnel expectations.

Summary

Accountability, consistency, credibility, and reproducibility are among the benefits that programs derive from the collection of standards developed for cardiac rehabilitation. To realize such positive results for their programs, professionals practicing in this well-established specialty need to understand the nature of standards, be familiar with the major standards documents and their sources, and apply expressed expectations in their daily patient care and program management. This chapter has attempted to provide background information and describe the current resources for meeting those needs. Realizing that standards express expectations—legal, professional, and functional—cardiac rehabilitation professionals are challenged to match their practice to standards. Recognizing that in today's health care environment compliance with standards may be used to judge quality and allocate shrinking health insurance dollars, programs are striving to meet standards. The standards discussed in this chapter are the culmination of over 2 decades of evolution in the specialty of cardiac rehabilitation.

Table 19.7 Program Issues Addressed in Current Standards Documents

Priority	Policy recommendations
Criteria for admission	Should identify appropriate candidates for cardiac rehabilitation, including • a list of indications encompassing a broad group of cardiac patients, • a list of contraindications to high-level exercise participation, and • a description of the intake process of referral and initial assessment.
Treatment plan	Should specify individualized services and include • a format for documenting patient needs and treatment plans, • tools for promoting patient participation in planning their own treatment, and • a method of comparing outcomes projected at entry to those actually measured upon discharge.
Exercise policy	Should emphasize the use of risk stratification to determine the extent of exercise monitoring and supervision for a given patient and include • a list of criteria for high-risk versus low-risk patients, • a process for determining stratification, • an outline of the program schedule indicating availability of both monitored exercise time and supervised exercise time.
Education policy	Should acknowledge the equal importance of education and exercise to rehabilitation success and include • a list of resources for behavior interventions and referrals, • methods and aids on basic cardiac education for patients and families, and • a process for documenting both teaching and learning.
Program time frame	Should outline optimal timing and flow of program events and include • referral to an outpatient program (within 1 to 2 weeks after hospital discharge), • the performance of symptom-limited graded exercise testing 3 to 4 weeks following illness or surgery, and • a statement of the length of the program (6 to 12 weeks) and exit criteria.

Note. Data compiled from references 35-37.

Table 19.8 Personnel Issues Addressed in Current Standards Documents

Issue	Policy recommendations
Competence	1. Initial job requirements must specify, and each personnel file must document: • valid, current state license for appropriate professionals, • type of academic background, • type and length of prior experience, • specific knowledge or skills required, (e.g., advanced cardiac life support), and • specialty training or internship expected. 2. Orientation checklist must itemize required job tasks and document satisfactory performance by each new employee.
Currency	1. An ongoing, individualized personnel development plan should include • employee-selected goals and projects, • annual performance evaluations, • documentation of continuing education, • participation in quality improvement activities, and • attendance at staff meetings. 2. Job descriptions should be reviewed and revised annually to reflect the latest standards and should include • an organizational chart • staff-patient ratios

Issue	Policy recommendations
Credentialing	Opportunities for advanced professional achievement should be encouraged, including • specialty certification through an appropriate discipline (e.g., the American College of Sports Medicine, the American Nursing Association, the American Physical Therapy Association) • academic coursework, • participation in research, • involvement in professional activities (e.g., membership, fellowship), and • publications and presentations.

Note. Data compiled from references 22, 34, 36, 37, and 78.

References

1. Berra, K. Cardiac and pulmonary rehabilitation: Historical perspectives and future needs. J. Cardiopul. Rehabil. 11(8):8-15; 1991.
2. Goss, J.E. Cardiac rehabilitation: Fad, ritual, or benefit? Practical Cardiol. 12(3):165-171; 1986.
3. Pollock, M.L.; Froelicher, V.F. The Journal of Cardiopulmonary Rehabilitation: Ten years in retrospect. J. Cardiopul. Rehabil. 11(1):5-7; 1991.
4. Wilson, P.K. Cardiac rehabilitation: Then and now. Phys. Sportsmed. 16(9):75-80; 1988.
4a. World Health Organization Expert Committee. Rehabilitation after cardiovascular diseases with special emphasis on developing countries. WHO Technical Report Series #831, Geneva: World Health Organization; 1993.
5. Committee on Exercise. Exercise testing and training of apparently healthy individuals: A handbook for physicians. New York: American Heart Association; 1972.
6. Neufeldt, V.; Guralnik, D.B. Webster's new world dictionary, 3rd college ed. New York: Simon & Schuster; 1988:1306.
7. Southwick, A.F. Negligence. In: The law of hospital and health care administration. Ann Arbor, MI: Health Administration Press; 1978:112-158.
8. Herbert, D.L.; Herbert, W.G. Standards of practice and competency. In: Legal aspects of preventive and rehabilitative exercise programs. 2nd ed. Canton, OH: Professional Reports Corporation; 1989:145-185.
9. Quigley, F.M. Legal issues in nursing—standards of care. Focus on Critical Care. 18(5):390-391; 1991.
10. North Carolina Heart Association. Organizational guidelines for myocardial infarction rehabilitation program. Chapel Hill, NC: The North Carolina Heart Association, Inc.; 1974.
11. Committee on Exercise. Exercise testing and training of individuals with heart disease or at high risk for its development: A handbook for physicians. Dallas: American Heart Association; 1975.
12. American College of Sports Medicine. Guidelines for graded exercise testing and exercise prescription. Philadelphia: Lea & Febiger; 1975.
13. Cardiac Rehabilitation Committee. Guidelines for cardiac rehabilitation centers. Los Angeles: American Heart Association, Greater Los Angeles Affiliate; 1978.
14. American College of Sports Medicine. Position statement: The recommended quantity and quality of exercise for developing and maintaining fitness in healthy adults. Med. Sci. Sports Exerc. 10:7-10; 1978.
15. Subcommittee on Rehabilitation. The exercise standards book. Dallas: American Heart Association; 1979.
16. American College of Sports Medicine. Guidelines for graded exercise testing and exercise prescription. 2nd ed. Philadelphia: Lea & Febiger; 1980.
17. American Nurses Association Division on Medical-Surgical Nursing Practice and American Heart Association Council on Cardiovascular Nursing. Standards of cardiovascular nursing practice. Kansas City, MO: American Nurses Association; 1981.
18. The Cardiac Rehabilitation and Exercise Committee. Guidelines for cardiac rehabilitation centers. 2nd ed. Irvine, CA: American Heart Association, Orange County Chapter; 1989.
19. North Carolina Department of Human Resources. Rules governing the certification of cardiac rehabilitation programs. Raleigh, NC: North Carolina Department of Human Resources; 1984.
20. Pollock, M.L.; Smith, L.K. Cardiac rehabilitation services—A scientific evaluation. New York: American Association of Cardiovascular and Pulmonary Rehabilitation; 1986.
21. American College of Cardiology. Position report on cardiac rehabilitation. J. Am. Coll. Cardiol. 7(2):51-453; 1986.
22. Executive Committee. Guidelines for cardiac rehabilitation. Boston: Massachusetts Society for Cardiac Rehabilitation; 1986.
23. American College of Sports Medicine. Guidelines for exercise testing and prescription. 3rd ed. Philadelphia: Lea & Febiger; 1986.
24. Subcommittee on exercise testing. Guidelines for exercise testing, a report of the joint American College of Cardiology/American Heart Association task force on assessment of cardiovascular procedures. Circulation. 74:653A-667A; 1986.

25. American Medical Association. Diagnostic and therapeutic technology assessment—coronary rehabilitation services. JAMA. 258(14):1959-1962; 1987.

26. American College of Physicians. Position paper—cardiac rehabilitation services. Ann. Intern. Med. 109:671-673; 1988.

27. Standards Committee. Standards for cardiac rehabilitation in California. Anaheim, CA: California Society for Cardiac Rehabilitation; 1988.

28. American College of Physicians. Position paper—evaluation of patients after recent acute myocardial infarction. Ann. Intern. Med. 110:485-488; 1989.

29. Leon, A.S. Position paper of the American association of cardiovascular and pulmonary rehabilitation—scientific evidence of the value of cardiac rehabilitation services with emphasis on patients following myocardial infarction: Exercise conditioning component. J. Cardiopul. Rehabil. 10(3):9-87; 1990.

30. American College of Sports Medicine. Position stand—the recommended quantity and quality of exercise for developing and maintaining cardiorespiratory and muscular fitness in healthy adults. Med. Sci. Sports Exerc. 22(2):265-274; 1990.

31. Miller, N.H.; Taylor, C.B.; Davidson, D.M.; Hill, M.N.; Krantz, D.S. Position paper of the American Association of Cardiovascular and Pulmonary Rehabilitation—the efficacy of risk factor intervention and psychosocial aspects of cardiac rehabilitation. J. Cardiopul. Rehabil. 10(6):198-209; 1990.

32. McHenry, P.L.; Ellestad, M.H.; Fletcher, G.F.; Froelicher, V.; Hartley, H.; Mitchell, J.; Froelicher, E.S. A position statement for health professionals by the committee on exercise and cardiac rehabilitation of the council on clinical cardiology of the American Heart Association. Circulation. 81(1):396-398; 1990.

33. Schlant, R.C.; Friesinger, G.C.; Leonard, J.J. Clinical competence in exercise testing: A statement for physicians from American College of Physicians/American College of Cardiology/American Heart Association task force on clinical privileges in cardiology. Circulation. 82(5):1884-1888; 1990.

34. North Carolina Department of Human Resources. Rules governing the certification of cardiac rehabilitation programs. Raleigh, NC: North Carolina Department of Human Resources; 1990.

35. Fletcher, G.F.; Froelicher, V.F.; Hartley, H.; Haskell, W.L.; Pollock, M.L. Exercise standards: A statement for health professionals from the American Heart Association. Circulation. 82(6):2286-2322; 1990.

36. American Association of Cardiovascular and Pulmonary Rehabilitation. Guidelines for cardiac rehabilitation programs. Champaign, IL: Human Kinetics; 1991.

37. American College of Sports Medicine. Guidelines for exercise testing and prescription. 4th ed. Philadelphia: Lea & Febiger; 1991.

38. Task Force on Cardiac Rehabilitation Nursing. The scope of cardiac rehabilitation nursing practice. Kansas City, MO: American Nurses Association; 1993.

38a. Smith, L.K.; Wenger, N.K.; Froelicher, E.S. Clinical practice guidelines for cardiac rehabilitation. Washington, DC: Agency for Health Care Policy and Research, Public Health Service, Department of Health and Human Services; 1994.

38b. American Association of Cardiovascular and Pulmonary Rehabilitation. Guidelines for cardiac rehabilitation programs (2nd ed.). Champaign, IL: Human Kinetics; 1995.

39. Jonas, S. Measurement and control of the quality of health care. In: Jonas, S. (ed.) Health care delivery in the United States. New York: Springer; 1977:374-409.

40. Hossack, K.F.; Hartwig, R. Cardiac arrest associated with supervised cardiac rehabilitation. J. Cardiac Rehabil. 2:402-408; 1982.

41. VanCamp, S.P.; Peterson, R.A. Cardiovascular complications of outpatient cardiac rehabilitation programs. JAMA. 256:1160-1163; 1986.

42. VanCamp, S.P. The safety of cardiac rehabilitation. J. Cardiopul. Rehabil. 11:64-70; 1991.

43. Oldridge, N.B.; Guyatt, G.H.; Fischer, M.E.; Rimm, A.A. Cardiac rehabilitation after myocardial infarction—combined experience of randomized clinical trials. JAMA. 260:945-950; 1988.

44. O'Connor, G.T.; Buring, J.E.; Yusuf, S.; Goldhaber, S.Z.; Olmstead, E.M.; Paffenbarger, R.S.; Hennekens, C.H. An overview of randomized trials of rehabilitation with exercise after myocardial infarction. Circulation. 80:234-244; 1989.

45. Blair, S.N.; Kohl, H.W.; Paffenbarger, R.S.; Clark, D.G.; Cooper, K.H.; Gibbons, L.W. Physical fitness and all-cause mortality—a prospective study of healthy men and women. JAMA. 262(17):2395-2401; 1989.

46. Blankenhorn, D.H.; Nessim, S.A.; Johnson, R.L.; San Marco, M.E.; Azen, S.P.; Cashen-Hemphill, L. Beneficial effects of combined colestipol-niacin therapy on coronary atherosclerosis and coronary venous bypass grafts. JAMA. 257:3233-3240; 1987.

47. Brown, G.; Albers, J.J.; Fisher, L.D. Regression of coronary artery disease as a result of intensive lipid-lowering therapy in men with high levels of apolipoprotein B. N. Engl. J. Med. 323:1289; 1990.

48. Ornish, D.; Brown, S.E.; Scherwitz, L.W.; Billings, J.H.; Armstrong, W.T.; Ports, T.A.; McLanahan, S.M.; Kirkeeide, R.L.; Brand, R.J.; Gould, K.L. Can lifestyle changes reverse coronary heart disease? Lancet. 336:129-133; 1990.

49. Wenger, N.K. Rehabilitation of the coronary patient: A preview of tomorrow. J. Cardiopul. Rehabil. 11(2):93-98; 1991.

50. Hall, L.K. Guidelines for cardiac rehabilitation: 1987-1190. J. Cardiopul. Rehabil. 11:79-83; 1991.

51. Wenger, N.K. Rehabilitation of the coronary patient in the 21st century: Challenges and opportunities. In: Wenger, N.K.; Hellerstein, H.K. Rehabilitation of the coronary patient. 3rd ed. New York: Churchill Livingstone; 1992.

52. DeBusk, R.F.; Kraemer, H.C.; Nash, E. Stepwise risk stratification soon after acute myocardial infarction. Am. J. Cardiol. 53:1161-1166; 1983.

53. DeBusk, R.F.; Blomquist, G.; Kouchoukos, N.T. Identification and treatment of low risk patients after acute myocardial infarction and coronary artery bypass graft surgery. N. Engl. J. Med. 314(3):161-166; 1986.

54. Herbert, W.G. An examination of the new exercise standards of the ACSM and the AHA. The Exercise Standards and Malpractice Reporter. 5(5):72-73; 1991.

55. Herbert, D.L. The development of standards for cardiovascular and pulmonary rehabilitation. The Exercise Standards and Malpractice Reporter. 4(2):20; 1990.

56. Creighton, H. The practice of nursing. In: Creighton, H. (ed.) Law every nurse should know. 5th ed. Philadelphia: Saunders; 1986.

57. Sol, N. Certification or licensure of fitness professionals—the debate begins. The Exercise Standards and Malpractice Reporter. 4(5):65-69; 1990.

57a. Gillespie, W.J. A model for licensure of exercise professionals. The Exercise Standards and Malpractice Reporter. 7(6):81-87; December, 1993.

58. Commissioner of Public Health. Emergency standards governing cardiac rehabilitation treatment (chapter 628, Acts of 1985). Boston: Massachusetts Department of Public Health; 1985.

59. Division of Health Care Quality. Standards governing cardiac rehabilitation treatment (regulation chapter 105-CMR). Boston: The Commonwealth of Massachusetts, Department of Public Health; 1988.

60. Blue Cross of Massachusetts. Cardiac rehabilitation program amendment (HA 31). 1988.

61. Commonwealth of Massachusetts. Directive to insurance commissioner (section 202). Boston: Author; 1991.

62. Feldstein, P.J. The market for health insurance: Its performance and structure. In: Fieldstein, P.J. (ed.) Health care economics. New York: Wiley; 137-145; 1979.

63. Public Health Service. Scientific evaluation of cardiac rehabilitation services. Federal Register. 50(158):32911; 1985.

64. National Center for Health Services Research and Health Care Technology Assessment. Health technology assessment report number 6—cardiac rehabilitation services. Pub. no. PHS 88-3427. Washington, DC: U.S. Department of Health and Human Services; 1987.

64a. Agency for Health Care Policy and Research. Health technology assessment reports—cardiac rehabilitation programs: Heart transplant, percutaneous transluminal coronary angioplasty, and heart valve surgery patients (# AHCPR 92-0015), Washington, DC: U.S. Department of Health and Human Services; 1991.

65. Greenland, P.; Chu, J.S. Efficacy of cardiac rehabilitation services. Ann. Intern. Med. 109:650-662; 1988.

66. Technology Management Department. Clinical recommendations for outpatient cardiac rehabilitation services. Chicago: Blue Cross and Blue Shield Association; 1988.

67. Wenger, N.K.; Alpert, J.S. Rehabilitation of the coronary patient in 1989. Arch. Intern. Med. 149:1504-1506; 1989.

68. Greenland, P. Efficacy of supervised cardiac rehabilitation programs for coronary patients: Update 1986 to 1990. J. Cardiopul. Rehab. 11(3):197-203; 1991.

69. Health Care Financing Administration. Cardiac stress testing and outpatient hospital cardiac rehabilitation programs (35-25). Medicare coverage handbook—Coverage issues appendix. Washington, DC: U.S. Department of Health and Human Services. May 1980.

70. Health Care Financing Administration: Cardiac rehabilitation programs (35-25, rev. 2). Medicare coverage issues—medical procedures. Washington, DC: U.S. Department of Health and Human Services. December 1985.

71. Medicare Communications. Medicare coverage of cardiac rehabilitation programs (hospital notice 87-27). Pittsburgh: Blue Cross of Western Pennsylvania; June 1987.

72. Health Care Financing Administration. Medicare coverage issues manual—cardiac rehabilitation programs (35-25, rev. 41). Washington, DC: U.S. Department of Health and Human Services. August 1989.

73. Smith, L.K. The realpolitik of rehabilitation. J. Cardiopul. Rehab. 10(9):307-311; 1990.

74. Division of Hospital Accreditation. Accreditation requirements for acute care hospitals. Chicago: American Osteopathic Association; 1992.

75. Commission on Accreditation of Rehabilitation Facilities. Standards manual for organizations serving people with disabilities. Tucson, AZ: Commission on Accreditation of Rehabilitation Facilities; 1988.

76. The Joint Commission. Ambulatory health care standards—strategies for quality care. Oakbrook Terrace, IL: Joint Commission on Accreditation of Healthcare Organizations; 1990:4.

77. The Joint Commission. Agenda for change. Oakbrook Terrace, IL: Joint Commission on Accreditation of Healthcare Organizations; 1986.

78. The Joint Commission. Accreditation manual for hospitals. Oakbrook Terrace, IL: Joint Commission on Accreditation of Healthcare Organizations; 1990:310.

79. Hall, L.K. Quality assurance in cardiac and pulmonary rehabilitation. J. Cardiopul. Rehab. 10:117-119; 1990.

80. The Joint Commission. Accreditation manual for hospitals. Oakbrook Terrace, IL: Joint Commission on Accreditation of Healthcare Organizations; 1993.

81. The Joint Commission. Ambulatory health care standards manual. Oakbrook Terrace, IL: Joint Commission on Accreditation of Healthcare Organizations; 1990.

82. The Joint Commission. Joint commission perspectives. Oakbrook Terrace, IL: Joint Commission on

Accreditation of Healthcare Organizations; May-June 1991.

83. Patterson, C.H.; Parsek, J.D. An introduction to joint commission nursing care standards. Oakbrook Terrace, IL: Joint Commission on Accreditation of Healthcare Organizations; 1991.

84. Hurley, M.L. What do the new JCAHO standards mean to you? RN. 54(6):42-47; 1991.

84a. The Joint Commission. Joint Commission perspectives—special issue on the 1994 accreditation manual for hospitals. Oakbrook Terrace, IL: Author; 1994.

85. Connecticut Society for Cardiac Rehabilitation. Standards of care. New Haven, CT: Author; 1983.

86. Standards and Issues Committee. Guidelines for cardiovascular and pulmonary rehabilitation. Columbia, MO: Missouri Association of Cardiovascular and Pulmonary Rehabilitation; 1991.

87. South Carolina Association of Cardiovascular and Pulmonary Rehabilitation. Program standards. Charleston, SC: Author; 1990.

88. Heggestad, J.C. Policies and procedures in the context of quality and risk management. The Exercise Standards and Malpractice Reporter, 7(6); December, 1993.

PART V

Special Considerations in Cardiac Rehabilitation

Chapter 20

Altitude and Cold

Kent B. Pandolf
Andrew J. Young

Millions of people worldwide live at high altitude or in cold geographical areas. In addition, there is an increasing trend for outdoor winter vacationing that involves recreational activities in the mountains and/or cold environments. The increase in life expectancy and the associated potential for developing coronary artery disease (CAD) means that more people with known or silent CAD might be at increased risk when exposed to the environmental extremes of high altitude and/or cold than in the past.

The issue of an added impairment for people with CAD who rest or exercise at high altitude is debatable because the published scientific literature is so limited. Grover (1) implies that as long as people with cardiovascular disease (CVD) recognize their limitations and maintain an exercise intensity within these limits, cardiac performance will not be compromised. However, West (2) recently advised a person who had apparently recovered from coronary artery bypass graft (CABG) surgery not to take part in a high-altitude trekking vacation in Nepal.

Exposure to a cold environment has been shown to aggravate angina pectoris in susceptible patients with CAD during either rest or exercise (3). Cold exposure provokes angina pectoris or lowers the threshold for exertional angina during whole-body cooling, limb cooling, facial cooling, and cold-air inhalation. Exposure to cold and high-intensity exercise or exercise involving the upper body, such as shoveling snow, would therefore likely put patients with CAD at even greater risk.

The interactive effects of cold and the hypoxic stress of high altitude during rest or exercise are not well understood because of a lack of experimental information (3). Cold and hypoxic stresses combined may decrease mental function, limit heat production, increase ventilatory demands, increase blood viscosity, and increase lactic acid production, therefore possibly producing an unhealthy situation for the normal, healthy person.

The added risks to people with disorders of the cardiovascular or pulmonary systems are obvious. This chapter reviews the separate and interactive effects of high altitude and cold on the physiological responses of people with CVD during rest or exercise.

High Altitude and the Cardiac Patient

Low-altitude residents are increasingly taking advantage of the improved accessibility of high-altitude regions. Some attend conventions or pursue business interests that involve relatively sedentary activities. Many others, however, engage in a variety of recreational activities requiring moderate to strenuous physical exertion. In 1984, for example, about nine million people skied in resorts located in the high altitudes of Colorado (4). Many of these visitors may have some degree (manifest or subclinical) of CAD (5), particularly since the incidence of this disease increases with age. A recent survey suggested that as many as half of the visitors to Keystone, Colorado (2,837 m), were between 40 and 60 years of age (6). Additionally, an estimated 10% of the persons trekking in Nepal are at least 50 years old (7).

Physiological Responses to High Altitude

Barometric pressure decreases with altitude, resulting in a reduction in the partial pressure of oxygen in inspired air (PiO_2), as seen in Figure 20.1. Persons from low altitudes exhibit physiological responses upon ascent to higher elevations that compensate for hypoxia. Whether these compensatory responses could constitute an excessive physiological strain for people with CAD will be considered next.

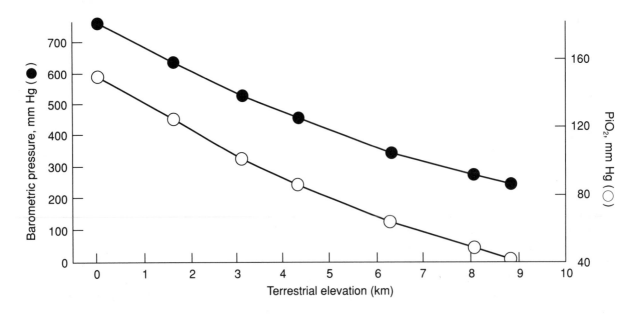

Figure 20.1   Relationship between altitude and both the barometric pressure and the partial pressure of oxygen in the inspired air (PiO₂).
Adapted from Reeves et al. (12).

Cardiac Output and Work Capacity at High Altitude

Acute hypoxia, that is, a PiO₂ less than about 110 mm Hg, which would occur at an altitude of about 2,800 m, stimulates ventilation during rest and exercise, but alveolar and arterial oxygen pressures and arterial oxygen content still fall below sea-level values (8,9). Tachycardia results from a sudden relocation to a high altitude, increasing the cardiac output ($\dot{Q}$) of the unacclimatized lowlander at rest or during any level of submaximal exercise (8,10, 11). Increased $\dot{Q}$ maintains systemic oxygen transport to muscles and submaximal oxygen uptake ($\dot{V}O_2$) the same for a given power output at altitude as sea level (10,11). Maximal $\dot{Q}$, however, is the same on arrival at altitude as at sea level, but is achieved at a lower exercise intensity. Therefore, maximal oxygen uptake ($\dot{V}O_2$max) is reduced at altitude, as seen in Figure 20.2 (8,10,11).

The reduction in $\dot{V}O_2$max with acute high-altitude exposure is proportional to the reduction in arterial oxygen content (C_aO_2) that results from arterial desaturation (8,11). There is little or no measurable decrement in $\dot{V}O_2$max between sea level and 1,000 m, but thereafter $\dot{V}O_2$max decreases by 8%-10% for every additional 1,000 m ascended (8,10). As seen in Figure 20.3, the reduction in $\dot{V}O_2$max with no change in $\dot{V}O_2$ elicited at a submaximal power output means that a given absolute exercise intensity corresponds to a greater relative intensity (i.e., percent of $\dot{V}O_2$max) at high altitude than at sea level (9-11).

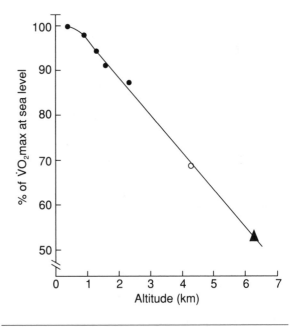

Figure 20.2   Decrement in maximal oxygen uptake ($\dot{V}O_2$max) at high altitude, expressed as a function of the elevation ascended above sea level.
Adapted from Grover et al. (10).

The higher $\dot{Q}$ required for a given intensity of submaximal exercise on arrival at high altitude as compared with sea level increases cardiac work and myocardial oxygen requirements, necessitating an increase in coronary blood flow (5). Even healthy persons experience more cardiovascular strain and reduced endurance for a given intensity

offset the reduction in C_aO_2 and maintain systemic oxygen delivery the same as at sea level. Thus, the higher the altitude ascended, the greater the increase in cardiac work. However, altitude appears to have no effect on the level of cardiac work that can be safely tolerated by people with CAD. The RPP at which angina or ST-segment depression is elicited is the same at high altitude as sea level, but these events occur at a lower intensity of exercise (14). Therefore, one approach to advising patients with known stable CAD is to estimate the activity level that will be safely tolerated by the patient, based on the altitude to which he or she plans to ascend, and then to compare this estimate with the patient's desired activities.

For example, a 55-year-old man whose GXT results indicate that he is at high risk desires to visit a mountain resort at 3,000 m. His $\dot{V}O_2max$ at sea level, measured or estimated using submaximal responses and the nomogram of Astrand and Rodahl (29), is 25 ml · kg^{-1} · min^{-1}. From Figure 20.2, it would be estimated that his $\dot{V}O_2max$ would decline to 21 ml · kg^{-1} · min^{-1} at 3,000 m. During the GXT at sea level, angina and ST-segment depression occurred at a HR of 120 beats/min and a $\dot{V}O_2$ (measured or estimated) of 17 ml · kg^{-1} · min^{-1} (about 5 METs [metabolic equivalents]), or 60% of his maximal capacity at sea level. The relationship between HR and the percentage of $\dot{V}O_2max$ does not change with altitude exposure (30). Therefore at 3,000 m, it would be estimated that the HR would reach 120 beats/min and angina and ST-segment depression would occur at a $\dot{V}O_2$ of about 13 ml · kg^{-1} · min^{-1} (less than 4 METs).

By consulting a table of energy expenditure requirements for various activities (31), it will be seen that activities such as fishing, horseback riding, and leisurely bicycling (< 5.5 mph) could probably be tolerated without adverse effects in this patient, while backpacking up hills, cross-country skiing and snowshoeing would exceed his capacity. The metabolic requirements of downhill skiing appear to be within the patient's tolerated range. However, Grover et al. (32) observed that the HR during downhill skiing is disproportionately high compared to other activities of similar metabolic intensity, possibly due to apprehension and the isometric component of this activity. Therefore, downhill skiing at 3,000 m may indeed elicit a sufficient increase in cardiac work to cause angina in this man.

Following the development of acclimatization, the altitude-induced increment in cardiac work abates. Therefore, the onset of angina and ST-segment depression would probably coincide with a higher intensity of exercise after a few days at altitude than on the first day. The magnitude of improvement varies among individuals and over different altitudes and therefore cannot be predicted before moving to altitude. All travelers, but especially those with CAD, would benefit by incorporating into their itinerary a one-day layover for acclimatization at an intermediate altitude (1,600 m) before continuing on to their ultimate high-altitude destination.

The analysis just described can help the physician advise patients whether the activities that they contemplate performing at a particular altitude might reasonably be expected to be sustained without producing ischemia. However, physicians should provide guidelines concerning activity not in terms of absolute exercise intensity, but rather in terms of HR (14). Travelers who intend to continue an aerobic exercise program at high altitude that was prescribed at sea level and employs ergometers, such as stair-stepping devices or electronic cycles, should be warned to exercise at a lower intensity than usual when they arrive at high altitudes. Most healthy people pace themselves at 35% to 45% of their $\dot{V}O_2max$ during prolonged aerobic activity at sea level (33) and unconsciously adjust their exercise intensity downward at high altitude to maintain a similar relative intensity (34). How people with CAD self-pace at high altitudes is not known.

Section Summary

Lowlanders sojourning at high altitude compensate for hypoxemia by increasing $\dot{Q}$. Systemic and pulmonary arterial pressure also rise. These responses increase cardiac work. Individuals with documented CAD are at higher risk of a coronary event than others at both sea level and high altitude. However, there is no evidence for an increased incidence of coronary events at high altitude. The increased cardiac work in the unacclimatized lowlander with CAD will probably result in increased symptoms, most notably a reduction in the exercise level that can be tolerated without producing angina or ST-segment depression. These effects may abate with acclimatization, so slow ascent is recommended. Increased sympathetic activity and elevated BP at high altitudes, among other changes, may necessitate an adjustment in medication, but this cannot be predicted at sea level. A target HR should be prescribed to guide the intensity of activity. Finally, individuals with CAD should be advised about expected effects of high altitude and encouraged to consult a physician immediately and/or to descend to a lower altitude upon experiencing a serious increase in symptoms. Although travel to high altitudes may not increase the risk of experiencing a coronary event, survival following a coronary event might be jeopardized by the lack of access to medical facilities.

Cold Exposure

Humans predominantly rely on such behavioral strategies as auxiliary heating devices, shelter, and warm clothes to protect themselves from the effects of exposure to the cold (35). If these approaches are inadequate, physiological mechanisms to defend body temperatures are elicited. Human physiological defenses to combat cold are mainly limited to altering peripheral circulation to reduce heat loss and increasing heat production. Before considering the effects of CAD on these physiological mechanisms, a brief review of the responses of normal, healthy individuals exposed to cold is appropriate. The interested reader can find more detailed information on this topic elsewhere (3,36,37).

Human Physiological Responses to Cold

Humans respond to cold stress with two major physiological adjustments: peripheral vasoconstriction, which reduces heat transfer from the deep body to the surface and thus limits loss of body heat to the environment, and involuntary muscular shivering, which increases metabolic heat production and offsets the loss of body heat to the environment (3,35). In addition, metabolic heat production increases with physical exercise and becomes greater as exercise intensity increases. As the exercise intensity increases, shivering is progressively suppressed (11,38), and the increased demand for muscle blood flow overrides the cold-induced vasoconstriction (36). Increased muscle blood flow during exercise facilitates body heat loss to the environment. Whether or not body temperatures decline during cold exposure depends on the balance between heat production and heat loss. Body heat loss is ultimately determined by the rate of heat transfer from the deep core to the surface and regulated by the specific environmental conditions. Moderate exercise easily results in a 10-fold increase in heat production and can be an effective counter to moderate cold stress, if carried out intelligently. The human regulatory adjustments to cold stress and their association with muscular exercise are further illustrated in Figure 20.6.

In comparison to air, water has a much higher thermal capacity (35,36). Therefore, heat conduction away from the skin is facilitated. For individuals exercising in water or wet clothing, moderately cool temperatures may result in body heat losses that cannot be balanced by the heat production achieved during most occupational or recreational activities (39). Many occupational and recreational activities sometimes require equal or greater use of the arms than legs. Heat loss is greater during arm exercise than leg exercise, particularly in cold water (36).

Cardiovascular and Thermoregulatory Responses to Cold

Body cooling results in marked systemic alterations (3,40). Peripheral vasoconstriction leads to a reduction in local circulation and also reduced perfusion to certain vascular beds, producing vascular stasis and local tissue anoxia. Upon initial exposure to cold, there is a paradoxical increase in HR, pulmonary ventilation ($\dot{V}_E$), and mean arterial pressure. As deep body temperature falls, HR, $\dot{V}_E$, and BP decline. Neurohumoral activation results in a release of the anterior pituitary hormones and catecholamines to further conserve body heat and possibly produce a slight nonshivering thermogenesis. Other than physical exercise, the major reflex responses for increasing heat production involve increased muscle tone and shivering. In certain situations, cold-induced vasodilation is observed in the superficial capillaries of limbs when mean skin temperature falls below approximately 18 °C (41). This nervous system reflex seems to act as a major mechanism in protecting peripheral tissues from freezing-cold injury.

During most recreational activities, people are more likely to encounter mild to moderate cold stress of a less prolonged nature (about 1 h) than more prolonged severe cold stress (3). Even mild cold stress alters cardiovascular performance and can result in circulatory alterations that tend to augment myocardial oxygen requirements. This places certain individuals at added risk, particularly while they are exercising. For example, in one study, mild cold stress (an ambient air temperature of 15 °C) during rest or light exercise resulted in a consistently higher total peripheral resistance (TPR), higher systemic arterial pressure, and greater left ventricular work in individuals with and without CAD (42). The increases in TPR were

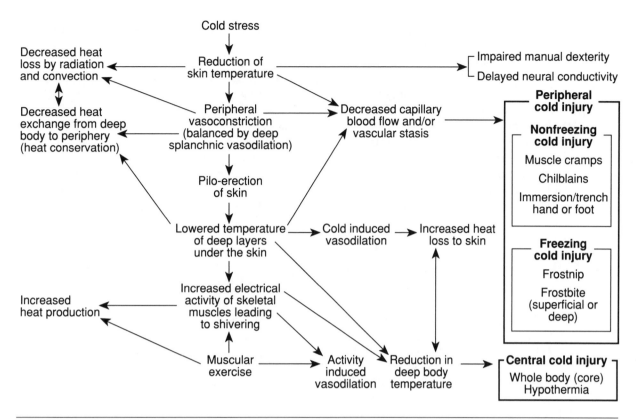

Figure 20.6   Mechanisms of thermoregulation during exercise and cold stress, and the causes of various peripheral or central cold injuries.
From Pandolf (3).

observed without any reflex bradycardia. In addition, $\dot{Q}$ and SV generally are not altered by cold exposure for a given $\dot{V}O_2$.

Facial exposure to moderate cold stress (4 °C) does result in bradycardia associated with a vagal reflex through trigeminal nerve stimulation (43). During facial exposure to cold, sympathetic nervous system stimulation causes a rise in both systolic and diastolic BPs. Therefore, facial and whole-body exposure to cold winds might be expected to precipitate angina in an individual with CAD. Physical exercise would likely accentuate this risk by demanding further increases in left ventricular work and myocardial oxygen demands (3).

Modifying Factors

Several factors influence physiological responses exhibited by normal, healthy people during cold exposure (3,35,43). Such anthropometric factors as body size, shape, and composition influence body heat loss. Smaller people, such as children and women, must maintain a relatively greater heat production to maintain thermal equilibrium for a given level of cold stress. In addition, for two persons of the same weight who differ in height, the

shorter person will lose less heat when cold stressed, primarily because he or she has less exposed surface area (shorter arms, legs, and trunk). In general, fatter people, who have thicker layers of adipose tissue and a smaller surface area–to–mass ratio, are more able to resist body cooling than leaner people (11,36) and are better able to tolerate colder temperatures without shivering. The advantages of increased subcutaneous fat are apparent for all types of cold exposure but are particularly important during cold-water immersion.

One's level of aerobic fitness appears to modify responses during cold exposure. Higher exercise intensities and the associated greater metabolic heat production are better sustained by aerobically fit individuals than by those less fit (36). In addition, aerobically fit individuals display a more sensitive and pronounced shivering response than those of lesser fitness (44).

Chronic or repeated cold exposure produces adaptations in human physiological responses to acute cold. However, the advantages that cold acclimation provides humans relative to their ability to maintain thermal balance during cold exposure are relatively small (37). Individuals seldom spend more than 2% to 10% of any given day outdoors; therefore, natural cold acclimation is not likely to occur (3). However, cold habituation is produced by a few short exposures (37).

Use of hot or alcoholic drinks produces peripheral vasodilation and a significant increase in heat loss from the hands. Alcohol is also thought to temporarily inhibit vasoconstrictor tone. In addition, alcohol increases the rate of deep body heat loss and could possibly enhance the risk of hypothermia (45).

Whether there are gender differences in response to cold air or cold-water immersion is debatable. Graham (46) concludes that women are less thermally sensitive than men to cold water, and men appear more metabolically sensitive during cold-air exposure when compared with women. In contrast, Pandolf and colleagues (47) suggest that water temperature, body mass, and exercise type and intensity are more critical factors to be considered in preventing a decline in deep body temperature during cold-water immersion than surface area–to–mass ratio and gender. This conclusion is more applicable to men and women matched for percent body fat and total skinfold thickness during exercise than at rest in cold water (47).

Obviously, clothing is a crucial factor in protecting people during exposure to the cold and should vary with the ambient temperature, wind velocity, solar load, and exercise intensity (3,39). Proper cold-weather clothing should be wind resistant but must also provide adequate ventilation to reduce sweat accumulation. A multilayered clothing system that can be opened or closed at the neck to eliminate or conserve heat is usually ideal for cold-weather use. Proper protection of the face and extremities may be of greater concern, particularly in the prevention of peripheral cold injuries.

Pathophysiology of Peripheral and Central Cold Injuries

The pathophysiology of peripheral and central cold injuries is not a major consideration of this chapter; cold-associated injuries are reviewed in detail elsewhere (48). Cold disorders are categorized as either non–freezing-cold injuries (muscle cramps, chilblains, immersion/trench hand or foot), freezing-cold injuries (frostnip and frostbite), and whole-body hypothermia. Frostnip and the more serious condition of frostbite result when exposure to cold air causes freezing of tissue, which can be superficial or deep; frostnip is limited

to the superficial skin layers, while frostbite extends through the skin and can involve subcutaneous tissues (48). Skin is known to freeze at tissue temperatures below −2 °C (49). Individuals with CAD may also have peripheral vascular disease (PVD) and therefore be more susceptible to incurring peripheral-cold injuries, since impaired circulation would predispose superficial regions to cool more rapidly. Whole-body (core) hypothermia occurs when the rate of heat production due to exercise and shivering is less than the rate of heat loss at the skin and via the respiratory tract. An individual is considered hypothermic when his or her deep body temperature drops below 35 °C.

The Cardiac Patient

Morbidity and Mortality in the Winter

The incidence of CAD is reported to be higher in the winter than in the summer (50). Figure 20.7 presents the relationship between the number of deaths from CAD reported in England and Wales during June and December from 1950 to 1962. CAD mortality varied more in the winter than in the summer, but was consistently higher in the winter over this 13-year period, with a minimum and maximum rise above comparative summer levels of 20% and 70%, respectively. Figure 20.8 displays the log monthly mortality index for CAD in relationship to the mean monthly temperature from 1958 to 1962 in this same study (50). These data illustrate that the drop in mean monthly temperature is associated with a significant rise in mortality. These authors conclude that the high correlation (r = −0.95) with coldness indicates that nearly all of the fluctuation in CAD mortality can be accounted for by environmental temperature variations.

However, another study (51) provides somewhat conflicting observations in its evaluation of CAD mortality from 1960 to 1974 in metropolitan Toronto during winter months. A significantly greater increase in CAD mortality only occurred in men under 65 years of age. The authors suggest that unusual physical activity, such as snow shoveling, or other factors may have been a more potent cause of CAD mortality in these individuals than the sudden drop in environmental temperature.

Type of Cold Exposure

Cold exposure results in systemic responses that are indicative of an activated sympathetic nervous system. For instance, exposure to cold generally

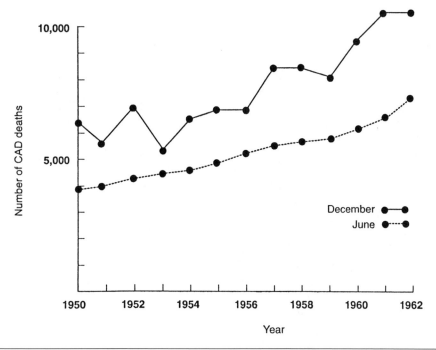

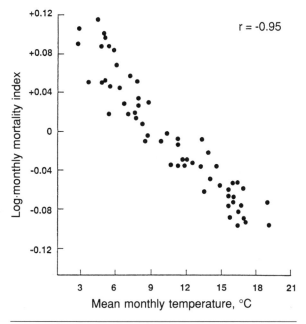

Figure 20.7 Number of deaths from coronary artery disease (CAD) in England and Wales during June and December from 1950 to 1962.
From Rose (50). Reprinted with permission.

Figure 20.8 Relationship between the logarithm of monthly mortality index from coronary artery disease and the average temperature for each month during the period of 1958-1962.
Adapted from Rose (50).

results in increased TPR, arterial pressure, myocardial inotropic state, and cardiac work during rest of exercise (3). Many of these altered responses are observed even during very mild cold stress,

whether the cold exposure is generalized (whole body) or localized. Therefore, both generalized and localized cold exposure can lower the threshold and provoke an attack of angina pectoris in individuals with CAD because of the consequent augmentation of increased myocardial oxygen demands.

Generalized Cold Exposure. Freedberg et al. (52) studied 22 CAD patients with angina pectoris during exercise in the cold (7.2° to 12.8 °C) and at room temperature (22.2° to 23.9 °C). Twelve of the 22 patients (55%) were able to perform more exercise before angina onset at the warmer temperature than when exposed to cold. In 10 patients (45%) with CAD, exercise tolerance was not affected by environmental temperature. The authors concluded that the majority of CAD patients experienced angina while exercising in the cold and that many of these same patients failed to develop angina at similar or greater intensities of exercise performed at a warmer room temperature. Epstein et al. (42) evaluated the circulatory responses of 6 CAD patients during rest and mild exercise at 15 °C and 25 °C. During both rest and exercise at 15 °C, the patients exhibited higher TPR, systemic arterial pressure, and left ventricular minute work than at 25 °C. Three patients (50%) experienced angina pectoris during exercise in the cold but not at the higher temperature. The authors concluded

that the increased myocardial oxygen requirements associated with cold exposure and exercise
would more readily provoke an angina attack in
CAD patients. More recently, Brown and Oldridge
(53) examined 9 male CAD patients with a history of effort angina during exercise in the cold
(–7.5 °C) or at temperate conditions (24 °C). At
this more severe level of cold stress, all 9 patients
experienced an earlier onset of angina compared to
the warmer environment. The authors concluded
that "at sub-zero environmental temperatures it is
advisable for CAD patients who are cold-intolerant
to dress appropriately and reduce their exercise
intensity or otherwise to exercise indoors." Rosengren et al. (54) studied 9 male CAD patients with
a history of both angina and ischemic exercise ECG
changes during exercise in the cold (mean temperature = –8.2 °C) and at a room temperature of
22 °C. SBP was higher in the cold, and 7 of the
patients displayed a greater ST-segment depression during exercise in the cold compared with the
same intensity at room temperature.

Localized Cold Exposure.   Neill and colleagues
(55) studied the coronary and systemic hemodynamic responses during facial cooling in 19 CAD
patients who displayed exertional angina pectoris.
Facial cooling was accomplished through the use
of a damp towel filled with ice chips that was
placed on the patient's forehead for 6 min. Figure
20.9 shows the systolic and diastolic systemic arterial pressures, HR, and coronary blood flow responses during facial cooling for the first 9 CAD
patients tested. Systemic arterial pressure and coronary blood flow rose to peak values in 1 min and
2 min, respectively, with a slight and more gradual
increase in HR. Facial cooling resulted in angina
in 5 patients, and chemical evidence of myocardial
hypoxia was seen in 7.

In addition to their experiments on whole-body
exposure to cold, Freedberg et al. (52) examined
the responses of the same 22 CAD patients during
exercise at room temperature while holding an ice
cube in one hand. All but 1 of the patients (95%)
experienced angina. Similar angina attacks were
produced after strapping ice on patients' thighs or
spraying their exposed backs with ethyl chloride.
Most of the patients experienced angina within 10
s of ice application, with the maximum effect 30
to 40 s after application.

Angina pectoris in CAD patients is also produced by cold-air inhalation during rest or exercise. Sorensen (56) studied 15 CAD patients with
known angina during the inhalation of cold air
(–14 °C) while they rested for 10 min at room temperature (20 °C). Under these conditions, 6 patients

(40%) suffered anginal pains, while only 1 showed
ECG changes. Hattenhauer and Neill (57) reported
that cold-air inhalation (–20 °C) of 4-min duration
at room temperature (20 °C) provoked angina in
4 of 17 CAD patients (24%) at rest and in 4 of 7
patients (57%) that were paced at a subanginal
HR level. Brown and Oldridge (53) contrasted the
onset of angina in 9 CAD patients during exercise
and with either generalized cold exposure or cold-
air inhalation. Figure 20.10 illustrates that, compared with exercising in a room temperature environment and breathing room temperature air,
angina onset time was reduced most (24%) when
patients breathed room temperature air in a cold
environment and reduced to a lesser extent (15%)
when patients breathed cold air in a cold environment. Cold-air inhalation at room temperature did
not significantly reduce exercise time to angina
onset when contrasted to the room temperature/
room inspired air condition.

Type and Intensity of Exercise

The type and intensity of exercise may modify the
risk that cold exposure poses for the CAD patient.
Occupational or recreational activities that greatly
involve the upper body or result in increased metabolic demands are of particular concern in the cold.

As discussed earlier, snow shoveling, which involves the muscles of the upper body, has been
associated with increased CAD mortality during
winter months (51). The use of the upper extremities during snow shoveling has a significant isometric component, which generally results in elevated systolic and diastolic BPs. In addition,
shoveling large loads of heavy snow results in respiratory effort (Valsalva maneuvers) that affects
circulation by decreasing venous return to the
heart and potentially causes significant cardiac ir-
regularities (58). Therefore, snow shoveling and
exposure to cold poses a potential danger for those
patients with known CAD, but an even greater
danger for people unaware of existing but silent
CAD (59). Balke (59) further stated that most CAD
patients would probably not venture out to shovel
snow during a cold morning after a winter storm.
However, people unaware of their existing CAD
and the threat posed by the combination of severe
cold and snow shoveling could trigger a cardiac
episode.

Recreational activities such as cross-country skiing could potentially pose hazards to CAD patients. Nilsson and Stanghelle (60) evaluated 33
CAD patients who participated on 52 occasions in

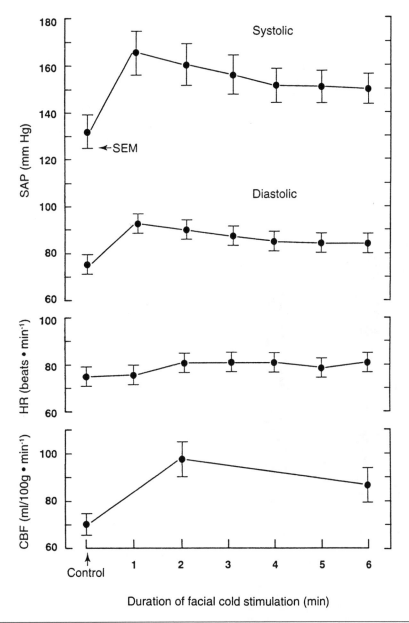

Duration of facial cold stimulation (min)

Figure 20.9 Systolic and diastolic systemic arterial pressures (SAP), heart rate (HR), and coronary blood flow (CBF) during 6 min of cutaneous facial cold stimulation in 9 CAD patients. (Values are mean ±SEM.) From Neill et al. (55). Reprinted with permission.

a 22-km cross-country ski race for impaired individuals. No complications were reported during these races. The authors concluded that cross-country skiing could be done by most CAD patients provided that extremes of cold and high-intensity exercise are avoided. However, it should be kept in mind that cross-country skiing increases metabolic demands and requires the use of the upper extremities in addition to the leg muscles. Pandolf et al. (61) have reported that walking over packed snow significantly increases energy requirements. The cross-country skiing surface at most recreational sites is soft pack over deep snow

which would likely further increase the energy cost for this type of locomotion (62).

The effects of swimming in cool or cold water may also pose a threat to CAD patients (63). In one study, 8 male CAD patients exercised in a swimming flume at water temperatures of 18 °C and 25.5 °C. Two patients reported experiencing angina while swimming in cool (25.5 °C) water and 1 in cold (18 °C) water. However, ST-segment depression was observed in 6 of the 8 patients at both water temperatures. The authors concluded that swimming in cool or cold water should be conducted with caution in CAD patients because

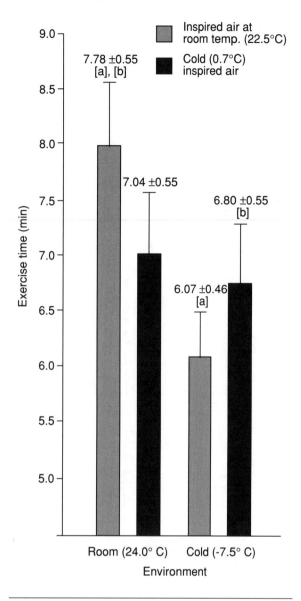

Figure 20.10 Exercise time to onset of angina as a function of environmental temperature and inspired-air temperature. (Values are mean ±SEM; *p* < 0.05 for comparisons [a] and [b].)
From Brown and Oldridge (53). Reprinted with permission.

many of these individuals fail to identify their ischemic symptoms and may put themselves at risk.

Section Summary

Cold exposure poses a potential hazard to the CAD patient. Both localized and generalized cold exposure during rest or exercise lower the threshold and can provoke angina in individuals with CAD. CAD patients should be reminded of the use of proper clothing during cold exposure. Clothing should be thick and multilayered and should provide adequate ventilation to keep it dry. All areas of the body (particularly the face, ears, neck, hands, and feet) should be adequately covered and kept warm. High-intensity exercise or exercise that mainly involves the upper extremities should be avoided by cardiac patients during cold exposure. Such recreational activities as canoeing and cross-country skiing can involve high-intensity exercise, which may be contraindicated for CAD patients during cold exposure. Physical activities like heavy lifting and snow shoveling involve the upper extremities and are contraindicated for many patients during exposure to cold. Caution should be exercised by patients at risk who employ swimming as a form as exercise. Swimming in unheated or improperly heated pools and in the ocean (50% of which is less than 20 °C) should be approached with caution (3). The degree of precaution during cold exposure will vary with the severity of the patient's CAD. When exposure to cold is expected, CAD patients should consult their physician as to the degree of precaution necessary.

High Altitude Combined With Cold Exposure

Air temperature and humidity generally decrease as one ascends mountainous terrain, and there are increases in wind velocity and solar radiation. Although much variation exists, air temperature decreases about 1 °C for every 150 m of ascent (64). The low humidity at high altitude increases heat loss by facilitating evaporative cooling. The low humidity combined with the greater pulmonary ventilation found at high altitudes may be associated with a significant increase in respiratory heat loss and serious performance consequences, particularly in the cold (65). The greater wind velocity observed in cold, mountainous terrain can increase the windchill factor and consequently increase the incidence of peripheral freezing-cold injuries. In addition, wind can penetrate clothing and disturb the trapped dead-air layer, decreasing the overall clothing insulation. Although precautions should be taken to prevent sunburn, the solar radiation at high altitude can provide an important source of heat gain (3). When high altitude is combined with cold exposure, it is important to wear dark colors because black clothing absorbs 88% of the solar radiation, khaki 57%, and white only 20% (64). Again, the importance of proper cold-weather clothing to minimize the effects of cold stress at altitude cannot be overemphasized.

For some of these reasons and others, Balke (59) concluded that altitude and cold "must be considered a greater hazard to the well-being of a heart patient than either of these stresses alone." However, because of a lack of scientific information, the interactive effects of cold and high altitude during rest or exercise are not well understood (3). The few published reports that evaluated human performance under the combined stresses of cold and high altitude did not evaluate CAD patients, but instead studied normal, healthy individuals. Grover et al. (32) reported observations from 149 men during recreational skiing above 3,100 m when the ambient temperature was -1 ± 3 °C. Five of the men (3% overall, or 5.6% of the 90 men over 40 years of age) developed abnormal ST-segment depression during or immediately after skiing. The authors concluded that the incidence of ST-segment depression during high-altitude skiing did not differ from that previously reported (4.9%-5.1%) during exercise at low altitude in the absence of cold or hypoxia. Further, this low incidence of ischemic ST-segment depression possibly reflected the high level of physical fitness reported by the subjects, who skied at high altitude in the cold. Shlim and Houston (7) reported no cardiac deaths among trekkers in Nepal to altitudes over 5,500 m during a 3.5-year period. Of the 148,000 persons who obtained trekking permits during this time, only 6 men required helicopter evacuation for "cardiac problems."

A number of factors have been suggested that could decrease human performance during cold exposure at altitude and ultimately affect CAD patients (3,64):

- Combined cold and hypoxic stress may decrease mental function and increase the risk for accidental injury.
- Since $\dot{V}O_2$max is reduced at high altitude, heat production is limited and a greater risk of cold injury exists.
- The increased $\dot{V}_E$ at high altitude results in a greater respiratory heat and water loss, which is a disadvantage during cold exposure.
- Both cold and chronic hypoxia are associated with hemoconcentration and a potentially additive effect on blood viscosity, which could lead to increased cardiac work and decreased blood flow, resulting in a compromised myocardium.
- Peripheral vasoconstriction (cold stress) and high blood viscosity could lead to an impairment of tissue perfusion, possibly tissue

necrosis, and a greater risk for peripheral cold injury. Since skin blood flow is reduced by vasoconstriction at high altitude under thermoneutral temperatures, this response could magnify the reduction in skin blood flow known to occur during cold stress.
- Combined cold and hypoxic stresses may increase lactic acid production at a given exercise intensity and possibly further compromise exercise performance.

Because these all pose a hazard for normal, healthy people during combined high altitude and cold, a CAD patient could well be at added risk when exposed to these two environmental extremes.

Summary

People with CAD are generally at higher risk than normal, healthy individuals at both sea level and high altitude, particularly while performing physical exercise. However, there is little scientific support for an increased incidence of coronary events at high altitude. Balke (59) has concluded that "moderate altitude should not necessarily be considered too great a risk for any patient with atherosclerotic heart disease." This conclusion is probably correct, assuming that exercise intensity is reduced in association with the known reduction in $\dot{V}O_2$max as one progressively ascends mountainous terrain. Elevations in BP and other cardiovascular alterations resulting from the hypoxia of high altitude may require adjustment in medication that is difficult to predict at sea level.

Cold exposure is known to present added risk to the CAD patient. Both localized and generalized exposure to cold have been shown to lower the angina threshold and provoke angina in individuals with CAD. High-intensity exercise and physical activities involving the upper extremities are contraindicated for CAD patients during cold exposure. Proper clothing is of utmost importance for patients at this environmental extreme. Brown and Oldridge (53) concluded that "at sub-zero environmental temperatures it is advisable for [CAD] patients who are cold-intolerant to dress appropriately and reduce their exercise intensity or otherwise to exercise indoors," which appears to be prudent advice.

Even though there is a lack of scientific information, it is probably safe to conclude that the interactive effects of high altitude and cold should be considered a potentially greater risk to the CAD patient than the single effects of either environmental extreme (3,59). When the potential exists for exposure to the environmental extremes of high altitude and/or cold, CAD patients should consult their physicians as to the degree of precaution necessary.

Acknowledgments

The authors gratefully acknowledge the assistance of Paul B. Rock, D.O., PhD, for his critical comments during the development of this chapter and of Ms. Edna R. Safran for her technical assistance in preparing the chapter.

The views, opinions, and findings in this report are those of the authors and should not be construed as an official Department of the Army position, policy, or decision, unless so designated by other official documentation. Approved for public release; distribution is unlimited.

References

1. Grover, R.F. Performance at altitude. In: Strauss, R.H. ed. Sports medicine and physiology. Philadelphia: Saunders; 1979:327-343.

2. West, J.B. The safety of trekking at high altitude after coronary bypass surgery. JAMA. 260:2218-2219; 1988.

3. Pandolf, K.B. Importance of environmental factors for exercise testing and exercise prescription. In: Skinner, J.S., ed. Exercise testing and exercise prescription for special cases-theoretical basis and clinical application. Philadelphia: Lea & Febiger; 1987: 77-98.

4. Moore, L.G.; Cymerman, A.; Huang S.-Y.; McCullough, E.R.; McCullough, R.G.; Reeves, J.T.; Rock, P.B.; Young, A.J.; Young, P.M.; Weil, J.V. Propranolol does not impair exercise oxygen uptake in normal men at high altitude. J. Appl. Physiol. 61:1935-1941; 1986.

5. Rennie, D. Will mountains trekkers have heart attacks? JAMA. 261:1045-1046; 1989.

6. Hultgren, H.N. Effects of altitude upon cardiovascular diseases. In: Syllabus of the first world congress on wilderness medicine. Point Reyes Station, CA: Wilderness Medical Society; 1991:247-258.

7. Shlim, D.; Houston, R. Helicopter rescues and deaths among trekkers in Nepal. JAMA. 261:1017-1019; 1989.

8. Fulco, C.S.; Cymerman, C. Human performance and acute hypoxia. In: Pandolf, K.B.; Sawka, M.N.; Gonzalez, R.R., eds. Human performance physiology and environmental medicine at terrestrial extremes. Indianapolis: Benchmark Press; 1988:467-495.

9. Young, A.J.; Young, P.M. Human acclimatization to high terrestrial altitude. In: Pandolf, K.B.; Sawka, M.N.; Gonzalez, R.R., eds. Human performance physiology and environmental medicine at terrestrial extremes. Indianapolis: Benchmark Press; 1988:497-543.

10. Grover, R.F.; Weil, J.V.; Reeves, J.T. Cardiovascular adaptation to exercise at high altitude. In: Pandolf, K.B., ed. Exercise and sport sciences reviews. New York: Macmillan; 1986:269-302.

11. Young, A.J. Energy substrate utilization during exercise in extreme environments. In: Pandolf, K.B.; Holloszy, J.O., eds. Exercise and sport sciences reviews. Baltimore: Williams & Wilkins; 1990:65-118.

12. Reeves, J.T.; Wolfel, E.E.; Green, H.J.; Mazzeo, R.S.; Young, A.J.; Sutton, J.R.; Brooks, G.A. Oxygen transport during exercise at altitude and the lactate paradox: Lessons from Operation Everest II and Pikes Peak. In: Holloszy, J.O., ed. Exercise and sport sciences reviews. Baltimore: Williams & Wilkins; 1992:275-296.

13. Balke, B. Cardiac performance in relation to altitude. Am. J. Cardiol. 14:796-810; 1964.

14. Morgan, B.J.; Alexander, J.K.; Nicoli, S.A.; Brammell, H.L. The patient with coronary heart disease at altitude: Observations during acute exposure to 3100 meters. J. Wilderness Med. 1:147-153; 1990.

15. Grover, R.F.; Lufschanowski, R.; Alexander, J.K. Alterations in the coronary circulation of man following ascent to 3100 m altitude. J. Appl. Physiol. 41:832-838; 1976.

16. Young, A.J.; Young, P.M.; McCullough, R.E.; Moore, L.G.; Cymerman, A.; Reeves, J.T. Effect of beta-adrenergic blockade on plasma lactate concentration during exercise at high altitude. Eur. J. Appl. Physiol. 63:315-322; 1991.

17. Fulco, C.S.; Cymerman, A.; Rock, P.B.; Farese, G. Hemodynamic responses to upright tilt at sea level and high altitude. Aviat. Space Environ. Med. 56: 1172-1176; 1985.

18. Fulco, C.S.; Larsen, R.; Rock, P.B.; Young, A.J.; Cymerman, A. The effect of spironolactone on the cardiocirculatory responses to upright tilt at sea level and at simulated high altitude. Aviat. Space Environ. Med. 57:787-791; 1986.

19. Fulco, C.S.; Cymerman, A.; Reeves, J.T.; Rock, P.B.; Trad, L.A.; Young, P.M. Propranolol and the compensatory circulatory responses to orthostasis at high altitude. Aviat. Space Environ. Med. 60:1049-1055; 1989.

20. Tuck, M. The sympathetic nervous system in essential hypertension. Am. Heart J. 112:877-886; 1985.

21. Inama, K.; Halhuber, M.J. Der herz-kreislaufkranke im hochgebirgs klima. Frankfurt: Deutsche Zentrale fur Volksgesundheitspflege; 1975.

22. Ward, M.P.; Milledge, J.S.; West, J.B. High altitude medicine and physiology. Philadelphia: University of Pennsylvania Press; 1989.

23. Hultgren, H.N.; Grover, R.F.; Hartley, L.H. Abnormal circulatory responses to high altitude in subjects with a previous history of high-altitude pulmonary edema. Circulation. 44:759-770; 1971.

24. Malconian, M.; Rock, P.; Hultgren, H.; Donner, H.; Cymerman, A.; Groves, B.; Reeves, J.; Alexander, J.; Sutton, J.; Nitta, M.; Houston, C. The electrocardiogram at rest and exercise during a simulated ascent of Mt. Everest (Operation Everest II). Am. J. Cardiol. 65:1475-1480; 1990.

25. Hackett, P.H.; Creach, C.E.; Grover, R.F.; Honigman, B.; Houston, C.S.; Reeves, J.T.; Sophocles, A.M.; Van Hardenbroer, M. High-altitude pulmonary edema in persons without the right pulmonary artery. N. Engl. J. Med. 302:1070-1073; 1980.

26. Froelicher, V.F.; West, J.B. Trekking in Nepal: Safety after coronary artery bypass. JAMA. 259:3184; 1988.

27. Hultgren, H.N. Coronary heart disease and trekking. J. Wilderness Med. 1:154-161; 1990.

28. Hultgren, H.N. The safety of trekking at high altitude after coronary bypass surgery. JAMA. 260:2218; 1988.

29. Astrand, P.O.; Rodahl, K.; editors. Textbook of work physiology. New York: McGraw-Hill; 1977.

30. Miles, D.S.; Wagner, J.A.; Horvath, S.M.; Reyburn, J.A. Absolute and relative work capacity in women at 758, 586, and 523 torr barometric pressure. Aviat. Space Environ. Med. 51:439-444; 1980.

31. McArdle, W.D.; Katch, F.I.; Katch, V.L. Exercise physiology. Philadelphia: Lea & Febiger; 1981:486-493.

32. Grover, R.F.; Tucker, C.E.; McGroarty, S.R.; Travis, R.R. The coronary stress of skiing at high altitude. Arch. Intern. Med. 150:1205-1208; 1990.

33. Levine, L.; Evans, W.J.; Winsmann, F.R.; Pandolf, K.B. Prolonged self-paced hard physical exercise comparing trained and untrained men. Ergonomics. 25:393-400; 1982.

34. Nag, R.K.; Sen, R.N.; Ray, U.S. Optimal rate of work for mountaineers. J. Appl. Physiol. 44:952-955; 1978.

35. Young, A.J. Effects of aging on human cold tolerance. Exp. Aging Res. 17:205-213; 1991.

36. Toner, M.M.; McArdle, W.D. Physiological adjustments of man to the cold. In: Pandolf, K.B.; Sawka, M.N.; Gonzalez, R.R., eds. Human performance physiology and environmental medicine at terrestrial extremes. Indianapolis: Benchmark Press; 1988:361-399.

37. Young, A.J. Human adaptation to cold. In: Pandolf, K.B.; Sawka, M.N.; Gonzalez, R.R., eds. Human performance physiology and environmental medicine at terrestrial extremes. Indianapolis: Benchmark Press; 1988:401-434.

38. Horvath, S.M. Exercise in a cold environment. In: Miller, D.I., ed. Exercise and sport sciences reviews. Philadelphia: Franklin Institute Press; 1981:221-263.

39. Gonzalez, R.R. Biophysics of heat transfer and clothing considerations. In: Pandolf, K.B.; Sawka, M.N.; Gonzalez, R.R., eds. Human performance physiology and environmental medicine at terrestrial extremes. Indianapolis: Benchmark Press; 1988:45-95.

40. Herrington, L.P. The range of physiological response to climatic heat and cold. In: Newburgh, L.H., ed. Physiology of heat regulation and the science of clothing. New York: Hafner Publishing; 1968:262-276.

41. Lewis, T. Observations upon reactions of vessels of human skin to cold. Heart. 15:177-208; 1930.

42. Epstein, S.E.; Stampfer, M.; Beiser, G.D.; Goldstein, R.E.; Braunwald, E. Effects of a reduction in environmental temperature on the circulatory response to exercise in man. N. Engl. J. Med. 180:7-11; 1969.

43. LeBlanc, J. Man in the cold. Springfield, IL: Charles C Thomas; 1975.

44. Bittel, J.H.M.; Nonotte-Varly, C.; Livecchi-Gonnot, G.H.; Savourey, G.L.M.J.; Hanniquet, A.M. Physical fitness and thermoregulatory reactions in a cold environment in men. J. Appl. Physiol. 65:1984-1989; 1988.

45. Goldman, R.F.; Newman, R.W.; Wilson, O. Effects of alcohol, hot drinks, or smoking on hand and foot heat loss. Acta Physiol. Scand. 87:498-506; 1973.

46. Graham, T.E. Thermal, metabolic, and cardiovascular changes in men and women during cold stress. Med. Sci. Sports Exerc. 20:S185-S192; 1988.

47. Pandolf, K.B.; Toner, M.M.; McArdle, W.D.; Magel, J.R.; Sawka, M.N. Influence of body mass, morphology, and gender on thermal responses during immersion in cold water. In: Bove, A.A.; Bachrach, A.J.; Greenbaum, L.J., eds. Underwater and hyperbaric physiology IX. Bethesda, MD: Undersea and Hyperbaric Medical Society; 1987:145-152.

48. Hamlet, M.P. Human cold injuries. In: Pandolf, K.B.; Sawka, M.N.; Gonzalez, R.R., eds. Human performance physiology and environmental medicine at terrestrial extremes. Indianapolis: Benchmark Press; 1988:435-466.

49. Pandolf, K.B.; Young, A.J. Environmental extremes and performance. In: Astrand, P.O.; Shepherd, R.J., eds. Sports and human performance. Oxford: Blackwell Scientific; 1992:270-282.

50. Rose, G. Cold weather and ischaemic heart disease. Br. J. Prev. Soc. Med. 20:97-100; 1966.

51. Anderson, T.W.; Rochard, C. Cold snaps, snowfall and sudden death from ischemic heart disease. Can. Med. Assoc. J. 121:1580-1583; 1979.

52. Freedberg, A.S.; Spiegl, E.D.; Riseman, J.E.F. Effect of external heat and cold on patients with angina pectoris: Evidence for the existence of a reflex factor. Am. Heart J. 27:611-622; 1944.

53. Brown, C.F.; Oldridge, N.B. Exercise-induced angina in the cold. Med. Sci. Sports Exerc. 17:607-612; 1985.

54. Rosengren, A.; Wennerblom, B.; Bjuro, T.; Wilhelmsen, L.; Bake, B. Effect of cold on ST amplitudes and blood pressure during exercise in angina pectoris. Eur. Heart J. 9:1074-1080; 1988.

55. Neill, W.A.; Duncan, D.A.; Kloster, F.; Mahler, D.J. Response of coronary circulation to cutaneous cold. Am. J. Med. 56:471-476; 1974.

56. Sorensen, E.W. Angina pectoris and exposure to cold. Acta Med. Scand. 179:329-331; 1966.

57. Hattenhauer, M.; Neill, W.A. The effect of cold air inhalation on angina pectoris and myocardial oxygen supply. Circulation. 51:1053-1058; 1975.

58. Lamb, L.E. Do you have the heart for shoveling snow? Health Letter. 18:11; 1981.

59. Balke, B. Altitude and cold: The cardiac patient. In: Pollock, M.L.; Schmidt, D.H., eds. Heart disease and rehabilitation. Boston: Houghton Mifflin; 1986:537-547.

60. Nilsson, S.; Stanghelle, J.K. Cross-country skiing in coronary patients. Int. Rehabil. Med. 5:206-208; 1983.

61. Pandolf, K.B.; Haisman, M.F.; Goldman, R.F. Metabolic energy expenditure and terrain coefficients for walking on snow. Ergonomics. 19:683-690; 1976.

62. Oldridge, N.B.; MacDougall, J.D. Cross-country skiing: Precautions for cardiac patients. Physician Sportsmed. 9:64-70; 1981.

63. Magder, S.; Linnarsson, D.; Gullstrand, L. The effect of swimming on patients with ischemic heart disease. Circulation. 63:979-986; 1981.

64. Ward, M. Mountain medicine: A clinical study of cold and high altitude. London: Crosby Lockwood Staples; 1975.

65. Baker, P.T., editor. The biology of high-altitude peoples. Cambridge: Cambridge University Press; 1978.

Chapter 21

Heat and Air Pollution

Lawrence J. Folinsbee

It has been predicted that the average temperature of the globe will increase substantially over the next century. This will be associated with increased numbers and severity of heat waves and, depending on the extent of control measures, could well result in increased levels of air pollution. Humans will cope with these thermal problems by using behavioral means, such as seeking locales that have shade, increased air movement, or air conditioning, and by physiological means that elicit increased peripheral blood flow and sweating.

This chapter will focus on the human physiological responses to heat stress, heat acclimatization, and exposure to air pollutants. Much of the data that will be discussed pertains to healthy subjects. The number of studies of cardiac patients exposed to these stresses is limited because of the risks inherent in stressing already compromised cardiac patients with heat and air pollutants. Nevertheless, several investigations of carbon monoxide exposure in patients with coronary artery disease (CAD) have been published recently. Most air pollutants have their primary effects on the lungs, and these responses will be discussed.

Environmental Heat Stress

The cardiovascular system is the primary effector system in the response to heat stress. An adequate cardiac reserve is essential to appropriate response to both acute and chronic heat stress. Not only do cardiac patients experience a loss of cardiac reserve because of disease, but there is also an age-related decline in both cardiovascular and pulmonary reserves.

Mortality During Heat Waves

About 200 excess deaths per year in the United States are attributed to extremes of heat exposure

(1). The true number of deaths caused by heat exposure is probably at least twice this figure, since many heat-related deaths may be misclassified as being due to cerebrovascular or cardiovascular disease (CVD). Excess deaths may exceed 1,500 in a year when heat waves are frequent; the increased mortality is usually correlated with the previous day's temperature. The greatest increase in risk is in the elderly population (Figure 21.1), in which a lower maximum $\dot{Q}$ may not permit adequate peripheral vasodilation, necessary to increase heat loss. In addition to advanced age, other risk factors include low socioeconomic status (presumably due to reduced access to air conditioning), male gender (mainly a risk in young men, among whom excess "machismo" or competitiveness may prevent them from drinking an adequate amount of water or seeking cool surroundings), chronic illness (including chronic pulmonary disease and CAD), prior history of heat illness, obesity (due to increased insulation, which prevents adequate heat loss), and the use of certain medications (such tranquilizers as phenothiazine, which impair thermoregulation, and such anticholinergic drugs as tricyclic antidepressants and antihistamines, which impair the sweating response). Severe heat stress represents a serious health threat that can lead to death.

Physiological Response to Heat Stress

Humans deal with heat stress through both physiological and behavioral means. Although this section will focus on physiological responses, the behavioral responses are equally important, particularly with the availability of air conditioning in our modern society. Simply moving from the outdoor environment of heat, humidity, and high radiant heat load into an air-conditioned building is an extremely effective means of dealing with heat exposure and one that is highly recommended for patients who have minimal reserve to handle the

327

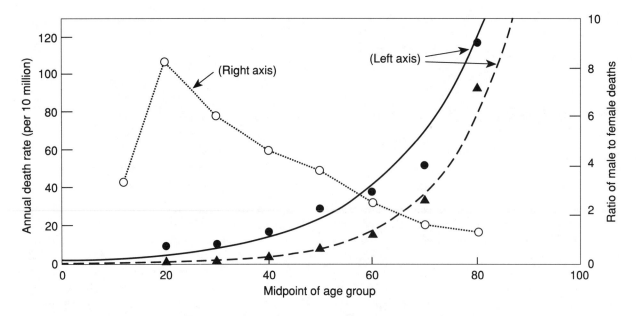

Figure 21.1   Annual death rate per 10 million population due to heat exposure in the United States from 1968 to 1980. The solid line represents males, the dashed line represents females, and the dotted line indicates the ratio of male to female deaths.
Data from Kilbourne, 1986 (1).

physiological demands of heat stress. Other behavioral means of dealing with heat stress include the use of loose fitting clothing or seeking increased air movement.

Changes in Core Temperature

During exercise, body temperature increases. Approximately 75% of the oxygen consumed goes into the production of heat. In order to maintain the core temperature, this heat must be dissipated so that there is no, or minimal, net heat storage. As seen in Figure 21.2, core temperature increases with increased energy production and falls when exercise is terminated. The steady state core temperature during exercise depends primarily on the relative exercise intensity (2) under a broad range of thermal conditions (the "prescriptive zone" in Figure 21.3). Heat storage and body temperature increase until a balance is achieved between heat production and heat dissipation. However, under moderate to high levels of heat stress, the steady state core temperature also increases with increasing heat stress. If the combination of metabolic heat production and ambient heat stress exceeds the capacity of the body to dissipate heat, the core temperature cannot be maintained at a steady state and ultimately either the exercise level or heat stress must be reduced. The ability to dissipate heat depends predominantly on the integrity of

the cardiovascular system, which may be compromised in cardiac patients. If the $\dot{V}O_2max$ is decreased, as often occurs in CAD patients, a given power output then requires a greater percentage of $\dot{V}O_2max$. Since the core temperature depends on relative exercise intensity, a low-fit individual or a patient with a reduced $\dot{V}O_2max$ will tend to have a higher core temperature for a given absolute amount of exercise than will a healthy fit person. Even though cardiac patients may perform at low intensity relative to healthy people, the intensity of exercise relative to their $\dot{V}O_2max$ is a more important predictor of core temperature.

The physiological responses to heat stress are listed here:

Variables that increase

- Heart rate (HR)
- Absolute stroke volume (SV)
- Cardiac output ($\dot{Q}$)
- Skin blood flow
- Venous compliance
- Insensible heat loss
- Body core and skin temperature
- Sweating

Variables that decrease

- Stroke volume (SV) (versus same cardiac output in cool environs)
- Splanchnic blood flow

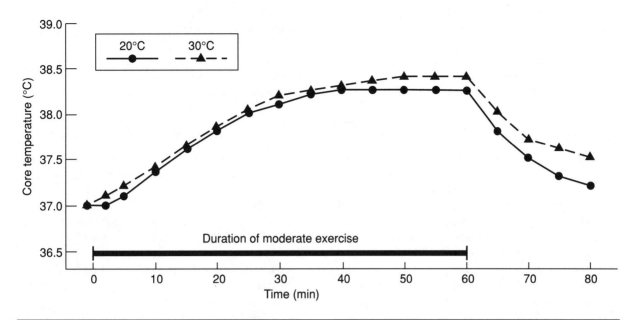

Figure 21.2   Change in core temperature during and after moderate exercise at two different ambient temperatures. Note the slightly higher but essentially similar core temperature at the normal (20 °C) and warm (30 °C) temperature and the somewhat slower cooling rate at the warmer temperature.
Based on data from Nielsen and Nielsen, 1962 (3).

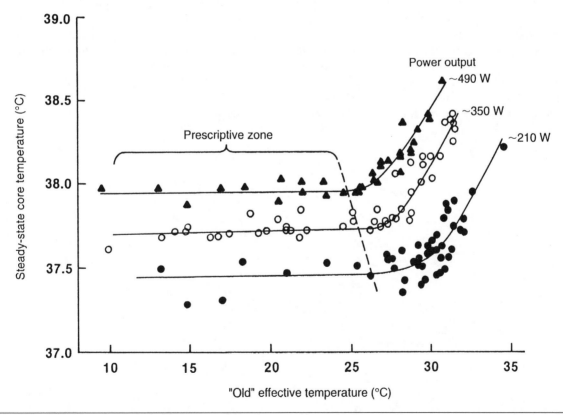

Figure 21.3   Change in steady-state core temperature at three different metabolic rates during exposure to different ambient temperatures. (The ambient temperatures are actually effective temperatures which take into consideration the air temperature, humidity, wind speed, and radiant temperature; they are appoximately equal to the wet-bulb globe temperature index at low wind speeds.) The prescription zone at a particular work load is the range of effective temperatures in which the core temperature remains relatively stable despite changes in ambient heat load.
From Sawka and Wenger, 1988 (4). Original data from Lind, 1963 (5,6).

- Renal blood flow
- Urine production
- Central blood volume
- Plasma volume
- Total body water

Cardiovascular Response to Exercise in the Heat

During heat stress, body heat is dissipated by increased blood flow to the skin. Heat loss is further facilitated by return of venous blood through superficial veins. As cutaneous heat loss is increased, retention of body heat is minimized and core temperature stabilized. Cutaneous blood flow may account for as much as one-fourth of $\dot{Q}$ during exercise in the heat; Rowell (7) suggests that this may reach up to 7 to 8 l/min. The increase in cutaneous blood flow is accomplished in part by redistribution of blood flow away from the renal and splanchnic circulations by vasoconstriction. Although cutaneous blood flow is primarily influenced by changes in core temperature and to a lesser extent by skin temperature, it is modified by other cardiovascular reflexes associated with postural change, exercise, and other factors that alter blood pressure (BP). Increased cutaneous blood flow is accompanied by increased cutaneous vascular volume due to increased venous compliance, which in turn leads to a drop in venous return. During exercise in the heat, venous constriction, which normally occurs during exercise, is still operative but it is modified by skin temperature and exercise intensity. Increased skin temperature and increased exercise intensity have opposing actions that increase or decrease venous compliance, respectively.

Heat Acclimatization

Repeated exposure to heat and exercise results in the process of heat acclimatization (7,8). Within a few days, daily heat exposure will result in a reduction of symptoms, such as headache, dizziness, cramping, or orthostatic hypotension. The physiological strain will also be markedly reduced by increased sweating, decreased HR, and reduced core temperature (Figures 21.4 and 21.5). With acclimatization, the sweating response is improved by the onset of sweating at a lower body temperature, a higher sustained maximum sweat rate, and less electrolyte loss. The cardiovascular response is improved by increased skin blood flow at lower core temperatures, improved SV, and increased plasma and blood volume relative to the unacclimatized state. In a humid environment, a higher skin-surface water vapor pressure and hence more skin wettedness is required for sufficient evaporation to provide adequate cooling. This leads to increased circulatory strain. Although acclimatization reduces the need for additional salt replacement, the need for water replacement is increased because of increased fluid losses via sweating.

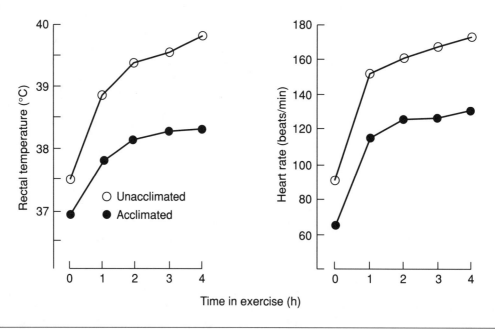

Figure 21.4   Change in heart rate (right) and rectal temperature (left) during four hours of exercise in humid heat illustrating the difference in response before and after heat acclimatization.
From Wenger (8). Original data from Wyndham et al. (15).

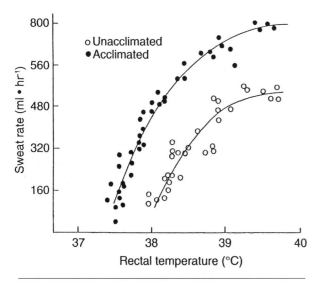

Figure 21.5 Rectal temperature and sweat rate relationships in acclimatized and unacclimatized subjects during exercise in humid heat. Note the onset of sweating at a lower rectal temperature and the higher peak sweat rate after acclimatization.
From Wenger (8). Original data from Wyndham (16).

The greatest improvements in response to heat stress occur over the first week of exposure, although acclimatization continues to improve with continued exposure. The amount of acclimatization is relative to the degree of heat and exercise stress imposed during the acclimatization period. Acclimatization is typically easier and more rapid in fit people and may be significantly impeded in people with poor fitness, especially those with inadequate cardiovascular responses to exercise. Heat intolerance is also more common in older adults. In addition to lack of acclimatization, tolerance to heat exposure may be impaired by sleep loss, fever associated with infection, obesity, alcohol or drug abuse, and dehydration or salt depletion.

Heat acclimatization, although quickly gained, is also quickly lost. Heat-acclimatized individuals who experience no heat exposure for a period of 2 to 3 weeks need to be reacclimatized. Daily exercise in the heat for a period of 7 to 10 days will result in acclimatization to the ambient temperature and humidity to which one is typically exposed. The degree of acclimatization is proportional to the amount of exercise performed during the acclimatization period (except that exercise durations in excess of 90 min do not add appreciably to the acclimatization process). Therefore, brief exercise bouts (of about 30 min) will confer less profound and less rapid acclimatization than longer exercise periods (up to about 90 min) (6).

However, longer exercise periods may not be well tolerated in unfit subjects or patients with compromised circulatory responses. Prior to initiating a heat acclimatization regimen, a period of aerobic training in which the body temperature is elevated (i.e., not swimming) is recommended to increase aerobic power and exercise tolerance. A training intensity of at least 50% of maximum will result in the most benefit during subsequent heat acclimatization.

In practical terms, one should exercise for about 1 h/day at about 50% of maximum for 8 to 10 days in the hot environment to become acclimatized. Completion of the exercise may be difficult on the first few days, and completion of the prescribed period should not be forced; a full exercise regimen should be easily accomplished after a week or so. An increase in the severity of heat exposure or in exercise intensity may require additional acclimatization.

Heat Stress and Exercise Prescription

The concept of the target HR (THR) for gauging relative exercise intensity is based on the assumption of a linear relationship between HR and relative exercise intensity (see chapter 17). However, this relationship may be perturbed by other factors, such as heat stress, dehydration, and food consumption. There is minimal information regarding the responses of cardiac patients to exercise training under adverse conditions of heat stress; thus, caution and prudence are advised when prescribing exercise that will be performed under other than optimal thermal conditions. There are two basic considerations with regard to exercise in the heat: (1) at any given work intensity relative to maximum, the HR will be higher and (2) at higher work intensities the cardiac strain will tend to be greater because of the decrease in ventricular filling pressure and the need for increased $\dot{Q}$.

Heat stress increases the HR independently of the exercise stress, as a result of the increased blood flow to the skin. During submaximal exercise, the increase in HR is associated with a decline in SV. However, $\dot{Q}$ is adequately maintained as long as venous return is not compromised. There is little effect of this increased HR on oxygen uptake ($\dot{V}O_2$) and hence the arteriovenous difference in oxygen content is not altered (9). After a period of acclimatization, as discussed previously, the HR increase associated with heat exposure is minimized. However, the reduced heat tolerance of older adults must also be considered in using HR as a predictor of relative exercise intensity (10). The most important aspect of exercise prescription for patients who will exercise in the heat is that, at a given exercise intensity, the cardiovascular strain for unacclimatized patients will be greater in a hot than in a thermoneutral environment.

For young adults exercising at a moderate exercise intensity, HR increases about 1 beat/min per 1 °C increase in ambient temperature above about 24 °C (75 °F) under hot, dry conditions (11). Raven (12) estimated that the effect of a 1 °C rise in ambient temperature in a hot, dry climate will be a HR increase of 1.5 beats/min, whereas in a hot, wet climate, HR will increase about 3.5 beats/min. Other factors that alter the relationship between HR and relative exercise intensity include dehydration (which should be avoided in a properly supervised program) and a high radiant (solar) heat load. Degree of acclimatization, level of heat stress, age, and adequacy of hydration should all be considered in the determination of the individual exercise prescription. Target HRs should be reevaluated on a seasonal basis.

Sheldahl et al. (13) studied CAD patients who exercised at 50% $\dot{V}O_2$ peak during moderate heat stress (ambient temperature 30 °C, relative humidity 50%, WBGT ≈ 75 °F). Although HR was higher and SV lower than under control conditions, there was no difference in $\dot{Q}$ or left ventricular ejection fraction. There was a slight decline in mean BP and LDEV (left ventricular end-diastolic volume). However, there were no increases in arrhythmias, EKG evidence of myocardial ischemia, or symptoms of angina as a result of exercise in the heat. These results suggest that cardiac function is not compromised in patients with uncomplicated CAD performing moderate aerobic exercise during moderate heat stress. It is nevertheless prudent to avoid excessive heat exposure and dehydration in exercising CAD patients.

Patrons of many fitness clubs have the opportunity to expose themselves passively to heat through saunas, steam baths, or hot tubs. Although exercise is not permitted under such situations, there is a risk of hyperthermia if a person does not allow for an adequate cool-down period after prior exercise. For elderly and cardiac patients especially, the increased venous compliance associated with passive heating may lead to orthostatic hypotension. However, Allison et al. (14) found no adverse response due to brief (15-min) passive heating in a hot tub at 40 °C. Passive heating of moderate duration (with a rise in core temperature of less than 1 °C) may be safe for patients who are stable enough for unsupervised exercise programs.

Fluid Loss and Replacement

During exercise in the heat, sweat losses may reach 1.5 l/min, and this may be further increased to as much as 2 to 3 l/min after acclimatization. Water losses can be easily approximated by changes in body weight; a 2% loss of body weight is approximately equal to a 3% decline in body water. A person can lose as much as 2% of body water before feeling thirsty. At body water deficits of 4 to 6%, headache and anorexia are common symptoms. Thus, adequate measures to prevent large fluid losses should not rely on thirst as an index of water deficit. Even modest levels of dehydration will lead to a relative increase in core temperature during heat exposure. As the body water deficit increases, the sweating rate at a given core temperature is decreased (Figure 21.6). The ability to maintain cardiovascular responses to heat exposure are compromised by dehydration. Regular intake of cooled fluids with a low glucose content (< 6% to 8%) is important for exercise in the heat. Plain cool water may be adequate in most situations. Hydration should begin prior to exercise using water or a balanced electrolyte beverage. Drinking should be encouraged every 15 to 20 min. Finally, fluids should never be restricted during exercise in the heat even as a voluntary measure to produce transient weight loss. Adequate fluid maintenance

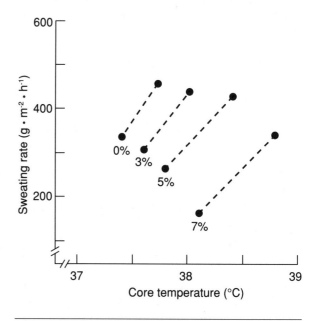

Figure 21.6 The effect of hydration state on the relationship between core temperature and sweat rate. Note the decrease in peak sweat rate and the lower sweat rate at a higher core temperature in subjects who are dehydrated.
From Sawka, 1988 (17).

is essential to optimal cardiovascular and thermoregulatory responses during heat exposure.

Characterizing the Environment

One relatively simple method of characterizing the physical environment's potential for heat stress is to use the wet-bulb globe temperature (WBGT) index, which combines the normal dry-bulb temperature (T_{db}), the wet-bulb temperature (T_{wb}), and the globe temperature (T_g):

$$WBGT \text{ index} = 0.7\ T_{wb} + 0.2\ T_g + 0.1\ T_{db}$$

When there is no appreciable solar radiation, the T_g term is dropped and the multiplier for T_{db} is increased to 0.3. Table 21.1 presents recommended WBGT ranges for exercise training.

Prevention of Heat-Related Problems and Illness During Exercise

There is a broad spectrum of heat-related disorders, which range from bothersome to life-threatening, including heat cramps, heat syncope, heat exhaustion, and heat stroke. *Heat cramps* are painful muscle cramps induced during exercise in the heat. There appears to be an individual susceptibility to this problem. Cramping is associated with sodium depletion and thus may be more common in the initial stages of heat acclimatization, but the exact mechanism of response and the factors associated with individual susceptibility are not

Table 21.1 Recommendations for Exercise Training Activities at Various Wet-Bulb Globe Temperature (WBGT) Index Ranges

Range of WBGT index	Recommendations
< 64°F	No limits on activity.
64°–76°F	Be alert for symptoms of heart stress.
73°–82°F	Active-exercise period for unacclimatized people should be shortened.
82°–86°F	Only well-acclimatized people should engage in activity.
> 86°F	All training should be canceled.

Note. Adapted from Hughson, R.L. Primary prevention of heat stroke in Canadian long-distance runs. Can. Med. Assoc. J. 122:1115-1116, 1980.

well understood. *Heat syncope* results when the baroreceptor reflexes appear to fail during periods of high skin–blood flow and increased venous compliance. It may be associated with inadequate acclimatization, hyperventilation, or fever and is accompanied by elevated core and skin temperature. *Heat exhaustion* is associated with water and electrolyte depletion caused by multiple days of heat exposure resulting in extreme fatigue, anorexia, tachycardia, and nausea. Hyperthermia is not usually excessive (core temperature typically below 39.5 °C, or 103 °F) and sweating may or may not be present. *Heatstroke* is a serious, life-threatening condition associated with core temperatures typically in excess of 40 °C (105 °F), lack of sweating, and tachycardia, possibly leading to seizures, coma, and, in many cases, death.

None of these problems should occur in a well-supervised exercise program where adequate provision is made for heat acclimatization, maintenance of water and electrolyte balance, and avoidance of excessive heat exposure. Individuals who have experienced previous heat-related problems may be at increased risk for subsequent heat illness, and this should be taken into consideration if exercise in the heat will be involved.

A position statement published by the American College of Sports Medicine (ACSM) (19) entitled "Prevention of Thermal Injuries During Distance Running" provides some general guidelines for the avoidance of heat problems during competitive running races. These guidelines provide good general principles for the avoidance of problems during various types of exercise in the heat and are essential reading for those who conduct exercise programs in the heat. When the WBGT index exceeds 82 °F (28 °C), heavy exercise should be avoided. Early morning and evening hours are usually much cooler than the temperatures at midday and these times are best for exercise programs in hot climates. However, unsafe heat stress conditions can also occur indoors in exercise facilities with excessive heating or inadequate ventilation or air conditioning. Use of loose-fitting, light-colored clothing made of natural fabric that will absorb sweat and facilitate its evaporation is recommended. Adequate hydration should be stressed and the use of impervious "sweat suits" should never be permitted.

Section Summary

Exposure of patients with CVD to the heat is not uncommon, except among those who live a relatively encapsulated existence. An adequate thermoregulatory response to heat exposure requires increased $\dot{Q}$ in order to provide for increased sweating and increased peripheral blood flow. The amount of impairment of the cardiovascular response to exercise and heat stress in the cardiac rehabilitation patient depends on numerous factors, including age, extent of cardiac damage, stage of rehabilitation, and stage of heat acclimatization. With acclimatization, adequate hydration, and common sense, exercise in the heat can be performed safely.

Exposure to Air Pollutants

Air pollution presents a public-health risk not only to the cardiac patient but also to the population as a whole. Indeed, increased levels of respirable particles are associated with increased mortality, especially in elderly patients with CVD and pulmonary disease. Air pollutants such as ozone (O_3), nitrogen dioxide (NO_2), sulfur dioxide (SO_2) acid aerosols, carbon monoxide (CO), and respirable particles, may be present at unacceptably high levels in suburban and rural areas, as well as in the more often maligned urban industrial complex. In addition to daily variation, ambient pollution concentrations vary with season and meteorological conditions (i.e., air stagnation and inversions). For example, ozone and acid aerosols are more prevalent in the summer months and may be transported over large distances. Nitrogen dioxide, carbon monoxide, and other toxic pollutants may also be present in indoor environments.

Physiological responses to air pollutants are influenced by the amount inhaled and subsequently delivered to lung and other tissues. The major determinants of the exposure dose are the pollutant concentration, exposure duration, and the volume of air inhaled (i.e., the ventilatory volume). Because inhaled volume increases proportionately with the intensity of exercise, the responses to air pollutants are increased in people who exercise.

Ozone

Ozone is a major urban air pollutant produced by the action of sunlight on vehicular and industrial emissions. A potent airway irritant, ozone, at levels that exist in ambient air, has been shown to cause marked effects on lung function and to impair exercise performance. Symptoms typical of ozone exposure include a cough, a laryngeal or substernal pain after taking a deep breath, a sore or irritated throat, and a feeling of chest tightness. Even in

healthy young adults, ozone can impair exercise performance. A study of high school cross-country runners in Los Angeles, California, indicated that lack of improvement in running performance was associated with increased ambient ozone concentrations. Following ozone exposure in healthy young men, reduced endurance time, inability to complete prescribed exercise regimens, and reductions in peak $\dot{V}O_2$ have been observed (20-22). These responses were accompanied by marked respiratory symptoms (including a cough and pain on a deep breath), a rapid, shallow breathing pattern, and marked decreases in lung function measurements. The reduction in exercise performance appears to be caused primarily by the associated respiratory symptoms. Changes in exercise performance have been observed after only 1 h of moderately heavy exercise at an ozone level as low as 0.18 ppm. Such levels are often observed in Los Angeles and Mexico City but occur less frequently in other major metropolitan areas. At higher ozone concentrations, the effects of ozone on exercise performance and lung function are substantially increased (Table 21.2).

Exposures to ozone levels as low as 0.12 ppm for 1 to 2 h is sufficient to induce significant effects on standard lung function tests. The magnitude of the decrease in forced expired volume in 1 s (FEV_1), for example, is roughly proportional to the inhaled dose of ozone, as seen in Figure 21.7. Increasing the ozone concentration, respiratory minute volume, or duration of exposure will increase the pulmonary function responses. Prolonged exposure (6.5 h) to ozone levels as low as 0.08 ppm, a level common in many cities, can induce small changes in lung function (31, 32). Ozone also causes the bronchial airways to become hyperresponsive to such bronchoactive drugs as methacholine or histamine. Increased epithelial permeability and inflammation of the airways resulting from damage to the airway epithelium may cause a patient to become more responsive to aeroallergens (33). Recovery from ozone-induced lung function and respiratory symptom responses typically occurs within a few hours.

The only controlled study of cardiac patients exposed to ozone during moderate exercise was performed by Superko et al. (34). These researchers found no effects of ozone on either pulmonary function or cardiovascular endpoints, such as time to onset of angina or ischemic electrocardiographic (ECG) changes, suggesting that there may be no direct effects of ozone on the cardiovascular system. Because exercise may be prescribed for patients with chronic obstructive pulmonary disease

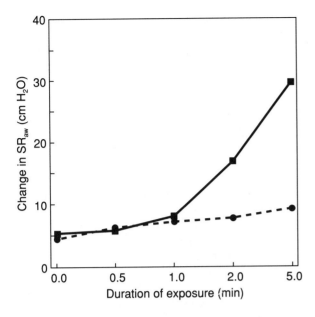

Figure 21.8 Change in airway resistance (SR_aw) in asthmatics exposed to 1.0 ppm sulfur dioxide (solid line) for up to 5 min, compared to clean air (dashed line). Note that symptom scores and resistance can more than double with only a 5-min exposure.
From Horstman et al. 1988 (40). Used by permission.

at rest, nearly all inspired sulfur dioxide is removed in the mouth or nose, but with increased mouth breathing during exercise there is increased delivery of the gas to the lower airway, resulting in greater bronchoconstriction. Exercise under cold, dry winter conditions in combination with sulfur dioxide exposure is the condition of greatest concern for the asthmatic patient. Cold, dry air exacerbates exercise-induced bronchoconstriction because of airway evaporative cooling and drying that lead to changes in osmolarity of airway surface fluids.

Common asthma medications, such as cromolyn sodium and β₂-sympathomimetics (albuterol, terbutaline), inhibit the effects of sulfur dioxide on airway resistance in a dose-dependent manner. Sulfur dioxide–induced bronchoconstriction is often self-limiting, and recovery, usually within 30-60 min, is typically spontaneous in mild asthmatics.

Carbon Monoxide

Of the commonly occurring air pollutants, carbon monoxide is the one that should be of greatest concern to the cardiac patient. Carbon monoxide binds reversibly with hemoglobin to form carboxyhemoglobin. Hemoglobin has a much greater affinity for carbon monoxide than for oxygen, a phenomenon that is important in clearing endogenously produced carbon monoxide from the tissues. Binding sites on the hemoglobin molecule that are occupied by carbon monoxide can no longer transport oxygen to the tissues. Thus, a blood level of 5% carboxyhemoglobin indicates a 5% loss in oxygen carrying capacity. The presence of increased carboxyhemoglobin levels also causes a shift in the hemoglobin-oxygen dissociation curve, which interferes with the unloading of oxygen at the tissue level. This can impair exercise performance by reducing $\dot{V}O_2$max (21,41) (Figure 21.9).

Carbon monoxide exposure occurs in urban areas (especially in places close to roadways), smoke-filled rooms, and poorly ventilated areas in which combustion sources (for example, parking garages and traffic tunnels) are found. Although carbon monoxide is produced endogenously through the breakdown of red blood cells, carboxyhemoglobin levels are normally less than 1% in nonsmokers, an indication that the above mechanism for the prevention of carbon monoxide accumulation works effectively. The normal process of carbon monoxide excretion via the lungs is reversed by even relatively low inspired levels of carbon monoxide (25 to 50 ppm), and carboxyhemoglobin levels increase rapidly.

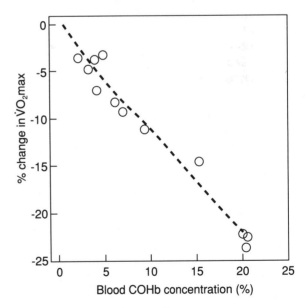

Figure 21.9 Change in maximal oxygen uptake ($\dot{V}O_2$max) as a function of blood carboxyhemoglobin (COHb) concentration. The dashed line is the linear regression from 5% to 20% COHb; the line was adjusted below 5% COHb to force an X-intercept at 0.7% COHb, the mean resting level in unexposed subjects.
Adapted with permission from Folinsbee and Raven (21).

Because of its high affinity for hemoglobin, the clearance of carbon monoxide from the blood is relatively slow; the half-time for excretion is some 2 to 4 h. Carbon monoxide can accumulate in the blood as a result of prolonged exposure to low concentrations (10 to 30 ppm) or brief exposure to high concentrations (> 100 ppm) of the gas. For example, 1 h of exercise near heavy traffic (mean levels of carbon monoxide 7 to 10 ppm with peak levels in excess of 100 ppm) can raise carboxyhemoglobin levels to 3% to 4%. Once carboxyhemoglobin is elevated, even relatively low levels of carbon monoxide (10 ppm) will slow the clearance of carbon monoxide from the blood by reducing the gradient for excretion across the alveolocapillary membrane.

$\dot{V}O_2$max is decreased by about 10% at sea level in nonsmokers as a result of increasing the carboxyhemoglobin level to about 10%. Carbon monoxide reduces $\dot{V}O_2$max primarily by reducing the oxygen carrying capacity of the blood; maximal $\dot{Q}$ is not appreciably altered. Although the relationship between exercise performance decrements and carboxyhemoglobin levels is essentially linear (21) (Figure 21.9), suggesting that even very low levels of carboxyhemoglobin should reduce $\dot{V}O_2$max, no statistically significant effects on maximal exercise performance have been observed below about 4% to 5% carboxyhemoglobin.

Although significant reductions in $\dot{V}O_2$max occur, moderate submaximal exercise performance (30% to 60% of maximum) is not impaired in healthy people. A compensatory increase in $\dot{Q}$ maintains tissue oxygen delivery with carboxyhemoglobin levels below about 15%. However, at exercise intensities achieved by elite athletes (75% to 95% of maximum), the cardiovascular system becomes unable to compensate for the reduced oxygen-carrying capacity of the blood, and submaximal exercise is limited. CVD patients may have difficulty increasing $\dot{Q}$ during submaximal exercise, in order to compensate for the additional burden of decreased oxygen carrying capacity due to elevated carboxyhemoglobin levels. Patients with intermittent claudication, a manifestation of peripheral arteriosclerotic vascular disease, demonstrate decreased time to onset of ischemic leg pain, presumably due to decreased oxygen delivery, with carboxyhemoglobin levels in the range of 2% to 3% (42).

Angina patients exposed to carbon monoxide showed a decrease in exercise time prior to the onset of exercise-induced angina and an increase in ischemic ECG changes (43, 44). These early studies (performed when automobiles emitted higher concentrations of pollutants) have recently been re-evaluated in a large multicenter trial of carbon monoxide exposure in 63 patients with angina and documented CAD (45). The decrease in exercise time prior to onset of ischemic changes was verified, although the change was much less than previously reported (Figure 21.10); there was approximately a 4% decrease in time prior to ischemic changes for each 1% increase in carboxyhemoglobin above the typical carboxyhemoglobin level of about 1%. Thus, at a carboxyhemoglobin level of 4%, a 12% decrease in time to onset of ischemic changes, as well as a 7% decrease in time to onset of angina, was observed. This level of carboxyhemoglobin may be achieved in freeway commuters (43), police officers, auto tunnel workers, and garage attendants (49). At slightly higher levels (6% carboxyhemoglobin), Adams et al. (47) found a reduced time to onset of angina, reduced duration of exercise, and a reduced ventricular performance indicated by reduced left ventricular ejection fraction (LVEF). However, at lower carboxyhemoglobin levels (3.8%), these investigators found no such responses (46).

Cardiac patients with electrical instability of the myocardium leading to frequent arrhythmias are at increased risk of sudden death. Despite the potentiation of ischemic changes by carbon monoxide exposure, there is a question of whether carbon monoxide causes an increase in resting or exercise-induced ventricular ectopic beats in patients with CAD (50,51). These observations were made at carboxyhemoglobin levels of 1% to 6%. Patients with significant numbers of ventricular ectopic beats at rest had the same absence of response to increased carboxyhemoglobin as those who had little or no baseline ectopy. A substantial increase in exercise-related arrhythmias, both single and multiple premature ventricular depolarizations, was seen in cardiac patients with 4% and 6% carboxyhemoglobin in another study (52). Although the evidence linking lethal arrhythmias to carbon monoxide exposure is still limited, cardiac patients should nevertheless be advised to avoid occupational, recreational, and exercise settings where carbon monoxide inhalation is a hazard. This suggestion is strongly supported by the observation of increased CAD mortality in traffic tunnel workers routinely exposed to 40 to 50 ppm carbon monoxide and daily rush hour peaks at higher concentrations (49).

Carbon monoxide can cause a fall in coronary sinus oxygen tension, leading to hypoxic tissue responses, as indicated by the presence of lactate

Chapter 22

Hypertension

Peter Hanson
Patricia Rueckert

Hypertension is the leading cardiovascular disease (CVD) in the industrialized nations of the world. Sustained hypertension is a major risk factor for coronary artery disease (CAD), stroke, and heart failure (1,2). Thus, the diagnosis and control of hypertension has been a major goal of public health efforts during the past decade (3).

The role of exercise in the diagnosis and management of hypertension is currently a topic of clinical interest. Exercise training has been recommended as a nonpharmacological approach, as well as a useful adjunct to pharmacological therapy, in controlling mild hypertension (4-6). This chapter will review the physiological basis and clinical guidelines for exercise testing, prescription, and training in hypertensive patients.

Epidemiological Considerations

Hypertension is defined according to population mean values of resting blood pressure (BP) summarized in Table 22.1. Normal BP includes all values below 130/85 mm Hg. Hypertension is classified as high normal (borderline), stage 1 (mild),

Table 22.1 Classification of Hypertension

| | Blood pressure (mm Hg) | |
	Diastolic	Systolic
Normal	< 85	< 130
High normal	85-89	130-139
Mild hypertension (borderline)	90-99	140-159
Moderate hypertension	100-109	160-179
Severe hypertension	> 109	> 179
Isolated systolic hypertension	(normal or borderline)	> 160

stage 2 (moderate), stage 3 (severe), and stage 4 (very severe). Elderly patients may exhibit *isolated systolic hypertension*, which is defined as systolic BP of greater than 160 mm Hg with normal or borderline diastolic values. The cutoff values for these classes may vary somewhat according to different sources (7-9).

Hypertension commonly begins in young adulthood and occurs in 5% to 10% of people aged 20 to 30 years (7). The incidence of hypertension continues to increase with age and is found in 20% to 25% of middle-aged adults and 50% to 60% of adults over 65 years of age (7,8).

A variety of risk factors contribute to the probability for development of hypertension. These include genetic, metabolic, and behavioral factors. In general, a family history of hypertension increases the probability for developing future hypertension (7). Males exhibit hypertension earlier than females (7). Overall, the black population in the United States shows a higher incidence of hypertension than Caucasian or Asiatic groups (10). The underlying reason for this is not understood.

Metabolic risk factors include obesity, insulin resistance, and glucose intolerance. These common clinical conditions produce abnormal regulation of vascular volume and peripheral resistance, which mediate the increase in BP (11).

Behavioral factors include repeated exposure to excessive environmental and social stress, leading to chronic (neurogenic) activation of the sympathetic nervous system (12,13). Other behavioral factors include excessive alcohol consumption (14) and recreational or ergogenic abuse of drugs, including stimulants (such as amphetamines and cocaine) and possibly anabolic steroids (15). The relationship of these ergogenic agents to the development of sustained hypertension is unclear but should be considered in competitive athletes. While smoking has not been shown to result in sustained hypertension, it can raise BP acutely (16).

Clinical Pathophysiology of Hypertension

For clinical purposes, hypertension is divided into two categories, primary and secondary hypertension.

Primary Hypertension

Primary hypertension accounts for over 95% of sustained high BP. Multiple regulatory mechanisms contribute to the evolution of primary hypertension: (1) abnormal neuroreflex and sympathetic control of cardiac output ($\dot{Q}$) and peripheral resistance, (2) abnormal renal and metabolic control of vascular volume and compliance, and (3) abnormal local smooth muscle and endothelial control of vascular resistance.

A detailed discussion of altered control mechanisms in primary hypertension is beyond the scope of this chapter. Briefly, the combined neurohumoral and metabolic abnormalities contribute to a gradual increase in systemic vascular resistance, which is characteristic of fully established primary hypertension. Activation of the sympathetic nervous system and pressor hormones, such as angiotensin, probably mediates the increase in vascular resistance. Increases in circulating catecholamines are seen most consistently in young patients with borderline or mild hypertension (17), and direct nerve recordings demonstrate increased sympathetic activity in these patients (18). Recent studies have implicated a primary defect in calcium and sodium balance in vascular smooth muscle as an underlying common defect in primary hypertension (19,20). Abnormalities in endothelial-derived vascular control factors may also be important (21,22). Structural changes within vascular smooth muscle ultimately develop so that the vascular resistance is self-maintained (23,24). Thus, the multiple factors that mediate the development of hypertension ultimately produce a sustained elevation of systemic vascular resistance. Finally, there is an alteration of arterial baroreceptor function, which allows a "resetting" of baroreflexes to permit a higher systemic arterial BP level (25).

Characteristic hemodynamic patterns vary with the stage or severity of hypertension. The early phase of mild, or borderline, hypertension is frequently characterized by an increased resting heart rate (HR) and $\dot{Q}$. Although vascular resistance is in the normal range for this group, it is inappropriately high for the corresponding $\dot{Q}$. In moderate hypertension, $\dot{Q}$ and HR are normal and vascular resistance is increased. With severe hypertension, there is a further increase in vascular resistance and varying depression of $\dot{Q}$ due to increased vascular afterload (26,27).

Secondary Hypertension

Secondary hypertension accounts for approximately 5% of sustained hypertension (1). The major causes of secondary hypertension are renal, endocrine, and vascular abnormalities. Secondary causes should be considered when hypertension develops in younger patients or develops rapidly in adult patients with no prior history of hypertension. In addition, secondary hypertension should be considered when elevated BP is poorly responsive to routine antihypertensive therapy.

Renal vascular disease causes an increased release of renin, which initiates the enzymatic conversion of plasma angiotensinogen to angiotensin-II. Angiotensin-II is a potent peripheral vasoconstrictor that stimulates the release of aldosterone, which promotes renal retention of sodium and water. Tumors of the adrenal medulla and cortex are less common causes of secondary hypertension. Pheochromocytoma is caused by a catecholamine-releasing adenoma within the adrenal medulla. Adrenal cortical adenomas may release cortisol or aldosterone, which produce a sustained hypertension. These renal-endocrine causes of secondary hypertension are successfully treated by surgery or medical management.

End-Organ Pathology

Regardless of cause, increased BP levels produce a predictable pattern of end-organ pathology within the cardiac chambers and vascular tree. Left ventricular hypertrophy (LVH) is nearly a universal response and is seen using echocardiographic measurements in borderline and mild hypertension (2,28). With sustained hypertension, concentric LVH increases and abnormal diastolic relaxation is seen. Vascular changes include hypertrophy and structural remodeling of the resistance vessels, as well as acceleration of atherosclerosis (29). The retinal and renal glomerular arterioles are exquisitely sensitive to hypertensive vascular degeneration. Vasodilator responses in the cerebral circulation are also impaired, and the risk for stroke increases significantly with untreated hypertension (29).

The end-organ damage from hypertension usually evolves over a period of years. However, rapid increases in BP that may occur in secondary hypertension may be poorly tolerated, while gradual increases in BP and isolated systolic hypertension in older patients may be surprisingly well tolerated for long periods without morbid events.

Blood Pressure Response to Exercise in Hypertensive Patients

Hypertensive patients with high resting BPs also have increased BPs during exercise; the mechanism of the increase in BP usually differs from that of normotensive individuals. The diagnosis of mild or borderline patients may be aided by characterizing their BP response to increased levels of activity.

Dynamic Exercise

With dynamic exercise, $\dot{Q}$ increases as a result of increased HR, stroke volume (SV), and cardiac contractility. Blood flow to working muscle is augmented by local vasodilation, while blood flow to nonworking muscle and visceral organs is diminished by sympathetic vasoconstriction. The net result is a rise in systolic BP with little change in diastolic BP and a decrease in vascular resistance (30).

In mild to moderate hypertension, $\dot{Q}$ increases normally; however, systolic and diastolic BPs and vascular resistance are higher at all levels of exercise compared with normotensive subjects (27). In patients with severe hypertension, $\dot{Q}$ is lower than in age-matched controls because of decreased SV. Systolic and diastolic BPs and vascular resistance are markedly increased (27).

Isometric exercise

The normal response to isometric exercise is a combined rise in systolic and diastolic BPs, commonly referred to as a pressor response. The pressor response is mediated by reflex increases in $\dot{Q}$ with little or no change in vascular resistance (31). The magnitude of the BP rise is proportional to the combined size of muscle mass and the percent of maximal effort used in performing the isometric contraction.

The increase in BP during isometric exercise may or may not be mediated by an increase in $\dot{Q}$ in individuals with hypertension. Rather, it has been observed that the pressor response is mainly associated with an increase in peripheral resistance.

This has been attributed to the inability to increase $\dot{Q}$ because of LVH (32) or a blunted β-adrenergic reactivity and predominance of α-adrenergic reactivity (33).

During both dynamic and isometric exercise, the peak systolic and diastolic BP achieved is substantially increased in hypertensive patients. However, the relative increase in BP (from resting values) is similar to normotensive control subjects. These findings suggest that BP is "reset" and maintained at higher levels throughout the spectrum of activity from rest to peak exercise. Figure 22.1 illustrates the general pattern of BP responses to exercise stress in mild hypertensive subjects. Note that hypertensive subjects exhibit greater systolic and diastolic BPs under conditions of treadmill exercise or isometric handgrip.

Exercise Testing in Diagnosis of Hypertension

Recent studies suggest that exercise BP responses may provide additional criteria for diagnosing and

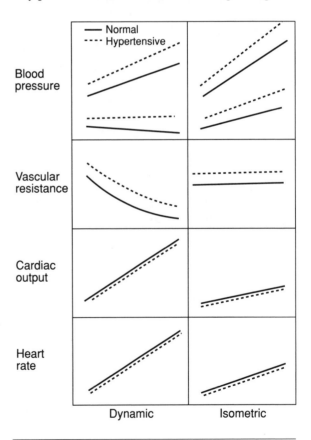

Figure 22.1 Comparison of hemodynamic responses to dynamic and isometric exercise in normal and hypertensive subjects. Axes are in arbitrary units. Note that hypertensive subjects show higher vascular resistance and blood pressure responses.

managing hypertension (34,35). A decision to begin earlier treatment may be made in those individuals who have borderline resting BPs but who exhibit elevated BP responses during periods of increased activity. This is especially important in athletes or recreational sport enthusiasts who spend more time exercising than the sedentary population. Optimal evaluation of the effectiveness of therapy would be done during either ambulatory BP monitoring or exercise.

BP values exceeding 180/120 mm Hg at 50% of maximum handgrip (90 s) and treadmill BP values exceeding 180/80 mm Hg at 50% intensity or 220/80 mm Hg at 100% intensity are usually defined as hypertensive responses (Table 22.2). Some patients with mild hypertension may show an early rise in systolic BP to levels of 180 to 200 mm Hg during submaximal exercise, and these values are maintained at maximal exercise. Such patients may exhibit an excessively high systolic BP with activities of daily living, although resting BP and peak exercise BP are within the normal range. Studies comparing echocardiographic measurements of cardiac hypertrophy with exercise BP and ambulatory BP monitoring indicate that patients with elevated BP responses during exercise or activity also show evidence of LVH (36) and are at greater risk for developing sustained hypertension (37).

Exercise Training in Hypertension

Epidemiological evidence overwhelmingly favors the concept that increased physical activity has a beneficial effect on cardiovascular risk factors. Active individuals tend to be leaner and have lower cholesterol levels, less glucose intolerance,

and lower BPs. This relationship is seen from adolescence to old age and is true for both women and men. One recent study specifically examined the association between leisure-time activities and BP in a group of older women. Resting BP levels decreased with each increase in reported activity intensity (38).

Interest in conducting controlled trials of the potentially positive effect of training on hypertension began in the 1960s (39,40) and continues to this day. Although some controversy remains, many studies have demonstrated that exercise training can lower BP in individuals with hypertension (41-50).

Dynamic Exercise

Most of the studies that have reported a favorable effect of dynamic exercise on BP have utilized training programs that involve moderate-intensity exercise, usually aerobics, jogging, or cycling. Significant decreases in BP have been seen as soon as 2 weeks after the initiation of training (51) and persist for years, as long as the active lifestyle is continued (46,47). When subjects stop training or participation in the exercise program, BPs often return to pretraining levels (46,47,52). It is noteworthy that higher intensity (46) or more frequent (45) exercise appears not to offer any advantage and may even be less effective (46) at lowering BP. Several reviewers suggest that studies showing no decrease in BP with training may have utilized overly intense exercise (53-55). Jost et al. (56) found that high-intensity interval training compared with endurance training increased the ratio of norepinephrine to epinephrine. Urata et al. (44) observed that mild exercise at the blood lactate

Table 22.2   **Blood Pressure Responses to Isometric Handgrip and Treadmill Exercise in Normal and Hypertensive Young Adults**

	Isometric handgrip, 50% of maximum	Treadmill exercise 50%	Treadmill exercise 100%
Normal	< 180/120[a]	≤ 180/80[a]	< 220/80[a]
Mild hypertension	$\frac{180\text{-}190}{120\text{-}130}$	$\frac{180\text{-}190}{80\text{-}90}$	$\frac{210\text{-}220}{80\text{-}90}$
Moderate hypertension	$\frac{>190}{130}$	$\frac{>190}{90}$	$\frac{>220}{90}$

[a]Values represent systolic/diastolic blood pressure in mm Hg.

Note. Data from Ward, A., Hanson, P., and Einerson, J. *Clinical Res.*, 1986; 34:3864.

threshold resulted in a drop in BP and a depletion in plasma volume without the activation of the renin-angiotensin-aldosterone system that may occur with more strenuous exercise. Thus, intense exercise may stimulate the sympathetic nervous and renin-angiotensin-aldosterone systems to an extent that overrides the hypotensive effect of milder exercise.

The failure of training to lower BP in some individuals has also raised the possibility that there exist subgroups of responders and nonresponders who may differ in baseline hemodynamic and neuroendocrine function. Kiyonaga et al. (43) found that the effectiveness of their training program was dependent on the initial value of plasma renin. In hypertensive patients with lower plasma renin, 10 to 20 weeks of exercise therapy tended to result in a greater reduction of BP than in the patients with higher renin. Duncan et al. (41) found that the reduction in BP with training was greater for their hypertensive patients with higher initial values of plasma norepinephrine. Kinoshita et al. (57) observed that responders to mild exercise therapy had a significantly higher cardiac index, higher ratio of serum sodium to potassium, and lower total peripheral resistance in pretraining than nonresponders.

Hagberg (54) performed a meta-analysis of 25 longitudinal studies of the antihypertensive effects of aerobic exercise training on patients with hypertension. The average reductions in systolic and diastolic BPs in this analysis were 10.8 and 8.2 mm Hg, respectively. It appeared that females, people with lower body weight, and those with higher diastolic BP tended to elicit greater decreases in systolic and diastolic BPs with exercise training. He also observed that the degree of reductions in systolic and diastolic BPs tended to be negatively correlated with exercise intensity.

Another meta-analysis of 118 published reports of exercise training and hypertension was recently reported by Spataro et al. (58). The results of this study, summarized in Table 22.3, indicate an overall reduction of 8 mm Hg of systolic BP and 5 mm

Hg of diastolic BP. They also found an increasing gradient of BP reduction from normal subjects to patients with mild to moderate sustained hypertension.

Recent studies have focused on the hypotensive effect of a single bout of dynamic exercise. A decrease in resting systolic and mean BP for at least 1 to 2 hours after a single bout of treadmill exercise has been described (Rueckert, P.A., Slane, P.R., and Hanson, P., unpublished data; 59) (see Figure 22.2). Most investigators find at least a transient decrease in BP following treadmill or bicycle exercise, although the reported hemodynamic changes are not consistent and may depend on baseline characteristics of the subjects and intensity of the exercise protocol (59-62). Floras et al. (63) utilized direct recording of sympathetic nerve traffic in the peroneal nerve of borderline hypertensive men before and after an exercise training session. In those subjects who had a decrease in BP, there was a substantial reduction in muscle sympathetic nerve activity recorded 60 minutes after the exercise. Whether the drop in BP persists once the subjects leave the test site is still a matter of debate. Pescatello et al. (64) showed that BP continued to decline in hypertensive patients over a period of 13 hours, whereas others found no evidence for sustained BP reduction (59,65).

Resistance Exercise

While most experimental designs have utilized dynamic exercise training, a small number of studies suggest that weight training may also be effective in lowering BP in hypertensive patients. Hagberg et al. (66) found that weight training with free weights or variable-resistance equipment 3 days/week was effective in maintaining a reduction in systolic BP in adolescents who had already completed an endurance exercise training program. In another study, 9 weeks of circuit weight training significantly reduced seated diastolic BP in 10 men

Table 22.3 Meta-analysis of Exercise Training Studies in Hypertension

	All	Control	Mild hypertension	Sustained hypertension
Δ SBP (mm Hg)	−8	−5	−13	−19
Δ DBP (mm Hg)	−5	−3	−8	−11

Note. 118 training studies with $n = 3,331$ experimental and $n = 2,316$ control subjects. SBP = systolic blood pressure; DBP = diastolic blood pressure. Data from reference 57.

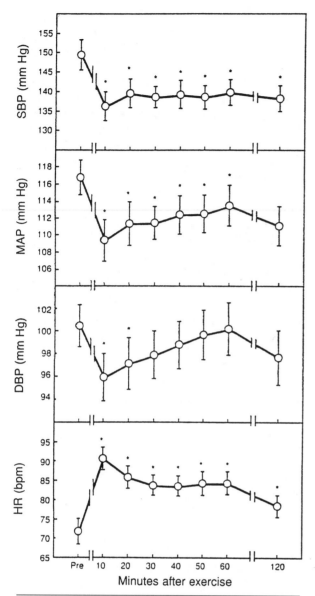

Figure 22.2 Ambulatory blood pressure recordings during and after a single bout of exercise training in hypertensive subjects. Note continuous decline in systolic (SBP), diastolic (DBP), and mean (MAP) after exercise. Reproduced from Rueckert et al. (59) with permission.

with mild hypertension (67). Kelemen et al. (50) observed a significant decrease in both systolic and diastolic BPs in men with mild hypertension consequent to exercise training consisting of 30 min of circuit weight training and 20 min of walking and jogging. They concluded that an exercise training program that includes circuit weight training appears to be safe in patients with mild hypertension. Animal studies have suggested that resistance training may not increase the risk for stroke (68) and that the concentric myocardial hypertrophy

that can result from resistance training does not appear to produce any adverse changes in left ventricular function (LVF) (69,70). More studies in humans seem warranted, however, before weight training alone is recommended as a means to lower BP or as an adjunct to antihypertensive therapy.

Mechanisms of Posttraining Decreases in Blood Pressure

A variety of mechanisms have been proposed to explain the reduction in BP following exercise training. These include reduced cardiac output (49), decreased activity of the sympathetic nervous system (41,43,44), reduced total peripheral vascular resistance (42,45), increased baroreflex sensitivity (51), and reductions in plasma volume (44).

Most studies have focused on hemodynamic and neurohumoral changes after exercise training. Many of these findings have been inconsistent. Nelson et al. (45) attributed the drop in BP in their patients to a decrease in total peripheral resistance, with $\dot{Q}$ increasing slightly. In a group of older hypertensives, the decrease in BP was also attributed to a decrease in total peripheral resistance (42). However, it has been observed that subjects with initially high $\dot{Q}$ values have lower $\dot{Q}$ values after training (49). Thus, age, duration of hypertension, the presence of LVH, and other factors probably influence the hemodynamic pattern contributing to the postexercise reduction in BP.

Catecholamine concentration and turnover rate have been studied in hypertensive patients undergoing exercise training programs. Circulating norepinephrine and epinephrine levels are variably reported to decrease (41,43,44) or remain unchanged (42). Nelson et al. (45) showed a significant reduction in circulating norepinephrine along with a decrease in peripheral resistance in middle-aged hypertensive patients who underwent 4 weeks of exercise training. Jennings et al. (71) have emphasized the difficulty in interpreting changes in circulating catecholamine concentration due to the competing effects of release versus reuptake. They measured the norepinephrine spillover rate as a more sensitive index of catecholamine activity and found a reduction in this parameter in 8 of 10 normotensive subjects after exercise training.

As discussed earlier, a decrease in muscle sympathetic nerve traffic follows a single bout of exercise, suggesting that an attenuation of sympathetic nerve activity may play an important role in mediating acute postexercise hypotension and possibly chronic posttraining lowering of BP. Ambulatory

BP data reveal that decreases in postexercise BP are often most evident during the day when sympathetic activity is normally high (72). Somers et al. (52) reported that endurance training lowered daytime BP during both rest and activity, but that it did not reduce sleep BP. They also reported an increase in baroreflex sensitivity and a decrease in set point with increased physical fitness in their subjects with mild and borderline hypertension.

A detailed discussion of other possible mechanisms contributing to BP reduction in exercise training is beyond the scope of this chapter. Direct as well as indirect mechanisms are discussed in several excellent reviews (4,53,73,74).

Exercise Prescription Guidelines for Hypertensive Patients

Exercise training should be prescribed as part of a comprehensive treatment plan for hypertensive patients.

Patient Selection and Evaluation

Younger patients with borderline hypertension or mild sustained hypertension who do not have an excessive BP response to exercise should be placed on a regimen of diet and exercise for an initial nonpharmacological treatment. This is especially important in patients with moderate obesity who will benefit most from weight loss.

Patients with moderate to severe hypertension should be thoroughly evaluated for the presence of CVD before participating in a regular exercise training program. In these patients, the presence of LVH, retinal vascular disease, CAD, or peripheral arterial disease should be identified for further treatment. Patients with combined hypertension and diabetes form a high-risk subgroup who frequently have retinopathy, depressed LVF, nonsymptomatic CAD, and peripheral microvascular insufficiency.

Patients with complicated end-organ involvement or with a history or symptoms of coronary, cerebral vascular, or peripheral arterial insufficiency should not engage in a routine exercise training program. Patients with secondary hypertension should also not engage in an exercise program until their BP is well controlled by medications or definitive surgical treatment.

Contraindications to exercise training in hypertensive patients are as follows (75).

Signs or symptoms detectable at rest:

• Uncontrolled resting BP (systolic BP > 180; diastolic BP > 110)

• End-organ damage, especially retinal or renal changes or severe LVH

• Unstable angina, cerebral ischemia, or uncompensated congestive heart failure (CHF)

Signs or symptoms occurring during exercise or recovery:

• Hypertensive values at the prescribed training intensity (systolic BP > 225; diastolic BP > 100)

• Exercise-induced angina or cerebral ischemia

• Adverse side effects of antihypertensive medications (hypotension, bradycardia, muscle weakness and cramps, bronchospasm)

Patients with symptoms at rest should have the contraindications resolved, if possible, before initiating a training program. Those patients with exercise-induced symptoms should stop training and be reevaluated for modification of their therapy. Table 22.4 summarizes the potential effects of the major classes of antihypertensive agents on exercise and sport participation.

Exercise Testing and Monitoring

A graded exercise test (GXT) is usually recommended for adults over the age of 40 years who plan to begin an exercise training program (75). However, clinical judgment based on individual patient history and risk factors should determine the need for formal exercise testing. Most patients with mild hypertension and no other risk factors may begin a walking exercise program without a maximal GXT. Patients with moderate to severe hypertension should be thoroughly evaluated with a GXT and possibly myocardial radionuclear imaging if electrocardiographic (ECG) evidence of LVH is present. Patients with both hypertension and insulin-dependent diabetes should routinely be evaluated with combined exercise testing and radionuclear imaging prior to engaging in exercise training programs (76).

A treadmill GXT should be performed using protocols that maintain a constant walking speed (77). This permits an accurate measurement of BP throughout the exercise. The Bruce protocol frequently requires patients to use hand rails for support, and this limits the measurement of BP.

Submaximal exercise monitoring also may be used to evaluate BP and HR responses over the

Table 22.4   Summary of Potential Effects of Major Classes of Antihypertensive Agents on Exercise and Sports Participation

Drug classes	Hemodynamic effects	Metabolic and CNS effects	Effects on exercise
DIURETICS			
Thiazide (hydrochlorothiazide)		• Urinary loss of K^+ and Mg^{2+}	During activity: • Hypovolemia • Orthostatic hypotension
Loop inhibitors (lasix)	• Decreased plasma volume • Decreased $\dot{Q}$ • Long-term decreased SVR (Note: These have little or no control of exercise hypertension.)	• Increases in plasma cholesterol, glucose, and uric acid	Long-term effects: • Hypokalemia • Hypomagnesemia • Muscle weakness and cramps • Possible rhabdomyolysis • Possible arrhythmias
Potassium sparing (triamterene amiloride)		• Reduced K^+ loss	
BETA-ADRENERGIC BLOCKING AGENTS			
Nonselective (β-1/β-2) (propranolol)	• 20%-30% decrease in HR • Decreased contractility • Increased SVR in muscle and skin	• Inhibition of lipolysis and glycogenolysis • Increased cholesterol (but reduced HDL cholesterol) • CNS depression (with lipophilic β-blockers)	• Significant loss of $\dot{V}O_2$max due to decreased $\dot{Q}$ and skeletal muscle flow • Impairment of substrate mobilization • Earlier fatigue and lactate threshold • Possible exercise bronchospasm
Selective (β-1) (atenolol, bisoprolol)	• Less effect on β-2 vasodilation	• Less impairment of glycogenolysis and lipolysis	• Less effect on bronchial smooth muscle
Combined (β/α-1) (labetalol)	• Decreased SVR • Less impairment of muscle blood flow		(Note: Combined β/α-1 may be best choice if β-blockade is necessary.)
ALPHA-ADRENERGIC BLOCKING AGENTS			
Peripheral (α-1) (prazosin, terazosin)	• Decreased SVR • Marked orthostatic BP increase after oral dose • Only limited control of exercise hypertension	• No major changes in energy metabolism	• $\dot{V}O_2$max preserved • No major effect on training or sports performance
Central (α-2) (clonidine, guanabenz)	• Decreased SVR • Minor decrease in HR	• No major changes in energy metabolism • Mild to moderate drowsiness • Dry mouth (minimized with transcutaneous preparation)	• $\dot{V}O_2$max preserved • No major effect on training or sports performance
VASODILATORS			
Direct (hydralazine, minoxidil)	• Decreased SVR • Increased HR • Reflex increase in $\dot{Q}$	• Headaches • Flushing • Fluid retention secondary to activation of renin-agiotensin system • Lupus erythematosus reaction possible	• Potential for competive "steal" of muscle blood flow due to generalized vasodilation

Drug classes	Hemodynamic effects	Metabolic and CNS effects	Effects on exercise
VASODILATORS (*continued*)			
Calcium channel blockers (nifedipine, diltiazem, verapamil)	• Decreased SVR • Increased HR (nifedipine) • Decreased HR (verapamil)	• Headaches • Flushing • Fluid retention (nifedipine) • Constipation (verapamil)	• $\dot{V}O_2$max generally preserved • Potential for competitive "steal" of muscle blood flow due to generalized vasodilation
ANGIOTENSIN-CONVERTING ENZYME INHIBITORS			
Captopril, enalapril, fosinopril, etc.	• Decreased SVR • No increase in HR	• No major effect on energy metabolism • Potential for increased K^+	• No impairment of $\dot{V}O_2$max, training, or competition

Note. BP = blood pressure; CNS = central nervous system; HR = heart rate; $\dot{Q}$ = cardiac output; SVR = systemic vascular resistance; $\dot{V}O_2$max = maximal oxygen uptake.

range of planned exercise training intensities in low-risk patients and in those patients who are known to have normal or nonobstructive CAD determined by recent (within 1 year) invasive or noninvasive studies.

The assessment of BP responses to isometric muscle contraction should also be evaluated if resistance training is incorporated into the exercise prescription. Isometric handgrip is usually performed at 50% of maximal handgrip strength for 90 s with BP measured at 30-s intervals in the contralateral arm. BP values exceeding 180/120 mm Hg are considered a hypertensive response (see Table 22.2).

Exercise Mode and Intensity

The exercise prescription should focus on dynamic exercise utilizing the legs or combined leg and arm exercise. Vigorous walking or interval walking and jogging are often the easiest modes for younger, active patients. Stationary ergometer exercise is also a conveniently prescribed mode of exercise. Patients may use a traditional cycle ergometer or combined arm-leg training using an Airdyne-type cycle or cross-country ski ergometer. These modes usually require access to a fitness center to avoid the considerable expense for purchase of this equipment. Other forms of dynamic exercise may include low-impact aerobic dance, circuit training calisthenics, swimming, and stair-climbing ergometers.

The selection of exercise mode will be strongly influenced by the aerobic capacity of individual patients. Some modes of exercise training, such as rope jumping and aerobic dance, may have baseline metabolic requirements that exceed the desired training intensity.

Aerobic training intensity should begin at a moderate level of 55% to 65% of estimated $\dot{V}O_2$max, which usually corresponds to 60% to 70% of maximal HR (HRmax) estimated from age or measured during exercise testing. The intensity may be progressed over a period of 4 to 6 weeks to a stable level of 65% to 70% of $\dot{V}O_2$max, which corresponds to 70% to 75% of HRmax. Ratings of perceived exertion (RPE) also provide a satisfactory guideline for exercise intensity (see chapter 17). An RPE of 12 to 14 on the 15-point Borg scale usually corresponds to the desired exercise prescription range.

Patients who use a walking program may not attain the higher range of training intensities (70% of $\dot{V}O_2$max, 75% of HRmax). They may be assigned a target HR goal of 25 to 30 beats/min above the standing, resting HR. Patients on beta-blockade therapy should attain a 10- to 15-beat/min increase in HR above the standing, resting level.

Resistive exercise training in the form of repetitive light weight lifting may be incorporated into the exercise prescription for patients who do not show an excessive BP rise during isometric BP testing described previously. Resistance or weight training should emphasize high repetitions of light free weights or equipment-mounted resistance weights. The selection of weights or resistance should be based on the ability to easily perform 10 to 15 repetitions at an RPE of 12 to 14. Studies by Kelemen (78) have indicated that the training weight should correspond to 30% to 50% of the single-lift maximum.

Duration and Frequency

The aerobic workout includes an initial 5- to 10-min warm-up phase. This is especially important in hypertensive patients so that muscle vasodilation is achieved. The aerobic phase should cover a minimum of 30 to 40 min at the prescribed training intensity. The aerobic training phase may be decreased if resistive or circuit weight training is included in the exercise prescription. Finally, a 10-min cool-down at 50% of $\dot{V}O_2$max should conclude each exercise session.

Exercise training should be performed 3 or 4 days/week. Less than 2 sessions/week is not effective and more than 5 sessions/week provides no additional benefit to controlling hypertension (45). Compliance with exercise programs is strongly influenced by the convenience and available time to exercise within the patient's daily routine. For some patients a combination of home exercise and monitored exercise in a cardiac training center may optimize the overall training program.

Clinical Outcomes

A reduction in resting BP should be observed over a period of 4 to 8 weeks. A further decline may be seen in obese patients who experience continued weight loss over time. As previously mentioned, the expected decrease in resting systolic BP is 10 to 15 mm Hg and in diastolic BP, 5 to 10 mm Hg. Decreases in submaximal exercise BPs may also occur and may be documented during monitored exercise sessions in those patients who perform exercise in a monitored cardiac exercise program.

Additional improvements in lipid and carbohydrate metabolism may occur. Typically, a reduction in fasting triglycerides and an increase in high-density lipoprotein (HDL) cholesterol occur in patients with moderate hypertriglyceridemia and depressed HDL cholesterol levels. Fasting glucose levels usually decline and hemoglobin-A_{1C} levels may decrease in Type II diabetic patients. The combination of exercise and weight loss both contribute to improving receptor insulin sensitivity (see chapter 23) (79).

Medications

Patients who have borderline or mild hypertension at rest and do not demonstrate excessive exercise BPs may be able to lower their BP by exercise alone. Patients with higher resting or exercise BPs should control their hypertension pharmacologically before starting an exercise training program. After several months of training and perhaps accompanying weight loss, it may be possible to decrease the dose of antihypertensive medication or even discontinue its use.

Patients on antihypertensive medications should be observed for potential side effects during exercise. The five major classes of antihypertensive agents and their potential side effects are summarized in Table 22.4. The following comments concern the most important potential complications in each class of antihypertensive agents.

Diuretics

Diuretics continue to be extensively used for treating primary hypertension, although the recommended dosage has been decreased substantially during the past decade (e.g., hydrochlorothiazide from 50 mg/day to 25 mg/day). The major side effect of long-term diuretic therapy is urinary loss of potassium, magnesium, and other cations. This leads to the potential complications of muscle weakness and cramps and cardiac arrhythmias (80). Occasionally, vigorous treatment with loop diuretics may produce intravascular volume depletion and orthostatic hypotension.

Beta-Adrenergic Blocking Agents

Beta-adrenergic blockade is also used for antihypertensive therapy in selected groups, especially younger adults with evidence of increased adrenergic activity. Most studies indicate a significant impairment of $\dot{V}O_2$max due to decreases in maximal $\dot{Q}$ and skeletal muscle blood flow (81). In addition, beta-blockade may impair mobilization of fatty acids and glucose during exercise (82). Finally, exercise bronchospasm may be aggravated in some patients on beta-blocking agents.

Alpha-Adrenergic Blocking Agents

Alpha-1 blocking agents (Prazosin) are occasionally used as a first-line antihypertensive agent. Although they have minimal effect on cardiovascular responses to exercise, many patients experience marked orthostatic hypotension within the first hour after the initial dose of an alpha-1 blocking drug. Transcutaneous clonidine is an effective, centrally acting alpha-2 agonist that minimizes the usual side effects associated with oral clonidine.

Vasodilators

Arterial vasodilators include direct-acting agents (hydralazine) and calcium channel blockers (e.g., diltiazem, verapamil, nifedipine). These agents may produce marked vasodilation with secondary reflex increases in HR. Postexercise hypotension due to combined metabolic vasodilation and pharmacological dilation may occur in some patients. Hypotension may be aggravated in patients who are treated with combined beta-blockade and vasodilators. Some studies have suggested that calcium channel blockers may interfere with regional vasoconstrictor mechanisms during exercise. This impairs the maximal shunting of cardiac output to active skeletal muscle, resulting in a relative "steal" of blood flow into nonexercise tissues (83).

Angiotensin-Converting Enzyme Inhibitors

A variety of angiotensin-converting enzyme inhibitors are now available. This class of drugs is frequently used in the treatment of mild, moderate, and severe hypertension. In general there is no major impairment in cardiovascular function for exercise training. Some patients may experience hyperkalemia due to increased renal potassium retention.

Summary

Exercise is effective for treating mild to moderate primary hypertension. Average reductions of 10 mm Hg in systolic BP and 5 mm Hg in diastolic BP can be expected.

Exercise training is best used in combination with weight loss and diet management in obese patients with mild hypertension. Patients with more severe hypertension must be carefully evaluated for potential complications associated with exercise. Exercise training alone is unlikely to correct BP in this patient group.

The exercise prescription should emphasize moderate intensity and aerobic training, but may also include low-level resistive exercise. There is no apparent benefit to increasing the intensity or frequency of exercise training sessions for reducing BP.

Some antihypertensive medications or combinations of antihypertensive agents may modify or complicate exercise training. Dose reduction or alternate medications may be necessary in these cases.

References

1. Stokes, J.; Kannel, W.B.; Wolf, P.A.; D'Agostino, R.B.; Cupples, L.A. Blood pressure as a risk factor for cardiovascular disease: The Framingham study—30 years of followup. Hypertension. 13[Suppl. 1]:I13-I18; 1989.
2. Julius, S.; Jamerson, K.; Mejia, A.; Krause, L.; Schork, N.; Jones, K. The association of borderline hypertension with target organ changes and higher coronary risk. JAMA. 264:354-358; 1990.
3. U.S. Preventive Services Task Force. Guide to clinical preventive services: An assessment of the effectiveness of 169 interventions. Baltimore: Williams & Wilkins; 1989.
4. Gordon, N.F.; Scott, C.B.; Wilkinson, W.J.; Duncan, J.J.; Blair, S.N. Exercise and mild essential hypertension. Recommendations for adults. Sports Med. 10(6):390-404; 1990.
5. Report. Physical exercise in the management of hypertension: A consensus statement by the world hypertension league. J. Hypertens. 9:283-287; 1991.
6. Chockalingam, A.; Abbott, D.; Bass, M.; Battista, R.; Cameron, R.; de Champlain, J.; Evans, C.E.; Laidlaw, J.; Lee, B.L.; Leiter, L.; Lessard, R.; MacLean, D.; Nishikawa, J.; Rabkin, S.; Thibaudeau, C.; Strachan, D. Recommendations of the Canadian consensus conference on non-pharmacological approaches to the management of high blood pressure. Can. Med. Assoc. J. 142:1397-1409; 1990.
7. The fifth report of the joint national committee on detection, evaluation, and treatment of high blood pressure. Arch. Intern. Med. 153:154-183; 1993.
8. Gifford, R.W.; Kirkendall, W.; O'Connor, D.T.; Weidman, W. AHA scientific council special report: Office evaluation of hypertension. Circulation. 79:721-731; 1989.
9. Lewin, A.; Blaufox, M.D.; Castle, H.; Entwisle, G.; Langford, H. Apparent prevalence of curable hypertension in the hypertension detection and follow-up program. Arch. Intern. Med. 145:424-427; 1985.
10. Subcommittee on Definition and Prevalence of the 1984 Joint National Committee. Hypertension prevalence and the status of awareness, treatment, and control in the United States: Final report of the subcommittee on definition and prevalence of the 1984 joint national committee. Hypertension. 7:457-468; 1985.
11. Peterson, H.R.; Rothschild, M.; Weinberg, C.R.; Fell, R.D.; McLeish, K.R.; Pfeifer, M. Body fat and the activity of the autonomic nervous system. N. Engl. J. Med. 318:1077-1082; 1988.
12. Egan, B. Neurogenic mechanisms initiating essential hypertension. Am. J. Hypertens. 2:3575-3625; 1989.
13. Esler, M.; Lambert, G.; Jennings, G. Increased regional sympathetic nervous activity in human hypertension: Causes and consequences. J. Hypertens. 8[Suppl. 7]:S53-S57; 1990.

14. MacMahon, S.W.; Norton, R.N. Alcohol and hypertension: Implications for prevention and treatment. Ann. Intern. Med. 105:124-125; 1986.

15. Freed, D.L.; Banks, A.J.; Longson, D.; Burley, D.M. Anabolic steroids in athletes: Crossover double-blind trial on weightlifters. Br. Med. J. 2:471-473; 1975.

16. Cryer, P.E.; Haymond, M.W.; Santiago, J.V.; Shah, S.D. Norepinephrine and epinephrine release and adrenergic mediation of smoking-associated hemodynamic and metabolic events. N. Engl. J. Med. 295(11):573-577; 1976.

17. Goldstein, D.S. Plasma catecholamines in essential hypertension: An analytical review. Hypertension. 5:86-90; 1983.

18. Anderson, E.A.; Sinkey, C.A.; Lawton, W.J.; Mark, A.L. Elevated sympathetic nerve activity in borderline hypertensive humans: Evidence from direct intraneuronal recordings. Hypertension. 14:177-183; 1989.

19. Aviv, A. Prospective review. The link between cytosolic Ca^{2+} and the NA^+-H^+ antiport: A unifying factor for essential hypertension. J. Hypertens. 6:685-691; 1988.

20. Resnick, L.M. Ionic basis of hypertension, insulin resistance, vascular disease, and related disorders. The mechanism of "syndrome X." Am. J. Hypertension; 6:1235-1345; 1993.

21. Lusher, T.F. Imbalance of endothelium-derived relaxing and contracting factors: A new concept in hypertension. Am. J. Hypertens. 3:317-330; 1990.

22. Raij, L. Hypertension, endothelium, and cardiovascular risk factors. Am. J. Med. 90[Suppl. 2A]:13S-18S; 1991.

23. Folkow, B. The fourth Volhard lecture: Cardiovascular structural adaptation: Its role in the initiation and maintenance of primary hypertension. Clin. Sci. Mol. Med. 55[Suppl. 4]:3S-22S; 1979.

24. Conway, J.A. A vascular abnormality in hypertension. A study of blood flow in the forearm. Circulation. 27:520-529; 1966.

25. Korner, P.I. Baroreceptor resetting and other determinants of baroreflex properties in hypertension. Clin. Exp. Pharmacol. Physiol. [Suppl. 15]:45-64; 1989.

26. Julius, S. Autonomic nervous system dysregulation in human hypertension. Am. J. Cardiol. 67:3B-7B; 1991.

27. Lund-Johansen, P. Hemodynamics in essential hypertension. Clin. Sci. 59:343-354; 1980.

28. Reichek, N.; Devereux, R.B. Left ventricular hypertrophy: Relationship of anatomic, echocardiographic and electrocardiographic findings. Circulation. 63:623-632; 1981.

29. Heistad, D.D.; Lopez, A.G.; Baumbach, G.L. Hemodynamic determinants of vascular changes in hypertension and atherosclerosis. Hypertension, 17[Suppl. III]:III-7-III-11; 1991.

30. Rowell, L. Human circulation regulation during physical stress. Cambridge: Oxford University Press; 1986:257-267.

31. Hanson, P.; Nagle, F. Isometric exercise, cardiovascular responses in normal and cardiac populations. Cardiol. Clin. 5:157-170; 1987.

32. Ewing, D.J.; Irving, J.B.; Kerr, F.; Kirby, B.J. Static exercise in untreated systemic hypertension. Br. Heart J. 35:413-421; 1973.

33. de Champlain, J.; Petrovich, M.; Gonzalez, M.; Lebeau, R.; Nadeau, R. Abnormal cardiovascular reactivity in borderline and mild essential hypertension. Hypertension. 17[Suppl. III]:III-22-III-28; 1991.

34. Chaney, R.H.; Eyman, R.K. Blood pressure at rest and during maximal dynamic and isometric exercise as predictors of systemic hypertension. Am. J. Cardiol. 62:1058-1061; 1988.

35. Wilson, N.V.; Meyer, B.M. Early prediction of hypertension using exercise blood pressure. Prev. Med. 10:62-68; 1981.

36. Devereux, R.B.; Pickering, T.G.; Harshfield, G.A.; Kleinert, H.D.; Denby, L.; Clark, L.; Pregibon, D.; Jasm, M.; Kleiner, B.; Borer, J.S.; Laragh, J.H. Left ventricular hypertrophy in patients with hypertension: Importance of blood pressure response to regularly recurring stress. Circulation. 68:470-476; 1983.

37. Pickering, T.G.; Harshfield, G.A.; Kleinert, H.D.; Blank, S.; Laragh, J.H. Blood pressure during normal daily activities, sleep and exercise: Comparison of values in normal and hypertensive subjects. JAMA. 247:992-996; 1982.

38. Reaven, P.D.; Barrett-Connor, E.; Edelstein, S. Relation between leisure time physical activity and blood pressure in older women. Circulation. 83:559-565; 1991.

39. Boyer, J.L.; Kasch, F.W. Exercise therapy in hypertensive men. JAMA. 211:1668-1671; 1970.

40. Johnson, W.P.; Grover, J.A. Hemodynamic and metabolic effects of physical training in four patients with essential hypertension. Can. Med. Assoc. J. 96:842-846; 1967.

41. Duncan, J.J.; Farr, J.E.; Upton, J.; Hagan, R.D.; Oglesby, M.E.; Blair, S.N. The effects of aerobic exercise on plasma catecholamines and blood pressure in patients with mild essential hypertension. JAMA. 254:2609-2613; 1985.

42. Hagberg, J.M.; Mountain, S.J.; Martin, W.H.; Ehsani, A.A. Effect of exercise training in 60–69-year-old persons with essential hypertension. Am. J. Cardiol. 64:348-353; 1989.

43. Kiyonaga, A.; Arakawa, K.; Tanaka, H.; Shindo, M. Blood pressure and hormonal responses to aerobic exercise. Hypertension. 7:125-131; 1985.

44. Urata, H.; Tanabe, Y.; Kiyonaga, A.; Ikeda, M.; Tanaka, H.; Shindo, M.; Arakawa, K. Antihypertensive and volume-depleting effects of mild exercise on essential hypertension. Hypertension. 9:245-252; 1987.

45. Nelson, L.; Esler, M.D.; Jennings, G.L.; Korner, P.I. Effect of changing levels of physical activity on blood-pressure and haemodynamics in essential hypertension. Lancet. 2:473-476; 1986.

46. Roman, O.; Camuzzi, A.L.; Villalon, E.; Klenner, C. Physical training program in arterial hypertension. A long-term prospective follow-up. Cardiology. 67:230-243; 1981.

47. Cade, R.; Mars, D.; Wagemaker, H.; Zauner, C.; Packer, D.; Privette, M.; Cade, M.; Peterson, J.; Hood-Lewis, D. Effect of aerobic exercise training on patients with systemic arterial hypertension. Am. J. Med. 77:785-790; 1984.

48. Martin, J.E.; Dubbert, P.M.; Cushman, W.C. Controlled trial of aerobic exercise in hypertension. Circulation. 81:1560-1567; 1990.

49. Hagberg, J.M.; Goldring, D.; Ehsani, A.A.; Heath, G.W.; Hernandez, A.; Schechtman, K.; Holloszy, J.O. Effect of exercise training on the blood pressure and hemodynamic features of hypertensive adolescents. Am. J. Cardiol. 52:763-768; 1983.

50. Kelemen, M.H.; Effron, M.B.; Valenti, S.A.; Stewart, K.J. Exercise training combined with antihypertensive drug therapy. Effects on lipids, blood pressure, and left ventricular mass. JAMA. 263:2766-2771; 1990.

51. Meredith, I.T.; Jennings, G.L.; Esler, M.D.; Dewar, E.M.; Bruce, A.M.; Fazio, V.A.; Korner, P.I. Time-course of the antihypertensive and autonomic effects of regular endurance exercise in human subjects. J. Hypertension. 8:859-866; 1990.

52. Somers, V.K.; Conway, J.; Johnston, J.; Sleight, P. Effects of endurance training on baroreflex sensitivity and blood pressure in borderline hypertension. Lancet. 337:1363-1368; 1991.

53. Tipton, C.M. Exercise, training and hypertension: An update. Exercise & Sport Science Reviews, 19: 447-505; 1991.

54. Hagberg, J.M. Exercise, fitness, and hypertension. Exercise, fitness, and health. C. Bouchard, R.J. Shephard, T. Stephens, J.R. Sutton, and B.D. McPherson (eds): Human Kinetics, Champaign, 1990; 455-466.

55. Hagberg, J.M.; Seals, D.R. Exercise training and hypertension. Acta. Med. Scand. [Suppl.] 711:131-136; 1985.

56. Jost, J.; Weiss, M.; Weicker, H. Sympathoadrenergic regulation and the adrenoceptor system. J. Appl. Physiol. 68(3):897-904; 1990.

57. Kinoshita, A.; Urata, H.; Tanabe, Y.; Ikeda, M.; Tanaka, H.; Shindo, M.; Arakawa, K. What types of hypertensives respond better to mild exercise therapy? J. Hypertens. 6[Suppl 4]:S631-S633; 1988.

58. Spataro, J.A. The effects of exercise on human hypertension: A meta-analysis of studies. Med. Sci. Sports Exerc. [Suppl.] 23(4):S83; 1991.

59. Rueckert, P.A.; Slane, P.R.; Hanson, P. Hemodynamics of the acute post exercise blood pressure decline in hypertensive subjects. Am. J. Hypertens. 6(5 Pt 2):31A, 1993.

60. Cleroux, J.; Kouame, N.; Nadeau, A.; Coulombe, D.; Lacourciere, Y. Aftereffects of exercise on regional and systemic hemodynamics in hypertension. Hypertension. 19:183-191; 1992.

61. Hagberg, J.M.; Montain, S.J.; Martin, W.H. Blood pressure and hemodynamic responses after exercise in older hypertensives. J. Appl. Physiol. 63(1):270-276; 1987.

62. Coats, A.J.S.; Conway, J.; Isea, J.E.; Pannarale, G.; Sleight, P.; Somers, V.K. Systemic and forearm vascular resistance changes after upright bicycle exercise in man. J. Physiol. 413:289-298; 1989.

63. Floras, J.S.; Sinkey, C.A.; Aylward, P.E.; Seals, D.R.; Thoren, P.N.; Mark, A.L. Postexercise hypotension and sympathoinhibition in borderline hypertensive men. Hypertension. 14:28-35; 1989.

64. Pescatello, L.S.; Fargo, A.E.; Leach, C.N.; Scherzer, H.H. Short-term effect of dynamic exercise on arterial blood pressure. Circulation. 83:1557-1561; 1991.

65. Somers, V.K.; Conway, J.; Coats, A.; Isea, J.; Sleight, P. Postexercise hypotension is not sustained in normal and hypertensive humans. Hypertension. 18: 211-215; 1991.

66. Hagberg, J.M.; Ehsani, A.A.; Goldring, D.; Hernandez, A.; Sinacore, D.R.; Holloszy, J.O. Effect of weight training on blood pressure and hemodynamics in hypertensive adolescents. J. Pediatr. 104:147-151; 1984.

67. Harris, K.A.; Holly, R.G. Physiological responses to circuit eight training in borderline hypertensive subjects. Med. Sci. Sports Exerc. 19:246-252; 1987.

68. Tipton, C.M.; McMahon, S.; Youmans, E.M.; Overton, J.M.; Edwards, J.G.; Pepin, E.B.; Lauber, C. Response of hypertensive rats to acute and chronic conditions of static exercise. Am. J. Physiol. 254: H592-H598; 1988.

69. Effron, M.B. Effects of resistive training on left ventricular function. Med. Sci. Sports Exerc. 21:694-697; 1989.

70. Fleck, S.J. Cardiovascular adaptations to resistance training. Med. Sci. Sports Exerc. 20:S146-S151; 1988.

71. Jennings, G.; Nelson, L.; Nestel, P.; Esler, M.; Korner, P.; Burton, D.; Bazelmans, J. The effects of changes in physical activity on major cardiovascular risk factors, hemodynamics, sympathetic function, and glucose utilization in man: A controlled study of four levels of activity. Circulation. 73(1):30-40; 1986.

72. Van Hoof, R.; Hespel, P.; Fagard, R.; Lijnen, P.; Staessen, J.; Amery, A. Effect of endurance training on blood pressure at rest, during exercise and during 24 hours in sedentary men. Am. J. Cardiol. 63:945-949; 1989.

73. McMahon, M.; Palmer, R.M. Exercise and hypertension. Med. Clin. North Am. 69(1):57-70; 1985.

74. Arakawa, K. Antihypertensive mechanism of exercise. J. Hypertension, 11:223-229; 1993.

75. American College of Sports Medicine. Guidelines for exercise testing and prescription. 4th ed. Philadelphia: Lea & Febiger; 1990:1-10.

76. Nesto, R.W.; Phillips, R.T.; Kert, K.G.; Hill, T.; Perper, E.; Young, E.; Leland, O.S. Angina and exertional myocardial ischemia in diabetic and non-diabetic patients: Assessment by exercise thallium scintigraphy. Ann. Intern. Med. 108:170-175; 1988.

77. Schauer, J.; Hanson, P. Usefulness of a branching treadmill protocol for evaluation of cardiac functional capacity. Am. J. Cardiol. 60:1373-1377; 1987.

78. Kelemen, M.H. Resistive training safety and assessment guidelines for cardiac and coronary prone patients. Med. Sci. Sports Exerc. 21:675-677; 1989.

79. Ekoe, J.-M. Overview of diabetes and exercise. Med. Sci. Sports Exerc. 21:353-368; 1989.

80. Hollifield, J.W.; Slaton, P.E. Thiazide diuretics, hypokalemia and cardiac arrhythmias. Acta. Med. Scand. [Suppl.] 647:67-73; 1986.

81. Lundborg, P.H.; Astrom, C.; Bengtsson, C.; Fellenius, E.; Von Schenck, H. Effect of β-adrenoreceptor blockade on exercise performance and metabolism. Clin. Sci. 61:299-305; 1989.

82. Kaiser, P. Physical performance and muscle metabolism during beta adrenergic blockade in man. Acta. Physiol. Scand. [Suppl.] 536:1-44; 1987.

83. Choong, C.Y.P.; Roubin, G.S.; Shen, W.F.; Harris, P.J.; Kelly, D.T. Effects of nifedipine on systemic and regional oxygen transport and metabolism at rest and during exercise. Circulation. 71:787-796; 1985.

Chapter 23

Diabetic Patients

Peter Hanson

Skeletal muscle is the largest tissue mass in humans and can potentially serve as a voluntary metabolic organ to increase utilization of glucose, fatty acids, and other substrates. For over a century exercise has been recommended as a means of facilitating control of glucose levels in diabetic patients. Studies by Allen et al. (1), prior to the availability of insulin, showed that glucose levels declined in diabetic subjects after acute exercise.

Several more recent reports have shown that acute and chronic exercise training increases the apparent sensitivity of skeletal muscle to circulating insulin and attenuates hyperglycemia in most diabetic patients (2-5). Current research focuses on the mechanisms of exercise-induced insulin sensitivity and the effects of exercise training on the long-term management of diabetes. This chapter will examine the beneficial, and potentially adverse, effects of exercise training in diabetic patients.

Pathophysiology

Diabetes mellitus is a complex metabolic disorder characterized by impaired uptake of glucose by the tissues resulting from insufficient pancreatic insulin production or loss of peripheral insulin sensitivity. The resulting high circulating-glucose levels are associated with widespread vascular and microvascular damage, especially in the retina, kidney, and coronary circulations. In addition, peripheral sensory and cardiovascular autonomic neuropathy is common. The clinical spectrum of diabetes includes insulin-dependent diabetes and non–insulin-dependent diabetes. The major characteristics of each of these are summarized in Table 23.1.

Insulin-dependent diabetes, or *Type I diabetes*, usually begins in childhood or after puberty and is probably due to viral or immunologic damage to pancreatic islet cells. A family history of diabetes is present in approximately 50% of cases. Insulin replacement is mandatory for avoiding acute hyperglycemia, osmotic diuresis, and ketoacidosis. Vascular and neuropathic complications develop early and frequently produce blindness, renal failure, atherosclerosis, and peripheral neuropathy within a period of 10 years. This process is accelerated by inadequate insulin therapy. The progression of vascular and neurologic complications is closely related to the rate of glycosylation of various structural proteins in target tissues and to the action of various growth factors that stimulate microvascular proliferative changes. Coronary artery disease (CAD) with silent myocardial ischemia is frequently seen in Type I diabetics, presumably due to cardiac autonomic neuropathy.

Non–insulin-dependent diabetes, or *Type II diabetes*, typically occurs in adults over 40 years of age and is particularly common in sedentary, moderately obese men and women. The hyperglycemia found in Type II diabetes is usually associated with peripheral insulin resistance, especially in liver and skeletal muscle. Circulating insulin levels are initially increased due to persistently high glucose

Table 23.1 Comparison of Insulin-Dependent (Type I) and Non–Insulin-Dependent (Type II) Diabetes Mellitus

Characteristics	Type I	Type II
Frequency of occurrence (% of U.S. population)	0.5	4-5
Age of onset (years)	< 30	> 40
Genetic predisposition	Some	Fairly strong
Insulin production	None or trace	High in early years; low in later life
Pancreatic islet cell antibodies	Present	Absent
Association with obesity	Variable	Fairly strong
Complications	Frequent	Frequent

levels, which stimulate pancreatic insulin production. When pancreatic β-cell function is eventually exhausted, insulin levels decline. Thus, Type II diabetes includes a broad spectrum of early insulin resistance, progressive hyperglycemia with hyperinsulinemia, and an end stage of insulin deficiency.

Insulin resistance and hyperinsulinemia in Type II diabetes have recently been reported as common factors contributing to the combination of hyperglycemia, hypertension, and hyperlipidemia that frequently occurs in adults with central obesity (6,7). Impaired insulin sensitivity and corresponding high glucose levels facilitate hepatic overproduction of triglyceride-rich very low density lipoproteins (VLDLs), resulting in a mixed hyperlipidemia (8). Increased sympathetic tone and augmented intracellular Ca^{2+} in vascular smooth muscle are thought to contribute to hypertension (9,10). These metabolic risk factors have been called Syndrome-X and are associated with a higher incidence of coronary and peripheral vascular atherosclerosis (6,11).

Treatment of Diabetes

Type I diabetics require daily insulin supplements, usually administered as subcutaneous injections of a mixture of short-acting (peak time of 1 to 4 h) (regular) human insulin and an intermediate duration (peak time of 6 to 8 h) insulin (NPH). Most patients utilize a morning and evening dosing schedule and modify the insulin mixture according to self-monitored capillary blood glucose levels. Intensive therapy using more frequent (4 to 6) injections of regular insulin is recommended for some patients who exhibit poor glycemic control with twice-daily insulin regimes. Continuous insulin infusion pumps are also used to achieve optimum glycemic control in some patients who exhibit an inadequate response to subcutaneous insulin therapy.

Type II diabetics who are obese and insulin resistant are initially treated with a combination of diet and exercise to achieve weight loss and restore insulin sensitivity. Patients with inadequate insulin levels may respond to oral hypoglycemic agents, which act to stimulate β-cell insulin release. Subcutaneous insulin therapy is frequently required for advanced Type II diabetes with inadequate circulating insulin levels.

Metabolic Responses to Exercise

The metabolic responses to exercise are closely regulated by neuroendocrine control mechanisms to assure the availability of glucose and fatty acid substrates for muscle metabolism while also maintaining adequate glucose levels for dependent organs such as the brain. In diabetic patients the precise regulation of glucose release and peripheral uptake is variably limited by inadequate pancreatic insulin release (Type I diabetes) or diminished peripheral insulin sensitivity (Type II diabetes).

Normal Subjects

During exercise, skeletal muscle substrate uptake varies according to intensity, that is, the percentage of the maximum oxygen uptake ($\dot{V}O_2max$), and duration of work. At rest, free fatty acids (FFAs) are the primary energy source. Glucose and FFAs are both used during the initial phase of submaximal exercise, whereas FFAs become the dominant substrate during prolonged submaximal (50% to 60% $\dot{V}O_2max$) exercise. Circulating glucose levels are maintained from hepatic glycogen stores. However, small amounts of glucose from skeletal muscle glycogen stores are also required for both the initial phases and maintenance of prolonged exercise, and the depletion of these stores results in prompt muscle fatigue (12).

The release of hepatic glucose and adipose-tissue FFAs is mediated by a characteristic pattern of neurohormonal and hormonal response (Figure 23.1). The control of insulin levels is pivotal in maintaining the balance between hepatic glucose production and increased non–insulin-dependent muscle glucose uptake during exercise. In normal subjects, pancreatic insulin release is effectively inhibited by increased catecholamine levels, while hepatic glycogenolysis and gluconeogenesis are stimulated by increased levels of glucagon, epinephrine, and possibly growth hormone and cortisol. Plasma FFA levels also increase because of catecholamine-mediated lipolysis. Skeletal muscle uptake of glucose is simultaneously increased through non–insulin-dependent transport mechanisms. Circulating glucose levels remain stable or decline only slightly, although with prolonged exercise, hypoglycemia may occur in normal subjects (13). In the postexercise recovery state, muscle glucose uptake continues due to nonoxidative restoration of glycogen stores (14,15).

Type I Diabetes Mellitus

Insulin-dependent diabetics, who have absent or insufficient insulin levels and are hyperglycemic

Normal

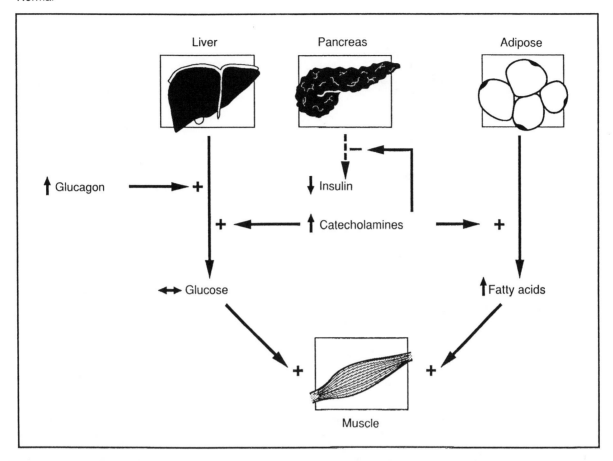

Figure 23.1   Hormonal control of glucose release and uptake during exercise in normal subjects. Increased skeletal muscle glucose uptake is balanced by increased hepatic glucose release stimulated by glucagon. Insulin secretion is inhibited by an increase in circulating catecholamines.

at rest, frequently respond to acute exercise with marked increases in plasma, glucose, FFAs, and ketone levels. This response is stimulated by excessive release of catecholamine, glucagon, and growth hormone (Figure 23.2).

With exogenous insulin replacement, Type I diabetics may exhibit relatively normal patterns of glucose and FFA in response to short-term exercise (Figure 23.3). When activity is performed shortly after a meal, high circulating glucose levels are reduced by non–insulin-dependent uptake by skeletal muscle. Accordingly, exercise training is most effective in modulating postprandial hyperglycemia in Type I diabetics.

Type I diabetic patients who take longer acting insulin preparations may experience hypoglycemia when exercise is performed 4 or more hours after a meal. Since exogenous insulin release is not suppressed by catecholamines, relatively high levels of exogenous insulin may inhibit hepatic

glucose release. Continued glucose uptake by skeletal muscle may then induce hypoglycemia (13). This continued glucose uptake is primarily directed to resynthesis of glycogen and has been termed "nonoxidative" (14). Late-onset (> 4 h) postexercise hypoglycemia has been reported to occur in approximately 16% of young Type I diabetics after unusually strenuous or prolonged exercise (15).

Type II Diabetes Mellitus

Non–insulin-dependent diabetics exhibit a variable spectrum of peripheral insulin resistance, hyperglycemia, and either increased or reduced insulin levels. Recent studies have shown that skeletal muscle is the major site of insulin resistance in Type II diabetes (16). This is manifested as impaired nonoxidative uptake of glucose for glycogen synthesis during insulin clamp studies (17).

Type I diabetes, without insulin

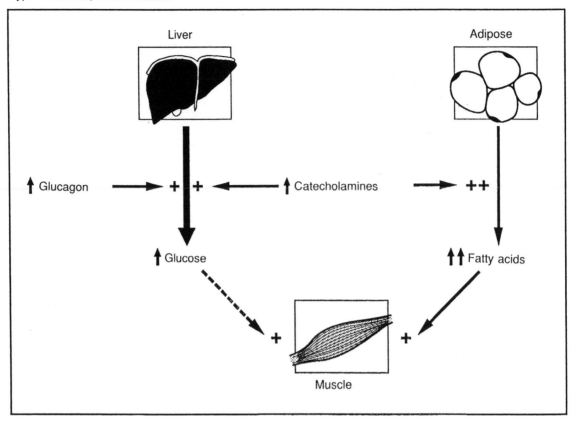

Figure 23.2 Hormonal control of glucose release and uptake during exercise in Type I diabetic subjects (without insulin replacement): Skeletal muscle glucose uptake is impaired and hepatic glucose release is excessive, due to more intense activity of glucagon and other counterregulatory hormones. Circulating glucose and free fatty acid levels rise, and ketosis may develop in some individuals.

During exercise, glucose levels usually decrease gradually because of enhanced oxidative utilization by skeletal muscle (Figure 23.4). Hepatic glucose production may be inhibited in the presence of high circulating insulin levels, and in some patients hypoglycemia may occur during or after extended exercise (17). This response may be aggravated in Type II diabetics who are treated with oral sulfonylurea agents (18).

Studies of Exercise Training in Diabetics

Most training studies involving diabetics have used traditional aerobic exercise prescription formats: an intensity of 70% to 80% $\dot{V}O_2max$ or 75% to 85% maximum heart rate (HRmax), for 30 to 60 min 3 to 5 times weekly for 6 to 12 weeks or more (see Table 23.2).

Type I Diabetics

Significant increases in $\dot{V}O_2max$ are generally achieved in subjects with uncomplicated Type I diabetes. These responses are accompanied by evidence of increased peripheral insulin sensitivity but with variable or limited improvement in glucose regulation (as measured by fasting glucose), 24-h urinary glucose excretion, oral glucose tolerance, intravenous glucose tolerance, and hemoglobin-A_{1c} (HbA_{1c}).

Exercise training studies by Soman et al. (2) showed increased insulin sensitivity (euglycemic clamp method) but no change in fasting glucose levels. Peterson et al. (3) subsequently showed significant decreases in mean glucose and HbA_{1c} levels and reduction in muscle capillary basement membrane thickness. Wallberg-Henricksson et al. (5) found increased insulin sensitivity and muscle oxidative enzyme activity but no change in 24-h urinary glucose excretion or HbA_{1c}. In contrast,

Diabetes and insulin

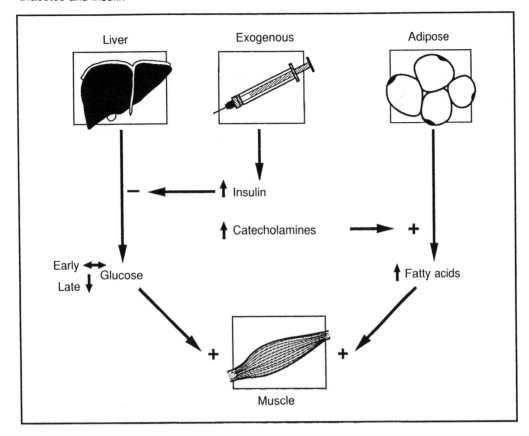

Figure 23.3 Hormonal control of glucose release and uptake during exercise in Type I diabetic subjects (with insulin replacement): Skeletal muscle glucose uptake and hepatic glucose release are normalized. However, hypoglycemia may occur during or after prolonged exercise due to the dual effects of exogenous insulin on hepatic glucose release and skeletal muscle glucose uptake.

Campaigne et al. (19) reported a reduction in fasting glucose and HbA$_{1c}$ in younger Type I diabetics after vigorous exercise for 12 weeks.

These findings probably reflect the marked heterogeneity of this population and emphasize the necessity for individual evaluation and follow-up monitoring to determine the effects of exercise on glucose control.

Type II Diabetics

Most exercise-training studies with Type II diabetic subjects, who are usually obese and sedentary, also show increased peripheral insulin sensitivity and improved glycemic control. The degree of improvement, however, may vary with the intensity, duration, and frequency of exercise training and is further influenced by diet and simultaneous weight loss.

Barnard et al. (20) reported significant decreases in fasting glucose and requirements for oral hypoglycemic agents or insulin therapy after a 26-day rigid-diet and exercise program. Reitman et al. (21) found decreased fasting glucose and improved oral glucose tolerance, and Trovati et al. (22) found decreases in fasting glucose, intravenous glucose tolerance, and HbA$_{1c}$ after 6 to 10 weeks of training. Leon et al. (23) recently reported no change in fasting or oral glucose tolerance or insulin levels in Type II diabetics who trained for 12 weeks without weight loss. These findings indicate a generally predictable trend toward improved glucose levels in Type II diabetics who follow prescribed exercise. Simultaneous weight loss, however, may be a major factor in this response.

The improvement in glycemic control following exercise training in Type II diabetes appears to be an acute and transient effect. Recent studies in several laboratories have demonstrated improved glucose tolerance and insulin sensitivity following a single bout of exercise (24). These favorable effects are maintained as long as regular exercise training continues. Rogers et al. (25) reported significant correction of oral glucose tolerance

Hyperinsulinemia

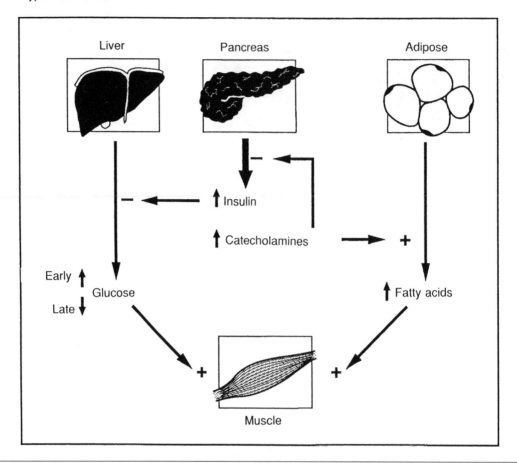

Figure 23.4 Hormonal control of glucose release and uptake during exercise in Type II diabetic subjects with hyperinsulinemia: Skeletal muscle glucose uptake is partially impaired by insulin resistance. Circulating glucose levels may increase initially, then decrease with prolonged exercise or during postexercise recovery.

response and hyperinsulinemia after 7 consecutive days of moderate-intensity exercise training in Type II diabetic subjects, who showed no change in $\dot{V}O_2$max or weight loss. The improved oral glucose tolerance was absent on follow-up testing after cessation of exercise training. Thus, frequent moderate exercise training appears to achieve and maintain improved glycemic control within a short period; however, these effects regress rapidly within several days following a period of nontraining.

Guidelines for Exercise Training

Patients with diabetes may exhibit a wide spectrum of pathological changes in various end organs ranging from near normal to diffuse multisystem abnormalities. Thus, it is essential to carefully evaluate all diabetic patients who wish to participate in prescribed exercise training.

Patient Evaluation and Testing

Evaluation of patients for prescribed exercise training should include a thorough review of diabetic control status. Cardiovascular screening should consider the following:

- Duration of diabetes
- Additional CAD risk factors
- Autonomic neuropathy
- Peripheral macrovascular or microvascular disease
- Abnormal electrocardiograph (ECG)
- Silent myocardial ischemia
- Low exercise tolerance

Type I patients with extensive retinopathy, autonomic neuropathy, or microvascular complications are poor candidates for exercise training and may experience repeated adverse effects during sustained exercise. Type II patients usually have

Table 23.2   Recent Exercise Training Studies Involving Diabetics

Study	Training conditions	Findings
Insulin-dependent (Type I) diabetes		
Pederson et al. (3)	Cycle ergometer 70% HRmax 35 min, 3 times/week, 8-10 months	↓ mean glucose ↓ HbA$_{1c}$ ↓ muscle cap basement membrane
Wallberg-Henricksson et al. (5)	Jogging and games 1 h, 2-3 times/week, 16 weeks	↑ insulin sensitivity ↑ muscle enzyme activity → glucose regulation → HbA$_{1c}$
Campaigne et al. (19)	Running and games HR ≥ 160 beats/min 12 weeks	↓ fasting glucose ↓ HbA$_{1c}$ (no change in controls)
Non–insulin-dependent (Type II) diabetes		
Barnard et al. (20)	Walking 75%-85% HRmax 30-45 min, 7 times/week, 26 days	↓ fasting glucose ↓ lipids ↓ oral hypoglycemic agents
Reitman et al. (21)	Cycle ergometer 60%-90% V̇O$_2$max 20-40 min, 5-6 times/week, 6-10 weeks	↓ fasting glucose Improved oral glucose tolerance ↓ or → fasting insulin and insulin oral glucose tolerance
Trovati et al. (22)	Cycle ergometer 50%-60% V̇O$_2$max 60 min, 7 times/week, 6 weeks	↑ insulin sensitivity ↓ free glucose ↓ HbA$_{1c}$ Improved intravenous glucose tolerance
Leon et al. (23)	Treadmill walking 50%-70% V̇O$_2$max 30-60 min, 2-4 times/week, 12 weeks Constant body weight	→ free glucose Unchanged oral glucose tolerance → insulin → HbA$_{1c}$ → lipids
Lampman et al. (26)	Walk-jog 75% HRmax 30 min, 4 times/week, 12 weeks	↑ insulin sensitivity Improved oral glucose tolerance (on oral hypoglycemics)
Rogers et al. (25)	Walking, cycling 68% V̇O$_2$max 50-60 min for 6 days, 50% HRmax for 1 day	Improved oral glucose tolerance ↓ insulin response

Note. HbA$_{1c}$ = hemoglobin A$_{1c}$; HR = heart rate; HRmax = maximal heart rate; V̇O$_2$max = maximal oxygen uptake; ↑ = increase; ↓ = decrease; → = no change.

multiple risk factors for atherosclerosis, which also require evaluation and treatment prior to initiating exercise training.

Exercise testing is generally recommended for all diabetic patients prior to starting a supervised or unsupervised exercise at intensities above 60% of V̇O$_2$max. A standard ECG monitored graded exercise test (GXT) may be adequate if baseline ECG changes are absent (i.e., no hypertrophy, prior myocardial infarction [MI], bundle branch block, nonspecific ST or T changes). Radionuclear-based exercise testing is necessary for patients who have an abnormal baseline ECG or a prior history of CAD or coronary artery bypass graft (CABG) surgery. Silent ischemia is frequent in Type I diabetes, and this finding on standard ECG exercise testing should also be reevaluated with radionuclear perfusion studies (27).

Hemodynamic responses to exercise are frequently abnormal in diabetic patients who have evidence of autonomic neuropathy. Heart rate (HR), blood pressure (BP), cardiac output (Q̇), and peripheral blood flow responses to dynamic and static exercise are typically attenuated, presumably because of combined effects of impaired sympathetic drive and diabetic cardiomyopathy. Postural hypotension and postexertional orthostatic hypotension are also common in diabetics with autonomic vasomotor neuropathy (28,29). Patients who exhibit one or more of these abnormalities are unlikely to benefit from conventional exercise training. Such patients may be able to participate in lower level activities that emphasize flexibility and muscle toning.

Exercise Prescription

Exercise prescription should initially emphasize moderate-intensity aerobic exercise combined with more frequent training stimulus in order to maximize the cumulative daily effect of exercise on muscle insulin sensitivity and postexercise glucose uptake (24,25). Training intensity of 60% to 70% of estimated $\dot{V}O_2$max and 70% to 75% of peak HR attained during the GXT is appropriate; these values are approximately 10 percentage points below the respective ranges currently recommended for cardiac rehabilitation. The duration and frequency of training may begin with 20- to 30-min sessions 3 times weekly and progress to 30 to 40 min at least 5 times weekly. Some out-of-shape patients may initially require training intervals of 5 to 10 min with several minutes of rest between intervals. Training duration can be gradually extended as tolerance increases.

Exercise training modes may include vigorous walking, stationary cycling, ergometer rowing, and ergometer stepping. A circuit training format with a combination of aerobic and light resistance training or weight lifting may be suitable for increasing muscle strength in previously sedentary patients. Jogging or running may be appropriate for low-risk Type I or Type II diabetic patients, but should not be recommended for those who have evidence of peripheral neuropathy or lower-extremity microvascular disease. Weight lifting or intensive resistance training should be avoided in patients with proliferative retinopathy because of the potential for retinal hemorrhage (30).

Monitoring and Follow-Up

Signs or symptoms of exercise or postexercise hypoglycemia should be anticipated in Type I diabetics. Therefore, high-intensity (> 75% $\dot{V}O_2$max)

and long-duration (> 60 min) training should be avoided. Blood glucose levels must be monitored prior to exercise and during the first 30 min of recovery after training. Additional glucose monitoring may be necessary after 4 to 6 h to detect late-occurring hypoglycemia due to continued nonoxidative glucose uptake in muscle. Appropriate adjustments in insulin dose, injection site, caloric intake, and the timing of exercise may be used to correct hypoglycemic responses (31).

Daily insulin requirements may decrease by 15% to 20% or more on exercise days. Patients who exercise in the morning hours should reduce or withhold regular insulin injection. The morning intermediate-duration insulin dose should be reduced in anticipation of afternoon exercise. Insulin should be injected at subcutaneous sites over nonexercising muscle to avoid overly rapid absorption (32) (but note that the importance of this strategy still is debated). Carbohydrate intake should be increased before exercise, using 1 bread exchange (15 g carbohydrate) for each 30 min of anticipated exercise. The need for increased caloric intake may be alleviated by exercising shortly after a meal. Monitor blood glucose levels routinely to verify the outcome of changes in insulin and diet.

Type II diabetics may experience hypoglycemia due to improved insulin sensitivity following exercise training. Oral hypoglycemia agents aggravate this adverse response and may require a reduced dosage or cessation of these drugs on exercise days (18). Finally, patients should be reminded to maintain proper foot care. Other potential adverse effects of exercise training in diabetic patients include

- ketosis,
- silent myocardial ischemia,
- cardiomyopathy,
- hypertension,
- hypotension,
- microvascular trauma (especially feet),
- retinal hemorrhage, and
- proteinuria.

In many medical centers diabetes nurse clinicians are responsible for coordinating patient follow-up. They are a valuable resource for the exercise training specialist to consult for additional guidelines.

Summary

Exercise training is generally recommended for stable Type I and Type II diabetic patients. Both groups may show improvements in functional capacity and feelings of well-being. Type I patients often require readjustment of insulin therapy and carbohydrate intake to avoid hypoglycemia during or after exercise. Type II patients may also benefit from increased postexercise insulin sensitivity and weight loss, which frequently help to correct glucose intolerance. Both groups of patients must be adequately evaluated prior to exercise training to identify potential complications that may occur during exercise or postexercise recovery.

References

1. Allen, F.M.; Stillman, E.; Fritz, R. Total dietary regulation in the treatment of diabetes. In: Exercise. New York: Rockefeller Institute; 1919:chap. 5 (Monogr. 11).

2. Soman, V.R.; Koivisto, V.A.; Deibert, D.; Felig, P.; DeFronzo, R.A. Increased insulin sensitivity and insulin binding to monocytes after physical training. N. Engl. J. Med. 301:1200-1204; 1979.

3. Pedersen, O.; Beck-Nielsen, H.; Heding, L. Increased insulin receptors after exercise in patients with insulin-dependent diabetes mellitus. N. Engl. J. Med. 302:886-892; 1980.

4. Koivisto, V.A.; Felig, P. Effects of leg exercise on insulin absorption in diabetic patients. N. Engl. J. Med. 298:78-83; 1978.

5. Wallberg-Henricksson, H.; Gunnerson, R.; DeFronzo, R.; Felig, P.; Ostman, J.; Wahren, J. Increased peripheral insulin sensitivity and muscle mitochondrial enzymes but unchanged blood glucose control in type I diabetics after physical training. Diabetes. 31:1044-1050; 1982.

6. Fuh, M.M.-T.; Shieh, S.-M.; Wu, D.-A.; Chen, Y.-D.; Reaven, G.M. Abnormalities of carbohydrate and lipid metabolism in patients with hypertension. Arch. Intern. Med. 147:1035-1038; 1987.

7. Peiris, A.N.; Mueller, R.A.; Smith, G.A. Splanchnic insulin metabolism in obesity: Influence of body fat distribution. J. Clin. Invest. 64:1648-1657; 1986.

8. Olefsky, J.M.; Farquher, J.W.; Reaven, G.M. Reappraisal of the role of insulin in hypertriglyceridemia. Am. J. Med. 57:551-560; 1974.

9. Sowers, J.R.; Standley, P.R.; Ram, J.L.; Zemel, M.B.; Resnick, L.M. Insulin resistance, carbohydrate metabolism and hypertension. Am. J. Hypertens. 4:466S-472S; 1991.

10. Sowers, J.R. Relationship between hypertension and subtle and overt abnormalities of carbohydrate metabolism. J. Am. Soc. Nephrol. 1:S39-S47; 1990.

11. Reaven, G.M. Roles of insulin resistance in human disease. Diabetes. 37:1595-1607; 1988.

12. Felig, P.; Wahren, J. Fuel homeostasis in exercise. N. Engl. J. Med. 293:1078-1084; 1975.

13. Felig, P.; Cherif, A.; Minagawe, A.; Wahren, J. Hypoglycemia during prolonged exercise in normal man. N. Engl. J. Med. 306:895-900; 1982.

14. Richter, E.A.; Garetto, L.P.; Goodman, M.N.; Ruderman, N.B. Enhanced muscle glucose metabolism after exercise: Modulation by local factors. Am. J. Physiol. 246:E476-E482; June 1984.

15. McDonald, M. Post exercise late-onset hypoglycemia in insulin dependent diabetic patients. Diabetes Care. 10:584; 1987.

16. Shulman, G.I.; Rothman, D.L.; Jue, T.; Stein, P.; DeFronzo, R.; Shulman, R.G. Quantitation of muscle glycogen synthesis in normal subjects and subjects with non-insulin dependent diabetes by ^{13}C nuclear magnetic resonance spectroscopy. N. Engl. J. Med. 322:223-238; 1990.

17. DeFronzo, R.A.; Gunnarsson, R.; Bjorkman, O.; Olsson, M.; Wahren, J. Effects of insulin on peripheral and splanchnic glucose metabolism in non-insulin dependent (type II) diabetes mellitus. J. Clin. Invest. 76:149-155; 1985.

18. Kemmer, F.W.; Tacken, M.; Berger, M. Mechanism of exercise induced hypoglycemia during sulfonylurea treatment. Diabetes. 36:1178-1182; 1987.

19. Campaigne, B.; Gilliam, T.B.; Spencer, M.L.; Lampman, R.M.; Schork, M.A. Effects of a physical activity program on metabolic control and cardiovascular fitness in children with insulin-dependent diabetes mellitus. Diabetes Care. 7:57-62; 1984.

20. Barnard, R.J.; Lattimore, L.; Holly, R.G.; Cherny, S.; Pritikin, N. Response of noninsulin-dependent diabetic patients to an intensive program of diet and exercise. Diabetes Care. 5:370-374; 1982.

21. Reitman, J.S.; Vasquez, B.; Klimes, I.; Nagulesparan, M. Improvement in glucose hemostasis after exercise training in noninsulin-dependent diabetes. Diabetes Care. 7:434-441; 1984.

22. Trovati, M.; Carta, Q.; Cavalot, F.; Vitali, S.; Banaudi, C.; Luccina, P.G.; Fioccli, F.; Emanuelli, G.; Lenti, G. Influence of physical training on blood glucose, glucose tolerance, insulin secretion, and insulin action in noninsulin-dependent diabetic patients. Diabetes Care. 7:416-420; 1984.

23. Leon, A.S.; Conrad, J.C.; Casal, D.C.; Serfass, R.; Bonnard, R.A.; Goetz, F.C.; Blackburn, H. Exercise for diabetics. Effects of conditioning at constant body weight. J. Cardiac Rehabil. 4:278-286; 1984.

24. Devlin, J.T.; Hirshman, M.; Horton, E.D.; Horton, E.S. Enhanced peripheral and splanchnic insulin sensitivity in NIDDM after a single bout of exercise. Diabetes. 36:434-439; 1987.

25. Rogers, M.A.; Yamamoto, C.; King, D.S.; Hagberg, J.M.; Ehsani, A.A.; Holloszy, J.O. Improvement in glucose tolerance after 1 wk of exercise in patients with mild NIDDM. Diabetes Care. 11:613-618; 1988.

26. Lampman, R.M.; Schteingart, D.E. Effects of physical training on glucose control, lipid metabolism and insulin sensitivity in hypertriglyceridemia and non–insulin-dependent diabetes mellitus. Med. Sci. Sports Exercise. 26:703-712; 1991.

27. Nesto, R.W.; Phillips, R.T.; Kett, K.G.; Hill, T.; Perper, E.; Young, E.; Leland, O.S., Jr. Angina and exertional myocardial ischemia in diabetic and non-diabetic patients: Assessment by exercise thallium scintigraphy. Ann. Intern. Med. 108:170-177; 1988.

28. Hilsted, J. Pathophysiology in diabetic autonomic neuropathy: Cardiovascular hormonal and metabolic studies. Diabetes. 31:730-737; 1982.

29. Hilsted, J.; Galbo, H.; Christensen, N.J. Impaired cardiovascular responses to graded exercise in diabetic autonomic neuropathy. Diabetes. 28:313-319; 1979.

30. Bernbaum, M.; Albert, S.G.; Cohen, J.D.; Drimmer, A. Cardiovascular conditioning in individuals with diabetic retinopathy. Diabetes Care. 12:740-742; 1989.

31. Jensen, M.D.; Miles, J.M. The roles of diet and exercise in the management of patients with insulin dependent diabetes mellitus. Mayo Clin. Proc. 61:813-819; 1986.

32. Koivisto, V.A.; Felig, P. Effects of leg exercise on insulin absorption in diabetic patients. N. Engl. J. Med. 298:79-83; 1978.

Chapter 24

Sexual Relations

James S. Skinner

It is obvious from reviewing the literature on sexual activity that we know more about the effects of physical activity on humans in space, underwater, and on the athletic field than in the bedroom. There is even less information about the effects of sexual activity on patients with coronary artery disease (CAD).

Sexual activity is not easy to study, however, because there are various physiological, psychological, and ethical matters to consider. For example, sex cannot be studied merely as physical activity. The subjects are generally in a body position (lying down) different from that of other activities, use muscle groups different from those used while walking or cycling, are not in a metabolic steady state (especially during the brief period of orgasm), and may be doing a combination of isotonic and isometric work. All of these factors make it difficult to quantify the physiological effects of sex. In addition, autonomic and emotional factors tend to accentuate the physiological reactions in a variable manner. Nevertheless, a close look at the available evidence indicates more agreement than disagreement about sexual activity in general and for patients with CAD in particular.

Before narrowing our viewpoint to patients with CAD, looking at the overall population can yield a better perspective. First, it should be stated that much less is known about the sexual responses of women in part because the male response is more visible and quantifiable.

Since CAD patients are most often over 40 years old, one needs to look at the general effect of the aging process on sexual activity. According to Kinsey et al. (1), men show a decrease in the frequency of sexual intercourse with age and an increase in impotence after the age of 35 years (Figure 24.1). On the other hand, continued sexual activity appears to reduce the drop-off in performance in the man.

In both sexes, it is clear that the demand for or need for orgasm is reduced with advancing age (2). Mulligan and Moss (3) surveyed male veterans aged 30 to 99 years and found that although interest in sex declined over this age range, it was still present in the older men. When a partner was available, there was close agreement between a respondent's interest and that of his partner. In women, Masters and Johnson (4) noted little loss in orgasmic responsiveness with age; a woman's reduced frequency of intercourse seemed to be more related to the sexual activity of her mate.

Mulligan and Moss (3) found that the reported frequency of all forms of sexual activity decreased with age. Men aged 30 to 39 years reported having intercourse more than once weekly; men 90 to 99 years old, less than once a year. The researchers found that the frequency, duration, and rigidity of erections dropped significantly with age and that the ability to regularly achieve orgasm decreased from 82% in the youngest age group to 21% in the oldest.

Such trends suggest that it can be difficult to determine the effects of CAD on sexual function because there is also a high rate of sexual dysfunction in the normal population (5). Frank et al. (6) found that 40% of men in "happily married couples" had erectile or ejaculatory problems. Kolman (5) theorized that this rate may be even higher in men who subsequently have a myocardial infarction (MI), as Wabrek and Burchell (7) showed that two thirds of MI patients had sexual difficulties before their heart attack. A different interpretation can be found in the results of Dhabuwala et al. (8), however. They found no significant differences in sexual dysfunction between a group of 50 patients who had had an MI and a matched group of outpatients from a urology clinic. Sexual and erectile dysfunction was seen in 76% and 42% of the MI group, respectively. The corresponding values were 68% and 48% in the control group.

While there are many possible causes of dysfunction, two factors common in older people have been shown to have an effect. Depression, which is a common occurrence after an MI, can reduce libido in many patients (9). Of alcoholic men, 4%

367

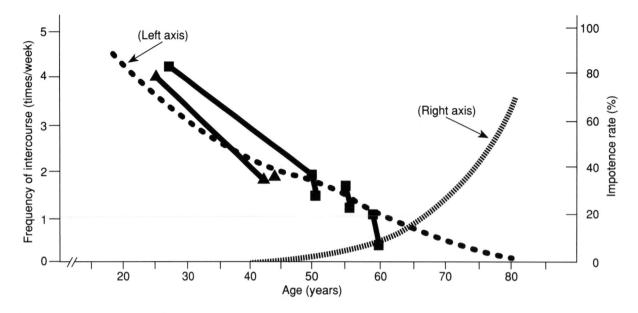

Figure 24.1 Frequency of sexual intercourse among married men (•••) and percentage of impotence among men (ıııııı) according to age (1). Included are results from CAD patients (■) and coronary-prone men (▲) from other studies (14,15,22).

are impotent and another 5% to 10% have ejaculatory problems (10).

Psychological Aspects

In addition to the effects of aging, the CAD patient has extra difficulties associated with a compromised cardiovascular system. This fact, plus the psychological trauma associated with an MI (fear, anxiety, depression, and so forth), puts the patient in a very dependent state. In addition to the aforementioned problems, Hackett and Cassem (11) report that post-MI patients have a decreased ego strength, a sense of "emasculation," and a feeling of fatigue and weakness. All of these problems cause patients to doubt their ability to engage in normal physical activity, much less to perform sexually on demand. Rosen and Bibring (12) describe the "middle-age crisis" of men aged 50 to 60 years who are already in conflict over the shift from an active to a more passive lifestyle. An MI during this period accentuates the impact of aging and may increase fears of sexual inadequacy.

Since many men already have psychological problems because of the mythology surrounding the penis and its relationship to their masculinity, this becomes an important question to them. The very words *potent* and *impotent* have connotations about a man's entire life and his ability to cope. If the patient begins to worry about impotence, this

concern itself can create problems. As Broderick (13) states, "There is nothing more recalcitrant than a recalcitrant penis." That is, if the patient thinks he will be impotent, he probably will be; a self-fulfilling prophecy is thus created.

Interaction of Age and CAD

Referring once again to Figure 24.1, one can observe the effects of aging and CAD. Hellerstein and Friedman (14) asked 48 randomly selected CAD patients to recall their frequency of intercourse at age 25 or during their first year of marriage, during the year before their MI (mean age = 48.5 years), and 1 year following an MI. Likewise, a group of 43 normal men considered to be coronary-prone were asked to record their frequency of intercourse at age 25 or during their first year of marriage, upon entering a physical reconditioning class (mean age = 42.3 years), and approximately 1 year thereafter. Although recall from 15 to 25 years earlier may have been difficult and although the actual frequency may have been slightly high, given that it was the first year of marriage, the data for the two groups are not very different from those of Kinsey et al. (1). In the MI group, there was a drop from 2.1 times/week to 1.6 times/week in the period before MI to the period after MI. Bloch et al. (15) found similar results in a group of 100 CAD patients from Switzerland (88 men and 12 women, average age = 58 years), that is, a reduction in frequency from 1.2 times/week to 0.6/week.

These data agree with those of other investigators (16-18). Tuttle et al. (16) found a reduction of at least 50% in the frequency of intercourse following an MI in two-thirds of the patients studied. In a sample of 20 patients 3 to 4 years following an MI, Klein et al. (17) found that 5 had maintained normal relations, 8 had diminished sexual activity, and 7 had totally abstained. In these studies, there was no relationship between frequency of intercourse and physical working capacity (15), or between frequency of intercourse and age of the patient or severity of the disease (17).

Data on women in this regard are practically nonexistent, except for those of Abramov (18), who studied the sexual life of 100 female patients aged 40 to 60 years at the time of hospitalization for acute MI. Sexual frigidity and dissatisfaction were found in 65% of the CAD patients compared with 24% in a control group of 100 patients of the same age who were hospitalized for other reasons. The most common cause of dissatisfaction (20%) was premature ejaculation and male impotence. Only 4% attributed the dissatisfaction to the disease of the patient herself. As Kolman (5) correctly points out, however, the incidence of MI in women (as in men) is associated with the Type A personality. Thus, the sexual problems may have been the result of the same personality traits that had adversely affected the marriage. Supporting this is the fact that 77% of the women in Abramov's study (18) complained of sexual frigidity and dissatisfaction before their MI.

Reasons for Reduced Sexual Activity

Several studies (14,15,19) ascertained that the reasons for reduced sexual activity after an MI are primarily psychological. Interestingly, only 1 subject in one study and none in the other two studies claimed that reduced activity was due to impotence. According to the results of Kinsey et al. (Figure 24.1), values of at least 5% to 10% would have been expected. Whether this finding reflects a process of denial in the subjects of the post-MI studies, these results contrast with those of Dhabuwala et al. (8), Weiss and English (20), and Tuttle et al. (16), who found impotence in CAD patients of 42%, 32%, and 10%, respectively (Table 24.1).

In a study by Dorossiev et al. (21) in Bulgaria on 59 MI patients and 41 patients who had had heart surgery, about 50% of the patients up to age 50 had decreased libido and potency (Table 24.2).

Table 24.1   Reasons Given by CAD Patients for Reducing Sexual Activity

Study	n	Reasons
Bloch et al. (15)	100	• Loss of desire • Depression • Fear, anxiety • Wife's decision • Symptoms, fatigue • Impotence (1%)
Hellerstein and Friedman (14)	12	• Loss of desire • Wife's decision • Symptoms • Fear • Impotence (0%)
Weiss and English (20)	—	• Impotence (32%)
Tuttle et al. (16)	—	• Impotence (10%)

After age 50 this proportion increased to 95%. In another group of 100 patients, only 21% had normal sexual activity following MI or surgery, whereas 69% reported that they had stopped all sexual activity because of their disease. Although it may be argued that one should not consider surgical and post-MI patients as one group, the results do indicate that sexual troubles are frequent in patients with CAD.

Johnston et al. (22) sent questionnaires to 130 exercising patients inquiring about their sexual activity; 87 patients (mean age = 54 years) responded. Frequency of intercourse declined significantly from 1.6 times/week to 1.2 times/week in 68 post-MI patients, who waited a mean of 9.4 weeks before resuming sexual activity. The 19 postrevascularization patients had an insignificant reduction in frequency, from 2.1 times/week to 1.9/week and waited only 5.7 weeks to resume. Their results concur with those of Hellerstein and Friedman (14): The longer the delay before resuming coitus after a cardiac event, the lower the frequency. These studies also suggest that the higher the frequency before the cardiac event, the smaller the decrease in frequency afterward.

Physiological Aspects

As mentioned previously, relatively little is known about the physiological effects of sexual activity. Studies done once in a laboratory setting with

Table 24.2   Percent of Patients (59 Post-MI, 41 Post–Heart Surgery) Reporting Various Degrees of Sexual Activity and Potency/Libido

| | Age (years) | | | |
Parameter	≤ 40 (*n* = 48)	40-50 (*n* = 32)	> 50 (*n* = 20)	Total (*n* = 100)
Sexual activity				
Normal	17	28	20	21
None (libido[a])	15	6	5	10
None (coronary artery disease[b])	68	66	75	69
Potency/libido				
Same or more	48	50	5	40
Lost or less	52	50	95	60

[a]Decreased libido cited by patients as the reason for no sexual activity.

[b]Presence of coronary artery disease cited by patients as the reason for no sexual activity.

From Dorossiev et al. (21).

young, healthy subjects have little relevance to repeated sexual relations in the privacy of the bedroom between two older people, one of whom has had an MI. Nevertheless, by studying the former, insight about the latter can be gained.

Physiological Responses to Sexual Activity

The sexual act can be divided into four phases: (1) arousal (contemplation, libido, erection), (2) intromission-plateau, (3) orgasm, and (4) resolution. In the absence of cerebrovascular problems, extensive occlusive disease of the iliac arteries, or interruption of the nervous connections involved, there should be no physiological reason for most people to have problems with arousal. In one of the first sexuality studies (1930), Scott (23) investigated the arousal phase and found that nearly all students had an increased systolic blood pressure (SBP) after sexual arousal while watching an erotic film. Since that time, most studies have dealt with the last three phases.

The normal responses to sexual intercourse are increases in heart rate (HR), SBP, and pulmonary ventilation ($\dot{V}_E$). These parameters generally rise progressively during arousal and intromission, increase rapidly in the minute preceding orgasm, peak briefly during orgasm, and then rapidly decline to baseline within 2 to 3 min (24).

In 1932, Boas and Goldschmidt (25) reported on the HR response of young men and women volunteers following their normal daily routines while locked in a hospital room. Although they knew they were being monitored, one couple had sexual relations with an average peak HR of 148 beats/min during orgasm. Klumbies and Kleinsorge (26) studied the effects of auto-arousal on two subjects, one male and one female. While remaining inactive, the woman brought herself to orgasm via erotic fantasy. Her HR rose from 60 beats/min to 103 beats/min and her SBP increased from 110 mm Hg to 160 mm Hg. Similar results were shown by the man, who masturbated to orgasm (peak HR = 142 beats/min). In both cases, there was a rapid drop in HR and SBP after orgasm; the man took only 4 s to bring his HR back to 67 beats/min. Bartlett (27) determined the HR and $\dot{V}_E$ of three married couples aged 22 to 30 years on three different occasions in a laboratory setting. The total duration of coitus was 9 to 10 min, with both partners showing an increase in HR and $\dot{V}_E$ during coitus and especially at orgasm. As stated in the article, an HR approaching 170 beats/min was obtained in one female. Although the actual figures are not given, an estimate of the HR responses from the graphs reveals the following: for women, the average HR at orgasm was about 135 to 140 beats/min and ranged from 100 to 170 beats/min; in men, the average HR at orgasm was about 150 beats/min and ranged from 130 to 160 beats/min. Considering, however, that the subjects were wired, wore a nose clip, breathed through a mouthpiece, and performed in a laboratory room next to that of the researcher, it is hard to know how representative these values are.

Should sexual activity be considered "strenuous"? Masters and Johnson (4) reported a range in HR at orgasm of 110 to 180 beats/min, without stating the average value, how many people were measured, how many attained the high HR, the ages of the subjects, or other variables. Reporting respiratory rates of "up to 40 per minute" and increased SBPs, they indicated that sex may be considered a strenuous activity. Unfortunately, because of the lack of actual data, it is not possible to evaluate their statements.

Masters and Johnson (4) also stated that the physiological response was approximately the same whether the sexual activity was heterosexual or autoerotic in nature. It is likely that the physiological effects of homosexual activity are similar, although there is a suggestion of an increased risk of cardiac arrhythmias with stimulation of the anal sphincter and the rectal mucosa (28).

With the advent of the portable tape recorder, it has been possible to eliminate the contrived laboratory setting and to substitute the more natural setting of the private bedroom. One of the earliest studies to use this approach was that of Hellerstein and Friedman (14). The subjects described previously (Figure 24.1) were asked to wear a portable electrocardiogram (ECG) tape recorder during their usual activities, with no mention of sexual activity. Of the 91 subjects monitored, 14 did engage in sexual activity. The mean peak HR at orgasm was 117 beats/min (range = 90 to 144), with an average HR of 87 beats/min 2 min before, 101 beats/min 1 min before, 97 beats/min 1 min after, and 85 beats/min 2 min after orgasm. The average time between going to bed and reaching orgasm was 16 min, with a range of 10 to 30 min. Thus, these data suggest that sexual activity done in privacy by a married, middle-aged couple does not represent strenuous activity. In fact, several subjects had higher HRs during their regular daily activities. Similarly, Jackson (29) obtained 24-h ECGs on 14 patients before and after administration of beta-blockers. Before blockade, the average peak HR over a 24-h period was 124 beats/min, compared with 122 beats/min during intercourse. After blockade, both HRs were reduced to 82 beats/min.

In order to estimate the energy cost of sexual activity in their patients, Hellerstein and Friedman (14) looked at the data obtained when the subjects described above performed an exercise test on a cycle ergometer. During the test, HRs of 117 beats/min (the peak HR at orgasm) and 97 beats/min (average HR for the period 2 min before to 2 min after orgasm), the subjects' oxygen intakes ($\dot{V}O_2$) were 16 ml · kg^{-1} · min^{-1} and 12 ml · kg^{-1} · min^{-1},

or 4.5 and 3.4 METs (metabolic equivalents), respectively. (A MET is a multiple of the resting metabolism or the $\dot{V}O_2$ at rest, generally estimated to be 3.5 ml · kg^{-1} · min^{-1}.) Bohlen et al. (24) measured the HR, rate-pressure product (RPP, which is HR × SBP), and $\dot{V}O_2$ of healthy young men in different coital positions and found a maximal energy cost of 3.3 METs. There was a large variation in the maximal values for RPP, with a mean of about 20,000 and a standard deviation of about 6,000. Douglas and Wickes (30) measured $\dot{V}O_2$ and found peak values of 4.7 to 5.5 METs for a few seconds at orgasm.

Littler et al. (31) measured the direct arterial BP and ECG over a 24-h period in 72 subjects. Seven normotensive subjects (6 men and 1 woman) had coitus at home with their partners during this time. The duration of intercourse was 8 to 20 min. In their summary, the authors stated that SBP rose by 25 to 120 mm Hg, DBP increased by 25 to 48 mm Hg, and HR increased by 20 to 87 beats/min. Unfortunately, this is a misleading statement. Closer scrutiny reveals that the HR was 100 to 120 beats/min in four of the men at orgasm, and the woman did not experience orgasm (peak HR was 96 beats/min). Likewise, the SBP was 150 to 190 mm Hg in the four men and 120 mm Hg in the woman. Only the other two men showed the marked elevations in SBP and HR reported in the article; one of them was an unmarried 20-year-old man whose partner was his girlfriend and not a wife of many years.

Nemec et al. (32) used a portable ECG tape recorder and an automatic ultrasonic recorder to study the HR and BP responses of 10 men (24 to 40 years of age) during four episodes of sexual intercourse with their wives. Two sessions were with the man on top and two sessions were with the man on the bottom. Both positions were used because many physicians counsel their cardiac patients to assume a more passive position in order to avoid overexertion; the man-on-bottom position was one of the passive positions suggested. As can be seen in Figure 24.2, there was essentially no difference in HR, SBP, or DBP in the various phases of intercourse, and the HRs of 117 and 114 beats/min are similar to those found by Hellerstein and Friedman (14). An average BP of 162/79 mm Hg at orgasm is also less than usually reported.

A similar approach was used by Stein (33) with a group of 16 men (aged 46 to 54 years) who underwent a 16-week cycle ergometer training program 12 to 15 weeks after their first MI. Coital HR was measured twice before and twice after training by means of a portable ECG tape recorder. Peak HR

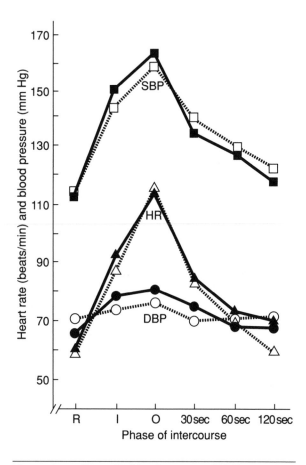

Figure 24.2   Diastolic blood pressure (DBP), systolic blood pressure (SBP), and heart rate (HR) during various phases of sexual intercourse with the man on top (solid figures) and on bottom (open figures) (32). R = rest; I = intromission; O = orgasm.

during coitus by 24-h ambulatory ECG monitoring, they found no significant differences between male and female patients in the respective values for peak HR (111 beats/min versus 104 beats/min), duration of intercourse (17.3 min versus 16.5 min), or time of recovery (3.1 min versus 2.6 min). Four female patients had the lowest peak HR (87 beats/min) during their first intercourse after MI. This rose to 115 beats/min during their second experience, which occurred after 15 days of rehabilitation and when there was less fear. Thus, it is probable that women and men have similar physiological responses, the difference being that women are multiorgasmic and can obtain sexual pleasure without an erection.

Medical Aspects

Since for most couples in a long-standing marriage the average frequency of intercourse is less than two times/week, the mean duration of intercourse is 5 to 20 min (the period of significantly increased HR less than 5 to 10 min), and its intensity (peak and average) is moderate, intercourse does not appear to be a major medical problem. According to Green (36), the average American man spends 2% of his day in strenuous effort and 33% to 50% in mild to moderate effort; coitus would be included in the latter category. On the other hand, if the activity is dangerous, then this fact should be reflected in data on morbidity and mortality. Again, there appear to be few factual data.

Sex-Related Morbidity and Mortality

The one study most often cited is that of Ueno (37), who reported on 5,559 sudden deaths in Japan, of which 34 (0.6%) were associated with coitus. Eighteen deaths (0.3%) were related to CAD. Upon closer examination, he noted that 27 of the 34 deaths (80%) were associated with extramarital sexual activity, that there were no deaths of women or men over 60 years of age, that most of the men were 40 to 50 years old and at least 20 years older than their partners, and that these men had been eating rich food and drinking alcohol beforehand. It is probable that even this low incidence of death related to coitus is still higher than the incidence of coital deaths at home with a spouse. Being away from home with a younger woman and possibly having too much to eat and drink, combined with the psychological problems of guilt, fear of im-

was 127 beats/min before training and 120 beats/min after training. In a control group of 6 men who did not train, peak HR remained unchanged at 128 beats/min.

Looking at all of the studies on middle-aged men, with or without MI, it is obvious that peak HR rarely exceeds 130 to 140 beats/min. Although the SBP during intercourse may be somewhat higher than that obtained at a comparable HR on a treadmill, cycle ergometer, or stair-climbing test (34), the relatively short period of peak intensity suggests that sexual intercourse in this group of men is not a strenuous activity.

Unfortunately, little information is available on the reactions of women. In the few studies on younger women (e.g., Bartlett [27]), the HR of women during coitus was not very different from that of their partners, even though there was a great deal of variation with both genders. García-Barreto et al. (35) studied 13 men and 10 women who had had an MI. Comparing the data obtained potence, and fear of being caught, may have created too much stress for these men.

Although Ueno reported additional deaths related to extramarital sex (37), the real issue, according to Scheingold and Wagner (38), is not the morality of the situation but the familiarity of the partner and the setting. During intercourse with a new partner, increases in HR, BP, and the like are greater. Johnston et al. (22) reported on 10 cardiac patients who had sexual intercourse with someone other than their regular partners. Two of these patients felt that their angina was more severe during intercourse with the new person. The increases would likewise be greater when resuming sexual activity with a spouse after a long period of abstinence. On the other hand, a man having sexual intercourse with his mistress of many years may have no difficulty. Thus, a patient with cardiovascular limitations who undertakes a sexual relationship with a new person should be told of the increased risks. Even in the extramarital situation, however, the risk of cardiac problems is still small.

Masters and Johnson (4) found that the lower the initial HR in the resting state before sexual intercourse, the lower the peak HR during sexual stimulation. Although endurance-trained athletes tend to have lower resting HRs, this fact is of almost no value in predicting fitness. Thus, the low resting HR probably reflects the emotional state rather than the fitness of the person before intercourse. If this conclusion is true, it would partly explain the higher HR and BP observed in such artificial settings as laboratories, hospital rooms, and hotels.

Unfortunately, there are no comparable data on coital deaths in older married couples. The spouse has the option of saying that his or her mate died while sleeping; this option is not available to the mistress in a hotel. The physician may not inquire or may change the cause of death out of deference to the family. Hellerstein and Friedman (14) state that after discussions with a local coroner, they gained the impression that the rate of coital death in Cleveland was about 3 per 500 CAD patients (0.6%).

Derogatis and King (39) correctly point out, however, that despite apparent research about coital death, they found only two empirical studies (14,37), one of which, Ueno's (37), was conducted in a different culture. For this and other reasons, Derogatis and King (39) consider the evidence insufficient to state that extramarital sex is more dangerous, especially when there is no information on the incidence of conjugal deaths.

Related to the problem of risk during physical activity, Rochnis and Blackburn (40) reported that the death rate associated with exercise testing is about 1 per 10,000 tests. The intensity and duration of activity during these tests are usually much greater than those found during intercourse. Therefore, sexual intercourse does not appear to be a high-risk activity for the majority of the population.

Signs and Symptoms Associated With Intercourse

Nevertheless, for some post-MI patients, especially men, sexual intercourse may exceed their limited tolerance. As well, Kolman (5) suggests that sex differs from other forms of exercise in its emotional impact. The resultant rise in adrenergic activity may increase the chance of developing arrhythmias. As a result, post-MI patients may have coital or postcoital angina, fatigue, or arrhythmias. Hellerstein and Friedman (14) found that 42% of 43 CAD patients in their study had one or more symptoms associated with coitus. Of these, 30% had tachycardia and 21% had angina. In comparison, only 12% of the coronary-prone men had any symptoms. According to Eliot and Miles (41) symptoms occur more often during the resolution phase. During sex, 4 patients (9%) had ST depression and 3 (7%) had ectopic beats; this result was comparable in frequency and severity to changes found during normal occupational activities. García-Barreto et al. (35) studied post-MI patients (13 men and 10 women) with 24-hour ECG monitoring. Of 11 patients (9 men and 2 women) with premature ventricular contractions (PVCs) before coitus, only 1 man had an arrhythmia during intercourse and 5 had a lower rate of PVCs while sleeping after intercourse.

Notwithstanding the importance of symptoms associated with coitus, it is possible that CAD patients are more psychologically sensitive than healthy persons to palpitations and high HRs. That is, although tachycardia is the usual result of orgasm, the healthy person accepts this fact as normal; only after an MI does he or she wonder whether it is dangerous and report it to the physician.

In a study of the sexual activity of post-MI patients, Kavanagh and Shephard (19) reported that angina was noted in 12.4% of the patients during intercourse, compared to 36% of the patients during a cycle ergometer test in the laboratory at HRs of 140 beats/min. The incidence of PVCs and dysrhythmia was 3.7% and 4.6%, respectively. This finding again suggests that the intensity of sexual activity is neither strenuous nor contraindicated for the majority of CAD patients who are able to join a physical reconditioning program. For those few who do develop angina or arrhythmias, proper prophylactic and therapeutic use of nitroglycerin, standard cardiac drugs, and perhaps tranquilizers are recommended (14,42,43). A good example of this is the study by Jackson (29). Of the 30 men and 5 women with angina, 19 (65%) had angina during intercourse and 4 complained of palpitations. With beta-blockade, the tachycardia was abolished and the 19 with angina were free of pain during intercourse after 6 months.

Energy Expenditure During Sex

According to the data presented on married, middle-aged couples, sexual intercourse requires an energy expenditure of about 3 to 4 METs before and after orgasm and 4 to 5 METs during the brief period of orgasm. In order to know whether a patient can exercise safely at this intensity, he or she should be given a graded exercise test (GXT). Assuming that the patient can perform safely at levels as high as 5 to 6 METs (New York Heart Association functional Class II; Table 24.3), there should be little problem with sexual activity. If he or she has a functional capacity greater than or equal to 7 METs (Class I), there should be little or no hesitation on the physician's part. If the patient still reports problems, however, the physician should look more carefully for nonphysical reasons. For patients in functional Classes III and IV, sexual activity can and usually will be limited by

Table 24.3 New York Heart Association Functional Classification

Class	Functional capacity (METs)	Symptoms
I	≥ 7	None
II	5-6	Occur with ordinary activity
III	3-4	Occur with less than ordinary activity
IV	≤ 2	Occur at rest

Note. The energy expenditure required for sexual activity is 3-4 METs (metabolic equivalents) before and after orgasm and 4-5 METs during orgasm.

a severely diseased myocardium. Patients with severe myocardial insufficiency or congestive failure cannot do many things and will probably be less interested in having sexual relations.

To give the reader a better idea of an energy requirement of 6 to 7 METs, so that this information may be useful in estimating whether or not a patient would have problems during intercourse, this energy level is required by the following activities: the Double Master step-test, Level 2 of the Bruce treadmill test, 600 to 750 kpm (kilopond meters) (100 to 150 Watts) on a cycle ergometer, walking 3 mph up a 10% grade, walking 4.5 mph on the level, cycling 10 mph on the level, cross-country hiking, square dancing, cross-country skiing 4 mph on the level, and carrying 50 to 60 pounds while walking 3 mph. Any patient able to engage in these activities without symptoms is in functional Class I or II and should have no trouble during sexual intercourse.

By performing GXTs, not only does the physician gain a better idea of the functional capacity of the patient and how he or she responds to a known amount of work, but the patient receives a better idea of his or her capacity to function physically and sexually.

Resumption of Sexual Activity

Many patients resume sex within 9 to 16 weeks after their MI (14,22). As there is no reason why patients must wait that long, Kolman (5) suggests that if patients were told they could resume sex after their discharge, the incidence of sexual dysfunction would be less. Stein (44) agrees, finding that patients who received counseling on the basis of a medical examination and a GXT resumed sexual activity sooner after MI than patients who were not counseled. Similarly, Dhabuwala et al. (8) found that patients who were counseled and informed when it was safe to resume sexual activity had much less apprehension. By using a portable ECG tape recorder, better counseling can be given to the patient who complains of angina, palpitations, or tachycardia during or after coitus.

When counseling a patient, the physician should include the spouse, who likely also has fears and anxieties about resuming sexual activity and significantly influences the patient's adaptation to a new lifestyle (45). In this regard, Johnston et al. (22) found that spouse restraint was the most commonly cited cause for sexual dysfunction. Scalzi and Dracup (46) suggest separate counseling sessions for the patient and the spouse, as well as a session together before discharge. The individual counseling sessions provide each partner with the opportunity to express personal concerns, and the joint session reinforces information given earlier.

According to Scalzi and Dracup (46), the goal of counseling is to provide patients with information they need to make their own choices. The general areas to be assessed are (1) previous patterns of sexual activity, (2) past experience with symptoms during sexual activity, (3) history of sexual difficulty 1 to 3 months before the MI, and (4) their degree of understanding of when they can resume sexual activity. Preliminary results by these authors also suggest that patients receiving appropriate sexual counseling returned to a precoronary level of sexual activity more quickly than patients receiving no counseling.

Boykoff (47) reviewed the literature on counseling and concluded that sexual dysfunction was largely attributable to psychological factors compounded by inadequate information. According to a study by Tuttle et al. (16), two-thirds of a sample of post-MI patients were given no advice at all about sexual activity. In the remaining one-third, only vague or nonspecific advice was given. They also found that 10% of the men became impotent. Patients are often the ones who must initiate discussions about possible or actual sexual dysfunction. One study (48) done in a VA hospital showed that physicians perceived that they themselves initiated these discussions more often than their patients thought they did.

Interestingly, Wabrek and Burchell (7) found that two-thirds of 131 male patients had had significant sexual problems before their MI. The implication of these findings is that returning the patient to the pre-MI level of sexual functioning may not always be sufficient.

Effect of Exercise Programs

In addition to counseling based on information from a GXT and possibly from portable tape recordings of the ECG during intercourse at home ("sexercise" tolerance test), the physician can suggest that the patient begin to increase his or her functional capacity with a properly supervised, controlled rehabilitative exercise program. More and more information is becoming available about the benefits of improved exercise capacity in CAD patients, as well as in normal persons (49).

In the study by Hellerstein and Friedman (14), most subjects reported little change in the frequency or quality of intercourse after an exercise program. On the other hand, 67% of the initially symptomatic subjects had few or no symptoms during intercourse after reconditioning. In the study by Stein (33) mentioned earlier, there was a significant reduction in peak coital HR, from 127 beats/min to 120 beats/min in the trained group, whereas the control group remained at 128 beats/min. This reduced HR lowers the myocardial oxygen demands and makes coitus even safer and, perhaps, more enjoyable for the CAD patient.

Kavanagh and Shephard (19) questioned post-MI patients participating in a physical training program about their sexual activities. After dividing the subjects into two groups according to sexual activity (group A, increased activity or no change; group B, decreased activity), they found that all 80 men in group A found sex as enjoyable as before, compared to only 55 of 81 men in group B. Although 69 men in group A made no change in the intensity of lovemaking, 11 said they became more active; none became more passive. This pattern is in contrast to that of the 29 men in group B who had more passive intercourse. Those in group A also attended the exercise classes more often, ran farther, and, as expected, had greater improvements in functional capacity.

In four of the studies already mentioned (14,19,33,51), subjects improved their self-image during the training program. Other studies have shown less depression in post-MI patients after reconditioning (11). Considering the importance of the psychological effects of MI on sexuality, self-image, ego, strength, fatigue, and helplessness mentioned earlier in this chapter, the positive effects of physical training should be emphasized to the physician and the patient.

Effects of Medications

Any discussion of the medical aspects of sexual activity for CAD patients would be incomplete without some mention of the medications that are prescribed for many of them. It appears that many drugs have secondary effects that may influence sexual activity. Among some of them that have been reported to reduce libido, increase impotence, or diminish ejaculation in the man or to affect libido in the woman are the following: digitalis, beta-blockers, antidepressants, some hypnotics and tranquilizers, alcohol, lipid-lowering agents (e.g., clofibrate), and several antihypertensive drugs (especially guanethidine, reserpine, methyldopa, and spironolactone) (28,41,52,53).

Unfortunately, many beliefs regarding medications and sexuality are based on inadequate research or incomplete data. For example, Papadopoulos (43) made a comprehensive summary of the sexual effects of cardiovascular drugs and presented the conclusions in an easy-to-read table. Unfortunately, the review paid little attention to methodology and reported only the findings. Moss and Procci (54) made a comprehensive literature review and found many examples of flawed methodology. Problems included the following:

- Complete information was lacking on sexual history and sexual functioning before treatment.
- Few studies included A-B-A research designs with placebo controls.
- Nonspecific terms were used to define sexual problems.
- Some studies used combinations of drugs before establishing the effects of single drugs.
- Little attention was paid to the effects of dosage, age, or chronicity of illness.

The placebo effect is especially important because "telling a patient that a drug can cause impotence may indeed cause it" (30). Moss and Procci (54) also found little or no data on drug-related sexual dysfunctions in women; this result was most disturbing to them in the case of antihypertensive drugs, since approximately 43% of hypertensives are women.

Most male patients with hypertension who can tolerate average doses of the commonly used antihypertensive agents will not have any special difficulty with impotence (55). The problem for many hypertensive persons is that they feel well and have no symptoms. Fortunately, the risk of increased medical problems during sexual activity is low in persons with hypertension, even when it is not well controlled (56). One special consideration for these patients (as well as for CAD patients) is the need to avoid isometric muscle contractions during sexual intercourse, for example, during periods of vigorous pelvic thrusting.

Summary

Sexual activity, at least as practiced by the majority of middle-aged and older men and women, is not a major problem in terms of increased risk of morbidity or mortality from CAD. Except for people who are limited by the severity of their disease to low-intensity activities, most patients should be able to perform sexually. The psychological and emotional effects of MI seem to be more important than the physiological effects in many patients. Specialists are beginning to realize that the tension generated by sexual frustration may be more harmful than the tension produced by sedate and relaxed intercourse (57). These facts reinforce the need for short-term psychotherapy (36) and counseling by the physician.

Sexual activity may be resumed after an MI in about the same way as other types of physical activity: gradually and carefully. That is, the return to work or to sexual activity is related to the presence or absence of symptoms. If the patient engages in self-monitoring to avoid symptoms or problems (assuming that he or she has been told what to expect and how to handle each situation), then there is little physiological reason for the physician to proscribe sexual activity for most patients. Thus, patients and their spouses should be able to continue having normal sexual relations.

References

1. Kinsey, A.C.; Pomeroy, W.B.; Martin, C.E. Sexual behavior in the human male. Philadelphia: Saunders; 1948: 218-263.
2. Weg, R.B. Physiology and sexuality in aging. In: Burnside, I.M., ed. Sexuality and aging. Los Angeles: USC Press; 1975: 7-12.
3. Mulligan, T.; Moss, C.R. Sexuality and aging in male veterans: A cross-sectional study of interest, ability, and activity. Arch. Sex. Behav. 20:17-25; 1991.
4. Masters, W.H.; Johnson, V.E. Human sexual response. Boston: Little, Brown; 1966: 174-175.
5. Kolman, P.B.R. Sexual dysfunction and the postmyocardial infarction patient. J. Cardiac. Rehabil. 4:334-340; 1984.
6. Frank, E.; Anderson, C.; Rubinstein, D. Frequency of sexual dysfunction in "normal" couples. N. Engl. J. Med. 299:111-115; 1978.
7. Wabrek, A.J.; Burchell, R.C. Male sexual dysfunction associated with coronary heart disease. Arch. Sex. Behav. 9:69-75; 1980.
8. Dhabuwala, C.B.; Kumar, A.; Pierce, J.M. Myocardial infarction and its influence on male sexual function. Arch. Sex. Behav. 15:499-504; 1986.
9. Spencer, R.F.; Raft, D. Depression and diminished sexual desire. Med. Asp. Hum. Sexuality. 11:51-61; 1977.
10. Lemers, F.; Smith, F.W. Alcohol-induced sexual impotence. Am. J. Psychiatry. 130:212-213; 1973.
11. Hackett, T.P.; Cassem, N.H. Psychological adaptation to convalescence in myocardial infarction patients. In: Naughton, J.; Hellerstein, H.; Mohler, I.,

eds. Exercise testing and exercise training in coronary heart disease. New York: Academic Press; 1973: 253-262.

12. Rosen, I.; Bibring, G.L. Psychological reactions of hospitalized male patients to a heart attack. Psychosom. Med. 28:808-821; 1966.

13. Broderick, C. Sexuality and aging: An overview. In: Burnside, I.M., ed. Sexuality and aging. Los Angeles: USC Press; 1975:1-6.

14. Hellerstein, H.K.; Friedman, E.H. Sexual activity and the post-coronary patient. Arch. Intern. Med. 125: 987-999; 1970.

15. Bloch, A.; Maeder, J.P.; Haissly, J.C. Sexual problems after myocardial infarction. Am. Heart J. 90:536-537; 1975.

16. Tuttle, W.B.; Cook, W.L.; Fitch, E. Sexual behavior in post-myocardial infarction patients. Am. J. Cardiol. 13:140-153; 1964.

17. Klein, R.F.; Dean, A.; Wilson, M.; Bogdonoff, M.D.; et al. The physician and post-myocardial infarction invalidism. JAMA. 194:143-148; 1965.

18. Abramov, L. Sexual life and sexual frigidity among women developing acute myocardial infarction. Psychosom. Med. 38:418-425; 1976.

19. Kavanagh, T.; Shephard, R.J. Sexual activity after myocardial infarction. Can. Med. Assoc. J. 116:1250-1253; 1977.

20. Weiss, E.; English, O.S. Psychosomatic medicine. Philadelphia: Saunders; 1957: 216.

21. Dorossiev, D.; Paskova, V.; Zachariev, Z. Psychological problems of cardiac rehabilitation. In: Stocksmeier, U., ed. Psychological approach to the rehabilitation of coronary patients. Berlin: Springer-Verlag; 1976:26-31.

22. Johnston, B.; Cantwell, J.D.; Watt, E.W.; Fletcher, G.F. Sexual activity in exercising patients after myocardial infarction and revascularization. Heart Lung. 7:1026-1031; 1978.

23. Scott, J.C. Systolic blood pressure fluctuations with sex, anger and fear. J. Comp. Physiol. Psychol. 10:97-113; 1930.

24. Bohlen, J.G.; Held, J.P.; Sanderson, O.; Patterson, R.P. Heart rate, rate-pressure product, and oxygen uptake during four sexual activities. Arch. Intern. Med. 144:1745-1748; 1984.

25. Boas, E.P.; Goldschmidt, E.F. The heart rate. Springfield, IL: Charles C Thomas; 1932.

26. Klumbies, G.; Kleinsorge, H. Circulatory dangers and prophylaxis during orgasm. Int. J. Sexol. 4:61-66; 1950.

27. Bartlett, R.G. Physiologic responses during coitus. J. Appl. Physiol. 9:469-472; 1956.

28. Tardif, G.S. Sexual activity after a myocardial infarction. Arch. Phys. Med. Rehabil. 70:763-766; 1989.

29. Jackson, G. Sexual intercourse and angina pectoris. Int. Rehab. Med. 3:35-37; 1981.

30. Douglas, J.E.; Wickes, T.D. Reconditioning cardiac patients. Am. Fam. Physician. 11:122-129; 1975.

31. Littler, W.A.; Honour, A.J.; Sleight, P. Direct arterial pressure, heart rate and electrocardiogram during human coitus. J. Reprod. Fertil. 40:321-331; 1974.

32. Nemec, E.D.; Mansfield, L.; Kennedy, J.W. Heart rate and blood pressure responses during sexual activity in normal males. Am. Heart J. 92:274-277; 1964.

33. Stein, R.A. The effect of exercise training on heart rate during coitus in the post-myocardial infarction patient. Circulation. 55:738-740; 1977.

34. Puksta, N.S. All about sex . . . after a coronary. Am. J. Nurs. 77:602-605; 1977.

35. García-Barreto, D.; Sin-Chesa, C.; Rivas-Estany, E.; Nieto, R.; Hernández-Cañero, A. Sexual intercourse in patients who have had a myocardial infarction. J. Cardiopulm. Rehabil. 6:324-328; 1986.

36. Green, A.W. Sexual activity and the post myocardial infarction patient. Am. Heart J. 89:246-252; 1975.

37. Ueno, M. The so-called coition death. Jpn. J. Leg. Med. 17:333-340; 1963.

38. Scheingold, L.D.; Wagner, N.N. Sound sex and the aging heart. New York: Human Sciences Press; 1974: 137-141.

39. Derogatis, L.R.; King, K.M. The coital coronary: A reassessment of the concept. Arch. Sex. Behav. 10: 325-335; 1981.

40. Rochnis, P.; Blackburn, H. Exercise tests. JAMA. 217:160-166; 1971.

41. Eliot, R.S.; Miles, R.R. Advising the cardiac patient about sexual intercourse. Med. Asp. Hum. Sex. 9:49-50; 1975.

42. Regestein, Q.R.; Horn, H.R. Coitus in patients with cardiac arrhythmias. Med. Asp. Hum. Sex. 12:108-125; 1978.

43. Papadopoulos, C. Cardiovascular drugs and sexuality. A cardiologist's view. Arch. Intern. Med. 140: 1341-1345; 1980.

44. Stein, R. Resuming sexual relations after myocardial infarction. Med. Asp. Hum. Sex. 10:159-160; 1976.

45. Mayou, R.; Foster, A.; Williamson, B. The psychological and social effects of myocardial infarction on wives. Br. Med. J. 1:699-701; 1978.

46. Scalzi, C.; Dracup, K. Sexual counseling of coronary patients. Heart Lung. 7:840-845; 1978.

47. Boykoff, S.L. Strategies for sexual counseling of patients following a myocardial infarction. Dimen. Crit. Care. Nursing. 8:368-373; 1989.

48. McLane, M.; Drop, H.; Mehta, J. Psychosexual adjustment and counseling after myocardial infarction. Ann. Intern. Med. 92:514-519; 1980.

49. Amsterdam, E.A.; Wilmore, J.H.; DeMaria, A.N. Exercise in cardiovascular health and disease. New York: Yorke Medical Books; 1977.

50. Soloff, L.A. Sexual activity in the heart patient. Psychosomatics. 18:23-31; 1977.

51. Roviaro, S.; Holmes, D.S.; Holmsten, R.D. Influence of a cardiac rehabilitation program on the cardiovascular, psychological, and social functioning of cardiac patients. J. Behav. Med. 7:61-81; 1984.

52. Gentry, W.O.; Williams, R.B. Psychological aspects of myocardial infarction and coronary care. St. Louis: Mosby; 1975:113.

53. Simpson, F.O. Beta-adrenergic receptor blocking drugs in hypertension. Drugs. 8:85-105; 1974.

54. Moss, H.B.; Procci, W.R. Antihypertensive drugs and sexual dysfunction. Psychosom. Med. 43:473-474; 1981.

55. Howard, E.J. Sexual expenditure in patients with hypertensive disease. Med. Asp. Hum. Sex. 7:82-92; 1973.

56. Page, L.B. Advising hypertensive patients about sex. Med. Asp. Hum. Sex. 9:103-104; 1975.

57. McCary, J.L. Sexual myths and fallacies. New York: Van Nostrand Reinhold; 1971:41.

Chapter 25

Drug Effects

David T. Lowenthal
Gregorio J. Guillen
Zebulon V. Kendrick

In a previous edition of this book it was emphasized how drugs affect exercise and, conversely, how exercise influences the mechanisms of drug kinetics and dynamics. Most studies were based on short periods of exertion, mostly covering drugs used to treat cardiovascular disorders, specifically hypertension (1). Since that edition, more data have been published regarding exercise and drugs for congestive heart failure (CHF), coronary artery disease (CAD), and hypertension.

Today, the goals of training while taking medication are still to allow normal physiological responses—such as increase in heart rate (HR), stroke index, cardiac index, and systolic blood pressure (BP), in addition to unaltered or decreased diastolic BP—in performing acute dynamic physical activity while on cardiovascular drugs. The following antihypertensive drugs permit normal dynamic exercise response:

Diuretics
Central alpha agonists

- Clonidine
- Guanabenz
- Guanfacine
- Methyldopa

Calcium entry blockers

- Diltiazem
- Nifedipine
- Verapamil

Angiotensin-converting enzyme (ACE) inhibitors

- Benazepril
- Captopril
- Enalapril
- Fosinopril
- Lisinopril
- Quinipril
- Ranapril

Peripheral alpha-blockers

- Doxazosin
- Prazosin
- Terazosin

Of equal importance are the following expected elevations in catecholamine, glucagon, insulin, potassium, renin, and aldosterone levels that occur during acute exertion and how these parameters are affected by cardiac medications (1):

- Increase in plasma catecholamine concentration
- Increase in plasma glucagon concentration
- Increase in plasma insulin concentration
- Increase in free fatty acid mobilization
- Increase in plasma potassium concentration
- Increase in renin activity
- Increase in plasma aldosterone concentration

The pressor responses to isometric activity may need to be blunted in the hypertensive patient, especially if heart failure or ischemic heart disease exist. The following antihypertensive drugs blunt the pressor response to static exercise:

Beta-blockers

- Propranolol
- Atenolol

ACE Inhibitors

- Captopril
- Enalapril

Central alpha agonists

- Clonidine
- Methyldopa

Peripheral alpha-blockers

- Prazosin

New data has since been published that refers to the chronic effects of cardiovascular drugs on exercise, mostly beta-adrenergic blocking agents (beta-blockers), ACE inhibitors, and calcium antagonists.

Diuretics

The hemodynamics in unmedicated trained mild hypertensives and normal people are summarized in Table 25.1. Diuretics are antihypertensive drugs; the hemodynamics of the diuretic effect have been studied by Lund-Johansen (2) (Table 25.2). It was found that not all diuretics have similar actions during exercise. Thiazides bring about a drop in exercise BP via a decrease in total peripheral resistance (TPR) and plasma volume. Thiazide-like diuretics, specifically chlorthalidone 100 mg/day, were shown to reduce BP during exercise by decreasing cardiac output ($\dot{Q}$). However, at doses of 200 mg/day there was a paradoxic increase in diastolic BP and HR (3), which was probably a reflection of marked volume contraction. Long-term thiazide dosing does not cause a drop in $\dot{Q}$.

Although studies involving the effects of drugs on exercise have included patients with heart failure who are taking furosemide, no studies dealing with this drug's direct effects on exercise parameters have been carried out. Additionally, as with any diuretic therapy, hypokalemia can become significant, resulting in moderate ST-segment depression, cardiac irritability, and skeletal muscle fatigue (4,5).

During vigorous exercise, serum potassium levels increase. The source is skeletal muscle. This result can occur with diuretic-induced hypokalemia; the response indicates that total body potassium stores are not depleted (6). However, to ensure against potassium loss, patients taking diuretics should receive potassium supplements. The much lower doses of diuretics employed now do not lower potassium significantly but can still elevate total and low-density lipoprotein (LDL) cholesterol, major cardiovascular disease (CVD) risk factors.

Second-generation drugs like indapamide, which share diuretic and hypotensive effects similar to the thiazides, but with less metabolic toxicity, are now widely used. However, hypokalemia remains a direct effect, though a less marked one

Table 25.1   Hemodynamics During Dynamic Exercise in Normal People and Unmedicated Trained Mild Hypertensives

	Normal	Hypertensives	Reason to explain differences
Heart rate	↑	↑ ↑	Greater adrenergic response and higher arteriovenous oxygen difference.
Stroke volume	↑ ↑	↑	Progressively falls with age, leading to submaximal cardiac output.
Cardiac index	↑ ↑	↑	(Same as for stroke volume.)
Total peripheral index	↓	↑ ↑	Higher at all ages and at all levels of work.
Blood pressure	↑	↑ ↑	Self-explanatory.
Arterial-venous oxygen difference	↑	↑ ↑	Safety mechanism for hypertensives to meet oxygen demand from skeletal muscle.

Note. ↑ = increases; ↑↑ = increases strongly; ↓ = decreases.

Table 25.2   Hemodynamics of Diuretics in Patients at Rest

	Heart rate	Stroke volume	Cardiac output	Total peripheral resistance	Blood pressure
Acute (single dose)	—	↓ ↓	↓ ↓	↑	↓
Chronic (multiple doses)	—	↓	↓	↓	↓

Note. ↑ = raised; ↓ = lowered; ↓↓ = lowered greatly; — = no change.

than that of any first-generation thiazides. Unlike thiazide medications, indapamide increases the release of the vasodilator prostaglandins PGE_2 and PGI_2, which effect might be beneficial in maintaining adequate BP response during exercise (7).

Finally, thiazide diuretics decrease urinary calcium loss (7). This may be of some usefulness in hypertensive postmenopausal women who exercise. It is conceivable that exercise and diuretic-induced calcium retention may synergistically work to help rebuild bone in osteoporosis (8).

Thus, diuretics result in a moderate decrease in the BP response to exercise and, with adequate potassium supplementation, should not cause any drug-related risks during physical activity. Exercise and diet can help readjust the short-term lipid changes.

Central Alpha Agonists

Many studies on the central alpha-agonist antihypertensive drugs have been performed. Clonidine, guanfacine, guanabenz, and methyldopa decrease central and/or peripheral outflow of catecholamines. This action results in reductions of plasma norepinephrine levels at rest and during exercise (9,10). Although all of these drugs can blunt the sympathetic response during exercise, the cardiovascular responses to exercise are normal, but the drugs have significantly different resting hemodynamic effects (Table 25.3).

Using cycle ergometers with mild hypertensive patients, methyldopa may decrease the BP and HR responses (11). TPR and Q may (12) or may not (13) decrease. On the contrary, work in our laboratory with normal persons taking methyldopa in multiple doses for 1 week demonstrated no decrease

Table 25.3 Hemodynamics of Central Alpha Agonists in Patients at Rest

Drug	Heart rate	Stroke volume	Cardiac output	Total peripheral resistance	Blood pressure
Guanfacine	sl ↓	sl ↑	—	↓	↓
Clonidine	↓	—	↓	↓	↓
Guanabenz	—	—	↓	↓	↓
Methyldopa	—	—	—	↓	↓

Note. sl↑ = raised slightly; ↓ = lowered; sl↓ = lowered slightly; — = no change.

in HR at rest or at peak exercise, yet systolic BP was reduced (14). Differences from clonidine may result from the peripheral effects of the false neurotransmitters of methyldopa.

Clonidine differs from methyldopa in that, in addition to reducing BP and HR during exercise, it decreases both the resting BP and the HR (15,16). The decrease in HR through central vagal stimulation results in a drop in Q (17). This decrease, however, is not considered a negative inotropic property, since after chronic use Q is normalized. Due to different molecular structures, guanabenz and guanfacine do not change HR at rest or with exercise as can clonidine or methyldopa.

Lowenthal et al. (10,14,16) found that serum potassium, renin, and aldosterone levels changed with exercise in normal volunteers after single and multiple doses of clonidine and methyldopa. Increases in potassium level during dynamic exercise in subjects taking clonidine or methyldopa were parallel to the response achieved with a placebo. The plasma renin concentration with both alpha agonists was suppressed at rest, and the expected increase in HR was blunted during exercise at maximum dosage. Plasma aldosterone levels apparently did not change significantly with the drugs when compared with the placebo, increasing during exercise in all groups. No significant ST-T wave changes on the electrocardiogram (ECG) occurred during exercise using these drugs. The rise in diastolic BP induced by isometric activity may be decreased with clonidine or methyldopa.

Alinidine (N-allyl-clonidine), a congener of clonidine not yet available in the United States, has been reported to improve exercise tolerance in patients with effort angina (18). The benefit is thought to be due to its bradycardic effect, which results in a prolongation of the diastolic filling time. Its beneficial effects have been compared to those of beta-blockers.

With the advent of transdermal clonidine patches, a recent study (19) found that in this form the drug was superior to oral atenolol in improving aerobic conditioning in a group of relatively young mild hypertensives. Atenolol acutely reduced endurance time by 35% and did not induce a better conditioning effect by the end of the 8-week training program, as demonstrated by comparing initial and final maximal oxygen uptake ($\dot{V}O_2max$).

Beta-Blockers

The most widely investigated hemodynamic changes during exercise are those associated with beta-adrenergic blocking agents (Table 25.4). Because of a reduction in myocardial contractility and HR, myocardial oxygen demand is reduced, thus allowing for a prolonged diastolic phase and improved coronary perfusion. Subjects with CAD have increased exercise capacity, fewer anginal episodes, and ST depression as a result of taking beta-blockers (19,20). These features constitute important advantages for patients requiring cardiac rehabilitation. Patients who undergo training while on propranolol for CAD or who have chronic atrial fibrillation improved exercise capacity by 31% (21,22) (Table 25.5).

Beta-blocker–induced alterations in hemodynamic responses during isometric and dynamic exercise have been studied at length, involving both cardioselective (beta$_1$) and nonselective

(beta$_1$/beta$_2$) beta-blockers (6,10,21-24). Comparing propranolol and metoprolol with placebo in graded exercise tests (GXTs), HR, systolic BP, and VO$_2$max were reduced at maximum exertion, but there were no major changes in diastolic BP or anaerobic threshold (23).

Lowenthal et al. (25) reported a reduction in resting and peak exercise diastolic BP during isometric exercise in normal volunteers given atenolol and propranolol. In addition, strength performance was not blunted with atenolol or propranolol given to young, healthy subjects (26). Recent data suggest that the changes in HR, systolic and diastolic BPs, and VO$_2$max on maximal exertion during a GXT are dose related, meaning there was no difference between placebo and 40 mg/day of propranolol administration, as opposed to

Table 25.4   Hemodynamics of Beta-Adrenergics in Patients at Rest

Drug	Heart rate	Stroke volume	Cardiac output	Total peripheral resistance	Blood pressure
B$_1$-B$_2$ (nonselective) Propranolol, timolol, nacolol	↓ ↓	↓	↓ ↓	↑ early ↓ later	↓
B$_1$ (selective) Atenolol, metoprolol, betaxolol	↓ ↓	↓	↓ ↓	↑ early ↓ later but less ↑ theoretically	↓
ISA only Pindolol	↓	↓	↓	sl ↑ early ↓	↓
ISA and B$_1$ Acebutolol	↓	↓	↓	sl ↑ early ↓	↓
Beta and alpha Labetalol	↓	↓	↓	↓	↓

Note. sl ↑ = raised slightly; ↓ = lowered; ↓↓ = lowered greatly.

Table 25.5   Duration and Work Load in Patients With Chronic Atrial Fibrillation Before and After Administration of Beta Blockade (Atenolol)

	Age < 60 years (mean = 53)		Age > 60 years (mean = 66)	
	Duration (s)	Work load (METs)	Duration (s)	Work load (METs)
Before	490 ±135	7.6 ±1.9	503 ±64	8.2 ±1.2
After	465 ±66	7.8 ±1.2	618 ±51*	10.0 ±1**

Note. All values are mean ± SD.

*$p < 0.05$. **$p < 0.01$.

160 mg/day and 320 mg/day, in which a significant difference was found (24).

Patients with borderline hypertensive heart failure defined by noninvasive criteria (enlarged cardiac silhouette on chest x-ray, M-mode echocardiography, and ECG changes), did not show suppressed elevations in BP during isometric exercise while taking metoprolol with or without prazosin (27), a peripheral alpha-blocker. Thus, it is important to keep in mind when prescribing an exercise program that responses in normal persons or mild hypertensives cannot be used as the barometer to forecast BP responses to isometric exercise in heart failure.

Like thiazide diuretics, beta-blocking drugs have numerous other metabolic effects, including an inhibition of lipolysis, glycogenolysis, catecholamine activity, and hyperkalemia. Propranolol in single and multiple doses causes a significant increase in serum potassium when compared to placebo in dynamic exercise (10) (Figure 25.1). The hyperkalemia may occur to a greater degree with nonselective beta-blockers and reflects a blockade of catecholamine action to drive potassium into the cells. In addition, beta-blockade with propranolol, 40 mg twice daily for 1 week, results in decreased levels of renin with changes in aldosterone,

both at rest and during peak exercise when compared with placebo (10); this is because during physical activity the rise in aldosterone is mediated through adrenocorticotropic hormone stimulation (25).

Propranolol and metoprolol augment the increase in catecholamines during rest, resulting in an accumulation of the plasma concentrations during light or heavy exercise (28-31). It has been hypothesized that vagal withdrawal and not an increase in sympathetic activity occurs until the HR rises above 30 beats/min (32). Patients with CAD can experience anginal attacks if suddenly withdrawn from beta-blockers. This is due to the rapid release of plasma catecholamines, which provokes hypertension and coronary vasoconstriction (23).

The influence of propranolol and atenolol on exercise-induced sweating remains controversial (34-36). Nonetheless, it has been found that beta$_1$-selective beta-blockers cause less disruption in thermoregulation than do nonselective beta-adrenergic antagonists. This is due to a diminished effect on peripheral vasoconstriction; the relatively greater vasodilation results in sweating. Lipid alterations are essentially similar for all beta-blockers, except that selective drugs produce less inhibition of exercise-induced lipolysis (37-39).

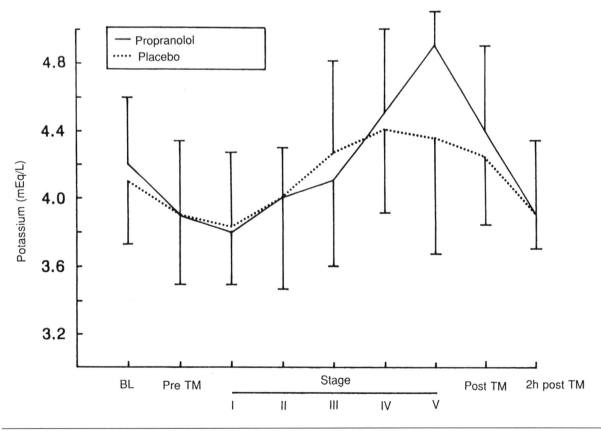

Figure 25.1 The effects of exercise and propranolol on plasma potassium.

It is known that beta-blockers prompt exertional fatigue in normal persons. The hypothesis is that the impairment of exercise-induced stimulation of glucose metabolism and lipolysis (40) is responsible for early exhaustion while on these drugs. Concomitantly, a rapid rise in glucagon levels was noted with these medications, probably owing to a decrease in muscle glycogenolysis, a process mediated by beta$_2$ adrenoreceptors. Propranolol is a stronger inhibitor of exercise-induced lipolysis when compared to selective beta-blocking agents (30,39).

Previous studies demonstrated that neither propranolol nor metoprolol decreases the ventilatory response to carbon dioxide during exertion (41,42). Furthermore, despite initial results showing a greater fall in $\dot{V}O_2$max with propranolol and atenolol when evaluating submaximal steady-state exercise, Jilka, et al. (43) found that, after a period of 9 days of dosing with either drug, there was less attenuation of $\dot{V}O_2$max, maximal pulmonary ventilation ($\dot{V}_E$max), and treadmill time, thereby suggesting a rapid adaptation to these drugs in normal individuals. These data are especially significant in the management of patients with chronic obstructive pulmonary disease (COPD), in whom these drugs do not worsen carbon dioxide retention at rest or during exercise but can readily provoke bronchospasm in patients with COPD. Once again, extrapolation of data from normal people to sick people can be misleading.

Plasma levels of propranolol and acebutolol increase significantly during exercise, probably owing to pH changes and their effect on hepatic metabolism during physical activity (44) or to an exercise-induced decrease in hepatic blood flow (45).

Virtually all studies published to date regarding the effects of beta-blockers on exercise (24) and how exercise alters the pharmacodynamics and kinetics of these drugs have been done in relatively young people. Recent research in healthy elderly volunteers has focused attention on the effects of 4 months of dynamic exercise training on propranolol kinetics and reveals no change in kinetic or protein binding characteristics of propranolol.

Despite the metabolic and circulatory changes reported with beta blockade, $\dot{V}O_2$max increases with aerobic exercise, especially with beta-selective drugs (atenolol, metoprolol, betaxolol); an overall training effect regardless of age can be obtained (24,36). However, it should be noted that in persons not limited by angina, the increase in $\dot{V}O_2$max is attenuated (24).

Vasodilators

The vasodilators are used adjunctively with other drugs in the treatment of hypertension; they include direct vasodilators such as hydralazine and minoxidil, indirect vasodilators such as the three peripheral alpha blockers, prazosin, terazosin, and doxazosin, and the calcium channel blockers (calcium channel blockers are discussed separately in a later section of this chapter). In normal volunteers, hydralazine decreases arterial BP, with a resultant reflex tachycardia. This tends to increase $\dot{Q}$ through an increase in sympathetic drive, which, in a compromised heart, may lead to myocardial ischemia with angina and/or myocardial infarction (MI) (46). However, the drug is useful as an afterload reducer in chronic heart failure patients (47).

Prazosin and its derivatives (terazosin, doxazosin) are closer to being atypical alpha antagonists than direct-acting vasodilators. Prazosin decreases mean arterial BP and TPR at rest (Table 25.6) and with dynamic work (48,49). In contrast to hydralazine, prazozin blunts any reflex increase in HR or pressor response during isometric exercise (49,50). During isometric activity, hydralazine neither improves skeletal muscle oxygen delivery in patients with heart failure (51) nor adequately attenuates increases in sympathetic activity (49,52).

In heart failure patients, vasodilators are of interest during exercise. During cycle ergometry while increasing $\dot{Q}$ by reducing afterload, hydralazine reduces both arterial and pulmonary wedge pressure and increases stroke volume (SV) (47). However, exercise tolerance as defined by left ventricular ejection fraction (LVEF) and peak $\dot{V}O_2$max appears not to improve unless nitrates are given concomitantly (51,53). The vasodilatory effect of hydralazine alone does not add to that of local metabolites that accumulate during exercise (51).

Table 25.6 Hemodynamics of Peripheral Alpha Agonists in Patients at Rest

Drug	Heart rate	Stroke volume	Cardiac output	Total peripheral resistance	Blood pressure
Prazosin, terazosin, doxazosin	—	—	—	↓	↓

Note. ↓ = lowered; — = no change.

Angiotensin-Converting Enzyme Inhibitors

Over the past few years the number of ACE inhibitors has burgeoned to seven. Hemodynamically these drugs have effects that are quite similar at rest and with exercise. None of them blunts the dynamic response to exercise. Enalapril (Table 25.7) has been shown to blunt the pressor response to static exercise and mental stress (54). Captopril and enalapril have been extensively studied as first-line drugs for the treatment of mild to moderate hypertension and as adjunctive therapy in heart failure. They are not only effective but well tolerated by the elderly (55-57). The effects of captopril and enalapril in dynamic exercise in hypertensive patients vary among investigators. While some authors found significant reduction in systolic and diastolic BPs during cycle exercise when compared with resting values (54,55,58), another found no difference in the same parameters during GXTs (59). Fagard et al. (56) reported that saralasin, a partial angiotensin-II antagonist, lowered BP in normotensive subjects during submaximal aerobic physical activity.

The reduction in angiotensin-II with captopril and saralasin, coupled with a varying response to blood pressure during exercise, indicates that angiotensin-II is not a major determinant of blood pressure regulation during exercise in hypertensive patients. In point of fact, angiotensin converting enzyme inhibition does not suppress plasma angiotensin-II increase during exercise in humans nor does it influence microalbuminuria with prolonged physical activity. This has significance in the management of the diabetic at rest or during exercise who has proteinuria as a manifestation of nephropathy wherein the converting enzyme inhibitor has been given to improve renal function.

Enalapril, a long-acting ACE inhibitor, has been shown to lower systolic BP response to submaximal and near-maximal exercise, an effect augmented when combined with hydrochlorothiazide

(57). These authors found no significant effect on HR, perceived exertion, exercise test duration, respiratory exchange ratio, or $\dot{V}O_2$max. It is unknown if these results would be the same after an exercise training period.

Both captopril and enalapril will improve exercise tolerance and cardiovascular capacity in patients with chronic CHF (60-64). Most patients receive concomitant treatment, including digoxin, diuretics, and nitrates. It is therefore imperative to realize that improvement in LVEF or peak exercise oxygen uptake ($\dot{V}O_2$) may reflect the addition of the ACE inhibitor to the regimen or a composite profile of all the drugs and their respective benefits.

After a short period of high dose captopril followed by dynamic exercise, angiotensin-II and plasma aldosterone levels were reduced significantly at rest and during exertion, plasma renin activity was higher than that attained with placebo, and norepinephrine and epinephrine concentrations were unaltered (55). ACE inhibitors also raise circulating levels of bradykinin (65), which stimulates production of vasodilator prostaglandins (66), therefore decreasing peripheral vascular resistance. Similar responses can be seen with all ACE inhibitors.

Since both exercise and ACE inhibitors independently raise serum potassium, there is always the possibility of hyperkalemia, but unlike hyperkalemia induced by beta-blockers, catecholamine action is not blunted and the likelihood of this interaction resulting in clinical consequences is remote. Fosinopril has been reported to show less change in potassium at rest with increase during exercise in contrast to changes in potassium seen with other ACE inhibitors and with nonselective beta blockers. This may be due to a more lipid soluble ACE inhibitor as a result of the phosphinic acid moiety unique to fosinopril (61).

Calcium-Channel Blockers

The clinical indications for calcium antagonist drugs (Table 25.8) vary according to their effects.

Table 25.7 Hemodynamics of Angiotensin-Converting Enzyme Inhibitors in Patients at Rest

Drug	Heart rate	Stroke volume	Cardiac output	Total peripheral resistance	Blood pressure
Captopril, enalapril, lisinopril, fosinopril, benazepril, ramapril, quinapril	—	—	—	↓	↓

Note. ↓ = lowered; — = no change.

Table 25.8   Hemodynamics of Calcium-Channel Blockers in Patients at Rest

Drug	Heart rate	Stroke volume	Cardiac output	Total peripheral resistance	Blood pressure
Verapamil	↓	↓	↓	↓	↓
Diltiazem	—	—	—	↓	↓
Nifedipine, nicardipine, nitrendipine, isradipine, felodipine	sl ↑	—	sl ↑	↓	↓

Note. sl ↑ = raised slightly; ↓ = lowered; — = no change.

While verapamil is usually prescribed as an antihypertensive and for supraventricular arrhythmias, nifedipine is used for hypertension and angina and after MI and coronary artery bypass graft (CABG) surgery to hinder further ischemia and to increase collateral myocardial flow (67).

During rest and treadmill exercise in normal volunteers, both nifedipine and verapamil had little or no effect on systolic and diastolic BPs. A mild blunting effect on diastolic BP or response to handgrip was observed with verapamil (68). In hypertensive patients though, both drugs were found to reduce systolic and diastolic BP during exercise, perhaps owing to a reduction in systemic vascular resistance (69,70), as has been reported for diltiazem and isradipine (71). Chronic treatment with newer drugs (i.e., isradipine and amlodipine) has been shown to lower blood pressure at rest and during exercise due to a reduction in systemic vascular resistance, similar to the same mechanisms of all calcium entry blockers.

An improvement in exercise tolerance was shown in patients with chronic angina who were using verapamil, nifedipine, or diltiazem (69, 70,72). The decrease in afterload produced by nifedipine, the improved left ventricular diastolic filling caused by verapamil, and the prolongation of exercise duration due to diltiazem diminish the myocardial oxygen demand, thus lowering the incidence of exercise-induced angina and ST-segment depression (69,70,72,73). A study using an exercise stimulus of bicycle ergometry and ambulatory 24-hour ECG monitoring for up to 8 weeks have indicated that in a randomized, crossover, double-blind study the effects of nifedipine or diltiazem, when added to beta blockers and nitrates, improved ambulatory and exercise tolerance in patients with severe yet stable angina due to multivessel coronary disease. Benefits included further prolongation of exercise duration, timed to 1 mm ST segment depression and to onset of angina, and a reduction in the sum of ST segment depressions at maximal identical load in ergometry.

Neither verapamil nor nifedipine affected the rise in potassium levels when compared to placebo during isometric exercise. Moreover, these drugs do not alter potassium levels significantly during aerobic activity (68). Once again, this is because these drugs do not blunt catecholamine action as do the beta-blockers.

Calcium antagonists are of value for cardiac patients who undergo training periods, since there is less risk of increased BP or serum potassium levels as compared to placebo. Also, these medications are beneficial for patients with bronchospastic pulmonary disease and insulin-dependent diabetes mellitus and those in whom beta-blockers induce fatigue or are contraindicated.

Nitrates

The oldest antianginal medications in use are the nitrates. Nitrates are prodrugs that enter the vascular smooth muscle, where they are denitrated to form the active agent, nitric oxide (75). Nitric oxide activates guanylate cyclase, which results in cyclic guanosine monophosphate production and vasodilation as a result of reuptake of calcium by the sarcoplasmic reticulum. Nitric oxide is identical to endothelium-derived relaxing factor, which induces vasodilation, inhibits platelet aggregation, reduces endothelium adhesion, and has anticoagulant and fibrinolytic properties (75). It is apparent that nitrates act to reduce ischemia as vasodilators but also may affect the atherosclerotic process.

Today there are various preparations of the drug, including the short- and long-acting (isosorbide dinitrate) forms and its major metabolite, isosorbide mononitrate. Owing to their numerous hemodynamic effects, patients with effort-induced angina can better tolerate exercise. Nitrates increase venous capacitance and subsequently decrease cardiac filling and mean arterial pressure, while reflexly increasing HR (74). Aerobic activity does not cause a decrease in Q̇, since all these hemodynamic parameters compensate for each other, as demonstrated by exercise radionuclide angiography (RNA) (75). In patients with angina pectoris it is advisable to avert *sustained* isometric activity, because this can induce left ventricular dysfunction (LVD), which is, however, reversible upon completion of the exercise.

Nitroglycerin lowers the triple product (systolic BP × HR × ejection period) at any level of exercise, an example of the mechanism by which it improves exercise tolerance, namely, reducing myocardial oxygen consumption (76). One sublingual nitroglycerin tablet can improve a patient's functional capacity by 1 MET (metabolic equivalent) during treadmill exercise (77). Nitrates decrease preload and therefore lower left ventricular end-diastolic pressure, which in turn determines myocardial wall tension and oxygen consumption (75), an effect that was also noted during isometric exercise (78).

Isosorbide dinitrate, a long-acting nitrate, did not improve exercise tolerance initially in patients with CHF, but at the end of a 3-month treatment period there was an improvement in peak V̇O₂ when compared to a placebo group (79). Such an outcome was believed secondary to increased peripheral use of oxygen, enhanced over time by the drug. When administered short-term, isosorbide dinitrate had no effect on the blunted vasodilation of exercising muscles in the patient with coronary heart failure (9). As previously indicated, long-acting nitrates combined with hydralazine have an added beneficial affect by increasing peak myocardial oxygen consumption (53).

Nitrates decrease ST-segment changes during physical activity in patients undergoing a program of cardiac rehabilitation.

The major problem with organic nitrates in the management of patients with angina pectoris is the clinical phenomenon of nitrate tolerance. It is thought that this may be as a result of sulfhydryl depletion as well as neurohumoral activation with increased plasma volume. N-acetylcysteine and angiotensin-converting enzyme inhibitors such as captopril or diuretics have not been shown on a persistent basis to prevent nitrate tolerance. The only acceptable way to prevent nitrate tolerance is with intermittent nitrate therapy by having a period of 8 to 12 hours of nitrate-free interval.

Another more recently marketed drug, isosorbide-5 mononitrate, given at 8 o'clock in the morning and 3 o'clock in the afternoon has been shown to decrease the number of episodes of angina without any augmentation of angina during the nitrate-free period and been shown to improve exercise tolerance.

Digitalis

In subjects with normal coronary arteries, digitalis produces ST-segment depression during exercise (20). Despite previous reports that digitalis did not improve exercise tolerance in patients with heart failure (80), it has been shown that digitalis does, in fact, improve work performance in such patients (81-84), though ACE inhibitors may have the same effect (85,86). Digitalis decreases left ventricular size and myocardial oxygen consumption at baseline, while during exertion it lowers left ventricular end-diastolic pressure (87,88). None of these studies, however, were done after long-term training.

Digitalis-induced arrhythmias can be exacerbated by exercise, especially if accompanied by diuretic-prompted hypokalemia and/or hypomagnesemia. Therefore, such patients should have electrolyte values and the potential for ectopic activity carefully monitored.

Digoxin plasma concentrations may vary from day to day in active persons. The most probable reason for these changes in the pharmacokinetics is a previously described increase in binding of digoxin to exercising muscles. There is reason to believe that the daily physical activity performed by digoxin treated patients will determine to some extent the body content of digoxin. Thus, physical exercise causes a redistribution of digoxin resulting in a fall in serum digoxin concentration with an increase in skeletal muscle digoxin concentration. The well-described quinidine-digoxin interaction could further affect the exercise induced redistribution of digoxin by reducing skeletal muscle binding of digoxin during quinidine administration. This has been attributable to a saturation of digoxin binding sites secondary to an increase in the total body load of digoxin at steady state rather than a direct effect of quinidine on digoxin binding. Quinidine did not interfere with the effect of physical exercise in causing a redistribution of digoxin between serum and skeletal muscle.

Antiarrhythmics

Originally, Gey et al. (89,90) reported no variation in patients' HR or V̇O₂ and only a slight drop in systolic BP during dynamic exercise while they were under the pharmacological effects of procainamide or quinidine. In the same study, exercise-induced arrhythmias were reduced in number and severity. Fenster et al. (91) found that quinidine increased HR both at rest and at low levels of exercise. They inferred that this effect was due to the vagolytic and alpha-adrenergic blocking action of the drug. On the other hand, procainamide and quinidine can mask exercise-induced ST-segment depression and produce false-negative ECG GXT results (92,93).

Plasma procainamide and its metabolite N-acetyl procainamide were quantified in healthy young volunteers during 4 hours of playing basketball. While the rate of acetylation was not affected by the intense exercise, which corresponded to a submaximal workload, urinary excretions of procainamide and the N-acetylated metabolite were decreased as a result of physical activity. This is very likely due to the renal clearance of procainamide being decreased commensurate with the reduction in glomerular filtration rate during physical activity. Plasma concentrations in rapid and slow acetylators of procainamide rose during exercise to a greater degree than concentrations measured over a 4-hour period of bedrest with the slow acetylators having a greater rise during the exercise phase than corresponding timepoints at bedrest. Correlation with electrocardiographic evidence of any added pharmacodynamic effect of procainamide was missing from this particular study. (In patients with demonstrable ectopy during physical activity not corrected by overdrive suppression, quinidine and procainamide may be effective in preventing symptomatic exercise-induced arrhythmias.) Tocainide has been reported as effective in blunting ectopic activity (94), but these data may reflect the selection of patients with refractory arrhythmias. Tocainide is used less today than 5 years ago because of hepatic and bone marrow toxicity. Furthermore, the safety of encainide and flecainide for routine use in the treatment of arrhythmias, especially in patients with CAD, has been challenged, proven and now virtually discontinued (95).

Summary

When tailoring an exercise program for patients taking drugs that affect the cardiovascular system, initial screening with GXTs or cycle ergometry must be combined with an understanding of how

these drugs influence expected changes in hemodynamic and biochemical parameters. Thus, drug therapy for CVD is not necessarily contraindicated in acute or chronic exercise if the mechanisms by which the former affects the latter are clearly understood.

Of all medications prescribed for hypertension, ischemic heart disease, and arrhythmias, only the beta-adrenergic blocking agents have been shown to partly limit an adequate hemodynamic response to exercise thereby affecting performance. A reduction in HR, which can limit $\dot{Q}$ and lower carbohydrate and lipid substrate availability and utilization by the working skeletal muscle causes an early perception of fatigue during exercise (96). Selective beta-blockers may thus be better tolerated (24).

Finally, lurking behind poor performance resulting from alleged medication usage may be the abuse of alcohol, excessive caffeine, anabolic steroids, or other purported ergogenic aids, such as amphetamines, cocaine, and marijuana. All of these abuses adversely alter BP, cardiac contractility, and conduction (97).

References

1. Lowenthal, D.T.; Stein, D.T. Drug effects: Exercise testing and training. In: Pollock, M.; Schmidt, D.H., eds. Heart disease and rehabilitation. Philadelphia: Wiley Medical; 1986:597-608.
2. Lund-Johansen, P. Hemodynamic changes in long-term diuretic therapy of essential hypertension. A comparative study of chlorthalidone, polythiazide and hydrochlorothiazide. Acta Med. Scand. 187:509-518; 1970.
3. Ogilvie, R.I. Cardiovascular response to exercise under increasing doses of chlorthalidone. Eur. J. Clin. Pharmacol. 9:339-344; 1976.
4. Knochel, J.P.; Vertel, R.M. Salt loading as a possible factor in the production of potassium depletion rhabdomyolysis and heat injury. Lancet. 1:659-665; 1967.
5. Bergstrom, J.; Hultman, S. The effect of thiazides, chlorthalidone and furosemide on muscle electrolytes and muscle glycogen in normal subjects. Acta Med. Scand. 180:363-376; 1965.
6. Falkner, B.; Onesti, G.; Lowenthal, D.T.; Affrime, M.B. Effectiveness of centrally acting drugs and diuretics in adolescent hypertension. Clin. Pharmacol. Ther. 32:577-583; 1982.
7. Clarke, R.J. Indapamide: A diuretic of choice for the treatment of hypertension. Am. J. Med. Sci. 301(3): 215-220; 1991.
8. La Croix, A.Z.; Wienpahl, J.; White, L.R.; Wallace, R.B.; Scherr, P.A.; George, L.K. Thiazide diuretic

agents and the incidence of hip fracture. N. Engl. J. Med. 322:288-290; 1990.

9. Virtanen, K.; Janne, J.; Frick, M.H. Response of blood pressure and plasma norepinephrine to propranolol, metoprolol and clonidine during isometric and dynamic exercise in hypertensives patients. Eur. J. Clin. Pharmacol. 21:275-279; 1982.

10. Lowenthal, D.T.; Affrime, M.B.; Falkner, B.; Saris, S.D.; Hakki, H. Potassium disposition and neuroendocrine effects of propranolol, methyldopa and clonidine during dynamic exercise. Clin. Exp. Hypertens. Theory Prac. A4(9,10):1895-1911; 1982.

11. Sannerstedt, R.; Varnanskes, E.; Werko, L. Hemodynamic effects of methyldopa (Aldomet) at rest and during exercise in patients with arterial hypertension. Acta Med. Scand. 171:75-82; 1962.

12. Lund-Johansen, P. Hemodynamic changes in long-term alpha methyldopa therapy of essential hypertension. Acta Med. Scand. 192:221-226; 1972.

13. Chamberlain, D.A.; Howard, J. Guanethidine and methyldopa: A haemodynamic study. Br. Heart J. 26:528-536; 1964.

14. Rosenthal, L.; Affrime, M.B.; Lowenthal, D.T. Biochemical and dynamic physical activity. Clin. Pharmacol. Ther. 32:701-710; 1982.

15. Lund-Johansen, P. Hemodynamic changes at rest and during exercise in long-term clonidine therapy of essential hypertension. Acta Med. Scand. 195:111-117; 1974.

16. Lowenthal, D.T.; Affrime, M.B.; Rosenthal, L.; Barruso, J.; Falkner, B. Dynamic and biochemical responses to single and repeated doses of clonidine during dynamic physical activity. Clin. Pharmacol. Ther. 32:18-24; 1982.

17. Onesti, G.; Schwartz, A.B.; Kim, K.E.; Paz Martinez, V. Antihypertensive effect of clonidine. Circ. Res. 2[Suppl.]:53-69; 1971.

18. Ferro, G.; Sinelli, L.; Duilio, C.; Spadafora, M.; Cinquegrana, G.; Condorelli, M. Alinidine in chronic stable angina: The effect on diastolic perfusion time. Cardiology. 77(4):287-294; 1990.

19. Davies, S.F.; Graif, J.L.; Husebye, D.; Maddy, M.M.; McArthur, C.D.; Path, M.J. Comparative effects of transdermal clonidine and oral atenolol on acute exercise performance and response to aerobic conditioning in subjects with hypertension. Arch. Intern. Med. 149:1551-1556; 1989.

20. Ellestad, M.H. Stress testing. Principles and practice. 3rd ed. Philadelphia: Davis; 1980:77-96.

21. Pratt, C.M.; Welton, D.E.; Squires, W.G., Jr.; Kirby, T.E. Demonstration of training effect during chronic beta-adrenergic blockade in patients with coronary artery disease. Circulation. 64(6):1125-1129; 1981.

22. Hare, T.W.; Lowenthal, D.T.; Hakki, H.H.; Goodwin, M. The effect of exercise training in older patients on beta adrenergic blocking drugs. Ann. Sports Med. 2:36-40; 1984.

23. Sklar, J.; Johnston, D.G.; Overlie, P.; Gerber, J.G. The effects of a cardioselective (metoprolol) and a nonselective (propranolol) beta-adrenergic blocker on

the response to dynamic exercise in normal men. Circulation. 65(5):894-899; 1982.

24. Pollock, M.; Lowenthal, D.T.; Foster, C.; Pels, A.E., III; Rod, J.; Schmidt, D.H.; et al. Acute and chronic responses in patients treated with beta blockers. J. Cardiopul. Rehabil. 11:132-144; 1991.

25. Lowenthal, D.T.; Saris, S.D.; Packer, J.; Haratz, A.; Conry, K. The mechanisms of action and clinical pharmacology of beta adrenergic blocking drugs. Am. J. Med. 77:119-127; 1984.

26. Yorko, J.; Kendrick, Z.V.; Kimuia, I.F.; Van Oort, G.; Paran, E.; Hare, T.W.; Lowenthal, D.T. Effect of B-blockade on strength performance. Ann. Sports Med. 5:176-180; 1990.

27. Nelson, G.I.C.; Donnelly, G.L.; Hunyor, S.N. Haemodynamic effects of sustained treatment with prazosin, and metoprolol, alone or in combination, in borderline hypertensive heart failure. J. Cardiovasc. Pharmacol. 4:240-245; 1982.

28. Laustiola, K.; Uusitalo, H.; Kovula, T.; Sovilijarvi, A.; Seppala, L.S.; Nikkari, T.; Vapaatalo, H. Divergent effects of atenolol, practolol and propranolol on the peripheral metabolic changes induced by dynamic exercise in healthy men. Eur. J. Clin. Pharmacol. 225:293-297; 1983.

29. Lundborg, P.; Astrom, H.; Bengtsson, C.; Fellenius, E.; von Schenk, H.; Svensson, L.; Smith, U. Effect of beta-adrenoreceptor blockade on exercise performance and metabolism. Clin. Sci. 61:299-305; 1981.

30. Franz, I.W.; Lohmann, F.W.; Koch, G.; Quabbe, H.J. Aspects of hormonal regulation of exercise: Effects of chronic beta-receptor blockade. Int. J. Sports Med. 4:14-20; 1983.

31. McLeod, A.A.; Brown, J.E.; Huhn, C.; Kitchell, B.B.; Sedor, F.A.; Williams, R.S.; Shand, D.G. Differentiation of hemodynamic, humoral, and metabolic responses to beta$_1$ and beta$_2$-adrenergic stimulation in man using atenolol and propranolol. Circulation. 67:1076-1084; 1983.

32. Christensen, N.J.; Brandsborg, O. The relationship between plasma catecholamine concentration and pulse rate during exercise and standing. Eur. J. Clin. Invest. 3:299-306; 1973.

33. Weiner, N. Drugs that inhibit adrenergic nerves and block adrenergic receptors. In: Gilman, A.G.; Goodman, L.S.; Rall, T.W.; eds. The pharmacologic basis of therapeutics, 7th ed. New York: Macmillan; 1985:198.

34. Freund, B.J.; Joyner, M.J.; Jilka, S.M.; Kalis, J.; Nittolo, J.M.; Taylor, J.A.; Peters, H.; Feese, G.; Wilmore, J.H. Thermoregulation during prolonged exercise in heat: Alterations with beta-adrenergic blockade. J. Appl. Physiol. 63:930-936; 1987.

35. Gordon, N.F. Effect of selective and non-selective beta-adrenoreceptor blockade on thermoregulation during prolonged exercise in heat. Am. J. Cardiol. 55:74D-78D; 1985.

36. Gordon, N.F.; Kruger, P.E.; van Rensburg, J.P.; van der Linde, A.; Kielblock, A.J.; Cilliers, J.F. Effect of beta-adrenoreceptor blockade on thermoregulation

during prolonged exercise. J. Appl. Physiol. 58:899-906; 1985.

37. Duncan, J.J.; Vaandrager, H.; Farr, J.E.; Kohl, H.W.; Gordon, N.F. Effect of intrinsic sympathomimetic activity on serum lipids during exercise training in hypertensive patients receiving chronic beta-blocker therapy. J. Cardiopulm. Rehabil. 9:110-114; 1989.

38. Lawlor, M.R.; Thomas, D.P.; Michele, J.; Jarey, R.A.; Paolone, A.M.; Bove, A.A. Effects of chronic beta-adrenergic blockade on hemodynamic and metabolic responses to endurance training. Med. Sci. Sports Exerc. 17:393-400; 1985.

39. Uusitupa, M.; Siitonen, O.; Harkonen, M.; Gordin, A.; Aro, A.; Hersio, A.; Johansson, G.; Korhonen, T.; Rauramaa, R. Metabolic and hormonal response to physical exercise during beta$_1$ selective and nonselective beta-blockade. Metabolism Research. 14:583-589; 1982.

40. Lundbeorg, P.; Astrom, H.; Bengtsson, C.; Fellenius, E. Effect of beta-adrenoreceptor blockade on exercise performance and metabolism. Clin. Sci. 61:299-305; 1981.

41. Leitch, A.G.; Hopkin, J.M.; Ellis, D.A.; Clarkson, D.M. Failure of propranolol and metoprolol to alter ventilatory responses to carbon dioxide and exercise. Br. J. Clin. Pharmacol. 9:493-498; 1980.

42. Pollock, M.L.; Wilmore, J.H. Exercise in health and disease: Evaluation and prescription for prevention and rehabilitation. 2nd ed. Philadelphia: Saunders; 1990:302.

43. Jilka, S.M.; Joyner, M.J.; Nittolo, J.M.; Kalis, J.K.; Taylor, J.A.; Lohman, T.G.; Wilmore, J.H. Maximal exercise responses to acute and chronic beta-adrenergic blockade in healthy male subjects. Med. Sci. Sports Exerc. 20:570-572; 1988.

44. Henry, J.A.; Iliopoulou, A.; Kaye, C.M.; Sankey, M.G. Changes in plasma concentrations of acebutolol, propranolol and indomethacin during physical exercise. Life Sci. 28:1925-1929; 1981.

45. Arends, B.G. Influence of physical exercise on the pharmacokinetics of propranolol. Eur. J. Clin. Pharmacol. 31(3):375-377; 1986.

46. Moyer, J.H. Hydralazine (Apresoline) hydrochloride. Pharmacological observations and clinical results in the therapy of hypertension. Arch. Intern. Med. 91:419-439; 1953.

47. Ginks, W.R.; Redwood, D.R. Haemodynamic effects of hydralazine at rest and during exercise in patients with chronic heart failure. Br. Heart J. 44:259-264; 1980.

48. Lund-Johansen, P. Hemodynamic changes at rest and during exercise in long-term prazosin therapy for essential hypertension. Postgraduate medicine, symposium on Prazosin: 1975 November; 45.

49. Lowenthal, D.T.; Dickerman, D.; Saris, S.D.; Falkner, B.; Hare, T.W. The effect of pharmacologic interaction on central and peripheral alpha-receptors and pressor response to static exercise. Ann. Sports Med. 1:100-104; 1983.

50. Lowenthal, D.T. Exercise in renal and hypertensive disease. In: Bove, A.A.; Lowenthal, D.T., eds. Exercise medicine: Physiologic principles and clinical applications. New York: Academic Press; 1983:292-301.

51. Wilson, J.R.; Untereker, W.; Hurshfeld, J. Effects of isosorbide dinitrate and hydralazine on regional metabolic responses to arm exercise in patients with heart failure. Am. J. Cardiol. 48:934-938; 1981.

52. O'Hare, J.A.; Murnaghan, D.J. Failure of antihypertensive drugs to control blood pressure rise with isometric exercise in hypertension. Postrgad. Med. J. 57:552-555; 1981.

53. Cohn, J.N.; Johnson, G.; Ziesche, S.; Cobb, F.; Francis, G.; Tristani, F.; Smith, R.; et al. A comparison of enalapril with hydralazine-isosorbide dinitrate in the treatment of chronic congestive heart failure. N. Engl. J. Med. 325:303-310; 1991.

54. Paran, E.; Neumann, L.; Cristal, N.; Lowenthal, D.T. Response to mental and physical stress before and during adrenoreceptor blocker and angiotensin converting enzyme inhibitor treatment in essential hypertension. Am. J. Cardiol. 68:1362-1366; 1991.

55. Manhem, P.; Bramnert, M.; Hulthen, U.L.; Hokfelt, B. The effect of captopril on catecholamines, renin activity, angiotensin II an aldosterone in plasma during physical exercise in hypertensive patients. Eur. J. Clin. Invest. 11:389-395; 1981.

56. Fagard, R.; Amery, A.; Reybrouck, T.; et al. Effects of angiotensin antagonism on hemodynamics, renin and catecholamines during exercise. J. Appl. Physiol. 43:440-444; 1977.

57. Leon, A.S.; McNally, C.; Casal, D.; Grimm, R.; Crow, R.; Bell, C.; Hunninghake, D.B. Enalapril alone and in combination with hydrochlorothiazide in the treatment of hypertension: Effect on treadmill exercise performance. J. Cardiopulm. Rehabil. 6:251-256; 1986.

58. Fagard, R.; Lijnen, P.; Amery, A. Hemodynamic response to captopril at rest and during exercise in hypertensive patients. Am. J. Cardiol. 49:1569-1571; 1982.

59. Pickering, T.G.; Base, D.B.; Sullivan, P.A.; Laragh, J.H. Comparison of anti-hypertensive and hormonal effects of captopril and propranolol at rest and during exercise. Am. J. Cardiol. 49:1566-1568; 1982.

60. The SOLVD Investigators. Effect of enalapril on survival in patients with reduced left ventricular exertion fractions and congestive heart failure. NEJM. 325:293-307; 1991.

61. Packer, M.; Medina, N.; Yshak, M.; et al. Hemodynamic patterns of response during long-term captopril therapy for severe chronic heart failure. Circulation. 68:803; 1983.

62. Kramer, B.L.; Massie, B.M.; Topic, N. Controlled trial of captopril in chronic heart failure: A rest and exercise hemodynamic study. Circulation. 67:807; 1983.

63. Creager, M.A.; Massie, B.M.; Faxon, D.P.; et al. Acute and long-term effects of enalapril on the cardiovascular response to exercise and exercise tolerance in

patients with congestive heart failure. J. Am. Coll. Cardiol. 6:163; 1985.

64. Cleland, J.G.F.; Dargie, H.J.; Ball, S.G.; et al. Effects of enalapril in heart failure: A double-blind study of effects on exercise performance, renal function, hormones, and metabolic state. Br. Heart J. 54:305; 1985.

65. Abrams, W.B. The role of ACE inhibition in cardiovascular therapy. Fed. Proc. 43:1314-1321; 1984.

66. Swartz, S.L. ACE inhibition and prostaglandins. Am. J. Cardiol. 49:1405-1409; 1982.

67. Stone, P.H.; Antman, E.M.; Muller, J.E.; et al. Calcium channel blocking agents in the treatment of cardiovascular disorders. Part II: Hemodynamic effects of clinical applications. Ann. Intern. Med. 93: 886-904; 1980.

68. Stein, D.T.; Lowenthal, D.T.; Porter, S.; et al. Effects of nifedipine and verapamil on isometric and dynamic exercise in normal subjects. Am. J. Cardiol. 54:386-389; 1984.

69. Subramanian, B.; Bowles, M.F.; Davies, A.B.; et al. Combined therapy with verapamil and propranolol in chronic stable angina. Am. J. Cardiol. 49:125-132; 1982.

70. Moskowitz, R.M.; Piccini, P.A.; Nacarelli, G.; et al. Nifedipine therapy for stable angina pectoris: Preliminary results of effects on angina frequency and treadmill exercise response. Am. J. Cardiol. 44:811-816; 1979.

71. Mayer, O.; Polivkova, H.; Rottenborn, J. Isradipine in the treatment of hypertension: Some additional effects observed during a one-year study. Am. J. Hypertens. 4:140S-143S; 1991.

72. Pool, P.E.; Seagren, S.C.; Bonanno, J.A.; et al. The treatment of exercise-inducible chronic stable angina with diltiazem. Effect on treadmill exercise. Chest. 78:234; 1980.

73. Bonow, R.O.; Leon, M.B.; Rosing, D.R.; et al. Effects of verapamil and propranolol on left ventricular function and diastolic filling in patients with coronary artery disease: Radionuclide angiographic studies at rest and during exercise. Circulation. 65:1337; 1982.

74. Goldstein, R.E.; Rosing, D.R.; Redwood, D.R.; et al. Clinical and circulatory effects of isosorbide dinitrate: Comparison with nitroglycerine. Circulation. 43:629-640; 1971.

75. Sorensen, S.G.; Ritchie, J.L.; Caldwell, J.H.; et al. Serial exercise radionuclide angiography. Validation of count-derived changes in cardiac output and quantitation of maximal exercise ventricular volume change after nitroglycerine and propranolol in normal men. Circulation. 61(3):600-609; 1980.

76. Georgopoulos, A.J.; Sones, F.M., Jr.; Page, I.H. Relationship between arterial pressure and exertional angina pectoris in hypertensive patients. Circulation. 23:892; 1961.

77. Markis, J.E.; Gorlin, R.; Mills, R.M.; et al. Sustained effect of orally administered isosorbide dinitrate on exercise performance of patients with angina pectoris. Am. J. Cardiol. 43:265; 1979.

78. Flessas, A.P.; Ryan, T.J. Effects of nitroglycerin on isometric exercise. Am. Heart J. 105:239; 1983.

79. Franciosa, J.A.; Goldsmith, S.R.; Cohn, J.N. Contrasting immediate and long-term effects of isosorbide dinitrate on exercise capacity in congestive heart failure. Am. J. Med. 69:559-566; 1980.

80. Glancy, D.L.; Higgs, L.M.; O'Brien, K.P.; et al. Effects of ouabain on the left ventricular response to exercise in patients with angina pectoris. Circulation. 43:45-57; 1971.

81. Vogel, R.; Kirch, D.; LeFree, M.; et al. Effects of digitalis on resting and isometric exercise myocardial perfusion in patients with coronary artery disease and left ventricular dysfunction. Circulation. 56: 355; 1977.

82. Guyatt, G.H.; Sullivan, M.J.J.; Fallen, E.L.; et al. A controlled trial of digoxin in congestive heart failure. Am. J. Cardiol. 61:371-375; 1988.

83. Sullivan, M.; Atwood, J.E.; Myers, J.; et al. Increased exercise capacity after digoxin adminstration in patients with heart failure. J. Am. Coll. Cardiol. 13: 1138-1143; 1989.

84. DiBianco, R.; Shabetai, R.; Kostuk, W.; Moran, J.; Schlant, R.C.; Wright, R. A comparison of oral milrinone, digoxin, and their combination in the treatment of patients with chronic heart failure. N. Engl. J. Med. 320:677-683; 1989.

85. The Captopril-Digoxin Multicenter Research Group. Comparative effects of therapy with captopril and digoxin in patients with mild to moderate heart failure. JAMA. 259:539-544; 1988.

86. Beaune, J. Comparison of enalapril versus digoxin for congestive heart failure. Am. J. Cardiol. 63:22D-25D; 1989.

87. Gross, G.J.; Waltier, D.C.; Hardman, H.F.; et al. The effects of ouabain on nutritional circulation and regional myocardial blood flow. Am. Heart J. 93: 487; 1977.

88. Parker, J.O.; West, R.O., Jr.; Ledwich, J.R.; et al. The effect of acute digitalization on the hemodynamic response to exercise in coronary artery disease. Circulation. 40:453; 1969.

89. Gey, G.O.; Levy, R.H.; Fisher, L.; et al. Plasma concentration of procainamide and prevalence of exertional arrhythmias. Ann. Intern. Med. 80:718-722; 1974.

90. Gey, G.O.; Levy, R.H.; Pettet, G.; et al. Quinidine plasma concentration and exertional arrhythmia. Am. Heart J. 90:19-24; 1975.

91. Fenster, P.E.; Dahl, C.; Marcus, F.I.; et al. Effect of quinidine on the heart rate and blood pressure response to treadmill exercise. A. Heart J. 104:1244; 1982.

92. Surawicz, B.; Lasseter, K.C. Effects of drugs on the electrocardiogram. Prog. Cardiovasc. Dis. 13:26-55; 1970.

93. Freedberg, A.S.; Riseman, J.E.F.; Speigel, E.D. Objective evidence of the efficiency of medical therapy in angina pectoris. Am. Heart J. 22:494-518; 1941.

94. LeWinter, M.M.; Engler, R.L.; Karliner, J.S. Tocainide therapy for treatment of ventricular arrhythmias: Assessment with ambulatory electrocardiographic monitoring and treadmill exercise. Am. J. Cardiol. 45:1045-1052; 1980.

95. Bigger, J.T., Jr. Implications of the cardiac arrhythmia suppression trial (CAST) for antiarrhythmic drug treatment. Am. J. Cardiol. 65(8):3D-10D; 1990.

96. Tarazi, R.D.; Dustan, H.P. Beta-adrenergic blockade in hypertension. Practical and theoretical implications of long-term hemodynamic variations. Am. J. Cardiol. 29:633; 1972.

97. Lowenthal, D.T.; Parmet, J; Paran, E.; Kendrick, Z. Drugs, exercise and the cardiovascular system. In: Strauss, R.H., ed. Drugs and performance sports. Philadelphia: W.B. Saunders; 1987:183-195.

Chapter 26

Patient Compliance

Neil B. Oldridge

Approximately 1 million people survived an acute myocardial infarction (MI) during 1990 in the United States (1). With an estimated rehabilitation population of 100,000 to 150,000 participating in outpatient cardiac rehabilitation programs (2,3), the annual costs of supervised cardiac rehabilitation in the United States would amount to between $180 million and $270 million, assuming a supervised rehabilitation cost of $1,800/patient, (2,4). The effectiveness of many current and emerging medical practices, however, has not been substantiated in adequately rigorous scientific studies (5), although there has been an increasing interest in outcomes research to provide "better information for physicians and patients to use in making decisions, improved guidelines for better medical practice, . . . and wiser decisions by health care purchasers" (5).

How and where best to spend scarce health-care resources should be decided at least partly on the probability that the intervention will be effective and on the impact the condition may have on health and on health-care resources. Thus, before clinical recommendations about alternative interventions can be made, research data on the efficacy of the intervention are needed, after which cost-effectiveness (direct costs of health care and lost earnings as well as indirect costs and such factors as mortality, disability, and quality of life) can be carried out. These analyses will allow sound decisions about clinical recommendations. However, analytic research often is compromised by bias. With limited resources and the demand for accountability, funding decisions about either analytic research into the efficacy of long-term interventions or clinical lifestyle intervention programs (e.g., for exercise) require careful and objective assessment of all potential biases.

Bias in analytic research that results from flaws in study design, data collection, analysis, or interpretation of the data will produce inaccurate interpretations. In a recent meta-analysis of physical activity in the prevention of coronary artery disease (CAD) (6) there is a clear difference in the outcome of the better-designed versus the less well designed studies. Compliance bias is one such potential bias important in executing any research or clinical intervention for long-term behavior change; that is, do patients drop out of the research protocol or the clinical intervention at different rates? Demonstration of the efficacy of long-term research interventions, such as cardiac rehabilitation, will depend on reducing compliance bias to a minimum; a likelihood of adequate compliance over extended periods of time will influence funding long-term trials of rehabilitation after an acute cardiovascular event (7,8).

The purpose of this chapter is twofold:

1. To examine compliance and other outcome data in randomized trials of cardiac rehabilitation services which have a follow-up of at least 12 months after myocardial infarction (MI)
2. To present some methodological issues in compliance-enhancing research

Cardiac Rehabilitation Services

The overall goals of rehabilitation in a chronic disease such as CAD, where the cause of the disease is uncertain and outcome variable, should be focused on quality of life as implied in the World Health Organization (WHO) definition of rehabilitation: "Rehabilitation is the sum of activity required to ensure the best possible physical, mental and social conditions so that patients may *by their own efforts regain* as normal as possible a place in the community and lead an active productive life" (9). The "sum of activities" referred to in the WHO definition is generally considered today to refer, with respect to the post-MI patient to education or counseling and risk factor management, including smoking cessation, altering blood lipid levels, reducing hypertension, initiating stress management

393

techniques, and increasing the level of regular physical activity.

Cardiovascular risk factor management strategies, such as serum cholesterol reduction, blood pressure (BP) control, smoking cessation, and exercise have a major impact on the decline in the incidence of CAD (10) and these same risk factors also have an impact in the rehabilitation, or secondary prevention, of CAD (11). Benefits of supervised cardiac rehabilitation include a reduction in cardiovascular disease (CVD) risk factors, a decrease in activity-induced symptoms, and an improved functional capacity (12,13). Improvements in psychosocial outcomes following cardiac rehabilitation have not been documented consistently (14). Meta-analyses of randomized clinical trials of cardiac rehabilitation (15,16) have demonstrated a 25% reduction in mortality after MI, although routine interventions such as thrombolysis and revascularization have a marked impact on early reinfarction, thus decreasing the probability of additional improvements in survival with rehabilitation (12).

At least four factors determine the success of such intervention programs as cardiac rehabilitation: (a) recognition of symptomotology and ill health, (b) correct diagnosis, (c) an adequate treatment plan, and (d) patient compliance with the treatment plan. Long-term compliance will most likely be achieved when the intervention or prescription is both attainable and attractive. As no intervention for health behavior change can work without adequate compliance, it is important to better understand why patients do not comply and how best to encourage compliance with presumably beneficial interventions (17-19). At the same time, successful rehabilitation requires adequate provision of information and services by the health professional, as well as adequate utilization of the proper services by the patient. Conceptually, the patient, health professional, and the intervention can each be targeted for possible compliance-enhancing strategies.

Compliance With Cardiac Rehabilitation Services

Unfortunately, many of the early studies of cardiac rehabilitation effectiveness were not designed rigorously and did not include a control group. Even when they did, compliance bias was a problem, as there often was a high dropout rate. To some degree, more recent studies have been better designed and the problem with compliance bias has

been less marked; perhaps awareness of this potential problem with poor compliance has resulted in the incorporation of compliance-enhancing strategies as part of the intervention protocols themselves.

Compliance in randomized trials of cardiac rehabilitation following MI (20-41) is generally considered to follow a negatively accelerating curve with a relatively large drop-out rate early in the program and randomized clinical trials with follow-up of at least 12 months duration will be presented to document compliance with cardiac rehabilitation services. The data on compliance with cardiac rehabilitation services (i.e., hypercholesterolemia and hypertension control, smoking cessation, reducing coronary prone behavior and increasing regular exercise habits) generally demonstrate that greater benefit from treatment is achieved with better compliance.

Education

It is important to distinguish between *patient education* in the strictly didactic sense of exchange of information, and *health education*, or patient counseling to facilitate adaptations of behavior conducive to health. A meta-analysis of education in chronic disease has demonstrated that true health education has a greater effect on the degree to which patients follow therapeutic advice as measured by compliance, therapeutic progress, and health outcomes than the didactic approach (42). However, in a recent review of selected studies in cardiac rehabilitation, the authors concluded that there was no conclusive evidence that either didactic teaching or health education were helpful after MI (43), and in a recent randomized trial comparing rehabilitation and patient counseling, the latter failed to show any benefit (40). While there may be great potential for health behavior education or counseling after MI, the challenge to communicate, bringing relevant, comprehensible, useful information to motivate, enable, or reinforce health behavior has not been fully realized.

Risk Factor Mangement

Such cardiovascular risk factor management strategies as serum cholesterol reduction, BP control, and smoking cessation have had a considerable impact on the observed decline in the incidence of CAD (10), and more recent evidence from meta-analyses has identified the importance of regular physical activity (6). Each of these risk factors also has a major impact in the secondary prevention of CAD (11).

Blood Cholesterol

As the excess risk attributable to increased serum cholesterol is 2 to 3 times greater among survivors of MI, reducing elevated serum cholesterol has been shown to prevent a significant number of recurrent events in these patients (11,44). In a landmark study, the Coronary Drug Project (45), where men with previous MI were assigned randomly to various medication treatment groups, poor 5-year compliance (defined as less than 65% of the protocol drug dosage taken) was seen in 44% of patients on niacin, 28% on clofibrate, and 26% on placebo, and more than 50% of the poorest compliers at 5 years demonstrated this pattern of behavior within the first 8 to 12 months of the intervention. Reinfarction rates at 5 and 15 years were reduced with intervention (45,46) but it is important to note that patients who took 80% or more of the protocol prescription during the 5-year follow-up period had a lower mortality rate than poor medication adherers (15.0% versus 24.6%; $p < 0.000$). On the other hand, it is important to note that similar findings for mortality rate were observed in the good and poor adherers in the placebo group (15.1% versus 28.3%; $p < 0.000$) (47). A review of studies investigating lowering cholesterol after MI suggests a 10% reduction in cholesterol is associated with reductions of 19%, 12%, and 15% in nonfatal, fatal, and all MI, respectively (44).

Reduced progression of atherosclerosis with adequate compliance to cholesterol-lowering medication and diet in patients with elevated low-density lipoprotein cholesterol and documented CAD has been demonstrated angiographically in at least two randomized clinical trials (48,49). In a randomized trial of exercise in survivors of MI, LaRosa et al. (50) reported that, although compliance was "adequate" in 73% of the exercise patients and in 69% of the control group, there were no differences in blood cholesterol levels between the exercise and control patients; no comparison of compliant and noncompliant subjects was carried out. Trials of dietary intervention that include compliance rates for patients after MI are rare; in one such randomized trial, patients in the treatment group, who complied with the 1-year protocol, demonstrated greater improvements in lipoprotein concentrations and body weight, with fewer recurrent coronary events than observed in the control group (51).

Hypertension

Antihypertensive treatment in patients with severe hypertension resulting in a 6 to 8 mm Hg decrease in diastolic BP is associated with a significant 12% reduction in CAD, and there is a borderline significant 9% reduction in patients with mild to moderate hypertension (52). In hypertensive patients, persistent reduction of diastolic BP, suggesting adequate compliance with treatment, is associated with a reduction in mortality (53).

Smoking

Smoking cessation may very well be the single most important risk factor modification for both primary (10,54,55) and secondary (11,56) prevention of CAD and, with modeling, has been shown to be cost-effective after MI (57). It would be unethical to carry out controlled trials of smoking cessation in secondary prevention of CAD, but evidence from representative observational studies demonstrates 43% compliance with smoking cessation over 72 months and a relative risk of mortality of 0.59 for men and women compared to continuing smokers (58), 46% compliance over 60 months with a relative risk of 0.46 in men, and 57% compliance over 60 months with a relative risk of 0.42 in women (59). The approximate 45% to 50% cessation rate has been substantiated in reports of comprehensive cardiac rehabilitation following MI (60,61).

Coronary-Prone Behavior

Coronary-prone behavior (the so-called Type A personality) does not appear to be associated with recurrent fatal or nonfatal cardiac events in survivors of an acute MI (62,63) and in fact has been associated with lower, not higher, CAD mortality in patients with documented MI (64). However, in the only randomized trial of counseling to reduce Type A behavior after MI there was a significantly higher 4.5 year recurrent event rate in patients who withdrew from behavioral counseling treatment during the study than that observed in patients who complied with treatment over the same period of time (65). There are intriguing recent data to suggest that, when compared to high-stress patients not receiving the intervention, high-stress patients who received stress-relieving strategies had relative risks of 0.49 (p = 0.051) for cardiac death rate during the year of intervention (66) and 0.36 (p = 0.006) over the next 5 years (67). Compliance with 1-year intervention was 88% among those experimental group patients who needed intervention (66,67). The results of both of these trials present intriguing possibilities for rehabilitation strategies following MI, but there is a need to reproduce them in order to corroborate the findings.

Multifactoral Rehabilitation

As previously mentioned, much of the data on compliance with multifactoral rehabilitation (exercise with and without other risk factor management) after MI are derived from randomized trials of the efficacy of cardiac rehabilitation and not from experimental investigations of compliance. This means that the compliance data are derived from studies that suffer from a number of basic methodological limitations, including a lack of a theoretical base, varied definitions of compliance, uncontrolled confounders, compliance bias, and incomplete follow-up. There has been little attempt to carry out hypothesis-testing research to determine causal mechanisms for dropout in cardiac rehabilitation with the objective of implementing optimally effective compliance-enhancing strategies (7,68,69). Health care services affect compliance through accessibility and acceptability of the services (70,71). Though dropout rates may be a useful measure of acceptability of service (7,70,71), other measures are necessary that complement and extend the concept of compliance/dropout as outcomes on a continuum. These measures might include program participation level, such as different levels of attendance, thus describing patterns of utilization over the duration of the prescribed intervention (7,70).

Dropout Rates. Dropout rates have been reported in many of the trials of rehabilitation following documentation of MI. Twenty-one randomized clinical trials of cardiac rehabilitation that meet the 12-month follow-up eligibility criterion have been identified (20-40); they had a total of 2,976 patients with a documented MI randomized to an active intervention, including an exercise prescription. The primary outcome in 10 of the trials was mortality (20-31), and was exercise tolerance, return to work, or psychosocial measures in the other 9 trials (32-40). Rates of compliance with intervention and follow-up are seen in Table 26.1.

In trials that lasted at least 12 months, the typical dropout curve in cardiac exercise rehabilitation is a negatively accelerating one, with the largest proportion of dropout occurring within 6 months. Paralleling the observations of a decreasing attendance in randomized trials of supervised exercise rehabilitation lasting 6 months (73-76), the mean 3-month dropout from 12-month trials was 25% to 30%, increasing to 40% to 50% by 6 to 12 months

(Figure 26.1). Daltroy (36) has extended these observations, reporting that 78% of their patients reported doing some exercise on their own although less than 10% were attending the supervised sessions at 11 months. This supports our own observations from clinical studies that dropout from supervised rehabilitation exercise programs does not automatically mean that the behavior change is not being maintained at some other more convenient supervised or unsupervised location (77). In a recently reported randomized trial, long-term follow-up of exercise behavior suggests a dropout as low as 0% over 4.5 years (31) when compared to earlier reports in similar trials after MI of a 45% to 70% dropout over 3.5 to 4.5 years (21,27); for comparison, data from long-term follow-up of hospital programs suggest a dropout of as little as less than 20% over 5 years (78) but also as high as 90% with "heavy exercise" after 6 to 9 years (79).

Patient Characteristics and Intervention Factors. Despite the methodological shortcomings inherent in nonexperimental and quasi-experimental studies, the following characteristics associated with a relatively high dropout rate have been identified: smokers (72,78,80-82); blue-collar occupation and low social class (in some [72,80,82] but not all studies [78]); few leisure exercise habits (72,79,82-84); symptoms of CAD, including angina (84); perceptions of little support (72) and other psychological factors, such as low self-motivation and more anxiety, depression, distress, and mood disturbance (84-86); there is little predictive value from the health belief model (80). To a considerable extent, these observations have been substantiated in one or more of the randomized trials noted previously (21,27,32,33,38,39).

Reasons for Dropout. As first suggested by Wilhelmsen et al. (21) and Bruce et al. (87) and later confirmed by us (27,71,80,88) and others (35,38,78, 79,83), the reasons for dropout from cardiac rehabilitation can be classified as avoidable reasons (e.g., staff, program, and prescription difficulties; inconvenience; and lack of motivation and interest) and unavoidable reasons (e.g., medical reasons and relocation). We have recently reported that about 40% of dropout occurred for avoidable reasons and that medical reasons accounted for almost 60% of unavoidable dropout (80). Awareness of the reasons for dropout may have important immediate, and potentially effective, consequences for program planning, in that many of the avoidable reasons for dropping out are often more amenable to change than patient characteristics. In this context, the relationships between compliance

Table 26.1   Compliance and Attendance Rates in Intervention Patients in Randomized Clinical Trials of Cardiac Rehabilitation Lasting at Least 12 Months

Reference	n	Intervention Duration (months)	Intervention Attendance (%)	Intervention Compliance (%)	Outcome follow-up Duration (months)	Outcome follow-up Compliance (%)
Trials in which mortality was the primary outcome:						
Kentala (20)	77	12	n/a	13 (@ ≥ 70%)	24	90
Wilhelmsen et al. (21)	158	48	63 (at 9 months)	30	48	100
Kallio et al. (22) and Hamalainen et al. (41)	188	3-12	n/a	n/a	36	100
Shaw (23) and Stern & Cleary (24)	323	36	n/a	48 (@ ≥ 50%)	36	93
Carson et al. (25)	151	3	n/a	69	25	100
Rechnitzer et al. (26) and Oldridge et al. (27)	379	48	n/a	54	48	93
Roman et al. (28)	93	42	76	77	56	77
Vermeulen et al. (29)	47	2	n/a	n/a	60	100
WHO (30)	705	2-36	(47% of centers reported at "high" level)	n/a	36	65
Marra et al. (31)	81	2	76 reported at "good" level	100	55	96
P.R.E. Cor. Group (40)	182	1.5	n/a	24	24	100
Total	2,384	1.5-48	72%	56%	24-60	92%
Trials with other primary outcomes:						
Mayou et al. (32)	43	2	n/a	76	18	96
Bengtsson (33)	81	3	n/a	64	14	54
Stern et al. (34)	42	3	81	88 (@ ≥ 66%)	12	90
Froelicher et al. (35)	72	12	76	82	12	82
Daltroy (36)	84	12	n/a	< 10	12	100
Burgess et al. (37)	89	3	n/a	86	13	76
Goble et al. (38)	166	2	n/a	65 (@ ≥ 75%)	12	70
Oldridge et al. (39)	99	2	n/a	82 (@ ≥ 75%)	12	91
Total	676	2-12	79%	58%	12-18	82%
Grand total	3,060	1.5-48	74%	57%	12-60	88%

Note. Figures with "@" in parentheses indicate the level of compliance at the stated attendance rate. n/a = not available.

and such factors as spouse support and patient-perceived spouse support—which are controversial, with both positive (8,72,89-92) and negative or neutral associations reported (72,93-95)—may have important implications for long-term compliance-enhancing strategies (7,8).

Section Summary

The evidence, largely derived from randomized clinical trials, demonstrates that the benefits of risk factor modification strategies to alter blood cholesterol, hypertension, smoking, and Type A behavior and lack of exercise are greatest in those patients actively complying with the prescribed intervention. Whether these benefits are then observed in routine clinical care depends on an adequate level of compliance maintained over extended periods of time. The challenge is therefore twofold; first, to motivate patients unwilling to take the initial step to alter modifiable cardiovascular risk factors, and second, to provide strategies to help patients maintain long-term compliance.

Compliance-Enhancing Research

While complete compliance by all patients would be ideal, the practicalities of cardiac rehabilitation

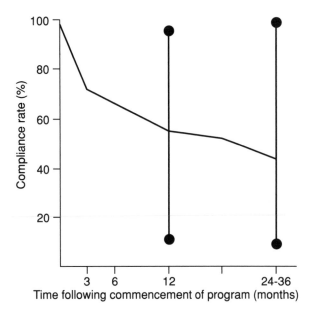

Figure 26.1 Compliance curves derived from randomized clinical trials of cardiac rehabilitation programs. The bars represent the maximum range in rates at 12 and 24 to 36 months.

after MI suggest that 75% to 80% compliance is probably the maximum that can be expected over an extended period of time. The evidence also suggests that the overall benefits of adequate compliance with a comprehensive exercise rehabilitation program are worth the costs and the patient's efforts, particularly if the program is initiated soon after the cardiac event. Compliance-enhancing strategies need to be studied prospectively in randomized controlled trials with groups of patients identified at a uniform point of their disease and followed up over an extended period of time in order to determine accurately the magnitude of noncompliance with the intervention. A number of issues in compliance research have been identified, and Sackett (96) has described these in detail. A review of these issues with reference to the cardiac rehabilitation and compliance literature is provided here.

Specification of the Problem

Sackett (96) states that the definition of *compliance* should be precise, unambiguous, and appropriate to both the research questions and the research setting; the key property of a definition as used in a trial must be its reproducibility by other researchers. However, the measure of compliance with cardiac rehabilitation in CAD has not been consistent

(7,68,69). *Compliers* have been defined as those patients either attending more than a given percentage of possible sessions or attending for a given time; *dropouts* are patients who miss more than a given number of consecutive sessions or do not complete the intervention; and *attendance* is the number of sessions attended out of all possible sessions.

Compliance-Enhancing Strategy

The experimental protocol must be precisely defined: who does what to which patients, why, where, how often, with what feedback, and with what expenditure of time and effort? This forces the investigator to be specific about the strategy, thus avoiding the confounding effect of multiple strategies. Others can then reproduce the trial or utilize it in a clinical setting. Precise definition of the experimental protocol should also include a description of who applies the strategy and a description of the appropriate control groups (96).

The content of the compliance-enhancing strategy must be precisely explained and the experimental protocol itself, the strategy (e.g., reinforcement, goal setting, and self-monitoring), and the objective of the strategy must be clear. The following system for evaluating and grading the methodological adequacy of the description of compliance-enhancing strategies has been developed:

- Top grade: complete description of the strategy that permits the reader to reproduce the strategy with precision
- Intermediate grade: incomplete description of the strategy
- Low grade: no description, or the strategy can only be inferred.

Bonus marks are given (for each category) if co-intervention with a second strategy or other treatment is precluded by study design or is noted when it occurs (97).

Describing the Sample

Sackett (96) suggests that because the major issue here can be summarized as "to which patients does the investigator wish to generalize the results?" the diagnostic and clinical characteristics of the study sample need to be carefully described. The diagnosis of CAD optimally should be as precise as possible (e.g., MI), and when there is more than one diagnosis (e.g., MI, CABG surgery, and angina) the proportion of patients in each group should be given. Other pertinent characteristics, such as sociodemographic and physiological factors, must also be specified, particularly if they are known to be associated with compliance, like smoking. This helps to answer whether the study sample is biased in ways that might distort the conclusions drawn about compliance.

Early dropout from cardiac rehabilitation is a problem, but if dropouts are omitted from analysis, invalid conclusions about the magnitude and determinants of compliance and the effectiveness of compliance-enhancing strategies may be drawn. It is important to indicate the proportion of a sample excluded from analysis and the time period during which "consecutive" patients were enrolled.

Randomization of the Sample

The objective of randomization is to reduce bias and maximize comparability of the experimental and control groups. Randomization is biased when allocation into groups of patients is done by hospital registration numbers or by some arbitrary date such as an admission date. Individual patient allocation to either the experimental or control group in a randomized trial should therefore be carried out by use of random number tables or computer programs that generate random numbers (96). Stratification is important, particularly if there is evidence that certain characteristics have been demonstrated to be associated with compliance.

Compliance Measures

A single measure of compliance, such as attendance, may be adequate, but, if possible, additional methods of assessing compliance should be used. The compliance measures used in the study must be relevant to the research question and be applicable to the wider population and the setting to which the results will be generalized. Compliance can be considered a dichotomous concept, since a patient either does or does not comply. However, information of much greater potential use may be derived when compliance is considered as a continuum (e.g., attendance at some number of sessions, which can be corroborated by other changes, such as fitness, weight loss, and psychosocial well-being) (70). Careful consideration must be given to the follow-up of dropouts, since they do, in fact, represent important end points in any given study.

Compliance and treatment goals should be correlated; in exercise rehabilitation programs, the specific treatment objective may be an improvement in exercise tolerance, while the overall rehabilitation goal may be an improved quality of life (39) or psychosocial well-being (32-34,37). Although these are subjective outcomes and as such may be questioned in terms of quantification, they can be quantified and so amenable to statistical analysis. These subjective, patient-oriented outcomes may be more important for the patient than, for example, a small, although statistically significant, change in oxygen uptake (12,13,39). If in a randomized trial of early rehabilitation, quality of life is the primary outcome, it must be tested for its correlation with compliance (39). The real benefit of cardiac rehabilitation may in fact be more related to improvements in psychological well-being and quality of life than to such changes in outcomes as exercise tolerance (12,39).

Monitoring for Decay

It is one thing to be able to maintain adequate compliance while patients are in a supervised program. It is quite a different thing either to sustain the momentum when patients are on their own, having either graduated from or dropped out of a supervised program, or to demonstrate that there is long-term behavioral change with the patient taking responsibility for his or her own actions. The effort should be taken to determine long-term compliance with the intervention (36,76).

Ethical Issues

In descriptive or analytic studies of compliance, does the informed-consent doctrine mean that patients must be told that their compliance will be measured in a specific way at some particular time? Not only might this bias a study of compliance, but it also raises the ethics of attempting to manipulate human behavior. To help control this, the following recommendations might be implemented: include measurements of patients' self-perceptions as well as their social and emotional function before and after the intervention; involve patients with nontrivial disorders only, and only where an intervention has been shown to be beneficial; and include all possible side effects of the intervention and strategy in the informed consent (96,97).

Collaboration

The investigation of the effectiveness of compliance-enhancing strategies in cardiac rehabilitation requires a multidisciplinary approach with extensive collaboration between individuals with expertise in wide-ranging subjects, such as epidemiology, physiology, psychology, statistics, and economics. For example, in a randomized trial of early cardiac rehabilitation, with health-related quality of life as the primary outcome measure and exercise tolerance and psychological measures as secondary outcomes (39), we designed the trial to include an economic evaluation of comprehensive cardiac rehabilitation (98). It is this multidisciplinary approach that makes compliance research an exciting, if at times frustrating, endeavor.

Section Summary

Compliance is a concern in complex treatment programs that require an extended duration. Arguably, an ideal, or maximum, compliance that can reasonably be expected in a group of patients is approximately 75% to 85%. Although some program dropout does occur early in the intervention, dropouts often continue to comply with the required behavior change. There are few studies of compliance-enhancing strategies in cardiac rehabilitation, compared with, for example, antihypertensive drug therapy (99). Two trials of compliance-enhancing strategies in cardiac rehabilitation

(36,87) and the variable degree to which they were useful and successful in increasing compliance have been examined in detail elsewhere (7).

Summary

Effective programs must provide relevant services when patients need them the most. Wenger has argued for a menu approach to individualized cardiac rehabilitation services in the future (100). A possible model to stratify patients and thereby optimize utilization of individualized cardiac rehabilitation services is outlined in Figure 26.2. This model assumes that education and cardiovascular risk factor management are integral components of cardiac rehabilitation and that lines of communication between patients and providers must be carefully nurtured at all times (69). Whether or not this will help to enhance either short- or long-term compliance with prescribed behavior changes needs examination.

Despite knowing that the success of lifestyle modifications in our daily lives depends entirely on our own decisions to comply with the modifications, few researchers have conducted descriptive and experimental studies of compliance in cardiac rehabilitation. One reason for this lack of interest

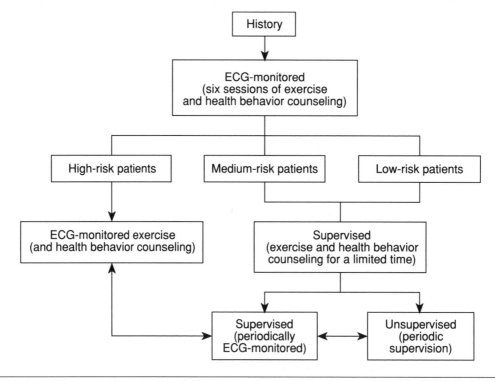

Figure 26.2 A model for stratification of patients into cardiac rehabilitation programs. (ECG = electrocardiographically.)

may be that compliance research is perceived to be based on "soft" rather than "hard" data, frequently collected where it cannot be observed by the investigator: It depends on what patients decide to do and what they report. One researcher's view, that "the worst of this widespread contempt for description is that it discourages people from even trying to analyze really complicated systems" (101), summarizes the discomfort with this kind of research and analysis. Even in clinical practice, compliance is frequently ignored by health care professionals.

The extent to which compliance with an intervention such as cardiac rehabilitation needs to be enhanced will obviously depend on a number of assumptions, including the safety and effectiveness of that intervention, the importance of the condition, the observed compliance with the intervention, and the strength of the source of evidence about effect and compliance. The safety of appropriately prescribed rehabilitation, including exercise, does not appear to be a concern, with few or no significant adverse effects reported in the trials examined in this chapter, and there is quite convincing evidence for greater improvement in outcome with greater compliance. It is apparent that the majority of the trials examined in this report were not investigations of compliance-enhancing strategies but rather investigations of intervention efficacy; therefore, inferences about compliance and compliance-enhancement should be made with caution. There can be little disagreement that with appropriate cardiac rehabilitation services and adequate compliance, there is a high likelihood of an accelerated (39,73-76,98) and possibly long-term (40,41,66,67) recovery with patients regaining as normal as possible a place in the community and leading an active productive life" (9).

Acknowledgments

This chapter is drawn with permission from the following publications: Oldridge, N.B. Cardiac rehabilitation exercise programme: Compliance and compliance-enhancing strategies. *Sports Med.* 6:42-55, 1988; and Oldridge, N.B. Compliance with cardiac rehabilitation services. *J. Cardiopulm. Rehabil.* 11:115-127, 1991.

References

1. American Heart Association. 1993 heart and stroke facts. Dallas: American Heart Association; 1993.

2. Wittels, E.H.; Hay, J.W.; Gotto, A.M. Medical costs of coronary artery disease in the United States. Am. J. Cardiol. 65:432-440; 1990.

3. American College of Chest Physicians. Cardiac rehabilitation services. Ann. Intern. Med. 109:671-673; 1988.

4. Byl, N.; Reed, P.; Franklin, B.; Gordon, S. Cost of phase II cardiac rehabilitation: Implications regarding ECG-monitoring practices [Abs]. Circulation. 78[Suppl. II]: 136; 1988.

5. Roper, W.L.; Winkenwerder, W.; Hackbarth, G.M.; Krakauer, H. Effectiveness in health care. An initiative to evaluate and improve medical practice. N. Engl. J. Med. 319:1197-1202; 1988.

6. Berlin, J.A.; Colditz, G.A. A meta-analysis of physical activity in the prevention of coronary heart disease. Am. J. Epidemiol. 132:612-628; 1990.

7. Oldridge, N.B. Cardiac rehabilitation exercise programme: Compliance and compliance-enhancing strategies. Sports Med. 6:42-55; 1988.

8. Oldridge, N.B.; Jones, N.L. Preventive use of exercise rehabilitation after myocardial infarction. Acta. Med. Scand. [Suppl.]. 711:123-129; 1986.

9. Rehabilitation of patients with cardiovascular disease: Report of a WHO expert committee. WHO Tech. Rep. Ser. 270: 1964.

10. Manson, J.E.; Tosteson, H.; Ridker, P.M.; Satterfield, S.; Herbert, P.; O'Connor, G.T.; Buring, J.E.; Hennekens, C.H. The primary prevention of myocardial infarction. N. Engl. J. Med. 326:1408-1416; 1993.

11. Siegel, D.; Grady, D.; Browner, W.S.; Hulley, S.B. Risk factor modification after myocardial infarction. Ann. Intern. Med. 109:213-218; 1988.

12. Wenger, N.K.; Alpert, J.S. Rehabilitation of the coronary patient in 1989. Arch. Intern. Med. 149:1504-1506; 1989.

13. Oldridge, N.B. Cardiac rehabilitation, self-responsibility, and quality of life. J. Cardiopul. Rehabil. 6:153-156; 1986.

14. Position paper of the American Association of Cardiovascular and Pulmonary Rehabilitation. The efficacy of risk factor intervention and psychosocial aspects of cardiac rehabilitation. J. Cardiopul. Rehabil. 10:198-209; 1990.

15. Oldridge, N.B.; Guyatt, G.H.; Fischer, M.E.; Rimm, A.A. Cardiac rehabilitation after myocardial infarction. JAMA. 260:945-950; 1988.

16. O'Connor, G.T.; Buring, J.E.; Yusuf, S.; Goldhaber, S.Z.; Olmstead, E.M.; Paffenbarger, R.S.; Hennekens, C.H. An overview of randomized trials of rehabilitation with exercise after myocardial infarction. Circulation. 80:234-244; 1989.

17. Feinstein, A. A "compliance bias" and the interpretation of therapeutic trials. In: Haynes, R.B.; Taylor, D.W.; Sackett, D.L., eds. Compliance in health care. Baltimore: Johns Hopkins University Press; 1979:309-322.

18. Horwitz, R.I.; Viscoli, C.M.; Berkman, L.; Donaldson, R.M.; Horwitz, S.M.; Murray, D.F.; Sindelar,

J. Treatment adherence and risk of death after a myocardial infarction. Lancet. 336:542-545; 1990.

19. Sackett, D.L.; Snow, J.C. The magnitude of compliance and noncompliance. In: Haynes, R.B.; Taylor, D.W.; Sackett, D.L., eds. Baltimore: Johns Hopkins University Press; 1979:11-22.

20. Kentala, E. Physical fitness and feasibility of physical rehabilitation after myocardial infarction in men of working age. Clin. Res. 4[Suppl. 9]:1-84; 1972.

21. Wilhelmsen, L.; Sanne, H.; Elmfeldt, D.; Grimby, G.; Tibblin, G.; Wedel, H. A controlled trial of physical training after myocardial infarction. Prev. Med. 4:491-508; 1975.

22. Kallio, V.; Hamalainen, H.; Hakklia, J.; Luurila, O.J. Reduction in sudden deaths by a multifactorial intervention programme after acute myocardial infarction. Lancet. ii:1091-1094; 1979.

23. Shaw, L.W. for the project staff. Effects of a prescribed supervised exercise program on mortality and cardiovascular morbidity in patients after a myocardial infarction. National exercise and heart disease project. Am. J. Cardiol. 48:39-46; 1981.

24. Stern, M.J.; Cleary, P. National exercise and heart disease project. Long-term psychosocial outcome. Arch. Intern. Med. 142:1093-1097; 1982.

25. Carson, P.; Phillips, R.; Lloyd, M.; Tucker, H.; Neophytou, M.; Buch, N.J.; Lawton, A.; Simpson, T. Exercise after myocardial infarction: A controlled trial. J. R. Coll. Physicians Lond. 16:147-151; 1982.

26. Rechnitzer, P.A.; Cunningham, D.A.; Andrew, G.M.; Buck, C.W.; Jones, N.L.; Kavanagh, T.K.; Oldridge, N.B.; Parker, J.O.; Shephard, R.J.; Sutton, J.R.; Donner, A.P. Relation of exercise to the recurrence rate of myocardial infarction in men. Ontario Exercise-heart Collaborative Study. Am. J. Cardiol. 51:65-69; 1883.

27. Oldridge, N.B.; Donner, A.; Buck, C.; Jones, N.L.; Andrew, G.M.; Parker, J.O.; Cunningham, D.A.; Kavanagh, T.K.; Rechnitzer, P.A.; Sutton, J.R. Predictors of dropout from the Ontario Exercise-heart Collaborative Study. Am. J. Cardiol. 1:70-74; 1983.

28. Roman, O.; Gutierrez, M.; Luksic, I.; Chavez, E.; Camuzzi, A.L.; Villalon, E.; Klenner, C.; Cumsille, F. Cardiac rehabilitation after acute myocardial infarction. 9-year controlled follow-up study. Cardiology. 70:223-231; 1983.

29. Vermeulen, A.; Lie, K.I.; Durrer, D. Effects of cardiac rehabilitation after myocardial infarction: Changes in coronary risk factors and long-term prognosis. Am. Heart J. 105:798-801; 1983.

30. World Health Organization. Rehabilitation and comprehensive secondary prevention after acute myocardial infarction. EURO Rep. Stud. 84:1-99; 1983.

31. Marra, S.; Paolillo, V.; Spadaccini, F.; Angelino, P.F. Long-term follow-up after a controlled randomized post-myocardial infarction rehabilitation programme: Effects on morbidity and mortality. Eur. Heart J. 6:656-663; 1985.

32. Mayou, R.; MacMahon, D.; Sleight, P.; Florencio, M.J. Early rehabilitation after myocardial infarction. Lancet. 2:1399-1401; 1981.

33. Bengtsson, K. Rehabilitation after myocardial infarction—A controlled study. Scand. J. Rehabil. Med. 15:1-9; 1983.

34. Stern, M.J.; Gorman, P.A.; Kaslow, P. The group counsel in exercise therapy study: A controlled intervention with subjects following myocardial infarction. Arch. Intern. Med. 143:1719-1725; 1983.

35. Froelicher, V.; Jensen, D.; Genter, F.; Sullivan, M.; McKirnan, M.D.; Wiztum, K.; Strong, M.L.; Ashburn, W. A randomized trial of exercise training in patients with coronary heart disease. JAMA. 252:1291-1297; 1984.

36. Daltroy, L.H. Improving cardiac patient adherence to exercise regimens: A clinical trial of health education. J. Cardiopul. Rehabil. 5:40-49; 1985.

37. Burgess, A.W.; Lerner, D.J.; D'Agostino, R.B.; Vokonas, P.S.; Hartman, C.R.; Gaccione, P. A randomized trial of cardiac rehabilitation. Soc. Sci. Med. 24:359-370; 1987.

38. Goble, A.J.; Hare, D.L.; Macdonald, P.S.; Oliver, R.G.; Reid, M.A.; Worcester, M.C. Effect of early programmes of high and low intensity exercise on physical performance after transmural acute myocardial infarction. Br. Heart J. 65:126-131; 1991.

39. Oldridge, N.B.; Guyatt, G.; Jones, N.L.; Crowe, J.; Singer, J.; Feeny, D.; McKelvie, R.; Runions, J.; Streiner, D.; Torrence, G. Effects on quality of life with comprehensive cardiac rehabilitation after acute myocardial infarction. Am. J. Cardiol. 67:1084-1089; 1991.

40. P.R.E. Cor. Group. Comparison of a rehabilitation programme, a counseling programme and usual care after an acute myocardial infarction: Results of a long-term randomized trial. Eur. Heart J. 10:55-62; 1989.

41. Hamalainen, H.; Luurila, O.J.; Kallio, V.; Knuts, L-R.; Arstila, M.; Hakkila, J. Long-term education in sudden deaths after a multifactorial intervention programme in patients with myocardial infarction: 10-year results of a controlled investigation. Eur. Heart J. 10:55-62; 1989.

42. Mazzuca, S.A. Does patient education in chronic disease have therapeutic value? J. Chronic Dis. 35:521-529; 1982.

43. Greenland, P.; Chu, J.S. Efficacy of cardiac rehabilitation services with an emphasis on patients after myocardial infarction. Ann. Intern. Med. 109:650-663; 1988.

44. Rossouw, J.E.; Lewis, B.; Rifkind, B.M. The value of lowering cholesterol after myocardial infarction. N. Engl. J. Med. 323:1112-1119; 1990.

45. The Coronary Drug Project Research Group. Clofibrate and niacin in coronary heart disease. JAMA. 231:360-381; 1975.

46. Canner, P.L.; Berge, K.G.; Wenger, N.K.; Stamler, J.; Friedman, L.; Prineas, R.J.; Friedewald, W.; for

The Coronary Drug Project Research Group. Fifteen year mortality in Coronary Drug Project patients: Long-term benefit with niacin. J. Am. Coll. Cardiol. 8:1245-1255; 1986.

47. The Coronary Drug Project Research Group. Influence of adherence to treatment and response of cholesterol on mortality in the Coronary Drug Project. N. Engl. J. Med. 303:1038-1041; 1980.

48. Brensike, F.J.; Levy, R.I.; Kelsey, S.F.; Passamian, E.R.; Richardson, J.M.; Loh, I.K.; Stone, N.J.; Aldrich, R.F.; Battaglini, J.W.; Moriarty, D.J.; Fisher, M.R.; Friedman, L.; Friedewald, W.; Detre, K.M.; Epstein, S.E. Effects of therapy with cholestyramine on progression of coronary arteriosclerosis: Results of the NHLBI type II coronary intervention study. Circulation. 69:313-324; 1984.

49. Blankenhorn, D.H.; Nessim, S.A.; Johnson, R.L.; Sanmarco, M.E.; Azen, S.P.; Cashin-Hemphill, L. Beneficial effects of combined cholestipol-niacin therapy on coronary atherosclerosis and coronary venous bypass grafts. JAMA. 257:3233-3240; 1987.

50. LaRosa, J.C.; Cleary, P.; Muesing, R.A.; Hellerstein, H.K.; Naughton, J. Effect of long-term moderate physical exercise on plasma lipoproteins. Arch. Intern. Med. 142:2269-2274; 1982.

51. Singh, R.B.; Rastogi, S.S.; Verna, R.; Laxmi, R.; Ghosh, S.; Niaz, M.A. Randomized trial of cardioprotective diet in patients with recent acute myocardial infarction: Results of one year follow-up. Br. Med. J. 304:1015-1019; 1992.

52. Hennekens, C.H.; Satterfield, S.; Hebert, P.R. Treatment of elevated blood pressure to prevent coronary heart disease. In: Higgins, M.W.; Luepker, R.V., eds. New York: Oxford University Press; 1988: 103-108.

53. Hypertension Detection and Follow-up Program Cooperative Group. Persistence of reduction in blood pressure and mortality of participants in the Hypertension Detection and Follow-up Program. JAMA. 259:2113-2122; 1988.

54. Fielding, J.E. Smoking: Health effects and control. N. Engl. J. Med. 313:491-498; 1985.

55. Fielding, J.E. Smoking: Health effects and control. N. Engl. J. Med. 313:555-561; 1985.

56. Mulcahy, R. The longterm care of the coronary patient. New York: Churchill Livingstone; 1990: 91-97.

57. Krumholz, H.M.; Cohen, B.J.; Tsevat, J.; Pasternak, R.C.; Weinstein, M.C. Cost-effectiveness of a smoking cessation program after myocardial infarction. J. Am. Coll. Cardiol. 22:1697-1702; 1993.

58. Hermanson, B.; Omenn, G.S.; Kronmal, R.A.; Participants in the Coronary Artery Surgery Study. Beneficial six-year outcome of smoking cessation in older men and women with coronary artery disease. N. Engl. J. Med. 319:1365-1369; 1988.

59. Perkins, J.; Dick, T.B.S. Smoking and myocardial infarction: Secondary prevention. Postgrad. Med. J. 61:295-300; 1985.

60. Sivarajan, E.S.; Newton, K.M.; Almes, M.J.; Kempf, T.; Mansfield, L.; Bruce, R. Limited effects of outpatient teaching and counseling after myocardial infarction: A controlled study. Heart Lung. 12:65-73; 1983.

61. Hedback, B.; Perk, J.; Perski, A. Effect of a post-myocardial infarction rehabilitation program on mortality, morbidity, and risk factors. J. Cardiopulm. Rehabil. 5:576-583; 1983.

62. Shekelle, R.B.; Gale, M.; Norusis, M. Type A score (Jenkins activity survey) and risk of recurrent coronary heart disease in the aspirin myocardial infarction study. Am. J. Cardiol. 56:221-225; 1985.

63. Case, R.B.; Heller, S.S.; Case, N.B.; the Multicenter Post-Infarction Research Group. Type A behavior and survival after acute myocardial infarction. N. Engl. J. Med. 312:737-741; 1985.

64. Ragland, D.R.; Brand, R.J. Type A behavior and mortality from coronary heart disease. N. Engl. J. Med. 318:65-69; 1988.

65. Friedman, M.; Thoresen, C.E.; Gill, J.J.; Ulmer, D.; Powell, L.H.; Price, V.A.; Brown, B.B.; Thompson, L.; Rabin, D.D.; Breall, W.S.; Bourg, E.; Levy, R.; Dixon, T. Alteration of type A behavior and its effect on cardiac recurrences in post myocardial infarction patients: Summary results of the Recurrent Coronary Prevention Project. Am. Heart J. 112:653-665; 1986.

66. Frasure-Smith, N.; Prince, R. The ischemic heart disease life stress monitoring program: Impact on mortality. Psychosom. Med. 47:431-445; 1985.

67. Frasure-Smith, N. In hospital symptoms of psychological stress as predictors of longterm outcome following acute myocardial infarction in men. Am. J. Cardiol. 67:121-127; 1991.

68. Martin, J.E.; Dubbert, P.M. Adherence to exercise. Exerc. Sport Sci. Rev. 13:137-167; 1985.

69. Oldridge, N.B. Compliance with cardiac rehabilitation services. J. Cardiopulm. Rehabil. 11:115-127; 1991.

70. Blodgett, C.; Pekarik, G. Program evaluation in cardiac rehabilitation III: Utilization assessment. J. Cardiopulm. Rehabil. 7:410-414; 1987.

71. Oldridge, N.B.; Ragowski, B.; Gottlieb, M. Use of rehabilitation services: Factors associated with attendance. J. Cardiopulm. Rehabil. 12:25-31; 1992.

72. Andrew, G.M.; Oldridge, N.B.; Parker, J.O.; Cunningham, D.A.; Rechnitzer, P.A.; Jones, N.L.; Buck, C.W.; Kavanagh, T.K.; Shephard, R.J.; Sutton, J.R.; McDonald, W. Reasons for dropout from exercise programs in post-coronary patients. Med. Sci. Sports Exerc. 13:164-168; 1981.

73. Miller, N.H.; Haskell, W.L.; Berra, K.; DeBusk, R.F. Home versus group exercise training for increasing functional capacity after myocardial infarction. Circulation. 70:645-649; 1984.

74. Hung, J.; Gordon, E.P.; Houston, N.; Haskell, W.L.; Goris, M.L.; DeBusk, R.F. Changes in rest and exercise myocardial perfusion and left ventricular function 3 to 26 weeks after clinically uncomplicated acute myocardial infarction: Effects of training. Am. J. Cardiol. 54:943-950; 1984.

75. DeBusk, R.F.; Haskell, W.L.; Miller, N.H.; Berra, K.; Taylor, C.B.; Berger, W.E.; Lew, H. Medically directed at-home rehabilitation soon after uncomplicated acute myocardial infarction: A new model for patient care. Am. J. Cardiol. 55:251-257; 1985.

76. Taylor, C.B.; Houston-Miller, N.; Haskell, W.L.; DeBusk, R.F. Smoking cessation after acute myocardial infarction: The effects of exercise training. Addict. Behav. 13:331-335; 1988.

77. Oldridge, N.B.; Spencer, J. Exercise habits and perceptions before and after graduation or dropout from supervised cardiac exercise rehabilitation. J. Cardiopul. Rehabil. 5:313-319; 1985.

78. Hedback, B.; Perk, J. 5-year results of a comprehensive rehabilitation programme after myocardial infarction. Eur. Heart J. 8:234-242; 1987.

79. Prosser, G.; Carson, P.; Phillips, R. Exercise after myocardial infarction: Long-term rehabilitation effects. J. Psychosom. Res. 29:535-540; 1985.

80. Oldridge, N.B.; Streiner, D. Health belief model as a predictor of compliance with cardiac rehabilitation. Med. Sci. Sports Exerc. 22:678-683; 1990.

81. Stegman, M.R.; Miller, P.J.; Hageman, R.K.; Irby, D.E.; Kositzky-Klutman, A.K.; Rajek, N.J. Myocardial infarction survival: How important are patients' attitudes and adherence behaviors? Am. J. Prev. Med. 3:147-151; 1987.

82. Conroy, R.M.; Cahill, S.; Mulcahy, R.; Johnson, H.; Graham, I.M.; Hickey, N. The relation of social class to risk factors, rehabilitation, compliance and mortality in survivors of acute coronary heart disease. Scand. J. Soc. Med. 14:51-56; 1986.

83. Kavanagh, T.; Shephard, R.J.; Chisolm, A.W.; Qureshi, S.; Kennedy, J. Prognostic indexes for patients with ischemic heart disease enrolled in an exercise-centered rehabilitation program. Am. J. Cardiol. 44:1230-1240; 1979.

84. Abbott, A.V.; Peters, R.K.; Vogel, M.E. Type A behavior and exercise: A follow-up study of coronary patients. J. Psychosom. Res. 34:153-162; 1990.

85. Miller, P.; Wikoff, R.; McMahon, M.; Garrett, M.J.; Ringel, K.; Collura, D.; Siniscalchi, K.; Sommer, S.; Welch, N. Personal adjustments and regimen compliance 1 year after myocardial infarction. Heart Lung. 18:339-346; 1989.

86. Giese, H.; Schomer, H.H. Life-style changes and mood profile of cardiac patients after an exercise rehabilitation program. J. Cardiopul. Rehabil. 6:30-37; 1986.

87. Bruce, E.H.; Frederick, R.; Bruce, R.A.; Fisher, L.D. Comparison of active participants and dropouts in CAPRI cardiopulmonary rehabilitation programs. Am. J. Cardiol. 37:53-60; 1976.

88. Oldridge, N.B.; Jones, N.L. Improving patient compliance in cardiac exercise rehabilitation: Effects of written agreement and self-monitoring. J. Cardiac. Rehabil. 3:257-262; 1983.

89. Taylor, C.B.; Bandura, A.; Ewart, C.K.; Miller, N.H.; DeBusk, R.F. Exercise testing to enhance wives' confidence in their husbands' cardiac capability soon after clinically uncomplicated acute myocardial infarction. Am. J. Cardiol. 55:635-638; 1985.

90. Miller, P.J.; Wikoff, R. Spouses' psychosocial problems, resources, and marital functioning postmyocardial infarction. Prog. Cardiovasc. Nurs. 4:71-76; 1989.

91. Daltroy, L.H.; Godin, G. The influence of spousal approval and patient perception of spousal approval on cardiac patient participation in exercise programs. J. Cardiopul. Rehabil. 9:363-367; 1989.

92. Ebbesen, L.S.; Guyatt, G.H.; McCartney, N.; Oldridge, N.B. Measuring quality of life in cardiac spouses. J. Clin. Epidemiol. 43:481-487; 1990.

93. Hilbert, G.A. Spouse support and myocardial infarction patient compliance. Nurs. Res. 34:217-220; 1985.

94. Dracup, K. A controlled trial of couples group counseling in cardiac rehabilitation. J. Cardiopul. Rehabil. 5:436-442; 1985.

95. Bramwell, L. Wive's experiences in the support role after husbands' first myocardial infarction. Heart Lung. 15:578-584; 1986.

96. Sackett, D.L. Methods for compliance research. In: Haynes, R.B.; Taylor, D.W.; Sackett, D.L., eds. Compliance in health care. Baltimore: Johns Hopkins University Press; 1979:323-333.

97. Haynes, R.B. Compliance with health advice: An overview with special reference to exercise programs. J. Cardiopul. Rehabil. 4:120-123; 1984.

98. Oldridge, N.; Furlong, W.; Feeny, D.; Torrance, G.; Guyatt, G.; Crowe, J.; Jones, N. Economic evaluation soon after myocardial infarction. Am. J. Cardiol. 72:154-161; 1993.

99. Gotto, A.M. Interactions of the major risk factors for coronary heart disease. Am. J. Med. 80[Suppl. 2A]:48-55; 1986.

100. Wenger, N.K. Future directions in cardiovascular rehabilitation. J. Cardiopul. Rehabil. 7:186-174; 1987.

101. Lorenz, K.Z. The fashionable fallacy of dispensing with description. Naturwissenschaften. 60:1-9; 1973.

Chapter 27

Returning the Patient to Work

Mary C. Gutmann
Lois M. Sheldahl
Felix E. Tristani
Nancy A. Wilke

Over 350,000 previously employed individuals in the United States survive a myocardial infarction (MI) or undergo coronary artery bypass graft (CABG) surgery or percutaneous transluminal coronary angioplasty (PTCA) each year (1). Despite major advances in medical and surgical management of coronary artery disease (CAD), there has been little or no improvement in return-to-work rates after a cardiac event. Reported rates of return to work vary from 49% to 93%, depending on the study population, treatment modalities, length of follow-up, and outcome criteria. On average, about 20% of previously employed individuals do not return to work following MI or CABG surgery. The large, multicenter Coronary Artery Surgery Study showed a consistent further annual decline in employment rate in both medically and surgically treated groups. At 1, 5, and 10 years after entry, 60%, 56%, and 34% of the surgical group were employed, compared with 66%, 50%, and 32% of the medical group (2). These results suggest that CABG surgery did not improve work resumption, and that many who initially resume work after medical or surgical intervention do not remain at work.

The failure of individuals with cardiovascular disease (CVD) to resume work has an enormous economic impact. Social Security disability payments for CVD total over $5 billion annually, and some people receive disability funds from other sources or take early retirement. Even an unnecessary delay in resuming work after a cardiac event can result in significant societal economic loss. Dennis et al. (3) showed that a focused work evaluation intervention designed to promote a timely return to work reduced the convalescence period by 32% and resulted in a savings of $2,102/patient based on earned income. Further assessment of a focused work evaluation program for MI patients

showed a savings of over $800 million nationally, including $160 million in medical cost savings and $675 million in additional earned income (4). Beside economic concerns, the social and psychological impact of occupational disability is immeasurable (5).

Thus, return to work is an important goal of cardiac rehabilitation and an appropriate measure of success in the treatment of CAD. This chapter reviews the variables associated with occupational outcome following MI and CABG surgery, describes a systematic approach to work evaluation, and discusses systemic factors that can facilitate the work resumption process, including interactions among the health care sector, industry, and organizations that grant disability funds.

Determinants of Return to Work

The decision to return to work is a complex process. No single variable can adequately explain the variance. The determinants of disability might best be conceptualized within a biopsychosocial model that takes into account factors related to disease, person and situation, and the interactions between patients and systems that affect occupational outcome (6).

Knowledge of medical and nonmedical factors that predispose patients to depart prematurely from the work place can be used to focus programs of intervention designed to preserve employment whenever appropriate. Many nonmedical factors contribute to the failure of patients to work until a normal retirement age, and some of these factors may be amenable to change through a multidimensional rehabilitation program designed to optimize return-to-work decisions.

Medical and Clinical Factors

The role of medical factors in determining return to work is equivocal at best (7-13). In a multivariable model for predicting 1-year work status after diagnostic cardiac catheterization, Mark et al. (11) found that medical factors accounted for only 20% of the predictive information at 1-year follow-up, whereas demographic and socioeconomic factors accounted for 45% and physical and emotional factors for 29%. Congestive heart failure (CHF) and extracardiac vascular disease were the only independent clinical predictors of 1-year work status in their multivariate analysis, although left ventricular ejection fraction (LVEF) and the number of diseased vessels were univariate predictors. In other studies, severity of disease was shown to have a weak but positive relationship to return to work following MI (12,14) and CABG surgery (15). The New York Heart Association's functional class designations and the extent of CAD were not found to predict return to work (7, 16, 17), but a history of prior MI was associated with failure to return to work in some patients (7,13,18). Preoperative index of disease severity have generally been nonpredictive of return to work, but success of revascularization (7,19,20) and functional improvement after surgery as evidenced by increased LVEF, maximum heart rate (HR), exercise tolerance, and symptomatic relief were associated with a greater likelihood of return to work (7,8,21-25).

The relief of angina pectoris appears to be a particularly salient factor. Relief from incapacitating angina is a common indication for CABG surgery. Approximately 70% to 90% of patients do obtain relief from disabling angina, suggesting that the majority of patients could be expected to return to work after surgery (2,25). The absence or presence of postoperative angina was shown to be predictive of follow-up employment status in some studies (16,26,27). However, Symmes et al. (27) found that improvement in work status (19%) did not match the percentage of patients in whom symptoms were relieved (80%) and that only 28% of patients reported symptoms as a reason for unemployment. Anderson et al. (28) reported that the effect of angina on reemployment was greater in younger patients. There was a 34% increase in return to work (from 49% to 83%) with relief of symptoms after CABG surgery among subjects 50 to 54 years of age compared with only a 9% (from 33% to 42%) increase among subjects 60 to 64 years of age. Thus, medical factors may play a greater role in decisions to return to work in younger patients,

whereas sociodemographic and employment factors may be more influential with patients closer to retirement age.

The type of intervention may also differ in its effects on return to work. Convalescent time is typically shorter after PTCA than after CABG surgery or MI. Some (9,16), but not all (11,29), investigators have also reported a higher rate of work resumption with PTCA. Yet over 10% of those employed at the time of PTCA fail to resume work, and many return to work after more than 1 month of convalescence (9,30).

Sociodemographic Variables

Nonmedical factors play a critical role and may in fact mediate the effects of physical and medical factors on the decision to return to work. Older age has consistently been shown to impact work resumption. Patients over 60 years of age are much less likely to return to work after an acute MI or CABG surgery (31,32). Some studies report a linear relationship between increasing age and failure to return to work (33,17), while others find a significant drop in return to work after age 55 or 60 (7,23,26). The effects of age may differ depending on the culture and country. American studies indicate age 60 as a threshold for increased retirement after surgery, while other countries, such as Spain, Ireland, and the Scandinavian countries, report a threshold for earlier retirement at age 50 or 55 (8). Shanfield (14) suggests that age reflects life cycle variables that affect decisions to return to work or retire.

Level of education and job classification have been shown to influence work resumption after an acute cardiac event (7,8,11,12,23,26,33). Many studies have shown that blue-collar workers return to work less frequently than white-collar workers (8,11-13,26). This could be related to several factors, including the physical work demands of the job, career goals, job satisfaction, job prestige, psychological stress, and decision latitude. One study of patients after CABG surgery reported an 81% return to work among professionals, 75% for administrators and executives, 61% for clerical and salespeople, 62% for skilled workers, and 34% for semiskilled workers (7).

There is relatively little data on the influence of gender on work resumption after a cardiac event, since most studies have focused on men. The current data suggest that women return to work less frequently and after a longer convalescent time than men (7,8,14,25,33,34). Women tend to be older, have less self-confidence in resuming work, express greater anxiety and depression, and have less economic incentives to return to work than men. With the increasing proportion of women entering the work force, greater attention needs to be directed at the effects of CVD on work resumption in this population.

The influence of ethnic background on work resumption has also received minimal attention. Race was found to be an independent predictor of work resumption in one study (11), although the authors speculated that the underlying factor may have been socioeconomic status.

Work-Related Factors

Preoperative work status, specifically, unemployment and the length of time out of work before a cardiac event, has been shown to be significantly related to the likelihood of work resumption (7,15,17,19,23,35-37). David (38) suggested that a period of "invalidism" greater than 6 months resulted in a 50% chance of permanent invalidism. Almeida et al. (7) cautioned that preoperative work status may reflect such additional factors as severity of disease, socioeconomic factors, and motivation and should not be considered an independent predictor of postoperative work status. However, this factor is unequivocally the most consistent finding across studies and can be a marker to identify individuals in need of intervention to prevent premature retirement or permanent disability.

A second major factor in determining return to work is the availability of disability compensation (8,23,33,34,35). Work resumption rates in the former West Germany are lower than in the United States, where disability compensation is more difficult to obtain (8). In the United States, determination of residual cardiac impairment is not a uniform process, so that some patients may qualify for disability funds with less severe cardiac impairment than others (10).

Some employers may be reluctant to restore cardiac patients to their work force because of liability risks. A survey in the Toronto Rehabilitation Center revealed that 10% of those who did not return to work cited employer attitudes as the reason for continued disability (24).

Other job-related factors that represent potential barriers to work resumption after a major cardiac event include high unemployment rates, the lack of alternative jobs or retraining opportunities, restrictive policies about return to work, and inflexible employer attitudes (8,14,24). The recent enactment of the Americans With Disabilities Act in the United States may reduce employment barriers, since it prohibits disqualification of workers or job applicants because of a history of CAD. An employer may, however, request a medical examination after a job offer has been made in occupations governed by law and safety regulations such as with airline pilots and truck drivers.

Psychological Factors

The psychological impact of an acute cardiac event can have a major influence in the patient's ability and desire to resume work. Approximately one-third of patients experience significant emotional distress after an acute MI or CABG surgery (14,23,39,40). In one study, 70% of the patients who experienced significant depression were still depressed 1 year later (41). Psychiatric difficulties are not only correlated with a lower return to work, but a longer convalescence period (14). In contrast the Type A behavior pattern is associated with earlier and higher rates of return to work (8,42).

Patients' perceptions of their health status and work tolerance can also have a major influence on their decision to resume work (23,32,37). Furthermore, their beliefs about the causes and consequences of CAD can determine their coping strategies, including decisions about work resumption (36). Gutmann et al. (23) found that 85% of cardiac patients believe that stress is a cause of their disease. Perceived job stress as a contributing factor significantly lowered the probability of work resumption (3,15). Likewise, job satisfaction and positive expectations for work resumption contributed to a higher rate of return to work (12,26,43). Thus, patient perceptions, expectations, and self-confidence interact with objective indexes of cardiovascular function to influence decisions about resuming work. Interventions to enhance positive expectations and self-confidence can facilitate work resumption and prevent self-imposed disability. Ewart and colleagues (44) have effectively demonstrated the influence of perceived self-efficacy in determining subsequent levels and types of physical activity. In a prospective study of 82 patients employed prior to PTCA, self-efficacy was found to be the strongest predictor of return to work 1 month after treatment (9).

Medical Advice

Physician attitudes and advice can have a major impact on patients' decisions regarding if and when to return to work. In three studies, 35% to

59% of patients cited physician advice as the reason for not working (7,24,45). The advice given to the patient by the physician can be influenced by several factors, including the medical information available to the physician, the patient's job requirements and the physician's understanding of these, patient and family expectations, and societal economic concerns. As discussed later, granting disability funds through the Social Security Administration in the United States is an administrative function of that agency. The physician's role is to document the degree of cardiac impairment (46).

Systematic Approach to Work Evaluation

Vocational assessment early in the rehabilitation process can provide objective information to patients, physicians, and employers about patients' capabilities and limitations and can build confidence in their decisions about work resumption. A systematic approach to work assessment is described in this section, along with a discussion of the interactions between health care professionals, industry, and disability support systems. The integration of biological, psychological, and social parameters ensures a comprehensive approach to this very complex, multifactorial problem and has the greatest potential for improving the occupational outcome of cardiac treatment and rehabilitation.

Vocational Assessment

Vocational assessment in a cardiac rehabilitation program has at least two goals: (1) determination of the feasibility and safety of work resumption for individual patients and (2) identification of potential problems related to work resumption. The results of the assessment will allow health professionals to give informed and more appropriate and specific recommendations on whether and when the patient can resume work and what changes, if any, need to be made in his or her work activities. Further, assessment results should suggest interventions for dealing with problems related to work resumption.

The assessment procedure should be initiated during the inpatient phase of rehabilitation, since early intervention tends to reduce the anxiety level of patients regarding their cardiac event. Since most patients can be reassured that they will be able to resume a meaningful and productive life, early intervention may help to prevent patients from adopting inappropriate disability perceptions and behaviors that, once developed, become difficult to reverse.

The assessment procedure during the inpatient phase begins with a clinical evaluation. Once the patient's condition is stabilized, other assessment procedures can be initiated while the patient is in the hospital. Some of the most important aspects of the vocational assessment include assessment of the patient's premorbid occupational requirements, emotional status, perceived psychological stressors, financial concerns, and response to exercise. The probability of returning to work can be discussed with the patient and family at the time of hospital discharge based on the information gathered from the inpatient assessment process. Before the final decision is made on whether or not to recommend that the patient return to work after MI and CABG surgery, the patient should be further evaluated. Determination of the patient's physical work tolerance at this time is quite beneficial in making decisions on the return to work. Some of the major assessment procedures will be discussed in greater detail in the following sections.

Clinical Assessment

The clinical assessment is an ongoing process that starts with the patient's admission to the hospital and continues throughout the rehabilitation process. In addition to evaluating the patient's cardiac function and associated cardiac complications, clinical assessment should cover other medical problems that could affect the patient's ability to participate in an exercise program or resume previous employment. A medical history, physical examination, resting electrocardiogram (ECG), and chest x-ray will usually uncover most abnormalities. Patients with significant cardiac symptoms may require further diagnostic work-up, which could include arrhythmia monitoring, rest and exercise cardiac imaging studies, and cardiac catheterization. Appropriate medical or surgical therapy may be required to improve symptoms before the patient is able to return to work.

Job Analysis

In evaluating the ability of a patient to return to work and in preventing disability disproportionate to disease, it is important to know the physiological and psychological demands of the patient's occupational work and his or her perceptions and concerns in these areas. This information is also important for referring selected patients for special programs, such as arm exercise training and stress management.

The major determinants of cardiovascular stress on the job are the type of work, energy demands, amount and length of work, environmental conditions, and job-related psychological stress. Several resource materials can be used in conjunction with a patient interview to assess the patient's work demands, including *Dictionary of Occupational Titles* (47), *Selected Characteristics of Occupations Defined in the Dictionary of Occupational Titles* (48), and energy cost tables (49-51).

Type of Physical Work

Physical work can be classified into two major types: dynamic and static. It is well established that the cardiovascular responses to these two types of work differ. Dynamic work produces primarily a volume load on the heart, whereas static work produces primarily a pressure load (52-54). Combined static-dynamic work may produce a combination of volume and pressure loads on the heart. A concern with dynamic work is that the circulatory demands may exceed appropriate limits for some cardiac patients; a concern with static work is that cardiac afterload may exceed acceptable levels. Laboratory graded exercise tests (GXTs) are available to evaluate dynamic, static-dynamic, and static effort (50,55,56).

Maximal oxygen intake ($\dot{V}O_2$max) with upper extremity work is typically 20% to 40% less than with lower extremity work (50,53). This is primarily attributed to lesser upper-extremity muscle mass. HR and arterial blood pressure (BP) at a given work load tend to be higher with upper-extremity work than with lower-extremity work.

Energy Requirements

In jobs requiring physical work, the energy expenditure requirements of job tasks represent the major determinant of myocardial oxygen demands. It should be noted, though, that several work-related factors, such as temperature stress, psychological stress, exercising in an awkward body position, and static work may have little effect on total body oxygen uptake $\dot{V}O_2$, but can significantly increase myocardial oxygen requirements. The approximate energy costs of selected

occupational tasks are shown in Table 27.1; more complete listings are available (49-51). It should be emphasized that the energy costs of activities presented in published tables are only approximations. The actual energy cost of work can vary with several factors, including the rate of work, the efficiency of the worker, and such personal characteristics as age, sex, fitness level, body size, and orthopedic disabilities. In using energy cost tables, it is important to note that the data is based principally on studies performed before 1960 (49,57-59). Increased automation and mechanization in the workplace since that time have significantly decreased the energy demands of some work tasks. Furthermore, most listings of energy costs are based on responses of workers without known CVD (50,60). Whether differences exist in workers with CVD is not clear (50). Recently, a few studies have reported on energy expenditure rates for selected job tasks in patients with CAD (61-68) and in the general working population (69,70).

Environmental Conditions

Many jobs require work to be performed under less than ideal temperature conditions. When work is combined with heat stress, especially when the environment is also humid, myocardial oxygen requirements may increase due to increased thermoregulatory blood flow requirements (71,72). When work is performed in a cold environment, patients may experience symptoms of angina pectoris at a lower level of effort than they would in a neutral environment. This may be the result of an increase in myocardial oxygen demand associated with a cold-induced rise in arterial BP or an increase in energy expenditure due to wearing heavier clothing, walking through snow, and possibly shivering (73). Based on ambulatory monitoring of left ventricular function during work in situations of moderate heat and cold stress, asymptomatic patients with relatively good functional work capacity do not show an alteration in LVEF compared with exercise at a comparable rate-pressure produce (RPP) in a neutral environment (62,74). Ventricular arrhythmias also do not seem to be increased by moderate warm and cold conditions (62,63,74). Physical work at high altitude will represent a higher relative cardiovascular stress than at sea level (if performed at the same absolute work output) because work capacity is reduced with lower air oxygen content (75).

Workers sometimes are exposed to other physical agents, like noise, vibration, and electricity, and

Table 27.1   Approximate Energy Requirements[a] for Various Occupational Work Loads

Expenditure	Occupation	Expenditure	Occupation
1.5-2 METs 2-2.5 kcal/min	Desk work Auto driving Typing Electric calculating machine operation	6-7 METs 7-8 kcal/min	Shoveling 10 times/min (4.5 kg or 10 lb)
2-3 METs 2.5-4 kcal/min	Auto repair Radio, TV repair Janitorial work Typing, manual Bartending	7-8 METs 8-10 kcal/min	Digging ditches Carrying 36.3 kg or 80 lb Sawing hardwood
3-4 METs 4-5 kcal/min	Brick laying, plastering Wheelbarrow (45.4-kg or 100-lb load) Machine assembly Trailer-truck in traffic Welding (moderate load) Cleaning windows	8-9 METs 10-11 kcal/min	Shoveling 10 times/min (6.4 kg or 14 lb)
4-5 METs 4-5 kcal/min	Painting, masonry Paper hanging Light carpentry	10+ METs 11+ kcal/min	Shoveling 10 times/min (7.3 kg or 16 lb)
5-6 METs 6-7 kcal/min	Digging garden Shoveling light earth		

[a]A major excess metabolic increase may occur due to excitement, anxiety, or impatience in carrying out some of these activities, and a physician must assess the patient's psychological reactivity.

Note. All expenditure values include resting metabolic needs. MET = metabolic equivalent, the energy expenditure at rest, equivalent to approximately 3.5 ml O_2/kg/min. The conversions into kcal/min are for a 70-kg person. Adapted from Fox, S.M., Naughton, J.P., Gorman, P.A.: Physical activity and cardiovascular health III: The exercise prescription, frequency and type of activity. *Mod. Concepts Cardiovasc. Dis.* 41:6, 1972. Published with permission.

to such chemical agents as carbon monoxide, lead, cadmium, nitrates, and organic solvents on the job (76). The impact of these types of exposure on the cardiovascular responses has received little attention. Low levels of carbon monoxide have been shown to reduce the exercise ischemic threshold (77). Arrhythmias have been reported to be increased (78) and unchanged (79) by exposure to carbon monoxide. (See chapters 20 and 21 for more details on the effect of environmental conditions on cardiac patients.)

Other factors in the work environment that may influence cardiovascular responses include rotating shift work and "job strain" (high psychological demands with low decision latitude). Reports (80-82) suggest that these conditions may adversely affect blood pressure and serum lipids.

Psychological Stress

In the analysis of a patient's job, the assessment of psychological factors should include assessment not only of psychological stress on the job, but also of the patient's perceptions and concerns regarding his or her ability to cope with the physical and emotional demands of the job. Psychological stress can significantly increase myocardial oxygen requirements, and excessive or prolonged psychological stress may increase cardiac risk. However psychological stress rarely justifies a recommendation that a cardiac patient not resume work (83). Recommending alternative employment, although occasionally useful, is more often ineffective or even counterproductive. Such a recommendation could ultimately become more stressful for patients if it were to lead to loss of employment, job dissatisfaction, or a reduction in salary. Even when successful, seeking and undertaking alternative employment is itself a stressful life event whose potential benefits need to be weighed. Tests are available to measure physiological responses to mental stress and may be beneficial in evaluating patients reporting symptoms with psychological stress (84).

Exercise and Work Testing

Various forms of exercise and work testing have proven to be of considerable value in helping physicians develop realistic vocational and avocational recommendations for patients after a major cardiac event (24,55,50,85,86). Such tests may help reassure the physician, patient, patient's family, and employer about the advisability of returning to work. The graded dynamic exercise test is the type of work testing most commonly performed for vocational assessment. However, simulated work testing and ambulatory monitoring may be recommended for selected patients.

Dynamic Exercise Testing

The value of a GXT in making return-to-work decisions is well established. Both a predischarge GXT and a symptom-limited GXT (SL-GXT) at about 4 to 8 weeks after MI and CABG surgery are helpful (86). One of the most important benefits of a SL-GXT for vocational assessment is determination of the patient's $\dot{V}O_2$max. In most clinical laboratories, $\dot{V}O_2$max is estimated from the peak work load attained rather than measured with specialized equipment (86-88). If estimated, it is important that the patients minimize their use of treadmill handrail supports, or not use them at all, since this can result in significant overestimation of $\dot{V}O_2$max.

When the patient's physical work tolerance has been determined, it can be compared to the expected oxygen demands of the patient's job. It is generally recommended that the average oxygen demands over an 8-hour working day should not exceed 40% of the patient's $\dot{V}O_2$max (24,50,69). This does not mean that all work tasks should be restricted to this level of effort; tasks carried out for shorter periods of time can be performed at higher relative intensities. The peak work intensity that should be recommended for the most demanding work tasks will depend upon the patient's conditions and the type of work, but probably should not exceed 70% to 80% of $\dot{V}O_2$max.

Although the $\dot{V}O_2$max of the patient is important in the initial return-to-work assessment, patients generally can assess the relative stress of work tasks more accurately when they return to work by monitoring pulse rate. This is the simplest and least costly form of ambulatory monitoring. The advantage of the pulse rate compared to METs (metabolic equivalents) is that HR reflects individual work patterns, including the rate of work and work efficiency. Furthermore, pulse rate monitoring provides the patients with tangible information

that may help them gain a greater sense of reassurance that the job is not too stressful. Patients should realize that there are work tasks, such as static exercise and arm work, for which a pulse rate based on dynamic exercise testing underestimates myocardial oxygen demands. In addition to pulse rate, patients should learn to gauge work intensity by perceived exertion (89).

A second benefit of the GXT in vocational assessment is that it helps to evaluate the adequacy of medical therapy and to identify the prognosis of patients (85,86). Separation of cardiac patients into high- and low-risk prognostic subgroups can be helpful in making return-to-work decisions (90). Patients considered to be at low risk for another major cardiac event in the immediate follow-up years should be able to return to work without unnecessary delays and without extensive diagnostic evaluation prior to work resumption. Patients at medium to high risk may require more extensive diagnostic evaluation and treatment before resuming work. More of the high-risk patients will not be able to resume work within a reasonable limit of cardiovascular safety.

A third benefit of the GXT in terms of work evaluation is that a satisfactory performance on the test often reassures the patient and others involved in the return-to-work decision, such as the patient's family, employer, and physician. Many patients are surprised at their work capacity, especially when it is discussed in relation to the energy demands of their job. This information may lead to an increase in patient confidence in returning to work (44), which in turn may reduce the number of patients who fail to return to work out of inappropriate fear and anxiety. It may also promote a more satisfying and productive experience for both the patient and the employer.

Finally, the results of the GXT can be used to develop individualized aerobic training programs for patients. This may be especially beneficial for work resumption in patients with low functional work tolerance or for those with jobs requiring relatively high energy demands.

Simulated Work Tests

For many cardiac patients, the GXT may be the only type of exercise test needed to make realistic return-to-work decisions. Yet for some patients, there are significant limitations in developing activity recommendations based on GXT results alone. One major limitation is that the type of work performed during a GXT is often quite different from the type of work required on the job. Many jobs, especially blue-collar jobs, require weight lifting or carrying, work combined with temperature stress, intermittent heavy work tasks, and work under such conditions of psychological stress as time pressure. Work tests can be designed to simulate these types of work tasks (24,55,90). Described below are two simulated work tests developed to simulate weight carrying and weight lifting. These tests are graded and designed so that one test applies to several similar types of work tasks, thus minimizing the time and cost of testing. The end points and monitoring are the same as for GXT, except that the test may be stopped prior to fatigue due to achievement of expected job demands.

In the *weight carrying test*, the purpose is to evaluate responses and tolerance for work requiring a static load added to light dynamic work (64,65). In the standard protocol, the patient's response to carrying weight loads of 20, 30, 40, and up to 50 lb are evaluated. The patient ambulates on a treadmill at a comfortable weight-carrying speed (mean = 2 mph) while carrying a specified weight load (e.g., dumbbell weights or a box) in either one or both hands for at least 2 min. A rest period of 3 min is interspersed between each weight-carrying stage. The initial load is 20 lb, with 10-lb increments added at each additional work stage. An upper load of 50 lb is used in the standard protocol, since this represents the peak weight-carrying load that is expected of persons in most occupational settings. However, if the patient is required to carry heavier loads on the job, the test can be extended to evaluate specific job requirements. The ECG is continuously monitored throughout the test, and the BP is taken at the end of each minute of weight carrying.

The *repetitive lifting test* is designed to evaluate the patient's ability to perform intermittent static effort added to light to medium dynamic work (66). It applies to many work tasks, including those performed by truck drivers, warehouse personnel, farmers, masons, and snow shovelers. The generalized protocol requires the patient to repetitively lift boxes weighing 30 to 50 lb over a 30-min period. The test is subdivided into three 8-min work stages with a 2-min rest interval between each stage. In the first work stage, the patient lifts 30-lb boxes up from the floor (or platform) to a table. A staff person or patient can return the boxes to the floor. During the second and third work stages, the box weights are increased to 40 and 50 lb, respectively. If the patient's job requires him or her to repetitively lift weights in excess of 50 lb or for a longer or shorter period, the test may be adjusted accordingly. Before the test, the patient is instructed to

set a pace of lifting that represents heavy work and can be sustained for a 30-min work period. An alternative approach would be to establish a set pace of lifting or to instruct the patient to work at the peak rate required on the job. The ECG is continually monitored during the test. BP is taken while the patient momentarily *holds* the weight at minute 2 and minute 8 of each work stage.

The responses to graded weight carrying, repetitive lifting, and the GXT differ (55,64,66). Peak diastolic BP typically is highest with heavy weight carrying, intermediate with heavy repetitive lifting, and lowest with heavy dynamic exercise. The pattern of the arterial BP response to weight carrying and repetitive weight lifting also differs in that BP remains elevated with weight carrying time but fluctuates significantly with repetitive lifting (66). HR and $\dot{V}O_2$ are highest with peak dynamic exercise, intermediate with repetitive lifting of 50 lb, and lowest with carrying 50 lb. The incidence of arrhythmias is similar for all three tests. Ischemic responses are less with static-dynamic testing than dynamic testing. As reviewed by others (54,91), patients with moderate to severe left ventricular impairment may show a greater rise in left ventricular end-diastolic pressure and more left ventricular wall motion abnormalities with static effort than normal people or patients with mild left ventricular impairment.

Many other testing procedures can be established to simulate job requirements (62,63,67, 68,74). Circuit weight equipment and the Baltimore Therapeutic Work Simulator can be used to simulate static-dynamic work. The latter can also be used to simulate many other job tasks (68). To evaluate tolerance for work combined with temperature stress, dynamic or static-dynamic testing can be performed in warm or cold air environments (62,63,74). Within industry, simulation tests can be set up to evaluate common tasks applicable to that industry.

Simulated work testing has several benefits. First, it provides more objective data for use in making realistic decisions on the patient's ability to return safely to work involving types of work not evaluated with the GXT. Second, the patient and the patient's family often gain confidence in the patient's ability to return safely to work through a satisfactory performance on a test that closely simulates the patient's peak work requirements. Third, the tests provide the employer with specific information on the patient's ability to resume such work tasks as how much weight the patient can lift or carry. Finally, simulated work testing provides an atmosphere that is conducive to instruction. If a patient has an excessive BP rise with static work, it is usually easier for the patient to understand why static work limitations are important. Proper methods of lifting objects and more efficient ways of performing work tasks can also be presented. The limitation of this type of testing is that it increases the cost to the patient. Although the cost-effectiveness of this type of testing remains to be determined, one must keep in mind not only the cost of the test but also the cost that would be incurred if the patient does not return to work due to inadequate information or if the patient becomes a less productive worker out of fear that the work is too stressful.

What criteria can be used to determine which patients are more likely to benefit from this type of testing? Experience suggests that the patients who seem to derive the most benefit from simulated work testing are (1) those with questionable physical tolerance for resumption of selected work tasks or home and leisure-time activities; (2) those whose employers or prospective employers have doubts regarding a patient's ability to perform a job or want specific guidelines, such as how much weight the patient can lift or carry on the job; (3) those who show considerable apprehension about resuming certain kinds of work; and (4) those within moderate- to high-risk prognostic categories. More investigation is required to delineate the value of simulated work testing and which patients gain the most from this type of testing in the return-to-work decision-making process.

Ambulatory Monitoring

Another assessment procedure that can be used to evaluate a patient's ability to return safely to work is ambulatory monitoring. Initially, the patient can keep a detailed diary of activities, with pulse rate monitoring and notations of any symptoms. If further information is necessary, ambulatory ECG and possibly BP monitoring may be performed. The advantage of ambulatory monitoring is that the patient's cardiovascular responses can be recorded while the patient follows a normal daily routine. Thus, the influence of environmental and emotional stress on arrhythmias, ischemia, HR, and BP can be assessed. The disadvantages of ambulatory monitoring are that it is a fairly expensive procedure and that not all patients are willing to wear a recorder while working.

Recommendations for Rehabilitation

As discussed in the previous section, the individual needs of the patient can be identified through a comprehensive medical and vocational assessment. The vocational goal of the cardiac rehabilitation team is to develop an individualized treatment plan for each patient based on this assessment information. Early identification of patients with occupational work potential can aid the team in developing a return-to-work goal for the patient, which, in turn, may help patients maintain a positive attitude about their ability to resume work.

Education

The patient and family need to be given the skills and framework necessary for their participation in the decision-making process. In order for patients to take an active role in rehabilitation, they need to have a basic understanding of CAD, the role of CAD risk factors, and the implications of these factors in resuming an active and meaningful life. In addition, education may serve as a starting point in the process of behavior change, and the satisfaction of being able to lead a healthy cardiovascular lifestyle may make the patient feel better physically as well as psychologically. The result may be a more satisfying work attitude.

The patient should be informed early in convalescence of the rather favorable statistics regarding returning to work after a major cardiac event. Anecdotes as well as contact with patients who have returned to work may engender and support an appropriately optimistic outlook. The patient's specific concerns regarding returning to work need to be addressed as part of the education process. The patient should also be told about the rather stringent requirements for qualifying for disability funds from many granting agencies such as the Social Security Administration. This may discourage the patient medically able to resume work from going through the long process of applying for disability benefits only to be rejected 6 months later.

Exercise Program

One of the major objectives of an exercise program in cardiac rehabilitation is to help patients return to work successfully by improving their physical work tolerance. The early postdischarge exercise program should help to gradually restore the patient's work tolerance so that he or she will be able to resume work within the appropriate recovery period.

Improved aerobic capacity with exercise training can enable patients to perform heavier dynamic work tasks. A reduction in HR and possibly systolic BP at a given submaximal workload may further allow individuals to resume work with less demand on the heart, since the RPP correlates closely with myocardial oxygen demands (92). This reduction in RPP can be especially beneficial to the patient who experiences angina pectoris at a relatively low workload, since angina pectoris, which typically occurs at the same RPP, may occur at a higher workload after training (93). Other benefits that may be derived from aerobic training include weight loss, reduction in BP, improved lipid profile, reduction in psychological stress, and improved confidence for exercise or work without cardiac-related problems.

If the patient is going back to a job that requires outdoor work, it may be advantageous to exercise outdoors during the early outpatient rehabilitation phase, especially when the outdoor air temperature is warm. Mild to moderate work in a warm environment promotes acclimation, which, over a period of a few days, can reduce cardiovascular demands of work in a warm environment (72).

Due to specificity of training, the exercise program for patients with jobs requiring arm or static-dynamic work should include these types of exercise as well as the traditional walking and cycling exercises (53,91). Until recently, static or static-dynamic exercise training was not encouraged for patients after a cardiac event. However, several recent reports have shown that circuit weight training can improve muscular strength in cardiac patients; appears to be safe, at least in uncomplicated patients; may add interest to an exercise program; and may promote self-confidence in resuming static or static-dynamic work tasks on the job (94-96). The relative value of this type of training on responses to static or static-dynamic work on the job needs to be assessed (53). A recent study (96) suggested that 12 weeks of circuit weight training had little or no benefit in lowering HR and BP with weight carrying, despite significant gains in upper body strength.

Psychological Intervention

Much of the psychological stress that people experience arises from habitual ways of perceiving and responding to situations. If the stress experienced is largely self-induced, it may not be effectively reduced by a change in job, but rather may require a change in the patient's perceptual and response patterns (97). Therefore, often a better intervention

is to identify the presence of job-related psychological stress through a job analysis and then recommend counseling or stress management training, as indicated, to help patients learn how to cope more effectively. This should be initiated early in the patient's recovery process. Monitoring and continued follow-up after the patient resumes work may be beneficial with some patients. Patients who are deemed medically able to resume work but who are reluctant to do so because of inappropriate fear may especially benefit from psychological intervention. As discussed by Blumenthal et al. (83), depression and anxiety after a cardiac event are common, but most cases are self-limiting. Less than 15% of patients need referral to trained professionals for treatment of depression and anxiety.

Work Resumption Process

The appropriate time to resume work after a cardiac event depends on the severity of the event and the patient's risk profile. Currently, the majority of patients who have had an MI or CABG surgery resume work within 6 to 12 weeks, while those who have undergone PTCA often return to work earlier. The return-to-work process can be quite complex, involving the interaction between the patient, the patient's family, the medical profession, industry, unions, insurance companies, vocational rehabilitation agencies, and disability agencies (24,98).

Interaction of Health Care Professionals and Industry

Employers may impose barriers or disincentives to the employment or reemployment of workers with known CAD 98,24,98-100). Several factors may contribute to this, including employers' lack of understanding regarding the recovery process after a cardiac event, inappropriate perception that those with CAD are "cardiac cripples," a fear that manpower flexibility and efficiency will be reduced if physical limitations have to be placed upon an employee, and perceived financial risk associated with increased insurance and compensation rates.

Health care professionals can also contribute to barriers to work resumption (10,24,98). They may concentrate on medical treatment and pay minimal attention to a patient's work-related matters. Some physicians will tell patients not to worry about work resumption at this time or give an evasive response if asked about work resumption soon after a cardiac event. Some may not provide employer-requested information regarding an employee's ability or disability following a cardiac event (such as information on appropriate limits for lifting and carrying), with the result that the employer may not be able to restore the patient to his or her job. Failure of health care professionals to understand employer policies or laws governing employability may contribute to the slow process of transferring advances in medicine to changes in administrative and legal employment guidelines. Minimal communication between health care professionals and industry may also result in failure to adopt employment policies that may aid the cardiac patient in resuming work—such policies as initial resumption of light duties, part-time transitional work, work site modifications, and change to another job position (98,101).

In large companies, an occupational physician may be available to assist in educating and influencing the employer to be more realistic about the cardiac patient's ability to perform a job safely. However, in the United States, small businesses predominate, and they often do not have an in-house medical program. To ensure that the employer receives accurate and sufficient information regarding a person's cardiac status, a member of the cardiac rehabilitation team should act as a liaison with the employer. Reporting the results from the assessment procedures to an apprehensive employer may help establish the person's ability to perform the job.

Clearly, more communication is needed between industry and the medical profession to enhance the employment or reemployment of those with CAD. Cardiac rehabilitation staff can afford to take a stronger role in providing to industry information on heart disease and occupational work capacity. In the future, it may become even more critical to reinstate medically able employees after a cardiac event rather than granting earlier retirement or disability funds (8,24). U.S. Census Bureau projections indicate that the percentage or workers between 45 and 64 years of age will substantially increase by the year 2020 and, since the incidence of CAD increases with age, more workers will likely have CAD. Medically able workers will be needed to meet the demands of the workplace as well as to maintain the solvency of disability and retirement funds for those medically unable to resume work.

The role that industry can play in informing their workers about risk factors for CAD and providing information to their workers on health promotion should also be discussed with employers (102,103). They can be informed, for example, of health care packages designed specifically for the workplace by the American Heart Association and other agencies. These packages contain information on nutrition, exercise, smoking cessation, stress management, and BP control. Films, demonstrations, and lectures may be suggested as other means to motivate workers to improve health habits. Improved health habits, in turn, may reduce employers' medical care costs and result in more satisfied workers.

Interaction of Health Care Professionals and Vocational Rehabilitation Agencies

Some patients do not have a job at the time of their event or need to find other employment. These patients may qualify for vocational rehabilitation services provided through a state vocational rehabilitation agency and funded by the state and federal governments. The extent of vocational services provided varies from state to state and may include psychological and vocational evaluations, counseling and training in job-seeking skills, job placement assistance, and work adjustment through skill training in rehabilitation facilities (104). If financial need is established, some state agencies will also provide training materials for proprietary instruction, correspondence study, or tutorial training. To be eligible for their services, two criteria must be met: (1) the person must be physically or mentally disabled to the extent that the disability interferes with employability and (2) there must be a reasonable expectation that the agency's services will benefit the person in terms of securing employment. Eligibility for services is established by a professionally trained rehabilitation counselor. Other private vocational rehabilitation programs are available in some communities.

It is important that a member of the cardiac rehabilitation team be aware of the services provided by vocational rehabilitation services and establish liaison with an appropriate counselor to facilitate referral for these services. Determining when to refer a patient depends to some extent on the facilities and expertise available to the cardiac rehabilitation team. A patient may be referred to vocational rehabilitation services early if it is anticipated that sufficient information and assessment will not be available to place the patient in his or her previous employment. A referral is also appropriate when it is anticipated that the patient may not be able to return to his or her previous work and that job retraining may be necessary.

Interaction of Health Care Professionals and Disability Support Systems

Some patients are not medically able to resume work after a cardiac event. Several programs are available to provide workers with disability funds (8,98,105). Sources include the Social Security Administration, private insurance companies, corporate retirement programs, state and municipalities, and the Department of Veterans Affairs. The criteria for granting disability income differs among these agencies. In general, criteria from the Social Security Administration are the most stringent, but this program is the most widely available source of disability funds for workers with heart disease (8,98,105). To qualify for Social Security disability funds, the worker must have impairments severe enough to result in death or to prevent substantial gainful activity for at least 12 months (106).

The Social Security Administration's criteria for each major disease category are published in *Disability Evaluation Under Social Security* (106). As indicated in this booklet, it is the responsibility of the medical profession to determine the degree of impairment based on anatomic and functional loss and evaluation of the patient's prognosis rather than to determine disability. The determination of disability is a function of the Social Security Administration that incorporates the medical evaluation along with other factors that can influence employability, such as age, education level, and economic environment. Anyone who advises cardiac patients on Social Security disability funds should be aware of the current criteria used by the administration for granting disability funds secondary to CAD. Otherwise, the patient may be advised to seek disability funds only to be denied at later date, by which time the patient may have adopted a "disability attitude," which can be difficult to reverse (98). It should be noted that in some states, "heart laws" provide less stringent criteria for obtaining disability funds from municipalities for fire fighters and police officers (10).

Some of the major issues regarding the insurability and employability of the patient with CAD were recently discussed by leading experts in a conference held at Bethesda, Maryland. Recognizing both the lack of uniformity within the Social Security Administration for determining residual impairment and the data indicating that many patients with impaired left ventricular function still retain good functional work reserve, it was suggested that a greater emphasis be placed on using functional work tolerance as a Social Security criterion for granting disability funds secondary to CAD (10,50). As a follow-up, the Social Security Administration recently published a proposed policy change, under which the administration would place a greater emphasis on functional work tolerance in granting disability for CAD (107). Provided this proposed change is accepted, the Social Security Administration will make provisions for the purchase of a GXT in clinically stable patients.

Some CAD patients may medically improve after being granted Social Security disability funds as a result of advances in the treatment of angina and other disabling cardiac conditions. For those who would like to determine whether they can resume work, the Social Security Administration provides opportunities for them to attempt work resumption without immediately losing their disability status. Under this "trial work" program, disability benefits can continue for up to 9 months while the patient tests his or her ability to work. After this period, a decision is made as to whether a person is capable of substantial gainful activity. If not, their disability payments continue. If the individual is able to achieve substantial gainful activity, benefits are paid for 3 additional months and then stopped. The Social Security Administration also provides an "extended period of eligibility," under which a person has special protection for at least 36 months following the "trial work" period. During this 36-month period, benefits are paid for each month in which the patient is disabled. Other benefits are available; a local Social Security office can be contacted for more information.

In some professions in which a cardiac event on the job may pose a danger to public safety—such as operators of public transportation, police officers, fire fighters, and operators of nuclear power plants—clinicians may be asked to "certify" that a patient can return to work or remain at work (85). Asymptomatic individuals within these professions may also be removed at a certain age as a precautionary measure. As others (24,50) have pointed out, inconsistencies exist in these regulations. Bruce and Fisher (108) found that exercise-enhanced risk assessment was more effective than mandatory age for removing workers at risk for sudden cardiac incapacitation.

Summary and Conclusions

The literature over the past 15 years has shown a remarkably consistent net loss from the work force after MI or CABG surgery, in spite of significant symptomatic relief and improved cardiovascular functioning. Nonmedical factors, including age, previous work status, patient beliefs and attitudes, and work conditions are more powerful predictors of return to work than objective indicators of disease severity or cardiovascular function. Women, older patients, blue-collar workers, and individuals who have been out of work 6 months or longer are at highest risk for early retirement or permanent disability.

Following an international conference on occupational cardiology, a consensus was reached on the need to increase the number of patients returning to work after an MI or revascularization (109). It was recommended that judgments on the possibility of returning to work be based on a clinical evaluation, a job evaluation, and an evaluation of the work environment.

The return-to-work process after a cardiac event can be complex, involving interactions among the patient, physician, other health care professionals, industry, and disability agencies. Increased communication among health care professionals, employers, and disability support systems may facilitate the process of returning to work and prevent premature retirement or unnecessary disability. Physician attitudes and advice can play a critical role. Advice based on a systematic approach to work evaluation that incorporates assessment of job requirements, evaluation of the patient's functional work tolerance, early identification and intervention of psychological and sociodemographic barriers to work resumption, and improved patient self-confidence in resuming work may decrease inappropriate disability after a cardiac event. The integration of biological, psychological, and social parameters ensures a comprehensive approach to this very complex, multifactorial problem and has the greatest potential for improving the occupational outcome of cardiac treatment and rehabilitation.

References

1. American Heart Association. 1991 heart & stroke facts. Dallas: American Heart Association: 1991.
2. Rogers, W.J.; Coggin, C.J.; Gersh, B.J.; Fisher, L.D.; Myers, W.O.; Oberman, A.; Sheffield, L.T. (for the CASS investigators). Ten-year follow-up of quality of life in patients randomized to receive medical therapy or coronary artery bypass graft surgery. The coronary artery study (CASS). Circulation. 82:1647-1658; 1990.
3. Dennis, C.; Houston-Miller, N.; Schwartz, R.G.; Ahn, D.K.; Kraemer, H.C.; Gossard, D.; Juneay, M.; Taylor, C.B.; De Busk, R.F. Early to work after uncomplicated myocardial infarction. JAMA. 260:214-220; 1988.
4. Picard, M.H.; Dennis, C.; Schwartz, R.G.; Ahn, D.K.; Kraemer, H.C.; Berger, III, W.E.; Blumberg, R.; Heller, R.; Lew, H.; DeBusk, R.F. Cost-benefit analysis of early return to work after uncomplicated acute myocardial infarction. Am. J. Cardiol. 63: 1308-1314; 1989.
5. Rost, K.; Smith, R. Return to work after an initial myocardial infarction and subsequent emotional distress. Arch. Intern. Med. 152:381-385; 1992.
6. Blackwell, B.; Knapp, D. Acute and chronic illness behavior in cardiac patients. Presented at the third annual symposium: multidisciplined approach to cardiac rehabilitation, cardiovascular disease and prevention. 1982 November; Louisville, KY.
7. Almeida, D.; Bradford, J.M.; Wenger, N.K.; King, S.B.; Hurst, J.W. Return to work after coronary bypass surgery. Circulation. 68 Suppl. II:205-213; 1983.
8. Davidson, D.M. Return to work after cardiac events: A review. J. Cardiac Rehabil. 3:60-69; 1983.
9. Fitzgerald, S.T.; Becker, D.M.; Celentano, D.D.; Swank, R.; Brinker, J. Return to work after percutaneous transluminal coronary angioplasty. Am. J. Cardiol. 64:1108-1112; 1989.
10. Guillette, W.; Judge, R.D.; Koehn, E.; Miller, J.E.; Palmer, R.K.; Tremblay, J.L.G. Committee report on economic, administrative and legal factors influencing the insurability and employability of patients with ischemic heart disease. J. Am. Coll. Cardiol. 14:1010-1015; 1989.
11. Mark, D.B.; Lam, L.C.; Lee, K.L.; Clapp-Channing, N.E.; Williams, R.B.; Pryor, D.B.; Califf, R.M.; Hlatky, M.A. Identification of patients with coronary diseases at high risk for loss of employment. A prospective validation study. Circulation. 86:1485-1494; 1992.
12. Smith, G.R.; O'Rourke, D.F. Return to work after a first myocardial infarction: A test of multiple hypotheses. JAMA. 259:1673-1677; 1988.
13. Hlatky, M.A.; Haney, T.; Barefoot, J.C.; Califf, R.M.; Mark, C.B.; Pryor, C.B.; Williams, R.B. Medical, physiological and social correlates of work disability among men with coronary artery disease. Am. J. Cardiol. 58:911-915; 1986.
14. Shanfield, S.B. Return to work after an acute myocardial infarction: A review. Heart Lung. 19:109-117; 1990.
15. Oberman, A.; Wayne, J.B.; Kouchoukos, N.T.; Charles, E.D.; Russell, Jr., R.O.; Rogers, W.J. Employment status after coronary artery bypass surgery. Circulation. 65 Suppl.II:115-119; 1982.
16. Laird-Meeter, K.; Erdman, R.A.; van Domburg, R.; Azar, A.J.; de Feyter, P.J.; Bos, E.; Hugenholtz, P.G. Probability of a return to work after either coronary

balloon dilatation or coronary bypass surgery. Eur. Heart J. 10:917-922; 1989.

17. Walter, P. Return to work after coronary artery bypass surgery. Eur. Heart J. Suppl.L:58-66; 1988.

18. Anderson, A.J.; Barboriak, J.J.; Hoffman, R.G.; Mullen, D.C. Retention or resumption of employment after aortocoronary bypass operations. JAMA. 243:543-545; 1980.

19. Danchin, N. Work capacity after myocardial revascularization: Factors related to work resumption. Eur. Heart J. 9 Suppl.L:44-47; 1988.

20. Gehring, J.; Koenig, W.; Rana, N.W.; Mathes, P. The influence of the type of occupation on return to work after myocardial infarction, coronary angioplasty and coronary bypass surgery. Eur. Heart J. 9 Suppl.L:109-114; 1988.

21. Frick, M.H.; Harjola, P.T.; Valle, M. Work status after coronary bypass surgery: A prospective randomized study with ergometric and angiographic correlations. Acta Med. Scand. 206:61-64; 1979.

22. Gohike, H.; Schnelbacker, K.; Steinrucken, H.; Samek, L.; Roskamm, H. Postoperative exercise performance determines return to work. In: Walter, P.J. ed. Return to work after coronary bypass surgery. Psychosocial and economic aspects. Berlin: Springer-Verlag; 1985: 102-107.

23. Gutmann, M.C.; Knapp, D.N.; Pollock, M.L.; Schmidt, D.H.; Simon, K.; Walcott, G. Coronary artery bypass patients and work status. Circulation. 66 Suppl.III:33-42; 1982.

24. Kavanagh, T.; Matosevic, V. Assessment of work capacity in patients with ischemic heart disease: Methods and practices. Eur. Heart J. 9 Suppl.L:67-73; 1988.

25. Zyzanski, S.J.; Rouse, B.A.; Stanton, B.A.; Jenkins, C.D. Employment changes among patients following coronary bypass surgery: Social, medical and psychological correlates. Public Health Rep. 97:558-565; 1982.

26. Stanton, B.A.; Jenkins, C.D.; Denlinger, P.; Savageau, J.A.; Weintraub, R.M.; Goldstein, R.L. Predictors of employment status after cardiac surgery. JAMA. 249:907-911; 1983.

27. Symmes, J.C.; Lenkei, S.C.M.; Berman, N.D. Influence of aortocoronary bypass surgery on employment. Can. Med. Assoc. J. 118:268-270; 1978.

28. Anderson, A.J.; Barboriak, J.J.; Hoffman, R.G.; Walker, J.A.; Mullen, D.C. Age- and sex-specific incidence and main factors. In: Walter, P.J. ed. Return to work after coronary artery bypass surgery. Psychosocial and economic aspects. Berlin: Springer-Verlag; 1985: 3-12.

29. Allen, J.K.; Fitzgerald, S.T.; Swank, R.T.; Becker, D.M. Functional status after coronary artery bypass grafting and percutaneous transluminal coronary angioplasty. Am. J. Cardiol. 65:921-925; 1990.

30. Ben-Ari, E.; Rothbaum, D.A.; Linnemeier, T.A.; Landin, R.; Tavel, M.; Steinmetz, E.F.; Hillis, J.S.; Hallam, C.C.; Noble, R.J., See, M.R.; Ball, M.; Martin, P. Return to work after successful coronary angioplasty. Comparison between a comprehensive rehabilitation program and patients receiving usual care. J. Cardiopul. Rehabil. 12:20-24; 1992.

31. Shapiro, S.; Weinblatt, E.; Frank, C.W. Return to work after first myocardial infarction. Arch. Environ. Health. 24:17-26; 1972.

32. Garrity, T.F. Vocational adjustment after first myocardial infarction: Comparative assessment of several variables suggested in the literature. Soc. Sci. Med. 7:705-717; 1973.

33. Allen, J.K. Physical and psychosocial outcomes after coronary artery bypass graft surgery: Review of the literature. Heart Lung. 19:49-54; 1990.

34. Hamilton, G.A. Recovery from acute myocardial infarction in women. Cardiology. 77 Suppl. 2:58-70; 1990.

35. Fitzgerald, S.T. Occupational outcomes after treatment for coronary heart disease: A review of the literature. Cardiovasc. Nurs. 25:1-6; 1989.

36. Knapp, D.; Gutmann, M.C.; Tristani, F.; Sheldahl, L.; Wilke, N. Returning the patient to work. In: Pollock, M.L.; Schmidt, D.H. eds. Heart disease and rehabilitation. New York: Wiley; 1986: 647-688.

37. Gutmann, M.C.; Knapp, D.N.; Pollock, M.L. Psychosocial predictor of work status. In: Walter, P.J. ed. Return to work after coronary bypass surgery. Psychosocial and economic aspects. Berlin: Springer-Verlag; 1985: 209-213.

38. David, P. Contributing factors preventing return to work of cardiac surgery patients. Cleveland Clin. Q. 45:177-178; 1978.

39. Cay, E.L.; Walker, D.D. Psychological factors and return to work. Eur. Heart J. 9 Suppl.L:74-81; 1988.

40. DeBusk, R.F.; Blomqvist, C.G.; Kouchoukos, N.T.; Luepker, R.V.; Miller, H.S.; Moss, A.J.; Pollock, M.L.; Reeves, T.J.; Selvester, R.H.; Stason, W.B.; Wagner, G.S.; Willman, V.L. Identification and treatment of low-risk patients after acute myocardial infarction and coronary-artery bypass graft surgery. N. Engl. J. Med. 314:161-166; 1986.

41. Stern, M.J.; Pascale, L.; Ackerman, A. Life adjustment post-myocardial infarction: Determining predictive variables. Arch. Intern. Med. 137:1680-1685; 1977.

42. Kornfield, D.S.; Heller, S.S.; Frank, K.A.; Wilson, S.N.; Malm, J.R. Psychological and behavioral responses. In: Walter, P.J. ed. Return to work after coronary artery bypass surgery. Psychosocial and economic aspects. Berlin: Springer-Verlag; 1985: 224-234.

43. Maeland, J.G.; Havik, O.E. Return to work after a myocardial infarction: The influence of background factors, work characteristics, and illness severity. Scand. J. Med. 14:183-195; 1986.

44. Ewart, C.K.; Taylor, C.B.; Reese, L.B.; DeBusk, R.F. Effects of early postmyocardial infarction exercise testing on self-perception and subsequent physical activity. Am. J. Cardiol. 51:1076-1080; 1983.

45. Wenger, N.K.; Almeida, D.; Bradford, J.M.; King, S.B.; Hurst, J.W. Return to work after coronary artery bypass surgery: Problems and prospects. In:

Walter, P.J. ed. Return to work after coronary artery bypass surgery. Psychosocial and economic aspects. Berlin: Springer-Verlag; 1985: 323-331.

46. DeBusk, R.F. 20th Bethsesda conference: Insurability and employability of the patient with ischemic heart disease. J. Am. Coll. Cardiol. 14:1008-1009; 1989.

47. U.S. Department of Labor. Dictionary of occupational titles (4th ed., revised) Indianapolis, IN: JUST Works, Inc.; 1991.

48. U.S. Department of Labor. Selected characteristics of occupations defined in the "dictionary of occupational titles." Washington, DC: U.S. Government Printing Office; 1981.

49. Passmore, R.; Durnin, J.V.G.A. Human energy expenditure. Physiol. Rev. 35:801-840; 1955.

50. Haskell, W.L.; Brachfeld, N.; Bruce, R.A.; Davis, P.O.; Dennis, C.A.; Fox, III, S.M.; Hanson, P.; Leon, A.S. Task force II: Determination of occupational working capacity in patients with ischemic heart disease. J. Am. Coll. Cardiol. 14:1025-1034; 1989.

51. Ainsworth, B.E.; Haskell, W.L.; Leon, A.S.; Jacobs, Jr., D.R.; Montoye, H.J.; Sallis, J.F.; Paffenbarger, Jr., R.S. Compendium of physical activities: Classification of energy costs of human physical activities. Med. Sci. Sports Exerc. 25:71-80; 1993.

52. Mitchell, J.H.; Wildenthal, K. Static (isometric) exercise and the heart: Physiological and clinical considerations. Ann. Rev. Med. 25:369-381; 1974.

53. Blomqvist, C.G. Upper extremity exercise testing and training. Cardiovasc. Clin. 15:175-183; 1985.

54. Hanson, P.; Nagle, F. Isometric exercise. Cardiovascular responses in normal and cardiac populations. Cardiol. Clin. 5:157-170; 1987.

55. Sheldahl, L.M.; Wilke, N.A.; Tristani, F.E. Exercise prescription for return to work. J. Cardiopul. Rehabil. 5:567-575; 1985.

56. Wilke, N.A.; Sheldahl, L.M.; Levandoski, S.G.; Hoffman, M.D.; Tristani, F.E. Weight carrying versus handgrip exercise testing in men with coronary artery disease. Am. J. Cardiol. 64:736-740; 1989.

57. Durnin, J.V.G.A.; Passmore, R. Energy, work and leisure. London: Heinemann Educational Books Ltd.; 1967: 47-95.

58. Ford, A.; Hellerstein, H. Work and heart disease. I. A physiologic study in the factory. Circulation. 18:823-832; 1958.

59. Ford, A.B.; Hellerstein, H.K.; Turell, D.J. Work and heart disease. II. A physiologic study in a steel mill. Circulation. 20:537-548; 1959.

60. Denolin, H.; Riviere, A. Physiological cost of vocational activities after myocardial infarction. Eur. Heart J. 9 Suppl.L: 54-57; 1988.

61. Aronov, D.M.; Rosykhodzhajeva, G.A. Energy expenditure and cardiovascular response to daily activities in patients with coronary heart disease of different functional classes. J. Cardiopul. Rehabil. 12:56-62; 1992.

62. Sheldahl, L.M.; Wilke, N.A.; Dougherty, S.M.; Levandoski, S.G.; Hoffman, M.D.; Tristani, F.E. Effect of age and coronary artery disease on response to snow shoveling. J. Am. Coll. Cardiol. 20:1111-1117; 1992.

63. Dougherty, S.M.; Sheldahl, L.M.; Wilke, N.A.; Levandoski, S.G.; Hoffman, M.D.; Tristani, F.E. Physiologic responses to shoveling and thermal stress in men with cardiac disease. Med. Sci. Sports Exerc. 25:790-795; 1993.

64. Sheldahl, L.M.; Wilke, N.A.; Tristani, F.E.; Kalbfleisch, J.H. Response of patients after myocardial infarction to carrying a graded series of weight loads. Am. J. Cardiol. 52:698-703; 1983.

65. Foss-Campbell, B.; Sheldahl, L.; Wilke, N.; Dougherty, S.; Levandoski, S.; Tristani, F.E. Effects of upper extremity load distribution on weight carrying in men with ischemic heart disease. J. Cardiopul. Rehabil. 13:37-42; 1993.

66. Sheldahl, L.M.; Wilke, N.A.; Tristani, F.E.; Kalbfleisch, J.H. Response to repetitive static-dynamic exercise in patients with coronary artery disease. J. Cardiac Rehabil. 5:139-145; 1985.

67. Sheldahl, L.M.; Levandoski, S.G.; Wilke, N.A.; Dougherty, S.M.; Tristani, F.E. Responses of patients with coronary artery disease to common carpentry tasks. J. Cardiopul Rehabil. 13:283-290; 1993.

68. Wilke, N.A.; Sheldahl, L.M.; Dougherty, S.M.; Levandoski, S.G.; Tristani, F.E. Baltimore therapeutic equipment work simulator: Energy expenditure of work activities in cardiac patients. Arch. Phys. Med. Rehabil. 74:419-424; 1993.

69. Astrand, I. Degree of strain during building work as related to individual aerobic work capacity. Ergonomics. 10:293-303; 1967.

70. Ahonen, E.; Venalainen, J.M.; Kononen, U.; Klen, T. The physical strain of dairy farming. Ergonomics. 33:1549-1555; 1990.

71. Brouha, L. Physiology in industry. Evaluation of industrial stresses by the physiological reactions of the worker. 2nd ed. New York: Pergamon Press; 1960:47-72.

72. Rowell, L.R. Cardiovascular adjustments to thermal stress. In J.T. Shepherd; F.M. Abboud; S.R. Geiger, eds. Handbook of physiology. The cardiovascular system. Peripheral circulation and organ blood flow. Bethesda, MD: Am. Physiol. Soc. 1983:967-1023.

73. Hall, R.J.C.; Bullock, R.E.; Albers, C. The effect of cold on patients with angina pectoris—a review. Postgrad. Med. J. 59 Suppl.2:59-61; 1983.

74. Sheldahl, L.M.; Wilke, N.A.; Dougherty, S.; Tristani, F.E. Cardiac response to combined moderate heat and exercise in men with coronary artery disease. Am. J. Cardiol. 70:186-191; 1992.

75. Balke, B. Cardiac performance in relation to altitude. Am. J. Cardiol. 14:796-810; 1964.

76. Petronio, L. Chemical and physical agents of work-related cardiovascular diseases. Eur. Heart J. 9 Suppl. L:26-34; 1988.

77. Alfred, E.N.; Bleecker, E.R.; Chaitman, B.R.; Dahms, T.E.; Gottlieb, S.O.; Hackney, J.D.; Pagano, M.;

Selvester, R.H.; Walden, S.M.; Warren, J. Short-term effects of carbon monoxide exposure on the exercise performance of subjects with coronary artery disease. N. Engl. J. Med. 321:1426-1432; 1989.

78. Dahms, T.E.; Younis, L.T.; Wiens, R.D.; Zarnegar, S.; Byers, S.; Chaitman, B.R. Effects of carbon monoxide exposure in patients with documented cardiac arrhythmias. J. Am. Coll. Cardiol. 21:442-450; 1993.

79. Sheps, D.S.; Herbst, M.C.; Hinderliter, A.L.; Adams, K.F.; Ekelund, L.G.; O'Neil, J.J.; Goldstein, G.M.; Bromberg, P.A.; Dalton, J.L.; Ballenger, M.N.; Davis, S.M.; Koch, G.G. Production of arrhythmias by elevated carboxyhemoglobin in patients with coronary artery disease. Ann. Intern. Med. 113:343-351; 1990.

80. Schnall, P.L.; Schwartz, J.E.; Landsbergis, P.A.; Warren, K.; Pickering, T.G. Relation between job strain, alcohol, and ambulatory blood pressure. Hypertension. 19:488-494; 1992.

81. Knutsson, A.; Akerstedt, T.; Jonsson, B.G.; Orth-Gomer, K. Increased risk of ischemic heart disease in shift workers. Lancet 2:89-92; 1986.

82. Romon, M.; Nuttens, M.C.; Fievet, C.; Pot, P.; Bard, J.M.; Furon, D.; Fruchart, J.C. Increased triglyceride levels in shift workers. Am. J. Med. 93:259-262; 1992.

83. Blumenthal, J.A.,; Bradley, W.; Dimsdale, J.E.; Kasl, S.; Powell, L.H.; Taylor, C.B. Task force III. Assessment of psychological status in patients with ischemic heart disease. J. Am. Coll. Cardiol. 14:1034-1042; 1989.

84. Steptoe, A.; Vogele, C.; Methodology of mental stress testing in cardiovascular research. Circulation. 83 Suppl.II:II-14-II-24; 1991.

85. Pryor, D.B.; Bruce, R.A.; Chaitman, B.R.; Fisher, L.; Gajewski, J.; Hammermeister, K.E.; Pauker, S.G.; Stokes, III, J. Task force I: Determination of prognosis in patients with ischemic heart disease. J. Am. Coll. Cardiol. 14:1016-1025; 1989.

86. Fletcher, G.F.; Froelicher, V.F.; Hartley, L.H.; Haskell, W.L.; Pollock, M.L. Exercise standards. A statement for health professionals from the American heart association. Circulation. 82:2286-2322; 1990.

87. Bruce, R.A.; Kusami, F.; Hosmer, D. Maximal oxygen uptake and nomographic assessment of functional aerobic impairment in cardiovascular disease. Am. Heart J. 85:546-562; 1973.

88. Haskell, W.L.; Savin, W.; Oldridge, N.; DeBusk, R. Factors influencing estimated oxygen uptake during exercise testing soon after myocardial infarction. Am. J. Cardiol. 50:299-304; 1982.

89. Borg, G. Physical performance and perceived exertion. Lund, Sweden: Gleerlup; 1962.

90. DeBusk, R.F.; Davidson, D.M. The work evaluation of the cardiac patient. J. Occup. Med. 22:715-721; 1980.

91. Franklin, B.A.; Bonzheim, K.; Gordon, S.; Timmis, G.C. Resistance training in cardiac rehabilitation. J. Cardiopul. Rehabil. 11:99-107; 1991.

92. Frick, M.H.; Katila, M. Hemodynamic consequence of physical training after myocardial infarction. Circulation. 37:192-202; 1968.

93. Robinson, B.F. Relationship of heart rate and systolic blood pressure at the onset of pain or angina pectoris. Circulation. 35:1073-1083; 1967.

94. Kelemen, M.H.; Stewart, K.J.; Gillilan, R.E.; Ewart, C.K.; Valenti, S.A.; Manley, J.D.; Kelemen, M.D. Circuit weight training in cardiac patients. J. Am. Coll. Cardiol. 7:38-42; 1986.

95. Stewart, K.J.; Mason, M.; Kelemen, M.H. Three-year participation in circuit weight training improves muscular strength and self-efficacy in cardiac patients. J. Cardiopul. Rehabil. 8:292-296; 1988.

96. Wilke, N.A.; Sheldahl, L.M.; Levandoski, S.G.; Hoffman, M.D.; Dougherty, S.M.; Tristani, F.E. Transfer effect of upper extremity training to weight carrying in men with ischemic heart disease. J. Cardiopul. Rehabil. 11:365-372; 1991.

97. Lazarus, R.S.; Folkman, S. Stress, appraisal, and coping. New York: Springer; 1984.

98. Hester, E.J. Disability and disincentives: Prospective models for change. In: Scheer, S.J., ed. Multidisciplinary perspective in vocational assessment of impaired workers. Rockville, MD: Aspen; 1990:205-218.

99. Naughton, J. Vocational aspects of rehabilitation after myocardial infarction. In: Wenger, N.K.; Hellerstein, H.K. eds. Rehabilitation of the coronary patient. New York: Wiley; 1978:283-294.

100. Sagall, E.L. Legal aspects of rehabilitation after myocardial infarction and coronary bypass surgery. In: Wenger, N.K.; Hellerstein, H.K. eds. Rehabilitation of the coronary patient. 2nd ed. New York: Wiley; 1984:493-511.

101. Social Security Administration/American Medical Association. Disability in transition: Cardiovascular impairment—a model. Washington, DC: U.S. Government Printing Office; 1984.

102. Eliot, R.S.; Bond, M.B.; Brandenburg, R.O.; Cooper, T.; Crumrine, J.L.; Glasser, M.A.; Hafner, D.; Herd, J.A.; Hollen, G.E.; Kerr, L.E.; Sherwin, R.; Resnekov, L.; Roberts, N.J.; Simmons, H.E.; Sparks, R.D.; Weiss, S.M. Task force 3: The physician in the work setting (industrial/occupational medicine). Am. J. Cardiol. 47:751-766; 1981.

103. Harris, J.S. The cost effectiveness of health promotion programs. J. Occup. Med. 33:327-330; 1991.

104. Demore-Taber, M.; Dohen-Siskind, B.M. The role of the vocational rehabilitation counselor. In: Scheer, S.J. ed. Multidisciplinary perspective in vocational assessment of impaired workers. Rockville, MD: Aspen; 1990:47-60.

105. Hester, E.J. Workers who become disabled. In: Scheer, S.J. ed. Multidisciplinary perspective in vocational assessment of impaired workers. Rockville, MD: Aspen; 1990:1-17.

106. U.S. Department of Health and Human Sciences. Disability evaluation under social security. SSA publication no. 64-039, 1992.

107. U.S. Department of Health and Human Services. Revised medical criteria for determination of disability, cardiovascular system. Federal Register 58:31268-31276, 1991.

108. Bruce, R.A.; Fisher, L.D. Strategies for risk evaluation of sudden cardiac incapacitation in men in occupations affecting public safety. J. Occup. Med. 31:124-133; 1989.

109. Denolin, H.; Feruglio, G.A.; Gobbato, F.; Maisano, G. Guidelines for return to work after myocardial infarction and/or revascularization. Eur. Heart J. 9 Suppl.L:130-131; 1988.

Chapter 28

Safety, Precautions, and Emergency Procedures

Steven P. Van Camp

Significant reductions in cardiovascular and total mortality have been reported for patients following acute myocardial infarction (MI) in meta-analyses of secondary-prevention trials of cardiac rehabilitation programs (1,2). Participants in cardiac rehabilitation programs have also achieved significant improvements in functional capacity (3), psychosocial characteristics (4), lipoprotein patterns (5), and myocardial perfusion and function (6). Even so, these participants are at risk for cardiovascular complications during exercise training. This risk depends upon a number of factors, including each participant's pathophysiological status and the type and intensity of exercise training.

Increasing numbers of patients with cardiovascular disease (CVD), in many cases severe and complex, will be undergoing cardiac rehabilitation in the future. It is critical to provide them with the benefits of exercise and cardiac rehabilitation without exposing them to significant and unnecessary risks. This chapter will address the potential cardiovascular complications of cardiac rehabilitation programs, identification of those who are likely to be at highest risk for these complications, and an approach to providing exercise safety in cardiac rehabilitation programs.

The goal of a cardiac rehabilitation program is to achieve physiological, symptomatic, psychological, and vocational benefits for patients at an acceptably low risk. This goal can be accomplished via careful patient evaluation, education, and supervision, as well as staff ability to quickly and properly administer emergency treatment as necessary. There are at least two key elements in this interrelated approach. The first is the stratification of patients according to their risk status—both their risk for an acute cardiovascular complication during exercise and their overall prognosis for event-free survival. Risk status is related primarily to the type of cardiovascular disease (CVD) and

its severity. Risk stratification is the basis for the guidelines on monitoring patients in cardiac rehabilitation programs that have been published by the American College of Cardiology (ACC) (7), the American College of Physicians (ACP) (8), and the American Association of Cardiovascular and Pulmonary Rehabilitation (AACVPR) (9).

The second, but equally important, element in cardiac rehabilitation programs involves the appropriate range of exercise intensity for a given patient. This is related primarily to the patient's pathophysiological status and the degree of supervision and monitoring needed during the exercise session.

The normal cardiovascular response to physical activity involves an increase in heart rate (HR), systolic and mean arterial blood pressures (BPs), and myocardial contractility. The resulting increase in myocardial oxygen consumption and the concurrent increase in serum catecholamine levels, and possible other metabolic changes, contribute to the increased likelihood of exercise-related cardiovascular problems.

Complications of Cardiac Rehabilitation Programs

The most serious complications of cardiac rehabilitation programs include cardiac arrest, MI, arrhythmias requiring cardioversion, pulmonary edema, pulmonary embolism, syncope, and unstable angina (10,11).

Studies in the 1970s (12,13) and in the early 1980s (14) reported risks of cardiac arrest ranging from one incident per 6,000 patient-hours to one incident per 15,000 patient-hours of exposure—relatively high by today's standards. In 1983 Shephard et al. (15) reported the Toronto Rehabilitation Centre's post-MI program to have an improved record of safety, with a cardiac arrest incidence of one per 113,583 patient-hours.

The largest surveys involving multiple cardiac rehabilitation centers were reported by Haskell (10) and our group (11). Haskell gathered data from 30 cardiac rehabilitation programs operating between 1960 and 1977. These centers reported 13,570 patients who exercised for an aggregate of 1,629,634 hours. Fifty patients experienced cardiac arrest, giving a cardiac arrest rate of one per 32,593 patient-hours. Of these, 42 (84%) were successfully resuscitated. Seven of these 42 experienced MIs, 2 resulting in fatalities. Four other fatal complications were recorded: 2 attributed to pulmonary embolism and 1 each as a result of pulmonary edema and cardiogenic shock. The total of 14 fatalities resulted in a fatality rate of one per 116,402 patient-hours. The 7 MIs resulted in an MI rate of one per 232,805 patient-hours.

Our study (11) reported the experience of 167 outpatient cardiac rehabilitation programs for the first 5 years of the 1980s. The programs were randomly selected from the cardiac rehabilitation directories of the American Heart Association (AHA), the California Society for Cardiac Rehabilitation, YMCArdiac Therapy Programs, and Cardiac Treatment Center programs. Data were gathered from these programs through questionnaires and follow-up telephone calls on 51,303 patients. The majority of the patients had coronary artery disease (CAD) as their primary diagnosis, but also included were patients with valvular heart disease,

cardiomyopathies, and primary arrhythmias. Table 28.1 summarizes the data of our study.

In order to evaluate the effect of ECG monitoring on complication rate, the programs were categorized by the extent of ECG monitoring provided during the exercise sessions: continuous monitoring, intermittent monitoring, and "graduated" monitoring (cardiac rhythm was monitored continuously for at least three sessions before progressing to intermittent monitoring). The three groups did not show any significant differences in frequency of cardiac arrest, fatalities, or MI.

Complication rates were also compared based on the size of the program. Programs were categorized as small, medium, or large, based on the number of patient-hours supervised during the 5-year study. There were no significant differences in frequency of cardiac arrest, fatalities, or MIs among these groups.

It has thus been documented that cardiac rehabilitation therapy is a highly safe procedure. The data from our study reveal a cardiac arrest rate approximately one fourth and a fatality rate approximately one seventh of the rates reported by Haskell (10). The risk of acute MI in our study was very similar to that reported by Haskell. Because the risk status of patients in the two studies is not known, strict comparisons between them is not appropriate. There is, however, a strong likelihood of improved safety in the practice of cardiac rehabilitation in the present era compared with the era of Haskell's study (1960 to 1977).

Table 28.1 Cardiovascular Complications of Cardiac Rehabilitation Programs

No. of programs studied: 167[a]
Period studied: January 1980 to December 1984
Total no. of patients: 51,303
Aggregate exercise hours: 2,351,916

Complications	Rate
21 cardiac arrests[b]	1 per 111,996 patient-hours
—3 fatalities	1 per 783,972 patient-hours
8 myocardial infarctions	1 per 293,990 patient-hours
—0 fatalities	—
29 major cardiovascular complications (total cardiac arrests and myocardial infarctions)	1 per 81,101 patients-hours

[a]The major cardiac complications indicated in the table occurred in only 23 of these programs.
[b]The 18 survivors of the cardiac arrests suffered no neurologic sequelae.

There is likely a multiplicity of factors responsible for the apparent improved safety in present-day cardiac rehabilitation therapy. Methods of risk stratification, including exercise ECG (16,17), stress thallium-201 myocardial perfusion imaging (18), and exercise radionuclide ventriculography (RNV) (19), are able to identify the patients at highest risk for cardiac events. These patients can then be treated more extensively prior to enrollment in cardiac rehabilitation programs. The treatment of patients with CVD during the period of our study compared with that of Haskell's study has also greatly improved. There have been major advances in, and there is now increased availability of, medical and surgical therapy, including beta-adrenergic blocking agents, long-acting nitrates, calcium antagonists, percutaneous transluminal coronary angioplasty (PTCA), thrombolytic therapy, and coronary artery bypass graft (CABG) surgery. Experience in management of cardiac patients during exercise sessions during the 1980s as compared with the period of Haskell's study also may have contributed to the improved safety.

The High-Risk Cardiac Rehabilitation Patient

The identification of "high-risk" patients has always been and remains one of the most important issues in cardiac rehabilitation. These are patients who are at high risk for cardiovascular complications during exercise training and who clearly require increased supervision and monitoring compared with those at lower risk.

Patients who experienced cardiac arrest in the Cardiopulmonary Rehabilitation Institute (CAPRI) Program from 1968 to 1981 were studied by Hossack and Hartwig (14). They reported on 2,464 participants who exercised for 374,616 hours under supervision at eight Seattle-area sites. Seventy percent of the participants had clinical evidence of CAD; the remainder had hypertension, multiple risk factors for CAD, or pulmonary conditions. Twenty-five cardiac arrests were reported, 16 during exercise and 9 during the recovery period. All cardiac-arrest victims were successfully resuscitated. Although 20% of the program participants were females, all of the cardiac arrests occurred in males. These arrests occurred in patients with clinical evidence of CAD, but only 1 had undergone previous CABG surgery. Three primary characteristics were found in the patients who experienced a cardiac arrest compared with those who

did not; cardiac-arrest patients had (1) an above-average exercise performance (10 METs [metabolic equivalents] versus 7 METs), (2) more marked ST depression during exercise testing (present in 68% versus 20%), and (3) poor compliance with prescribed training HRs (THRs).

High-risk cardiac rehabilitation patients were the focus of a follow-up study (20) of 21 patients who had experienced a cardiac arrest in the outpatient cardiac rehabilitation programs that were the subject of our original study (11). Clinical data regarding these patients were requested from the program directors and were obtained from all but one. Information gathered included the patient's age, sex, diagnosis, time involved in the cardiac rehabilitation program, activity at the time of the cardiac arrest, cardiac arrest rhythm, cardiopulmonary resuscitation results, history of compliance to exercise prescription, clinical history, exercise test results, and, if performed, cardiac catheterization findings.

Clinical data on the 20 patients in the study are summarized in Table 28.2. The range of ages, male sex predominance, and primary diagnoses probably reflect the frequency of these factors in the cardiac rehabilitation program participants in general. One or more clinical indicators (historical, graded exercise test [GXT], or cardiac catheterization) of poor prognosis in CAD were present in 16 (80%) of the 20 patients, and multiple indicators of poor prognosis were found in 10 (63%) of these 16. The four patients who did not have a clinical indicator of poor prognosis in CAD, however, did not have an entirely normal clinical picture. One patient had an unclear risk status due to a nondiagnostic GXT with Wolff-Parkinson-White pattern on his resting ECG. The other 3 patients had clinical situations that would make a cardiac arrest an understandable event. One had documented ventricular arrhythmias and missed his antiarrhythmic medication dose prior to his exercise session. Another experienced his cardiac arrest while changing a tire on his automobile after an uneventful exercise session. The third experienced an apparent vasovagal syncope.

Traditionally accepted risk factors for poor prognosis in persons with CAD (those related to poor left ventricular function, severe CAD, and electrical instability), while not present in all of the coronary arrest patients, did appear to identify patients at increased or high risk. The study supports the presently used risk stratification approach presented later in this chapter.

ECG monitoring in the programs was either continuous or intermittent. In an effort to evaluate the

Table 28.2 Clinical Characteristics of Patients Who Experienced Cardiac Arrest in Cardiac Rehabilitation Programs

No. of patients: 20
Sex: 18 males, 2 females
Age range: 40-80 years
Primary diagnosis: CAD, manifested as MI, MI with ventricular
fibrillation, prior CABG, prior CA, and angina, either alone or in combination.

Factor studied	Number of patients on whom information was available	Findings

Medical history	19	11 had histories indicative of poor prognosis in CAD patients:
		  4 had prior CA.
		  3 had prior ventricular tachycardia.
		  2 had CHF + prior ventricular tachycardia.
		  1 had CHF.
		  1 had CHF + prior CA.

Exercise ECG	18[a]	10 (56%) had markedly abnormal test results (3 had two of the following):
		  5 had poor exercise capacity (≤ 4.5 min using the Bruce protocol).
		  3 had ventricular tachycardia.
		  2 had ischemic ST-segment depression at an exercise HR < 120 beats/min.
		  2 had peak systolic BPs < 130 mm Hg.
		  1 had exertional hypotension.

Cardiac catheterization prior to in-program CA	14	4 had CABG.
		10 did not have CABG, of which data were available for 9:
		  6 had poor prognosis based on catheterization findings:
		    2 had triple-vessel CAD.
		    1 had LVEF < 40%.
		    2 had both triple-vessel CAD and LVEFs < 40%.
		    1 had 60% left main coronary lesions.
		  3 had significant CAD.

Clinical indicators for poor prognosis (any of the above)	20	Present in 16 patients (80%), of which 10 had multiple indicators

[a]17 performed maximal exercises tests; 1, submaximal.

Note. The patients studied were 20 of the 21 who experienced cardiac arrests during the rehabilitation programs noted in Table 29.1 (no data were available for the other patient). BP = blood pressure; CA = cardiac arrest; CABG = coronary artery bypass graft (surgery); CAD = coronary artery disease; CHF = congestive heart failure; HR = heart rate; LVEF = left ventricular ejection fraction; MI = myocardial infarction; SL-GXT = symptom-limited graded exercise test.

relative safety of these methods, patient profiles were compared; 9 patients were in continuous-ECG programs, 11 in intermittent-ECG programs. The patients who experienced a cardiac arrest in programs with continuous ECG monitoring were found to have a greater incidence of abnormal risk profiles. Patients participating in continuously monitored programs were more likely to have multiple indicators (20 in 9 patients versus 15 in 11 patients) when compared with subjects in intermittently monitored programs. (Additionally 3 of the 4 patients without clinical indicators of high-risk status happened to be participating in intermittently monitored programs.) In contrast, our earlier study did not find significant differences in frequency of cardiac arrest, fatalities, or MI in groups with differing ECG monitoring (11). The continuously monitored programs may have had higher risk patients in need of more monitoring than did the intermittently monitored and graduated programs, but this is not known for certain. In general, referrals to different programs are based on factors related to patient convenience and physician referral patterns, rather than to medical considerations regarding the need for monitoring. It is likely that programs with continuous ECG monitoring do provide increased safety, but also it is probable that most low-risk or even moderate-risk patients do not require them.

Although ECG monitoring of exercise training in the early outpatient period has been advocated and practiced, reported complications are not related to the time elapsed since the clinical event (10,12-14,20). In our study (20), patients experienced cardiac arrests with a great range of program experience, from the first session of cardiac rehabilitation after hospitalization to 10 years following entry into a program. These time periods may reflect an early vulnerability related to the events that led to entry into the program and a later vulnerability related to progression of CVD.

The time of greatest vulnerability during the exercise session is of concern. In general, it appears that most cardiac arrests occur during exercise sessions but that some do occur during the cool-down period. In the study of Hossack and Hartwig (14), 16 of the 25 cardiac arrests occurred during exercise. In our study (20), 12 of the 20 cardiac arrests occurred during the exercise session, 6 (30%) in the immediate cool-down period, and 2 (10%) between 30 and 60 min after the exercise session was completed.

Heart rhythm during cardiac arrest is generally thought to be ventricular tachycardia or ventricular fibrillation. Cardiac arrest rhythms were documented in 17 patients in our study (20) and were primarily ventricular in nature, as has been reported previously (12,14). In 4 patients, the rhythm was ventricular tachycardia; in another 4, ventricular tachycardia degenerating to ventricular fibrillation; in 2, primary ventricular fibrillation; and 6, an unknown rhythm possibly preceding the ventricular fibrillation found at the time of first monitoring. Additionally, 1 patient experienced a cardiac arrest due to bradycardia followed by asystole. This patient had a 20-year history of vasovagal syncope.

In contrast to the rather low frequency of successful resuscitation in out-of-hospital cardiac-arrest victims (21), most patients who experience a cardiac arrest at a cardiac rehabilitation program are successfully resuscitated. Successful resuscitation has been reported at 84% by Haskell (10), 100% by Hossack and Hartwig (14), and 86% in a study involving the 1980-1985 period (11). The prompt administration of emergency treatment in cardiac rehabilitation programs is likely to be a very important factor in the successful outcomes of cardiac arrest reported in cardiac rehabilitation programs.

Seventeen (85%) of the 20 patients who experienced a cardiac arrest in our study (20) were successfully resuscitated without any residual neurologic sequelae. Thirteen of the 17 were defibrillated, 1 was converted with administration of intravenous lidocaine, 1 was successfully "thumpverted," and 1 responded to cardiopulmonary resuscitation (CPR). The patient with bradycardia followed by asystole was resuscitated by administration of atropine, epinephrine, and CPR.

As noted previously, three of the cardiac arrests in this series resulted in fatal outcomes (20). Each of the victims would be considered to be very high risk. The first was a 43-year-old woman who experienced a cardiac arrest while driving home 30 min after an uncomplicated exercise session. Previous coronary angiography had revealed a 60% left main coronary artery lesion and a 60% left anterior descending lesion. Although she had consulted a cardiac surgeon, she did not undergo CABG surgery and continued to smoke cigarettes. The second was a 74-year-old man with multiple high-risk indicators, including a left ventricular ejection fraction (LVEF) of 20% by echocardiography, a history of congestive heart failure (CHF), and ventricular tachycardia. He experienced a cardiac arrest in the early stage of his first exercise session after hospitalization for ventricular tachycardia. The third victim was a 66-year-old man with triple-vessel CAD, abnormal left ventricular function, a previous exercise-related cardiac arrest and a reported tendency to overexert.

A number of program participants, in an effort to accelerate their recovery process, or for other reasons, may exceed their prescribed exercise intensity guidelines. Poor compliance to exercise intensity guidelines certainly places patients at increased risk and cannot be tolerated. The study by Hossack and Hartwig (14) identified poor compliance to exercise prescription to be a factor in the arrest of cardiac-arrest patients. In contrast, our study (20) reported only 1 cardiac-arrest victim out of 19 not to have had good compliance with exercise training guidelines. These data would indicate that good compliance, while very important, does not guarantee exercise safety.

Whereas most patients in the programs that have provided data for the published studies on cardiac rehabilitation program complications had CAD as their primary disease process, today's patients are more complex. They are less likely to be patients with myocardial ischemia as their only pathophysiological process. Today's patients may be older, have poor LVF, high-grade ventricular arrhythmias, and disease of multiple organ systems, including the pulmonary, renal, metabolic, and musculoskeletal systems. A number of patients have coexisting peripheral vascular disease (PVD), cerebrovascular disease, or both. They may be undergoing various forms of medical treatment, including multiple cardiovascular medications. They may have permanent pacemakers or implantable defibrillators. Many have had previous cardiac surgery, including CABG surgery, valvular repair or replacement, or both. Many patients have previously undergone PTCA and thus are at significant risk for restenosis and recurrent myocardial ischemia. Some patients in cardiac rehabilitation programs have undergone a heart transplant. In many cases, today's cardiac rehabilitation program patients have much more complex cardiovascular and medical pathophysiology than did their counterparts of 10 to 20 years ago. Thus, present programs require a more careful and well-planned approach to rehabilitation, so that they can provide exercise therapy at acceptably low risk levels.

How to Provide Exercise Safety in Cardiac Rehabilitation Programs

As can be seen from the data on the low risk of complications during cardiac rehabilitation programs, it has been established that exercise training in patients with CVD can be performed with a high level of safety. Five primary areas of evaluation and treatment are involved in this situation: (1) medical screening and assessment, (2) exercise prescription, (3) patient education, (4) patient supervision, and (5) emergency treatment.

Medical Screening and Assessment

The patient with CVD requires careful evaluation of functional capacity, left ventricular function (LVF), presence and extent of myocardial ischemia, and complexity of arrhythmias. A careful history

and physical examination combined with a maximal symptom limited exercise ECG are the minimum evaluation necessary prior to entry into a cardiac rehabilitation program. All patient data, including cardiac catheterization, echocardiography, ambulatory monitoring, signal-averaged ECG, and electrophysiological studies, if performed, should be used in the evaluation process.

The evaluation process will identify certain patients who are not eligible for entry because of a condition considered a contraindication to exercise training. Many of these patients can, *following* further evaluation and medical or surgical treatment to eliminate or reduce pathophysiological abnormalities, begin exercise training. The following are contraindications to exercise training identified by the AACVPR (9).

- Unstable angina
- Resting systolic BP over 200 mm Hg or resting diastolic BP over 110 mm Hg
- Significant drop ($\geq$ 20 mm Hg) in resting systolic BP from the patient's average level that cannot be attributed to medications
- Moderate to severe aortic stenosis
- Acute systemic illness or fever
- Uncontrolled atrial or ventricular arrhythmias
- Uncontrolled tachycardia (greater than 100 beats/min)
- Symptomatic CHF
- Third-degree heart block without pacemaker
- Active pericarditis or myocarditis
- Recent embolism
- Thrombophlebitis
- Resting ST displacement (> 3 mm)
- Uncontrolled diabetes
- Orthopedic problems that would prohibit exercise

Following evaluation, stabilization, and treatment, many of these patients will be allowed to exercise in a cardiac rehabilitation program.

The initial assessment will also stratify patients into high-, moderate-, and low-risk patient groups; the patients can then be supervised and monitored according to their risk status. The high-risk patient requires careful supervision and probably relatively extensive monitoring during exercise training; the low-risk patient theoretically requires less monitoring.

The ACC (7), ACP (8), and the AACVPR (9) have published recommendations on ECG monitoring of cardiac patients during cardiac rehabilitation programs. These recommendations are based on accepted clinical indicators of poor prognosis in

CAD (poor LVF, myocardial ischemia, and electrical instability).

The ACC's criteria for ECG monitoring are as follows (7):

- Severely depressed LVF (LVEF under 30%)
- Resting complex ventricular arrhythmias (Lown Type IV or V)
- Ventricular arrhythmias appearing or increasing with exercise
- Decrease in systolic BP with exercise
- Survivors of sudden cardiac death
- Patients following MI complicated by CHF, cardiogenic shock, and/or serious ventricular arrhythmias
- Patients with severe CAD and marked exercise-induced ischemia
- Inability to self-monitor heart rate due to physical or intellectual impairment

The ACP's position paper on cardiac rehabilitation services (8) recommends telemetry ECG monitoring for essentially the same group of patients. The AACVPR's *Guidelines for Cardiac Rehabilitation Programs* (9) recommends triaging of patients into continuous ECG-monitored and nonmonitored programs using risk stratification procedures, endorsing the above criteria of the ACC.

Data from our study (20) of patients who experience cardiac arrest during exercise training are consistent with the above recommendations for identifying and monitoring high-risk patients.

Research by Miller et al. (22) on small groups of post-MI patients has demonstrated that, in at least a short-term program (less than 6 months of training), low-risk patients can safely perform home exercise. These patients were identified as low risk by strict criteria: they were 70 years of age or under without CHF, unstable angina, moderately severe exercise-induced angina, valvular heart disease, atrial fibrillation, bundle branch block, previous stroke, limiting orthopedic abnormalities, PVD, chronic obstructive pulmonary disease, obesity, history of CABG surgery, or intercurrent noncardiac illnesses. Sixty-six patients meeting these criteria exercised in a home exercise program without supervision except for the use of HR monitors and twice-weekly transtelephonic ECG transmissions. Over a 26-week period after their initial MI, they did not experience any cardiovascular complications related to exercise. The exclusion criteria in these studies would significantly limit the number of patients eligible for home exercise programs. Such limitations, however, considering the potential risks involved, appear appropriate. Home

exercise programs do have the benefit of lower cost and greater convenience. However, they do not provide important educational, emotional, and social benefits of supervised group programs.

Following the initial evaluation and entry into the rehabilitation program, medical assessment should be performed regularly—following the first 12 weeks of the program and then at least on a yearly basis if a maintenance program is continued. Reevaluation will be performed more often as clinically indicated. It is also important to appreciate the potential for progression of disease, especially in patients who have undergone initially successful PTCAs, since they are at significant risk for restenosis.

Exercise Prescription

The exercise prescription is formulated with all the evaluation information available, especially with regard to exercise intensity. The appropriate exercise intensity should be below the threshold of myocardial ischemia or significant arrhythmia provocation. It is important for patients to appreciate that the exercise intensity should be high enough to achieve physiological benefits, but low enough to avoid cardiovascular and musculoskeletal problems and feelings of overexertion. It must also be understood by program personnel and participants that significant physiological benefits can occur at low levels of exercise intensity (< 45% maximal oxygen uptake [$\dot{V}O_2$max]) (23). For programs with only intermittent ECG monitoring available, it would appear prudent to lower exercise intensities for high-risk patients, so as to provide additional levels of safety.

While information from GXTs is important in determining an appropriate exercise intensity, some patients will have GXT findings that do not allow for the accurate determination of the presence of myocardial ischemia. Patients with nondiagnostic tests due to left ventricular hypertrophy (LVH), interventricular conduction delays (nonspecific or left bundle branch block), resting ST-T changes (including patients on digitalis), or permanent pacemakers must be accepted as having undetermined status based on their GXT. These patients' exercise intensities must therefore be based on other clinical information; an overall conservative approach would be appropriate.

The musculoskeletal exercises in a cardiac rehabilitation program are designed for patients who are likely to be deconditioned due to disease or inactivity. These patients may or may not have preexisting musculoskeletal problems. Musculoskeletal exercises can improve muscular strength and endurance and joint flexibility, but it is important to avoid any exercises that might aggravate preexisting conditions. (Guidelines and safety considerations regarding weight training for low-risk cardiac rehabilitation patients are addressed in chapter 17.)

Patient Education

Patients must understand the importance of compliance with their own exercise prescription, including general exercise guidelines on proper gradual warm-up and cool-down, progression of exercise, and their individual exercise intensity prescription. Attention to these factors will help avoid musculoskeletal and cardiovascular problems. Isometric exercise is generally discouraged, although patients without signs or symptoms of myocardial ischemia on a GXT at a level of 7 to 8 METs do not appear to have any difficulty with combined static and dynamic exercise compared with dynamic exercise alone (24).

Patients should be instructed to report any exercise-related problems or change in their typical symptoms. They must also be instructed to report any change in their medical regimen or whether they have forgotten to take any medication prior to their exercise session. Additionally, it is important for the staff to inquire about patients' general clinical status before each exercise session. All participants should avoid prolonged hot showers, steam baths, and saunas, since these may lead to peripheral vasodilation, hypotension, and possibly syncope. Any unusual behavior in a fellow participant should be reported by program participants to the medical staff. Patients should also learn to self-monitor HR and rhythm and to subjectively assess exercise intensity (level of perceived exertion).

Patient Supervision

As indicated previously, the degree of supervision depends on the risk status of the patient and the intensity of exercise prescribed. The most extensive supervision is clearly indicated for high-risk patients exercising at moderate to high intensities. The number of personnel and the extent of their training necessary for a cardiac rehabilitation program in general, and for attendance at specific exercise sessions, will depend on the risk status of the patients exercising and their exercise intensity.

AACVPR's *Guidelines for Cardiac Rehabilitation Programs* (9) states that all personnel must possess current certification in basic life support (BLS) from the AHA or equivalent and that at least one staff member certified in advanced cardiac life support (ACLS) and having the medicolegal authority to provide such care must be present whenever directly supervised rehabilitation exercise is provided for high- and intermediate-risk patients. These guidelines are generally appropriate, but should be interpreted for individual situations.

Patient supervision includes both observation of the patient's general appearance and monitoring of HR and rhythm. Monitoring can vary from continuous ECG monitoring to either intermittent ECG monitoring with quick-look paddles or self-monitoring by program participants with as-needed ECG monitoring. Patient supervision also includes enforcement of compliance with general and individual exercise guidelines. Significant variations of climactic conditions require exercise sessions to be adjusted appropriately (see chapters 20 and 21). Any games played during cardiac rehabilitation programs require adaptation of rules to discourage competition and high exercise intensity. Supervision must continue through the recovery period following exercise, as many cardiovascular complications occur during this time (14,20).

Program size has not been shown to correlate with any difference in complication rates among outpatient cardiac rehabilitation programs (11). It appears that programs of all sizes can provide cardiac patients with safe exercise. Obviously, personnel and monitoring requirements must be tailored to the number of patients being exercised and their risk status.

Emergency Treatment

The final important area in providing safe exercise for cardiac rehabilitation participants is emergency treatment. The resuscitation rate has been high in several studies, ranging from 84% to 100% (10,11,14). Cardiac arrhythmias with and without loss of consciousness, chest pain, CHF, hypertension or hypotension, hypoglycemia, dyspnea related to bronchospasm, seizures, transient ischemic attacks, and musculoskeletal problems are some of the emergencies that cardiac rehabilitation personnel must be able to handle. Emergency drugs, a defibrillator, personnel trained in CPR, and a well-practiced emergency plan are the basic requirements for emergency readiness.

A detailed approach to the management of emergencies, including emergency equipment, may be found in the *Guidelines for Cardiac Rehabilitation Programs* of the AACVPR (9).

Summary

The prevention of exercise-related complications involves both an awareness of potential problems and a careful preventive strategy and, if necessary, prompt emergency treatment. While it is reassuring that even patients with extensive CVD can exercise with a high level of safety, it must be remembered that such exercise is not inherently safe, but that safety results from careful planning and adherence to present standards of cardiac rehabilitation. The cardiovascular complications of cardiac rehabilitation programs generally occur in high-risk patients with traditional indicators of poor prognosis in CAD. Medical screening and assessment for the purpose of risk stratification, exercise prescription, and decisions regarding supervision and monitoring are critical initial steps for cardiac rehabilitation safety. Appropriate levels of monitoring and, if necessary, the administration of any necessary emergency treatment are the final factors in this important process.

References

1. Oldridge, N.B.; Guyait, D.H.; Fischer, M.E.; Rimm, A.A. Cardiac rehabilitation after myocardial infarction. Combined experience of randomized clinical trials. JAMA. 260:945-950; 1988.
2. O'Connor, G.T.; Buring, J.E.; Yusuf, S.; Goldhaber, S.Z.; Olmstead, E.M.; Paffenbarger, R.S., Jr.; Hennekens, C.H. An overview of randomized trials of rehabilitation with exercise after myocardial infarction. Circulation. 1989. 80(2):234-244; 1989.
3. Clausen, J.P. Circulatory adjustments to dynamic exercise and the effect of physical training in normal subjects and in patients with coronary artery disease. Prog. Cardiovasc. Dis. 18:459-495; 1976.
4. Stern, J.M.; Cleary, P. National exercise and heart disease project: Psychological changes observed in a low-level exercise program. Arch. Intern. Med. 141:1463-1467; 1981.
5. Hartung, G.H.; Squires, W.G.; Gotto, A.M. Effect of exercise training on plasma high-density lipoprotein cholesterol in coronary heart disease patients. Am. Heart J. 101:181-184; 1981.
6. Froelicher, V.; Jensen, D.; Genter, F.; Sullivan, M.; McKirnan, M.D.; Wiztum, K.; Scharf, J.; Strong, M.L.; Ashburn, W. A randomized trial of exercise training in patients with coronary heart disease. JAMA. 252:1291-1297; 1984.
7. Recommendations of the American college of cardiology on cardiovascular rehabilitation. J. Am. Coll. Cardiol. 7:451-453; 1986.
8. Health and Public Policy Committee, American College of Physicians. Cardiac rehabilitation services. Ann. Intern. Med. 109:671-673; 1988.
9. American Association of Cardiovascular and Pulmonary Rehabilitation. Guidelines for cardiac rehabilitation programs. Champaign, IL: Human Kinetics; 1991.
10. Haskell, W.L. Cardiovascular complications during exercise training of cardiac patients. Circulation. 57:920-924; 1978.
11. Van Camp, S.P.; Peterson, R.A. Cardiovascular complications of outpatient cardiac rehabilitation programs. JAMA. 256:1160-1163; 1986.
12. Mead, W.F.; Pyfer, H.R.; Trombold, J.C.; Frederick, R.C. Successful resuscitation of two near-simultaneous cases of cardiac arrest with a review of 15 cases occurring during supervised exercise. Circulation. 53:187-189; 1976.
13. Fletcher, G.F.; Cantwell, J.D. Ventricular fibrillation in a medically supervised cardiac exercise program. JAMA. 238:2627-2629; 1977.
14. Hossack, K.F.; Hartwig, R. Cardiac arrest associated with supervised cardiac rehabilitation. J. Cardiac. Rehabil. 2:402-408; 1982.
15. Shephard, R.J.; Kavanagh, T.; Tuck, J. Marathon jogging in post-myocardial infarction patients. J. Cardiac. Rehabil. 3:321-329; 1983.
16. McNeer, J.F.; Margolis, J.R.; Lee, K.L.; Kisslo, J.A.; Peter, R.H.; Kong, Y.; Behar, V.S.; Wallace, A.G.; McCants, C.B.; Rosat, R.A. The role of the exercise test in evaluation of patients with ischemic heart disease. Circulation. 57:64-70; 1978.
17. Theroux, P.; Waters, D.D.; Halphen, C.; Debaisieux, J.C.; Mizgala, H.F. Prognostic value of exercise testing soon after myocardial infarction. N. Engl. J. Med. 301:341-345; 1979.
18. Pitt, B.; Kalff, V.; Rabinovitch, M.A.; Buda, A.J.; Colfer, H.T.; Volgel, R.A.; Thrall, J.H. Impact of radionuclide techniques on evaluations of patients with ischemic heart disease. J. Am. Coll. Cardiol. 1:63-72; 1983.
19. Patterson, R.E.; Horowitz, S.F.; Eng, C.; Meller, J.; Goldsmith, S.J.; Pichard, A.D.; Halgash, D.A.; Herman, M.V.; Gorlin, R.A. Can noninvasive exercise test criteria identify patients with left main or three-vessel coronary artery disease after a first myocardial infarction? Am. J. Cardiol. 51:361-372; 1983.
20. Van Camp, S.P.; Peterson, R.A. Identification of the high-risk cardiac rehabilitation patient. J. Cardiopul. Rehabil. 9:103-109; 1989.
21. Cobb, L.A.; Hallstrom, A.P. Community-based cardiopulmonary resuscitation: What have we learned? Ann. NY Acad. Sci. 382:330; 1982.
22. Miller, N.H.; Haskell, W.L.; Berra, K.; DeBusk, R.F. Home versus group exercise training for increasing

functional capacity after myocardial infarction. Circulation. 70:645-649; 1984.

23. Blumenthal, J.A.; Rejeski, W.J.; Walsh-Riddle, M.; Emery, C.F.; Miller, H.; Roark, S.; Ribisl, P.M.; Morris, P.B.; Brubaker, P.; Williams, S.R. Comparison of high- and low-intensity exercise training early after acute myocardial infarction. Am. J. Cardiol. 61:26-30; 1988.

24. Hung, J.; McKillip, J.; Savin, W.; Magver, S.; Kraus, R.; Houston, N.; Goris, M.; Haskell, W.; DeBusk, R. Comparison of cardiovascular response to combined static-dynamic effort, postprandial dynamic effort and dynamic effort alone in patients with chronic ischemic heart disease. Circulation. 65:1411-1419; 1982.

Chapter 29

Legal Considerations

William G. Herbert
David L. Herbert

The number of personal-injury lawsuits filed in the United States today is believed by many to be out of control. The effects have been especially detrimental to the health care field. The annual number of large damage awards has driven medical malpractice insurance premiums to nearly unobtainable levels (1), a dilemma that has even caused an increasing number of physicians to leave their practices. Also disturbing is the fact that in many instances rising malpractice insurance premiums are passed directly on to patient fees, adding to what already are record-high costs of health care. An apparent predisposition to litigate may thus be driving up the cost of health care, as well as limiting the availability of providers.

Many have come to expect that lawsuits ought to serve as a method of early choice for resolving a variety of complex human issues, including how medical care is defined and administered. Many also have unreasonable expectations for medical treatment and of physicians, expecting cures even when faced with the most severe illnesses. When treatment outcomes are less than expected, many dissatisfied patients seek compensation. The public media is replete with accounts of how this scenario leads to lawsuits, including examples that seem blatantly frivolous. The seriousness of this problem has prompted ongoing legislative efforts to regulate damage awards and to call into question the effectiveness of the entire tort system (2).

While there has been scant media coverage of lawsuits involving cardiac rehabilitation, actions against providers in related medical areas, such as exercise testing, began to appear in the mid-1980s (3,4). Other negligence lawsuits directly involving cardiac rehabilitation providers are now in progress or have only recently been resolved. Thus, cardiac rehabilitation professionals need to understand their legal risks for negligence actions and what mechanisms are available to reduce these risks.

In general, professionals must address a variety of legally important concerns affecting both the design and delivery of clinical services, namely, writing program policies and procedures, utilizing appropriate equipment, employing and supervising qualified personnel, establishing and maintaining a legally acceptable informed-consent process, and supervising and documenting the delivery of appropriate care for the individual patient. Other legally important considerations include the development of emergency procedures and the related use of physician-developed "standing orders," counseling patients as to unsupervised physical activity, professional liability and other forms of insurance, waivers or prospective releases, incident reports, and communication and confidentiality issues. This chapter reviews fundamental medicolegal aspects of cardiac rehabilitation services. For extensive treatment of legal issues, interested readers are referred to other sources (5,6).

Historical Considerations

Cardiac rehabilitation is a relatively new health care specialization that is in some respects struggling for acceptance among health care professionals. In the 1950s, a few clinical trials were conducted; these demonstrated that controlled exercise was safe for low-risk cardiac patients who had at least a moderate exercise tolerance (> 6 to 8 METs [metabolic equivalents]). Thereafter, much debate ensued over matters of approach, patient eligibility, safety, and the effects on morbidity and mortality. Acceptance of these efforts improved substantially in the 1980s, both in the medical community and by the public, and cardiac rehabilitation gained considerable momentum. This may have been because "risk factor amelioration" techniques of cardiac rehabilitation were being viewed as consistent with concepts of preventive medicine that were gaining wide support nationally (7). Acceptance of cardiac rehabilitation services was also improved in the 1980s by the publication of findings from aggregated clinical trials that showed mortality reductions of 20% to 25% after patient participation in cardiac rehabilitation programs that included exercise (8,9).

Despite this progress, cardiac rehabilitation continues to be seriously challenged in the United States, both internally and externally. From within, there are controversies about appropriate treatment objectives, standards, cost control, the margin of safety, when to use technology, and the thresholds of competency and credentialing needed to practice. Several associations of health care providers with varying degrees of involvement in the practice continue to issue position papers without dialogue, and this tends to result in nonuniform standards of care (10,11). Governmental agencies and private organizations involved in third-party funding of services are constantly seeking means to modify the standards so as to reduce the scope of "medically necessary" reimbursable care (12). These forces have increased, in subtle ways, some of the legal risks inherent in providing care. The most important of these challenges are addressed in this chapter.

Cardiac rehabilitation services constitute a system of medical care. The fundamental objectives are to relieve symptoms, minimize loss of function, and optimize the recovery of life quality. Other features of the practice, including activities of diagnosis, prescription, and administration of treatment, evidence this medical character. Legally, practitioners need to remember that state statutes explicitly define who has the authority to deliver medical services. However, in the field of cardiac rehabilitation, a multidisciplinary staffing pattern has evolved in programs, and many specialized providers are not licensed. Moreover, it is common for both licensed and unlicensed providers, working under the authority of a physician in charge, to deliver many of the same patient services in different program settings. This may lead to serious problems for staff and programs when, in the event of an injury or death, the unlicensed professional is performing in a capacity reserved by law for the licensed provider. Therefore, an examination of the tort system and consideration of how the medical model applies to cardiac rehabilitation should be helpful to all those who seek to manage the legal risks attendant to their work.

General Liability Considerations

It is important to develop proper perspective on vulnerability for legal problems and the foundations on which risk management are formulated. To accomplish this objective, an overview of negligence, standards of care, and informed consent concepts will be presented. Some discussion of the standards most pertinent to the field of cardiac rehabilitation also will be presented in this section.

Negligence, Malpractice, and the Standard of Care

The tort system exists to resolve questions of civil wrongdoing. It examines conduct that may be intentional or negligent and seeks to determine if that conduct resulted in harm to another person. Legally defined, *negligence* is a failure to conform one's conduct to a generally accepted standard of conduct or duty. *Malpractice* is a special form of negligence applicable to a variety of professionals, including physicians and certain other health care providers. A cause of legal action for negligence is established by proof of a breach of duty proximately causing harm or damage to another. A cause of legal action for malpractice is essentially the same, except that proof of duty and breach of duty are provided by comparison to the applicable standard of care as established by the profession under examination. Proof of applicability of a given standard and failure to meet it are typically established through expert witnesses during the trial. Until the mid-1980s, determination of the appropriate standard in legal cases weighed heavily upon individual opinions of expert witnesses. Medically naive jurors often had to sort out conflicting interpretations by experts called either by defense or plaintiff counsels. This process increased legal exposure for physicians and their malpractice insurers. Many health care associations responded by developing consensus recommendations, guidelines, and standards to provide a more definitive and nationally applicable benchmark for practice. While these peer-promulgated standards tend to increase quality assurance for individual patients, unfortunately they also tend to limit the practitioner's latitude in clinical judgment (13). Furthermore, in immature specialty areas like cardiac rehabilitation, the standard-setting groups are more numerous and revisions come forth frequently. Difficulties then arise for the practitioner in terms of awareness of all these different standards and how to comply at the personal level when contradictory expectations exist.

Nevertheless, to provide quality care and reduce legal risks, practitioners should adopt the most up-to-date and authoritative standards possible. Several national organizations have issued such standards for cardiac rehabilitation in recent years. The most important and comprehensive statements are those of the American Heart Association (AHA), the American College of Sports Medicine (ACSM), the American College of Cardiology (ACC), and the American Association of Cardiovascular and Pulmonary Rehabilitation (AACVPR).

Standards of Care in Cardiac Rehabilitation

Professionals should recognize that the standards of these organizations are crucial to defining the elements of care that are professionally and legally owed to patients. They would most likely be used in a legal action to examine professional conduct. Before the fact, professionals can demonstrate that an appropriate standard is recognized and expected to guide services by citing such standards in written program policy and procedure manuals. Then, in specific challenges involving negligence claims, patient case notes showing the details of actual care delivered and staff annotations in program records can demonstrate fulfillment, which can link conduct to the manuals and the standard. Certain of these standards, as well as others not reviewed in this book, have already been used as reference points in the judicial setting (4). Thus, it is important to briefly describe the more important peer-developed standards (a more complete analysis and comparison of these is found in chapter 19).

American Heart Association

The AHA first developed cardiac rehabilitation guidelines for physicians in the early 1970s. These addressed exercise testing and physical activity prescription for management of heart disease patients (14). Later the AHA enlarged upon these guidelines in its *Exercise Standards Book* (15). This source emphasized physician control in all aspects of exercise evaluation, prescription, monitoring, and supervision. Although it recognized the roles of other professionals in delivery of exercise services, it implied a very high level of personal responsibility and involvement on the part of the physician. In 1990, the AHA published updated exercise standards that integrated information from recent research and clinical trials into a comprehensive set of recommendations (16). All cardiac rehabilitation practitioners should review this document for applicability to their programs.

American College of Cardiology

In 1986 the ACC published recommendations dealing primarily with admission and monitoring of exercise aspects of cardiovascular rehabilitation (11). Despite the adoption of these written statements, much is left to the individual determination and discretion of the physician. In the 1980s, with the rapid increase in the costs of cardiological care, the ACC formed a joint task force with the AHA to write consensus guidelines for physicians on appropriate uses of developing medical technology. Their published recommendations cover several expensive evaluation procedures, including ambulatory ECG (17) and exercise testing (10). The latter guidelines bear directly on patient evaluation in cardiac rehabilitation. In practice, serial graded exercise tests (GXTs) are the "cornerstone" for such key procedures as exercise prescription and risk stratification for exercise supervision. Yet, the ACC/AHA recommendations (10) conclude that routine serial GXTs within the framework of cardiac rehabilitation are not useful. This particular point contradicts the more recent guidelines of the AACVPR and demonstrates how legal uncertainty is created for programs and professionals when nonuniform guidelines coexist.

American College of Sports Medicine

The ACSM has developed a comprehensive set of guidelines for preventive and rehabilitative exercise programs. The guidelines have been updated at 4-year intervals, the latest set published in 1991 (18). The content is highly definitive and presents medically and scientifically based protocols for the full range of exercise services, from admission to exercise testing to supervision in exercise maintenance programs. In addition, ACSM guidelines are unique in specifying how exercise professionals should interact with physicians in the delivery of exercise services and include an extensive section that defines the competencies for rehabilitative exercise personnel. To support the implementation of these competency standards in the field, the ACSM maintains a national examination process that certifies as many as 500 Exercise Test Technologists, Exercise Specialists, and Program Directors each year. ACSM guidelines emphasize a multidisciplinary team approach for providing exercise (cardiac) rehabilitation services. Consequently, the roles and responsibilities for various personnel do not fully coincide with those of the AHA, particularly with regard to the physician (14,15). Such differences have the potential to create added legal concerns for some who practice outside the typical rehabilitation environment, especially in free-standing clinics, and for practitioners who do not operate under the legal authority of a licensed provider (generally a physician).

American Association of Cardiovascular and Pulmonary Rehabilitation

The AACVPR was formed in the mid-1980s to provide a national voice for the growing group of interdisciplinary clinicians who provide rehabilitative care for cardiovascular and pulmonary patients. The organization now represents a membership of nearly 3,000. In 1990, this association published its first comprehensive guidelines to define the minimum standards of care for cardiac rehabilitation (19). Issues addressed include, but are not limited to, risk stratification, electrocardiographic (ECG) monitoring, emergency procedures, staff-patient ratios, licensing and certification for personnel, and documentation of treatment outcomes. Although the first edition of the AACVPR's guidelines contains some topical "gaps" and incongruities in subject treatment, the contents would very likely be viewed today as highly applicable in the legal setting for resolving questions of professional duty and care owed to a particular patient (plaintiff).

Other Standards

A variety of other professional associations, as well as health insurance providers and governmental agencies, have published statements that may have important influences upon cardiac rehabilitation standards. In many cases, the guidelines of third-party payers are at odds with the standards of major associations, in that they tend to limit patient eligibility; duration of treatment; the application of such medically important areas as the nutritional, psychological, and educational; and the way in which physicians are expected to supervise individual patient care. The guidelines of the national Blue Cross and Blue Shield and of its affiliates in each state, as well as the Medicare guidelines for reimbursement of cardiovascular and pulmonary rehabilitation, are examples of these cost containment policies (20). Such measures often impose inordinate pressure to reduce the scope and quality of patient care, creating a dilemma for health care providers. Liability lawsuits are just now bringing questions before the courts on who may have responsibility for harm when cost containment measures corrupt medical judgment (21). These resource-conserving policies will continue into the foreseeable future. Professionals must weigh the need for compliance against their responsibility of providing reasonable care to patients and adhering to what may be contrasting standards prescribed by their peer associations.

Additional publications of governmental agencies and special interest groups may also have implications to the standard of care in special situations. For example, some of these address and specify certain expectations for hospital-operated programs (22), cardiovascular exercise maintenance facilities (23), and protocols utilized by physical therapists in providing cardiopulmonary rehabilitation treatment (24).

Informed Consent

Informed consent should be viewed as a protocol of communication between a qualified health care provider and a prospective patient. It is not legally sufficient merely to secure the patient's and practitioner's signatures on a form. The doctrine has a substantial history in medical case law (25), which is meant to safeguard a patient's legal rights of self-determination in all matters involving residual health and survival, and from which the elements of contemporary informed-consent procedures have evolved. Informed consent encompasses the patient's understanding of the risks associated with a particular treatment. Without such a legally effective informed-consent process, the performance of routine diagnostic and therapeutic procedures would cause medical practitioners to be liable for both civil battery and any harmful outcomes of treatment that might occur to the patient.

A legally sufficient informed-consent procedure implies clear communication, by the provider, of intent to test or treat and cognition of the patient concerning the procedure to be performed. It further implies the giving of permission, freely, by the patient (who must be a legally competent adult) that allows a provider to perform specified medical procedures. It requires that the patient be provided with information as to the purpose, nature, risks, and benefits of the procedure, as well as the applicable alternatives. Based upon these factors, the patient must voluntarily and knowingly agree to undergo the procedure, be given the opportunity to ask questions, and receive clear responses. Failures in the informed-consent process can result in litigation if harm to the patient occurs. *Hedgecorth v. United States* (26) is a case that demonstrates the question of liability due to provider failure in securing valid informed consent to conduct GXT at a Veterans Administration medical center. The elderly plaintiff had undergone a separate GXT at another location shortly before the GXT in question, but the results of the first test were not secured by the Veterans Administration facility or its physicians. The plaintiff complained of a loss of vision in his left eye and chest pain during the second GXT, at the Veterans Administration center. It was subsequently learned that he had suffered a stroke and blindness due to the stroke as a direct result of the second test. Although the plaintiff did sign an informed-consent document prior to the second test, the document did not contain a risk-disclosure provision as to the possibility of stroke occurring during the GXT. The court determined from the evidence presented at trial that the dangers of GXTs include the possibility that the patient will suffer a stroke. Furthermore, the court determined that the patient should have been warned of this possible outcome and, since he was not forewarned of the risk of stroke, he could not evaluate the danger of this specific risk in making his decision to undergo the test. As a result of this finding, the court held that the defendants were responsible for the plaintiff's "total and permanent disability." Damages approaching $1 million were awarded (26).

Traditionally, the informed-consent process would require only the disclosure of material risks that were historically evidenced through clinical experience of the profession. However, the law has begun to move toward requiring very broad risk disclosure to patients. While it is not possible to disclose all remotely possible risks and harmful outcomes, a trend is developing to require that patients be given more detailed and comprehensive information (27). In keeping with this trend, it is the contemporary practice in cardiac rehabilitation to provide separate informed-consent procedures for evaluation and treatment protocols. For each of the two consent procedures, the provider should specify the unique foreseeable risks, as well as the desired beneficial medical outcomes (see Appendixes A and B for sample forms).

Several additional considerations pertinent to informed consent need to be addressed, such as the dilemma of consent with the anxious patient (25,27) and use of prospective waivers of liability (5). Since the legal expectations for informed consent are changing rapidly, practitioners should secure periodic legal review of their informed-consent procedures and forms.

Key Liability Concerns and Risk Management

There are certain domains of service that, when considered within the context of standards and case litigation, should be emphasized for purposes of risk management in cardiac rehabilitation. This section addresses these domains and discusses risk-reduction procedures that may be helpful.

Exercise Testing and Exercise Prescription

Practices in exercise testing and prescription raise significant legal concerns for cardiac rehabilitation programs (28). These are clearly medical procedures. Consequently, material involvement of a licensed physician is critical at some level. State statutes mandate that only publicly licensed health care providers may perform procedures that are medical in nature. Cardiac rehabilitation undoubtedly meets the legal requirements of a medical-care specialty when its aims, tools, and protocols are compared against the statutory definitions of medical practice. Should any person engage in exercise testing or exercise prescription within the context of a medical model but not involve a licensed practitioner, then there is a risk of adverse consequences due to potential violations of both criminal and civil laws.

Virtually all states have enacted statutes making the unauthorized provision of medical care a criminal offense. Such statutes typically provide that the practice of medicine is "generally regarded as the diagnosis of an individual's symptoms to determine with what disease or illness he or she is afflicted, and then to determine on the basis of that diagnosis what remedy or treatment should be given or prescribed to treat that disease and/or relieve the symptoms" (5). A separate adverse consequence might occur for the nonphysician who is found to be engaged in the unauthorized practice of medicine. In such an event, the practitioner's conduct would be compared with the presumed conduct of a physician acting under the same or similar circumstances, a standard of care that cannot be met by nonphysicians. A finding of negligence is almost assured in such circumstances. Exercise testing in the medical setting has resulted in substantial instances of claim and litigation (see, for example, Edelman [27]).

Current legal mandates aside, there is considerable debate as to the professional need of having a physician present and in "visual contact" for every clinical GXT. Periodically, in efforts to delineate the "medically necessary" treatment, health insurance providers have sought to limit reimbursement for cardiac exercise rehabilitation services to those performed by a physician who is present and visually supervising the procedure. With respect to GXTs, Gibbons (29) has argued in support of physician presence on the basis of special diagnostic insight and ultimate responsibility for patient safety (see also Herbert [30]). Blessey (31) and DeBusk (32) have proposed that other professionals may effectively and safely provide this supervision in certain circumstances. From a legal perspective, each professional and program must examine relevant state statutes and regulations pertaining to authority for performance of medical procedures for direction in this matter. Some jurisdictions may allow certain licensed allied health care providers to act in narrowly defined and documented ways, as surrogates of the physician in charge. In certain program environments, these mechanisms may be used to effect valid physician supervision for such procedures as exercise testing, exercise prescription, and monitored exercise therapy.

The medical use of exercise testing has increased dramatically in recent years (33) and with this trend, questions have developed about its medical value with different patient populations. As utilization increases, no doubt so will the incidents of legal claim and suit (34,35). For these reasons, cardiac rehabilitation professionals should be particularly cautious about their legal exposure in this area. Concerted efforts should be made to be certain that sufficient physician control is maintained in every decision that requires a risk-benefit consideration for the individual patient. This is yet another area of concern for which individualized medicolegal advice is needed by each program.

Supervision of the Exercising Cardiac Patient

The monitoring of an individual patient's participation in rehabilitation, particularly for exercise, is sure to become an area of increasing claim and litigation in the years ahead. As cost considerations continue to reduce hospital stays for acute coronary patients, concerns about safety increase. This is particularly true for the post–myocardial infarction (MI) patient population, which suffers its highest mortality in the first 6 to 12 months after MI. New standards are evolving in cardiac rehabilitation to address this difficult problem (19). One strategy is to stratify patients for exercise supervision in accordance with the severity of their disease and risk for cardiovascular complications. Risk stratification is an imperfect process, and it remains to be seen whether application of the triaging criteria will conserve costs and still maintain a safe level of exercise supervision for moderate to severely diseased patients. Professionals should recognize that increased utilization of unsupervised, self-monitored programs for patients necessarily carries a greater potential for legal claim and suit (36).

Policy and Procedure Manual

Cardiac rehabilitation programs should develop individualized policies and procedure manuals to serve as blueprints for their operations. Such documents should be developed in conjunction with legal and medical consultation. These manuals should also reference the important standards from professional organizations and others to demonstrate how operations relate to peer expectations of quality and safety. Program policies and procedures will serve as the initial line of defense for program activity in the event of claim and suit. A caution is in order, however, because if the manual is not followed by the program's own personnel, proof of negligence may come from within the manual itself. Negligence or malpractice might be established by reference to program policies and breach thereof by program personnel, sometimes even without the requirement of expert testimony (37).

Communications and Record Keeping

Thorough and comprehensive communications and record keeping are important means for detection of clinical problems and for managing the progression of patient treatment. Legally, such functions also serve to demonstrate fulfillment of appropriate service within the mandates of written program policies. Detailed, legible, staff-signed records documenting patient treatment, progress, instruction, compliance, cautions, warnings, and referrals, are absolutely necessary to show defensible program activity. Many lawyers who represent injured parties say that if a file notation as to a particular procedure is not written within patient records, such an event did not happen. Those deciding these issues in malpractice cases sometimes agree. Thus, it is imperative for records of both negative and positive findings to be recorded and for a proper chronological sequence of documentation to be established in patient records. The time for record retention has traditionally been linked to so-called statutes of limitation, within which lawsuits might be filed. However, rapid changes in court rulings and new legislative enactments affecting this matter have created uncertainties, so it is best to keep these records as long as possible.

Liability Insurance

An essential component of risk management for health care providers and their employers is liability insurance. All those practicing in cardiac rehabilitation must secure and maintain such coverage or face exposure of their personal assets to claim and suit. Most professional associations participate in group insurance programs that allow their members access to professional liability insurance coverage at reasonable costs. Purchasers should be cautious, because the coverage available with certain policies may vary considerably. Therefore, before purchasing insurance it is essential to understand the qualifying criteria. Sometimes exclusions of certain categories of professional service or provisions affecting employees versus the self-employed can make such coverage invalid in the event of claim or suit.

Risk management is a series of proactive, ongoing activities designed to prevent harmful consequences of program services for patients and subsequent claims and suits. Effective risk management can minimize legal exposure and sometimes even allow providers to secure liability insurance at reduced premiums. Many medical malpractice lawsuits that are filed have recurring characteristics that result in contention. Prominent among these are inaccurate patient records, communication failure between provider and patient, and hostility attendant to fee collection procedures. Periodic administrative review of practices, especially in the aforementioned areas, constitutes one important risk-management strategy. Program audits by external consultants or representatives of peer associations can also provide objective evaluations of services. Audits typically assess compliance with industry standards in such areas as facilities, equipment, credentialing and maintenance of competencies of personnel, and documentation of

services. Implementation of risk-management recommendations can support the professional's primary service objective—providing better patient care—so these techniques should be adopted for all rehabilitative programs.

Summary

Complex legal questions arise for health care professionals who currently provide cardiovascular rehabilitation services in the United States. The legal risks involved, the medical nature of the services provided, and the applicability of laws in different jurisdictions make individual legal advice imperative for all programs. The foregoing overview of relevant civil-law concepts, malpractice issues, and risk-control strategies should sensitize practitioners to legal concerns. However, each professional must do more. We advise that program administrators regularly evaluate the legal risks inherent in the operation of services and act to manage these risks. This approach provides the best prospect for maintaining the expected standard of care and minimizing exposure to claim and suit.

References

1. Gest, T.; Work, C.P. Sky-high damage suits: The impact on consumers, business and professions. US News & World Report. 100:35-43; 1986.
2. Pollner, F. Tort reform: Liability crisis alive and kicking. Medical World News. (November):18-19; 1990.
3. Herbert, D.L. Informed consent and new disclosure responsibility for exercise testing: The case of Hedgecorth v. United States. The Exercise Standards & Malpractice Reporter. 1:30-32; 1987.
4. Herbert, W.G.; Herbert, D.L. Legal aspects of cardiac rehabilitation exercise programs. Phys. Sportsmed. 16:105-112; 1988.
5. Herbert, D.L.; Herbert, W.G. Legal aspects of preventive, rehabilitative and recreational exercise programs, 3rd ed. Canton, OH: Professional Reports Corporation; 1993.
6. Herbert, W.G.; Herbert, W.G. Legal aspects of cardiac rehabilitation exercise programs. Phys. Sportsmed. 16:105-112; 1988.
7. U.S. Department of Health and Human Services, Public Health Service. Promoting health/preventing disease: Year 2000, objectives for the nation. Washington, DC: U.S. Government Printing Office; 1989.
8. Oldridge, N.B.; Guyatt, G.H.; Fischer, M.E.; Rimm, A.A. Cardiac rehabilitation after myocardial infarction: Combined experience of randomized clinical trials. JAMA. 260:945-950; 1988.

9. O'Conner, G.T.; Burning, J.E.; Yusuf, S.; Goldhaber, S.Z.; Olmstead, E.M.; Paffenbarger, R.S.; Hennekens, C.H. An overview of randomized trials of rehabilitation with exercise after myocardial infarction. Circulation. 80:234-244; 1989.

10. American College of Cardiology/American Heart Association Task Force on Assessment of Cardiovascular Procedures. Special report: Exercise testing. JACC. 8:725-738; 1986.

11. American College of Cardiology. Recommendations of the American College of Cardiology on cardiovascular rehabilitation. Cardiol. 15:4-5; 1986.

12. Office of Health Technology Assessment. Public health service assessment: Cardiac rehabilitation services. DHHS publication no. (PHS) 88-3427. Springfield, VA; 1987.

13. Hornbein, T.F. The setting of standards of care. JAMA. 256:1040-1041; 1986.

14. American Heart Association. Exercise testing and training of individuals with heart disease or at high risk for its development: A handbook for physicians. Dallas: American Heart Association; 1972.

15. American Heart Association. The exercise standards book. Dallas: American Heart Association; 1980.

16. American Heart Association. Exercise standards: A statement for health professionals from the American Heart Association. Circulation. 82:2286-2322; 1990.

17. American College of Cardiology/American Heart Association Task Force on Assessment of Cardiovascular Procedures. Guidelines for ambulatory electrocardiography. JACC. 13:249-258; 1989.

18. American College of Sports Medicine. Guidelines for graded exercise testing and exercise prescription, 4th ed. Philadelphia: Lea & Febiger; 1991.

19. American Association for Cardiovascular and Pulmonary Rehabilitation. Guidelines for cardiac rehabilitation programs. Champaign, IL: Human Kinetics; 1990.

20. Meyer, G.C. Medicare guidelines for cardiovascular and pulmonary rehabilitation. The Exercise Standards & Malpractice Reporter. 2:71-74; 1988.

21. Herbert, D.L. Cardiac rehabilitation services and cost containment measures: Questions of patient safety and provider liability. The Exercise Standards & Malpractice Reporter. 2:1, 3-5; 1988.

22. Joint Commission on Accreditation of Hospitals. Accreditation manual for hospitals. Chicago: Joint Commission on Accreditation of Hospitals; 1990.

23. Fry, G.; Berra, K. YMCArdiac therapy. Chicago: National Council of the Young Men's Christian Associations of the United States; 1981.

24. Board for Certification of Advanced Clinical Competencies, Cardiopulmonary Specialty Council, American Physical Therapy Association. Specialty competencies in physical therapy: Cardiopulmonary. Manhattan Beach, CA: American Physical Therapy Association; 1983.

25. Banja, J.D. Informed consent: Historical development and relevance to exercise and cardiac rehabilitation programs. The Exercise Standards and Malpractice Reporter. 3:53-60; 1989.

26. Herbert, D.L. Informed consent and new disclosure responsibility for exercise stress testing: The case of Hedgecorth v. United States. The Exercise Standards and Malpractice Reporter. 1:30-32; 1987.

27. Edelman, P.S. The case of Tart v. McGann: Legal implications associated with exercise stress testing. The Exercise Standards and Malpractice Reporter. 1:21, 24-26; 1987.

28. Herbert, D.L. Risk disclosure in the informed consent process: Judging the adequacy of disclosure in light of the patients' need for information, an emerging trend. The Exercise Standards and Malpractice Reporter. 2:56-57; 1988.

29. Gibbons, L.W. The safety of maximal exercise testing. J. Cardiopul. Rehabil. 7:277; 1987.

30. Herbert, D.L. Is physician supervision of exercise stress testing required? The Exercise Standards and Malpractice Reporter. 2:6-7; 1988.

31. Blessey, R.L. Exercise testing by non-physician health care professionals: Complication rates, clinical competencies and future trends. The Exercise Standards and Malpractice Reporter. 3:69-74; 1989.

32. DeBusk, R.F. Exercise test supervision: Time for reassessment. The Exercise Standards and Malpractice Reporter. 2:65, 68-71; 1988.

33. Herbert, D.L. Trends: Dramatic increase in diagnostic testing for MI patients reported. The Exercise Standards and Malpractice Reporter. 2:28; 1988.

34. Herbert, D.L. Are GXTs required for screening of all men over 40? The Exercise Standards and Malpractice Reporter. 2:30; 1988.

35. Herbert, D.L. Exercise stress testing lawsuit results in defense verdict. The Exercise Standards and Malpractice Reporter. 4:23-34; 1990.

36. Herbert, D.L. Selected liability considerations of prescribed but unsupervised cardiac rehabilitation activities. The Exercise Standards and Malpractice Reporter. 2:89-94; 1988.

37. Herbert, D.L. Standard of care and deviation therefrom can be established without expert testimony. The Exercise Standards and Malpractice Reporter. 3:12; 1989.

Appendix A

Informed Consent for Exercise Testing of Patients With Known or Suspected Heart Disease

Name _____

1. Purpose and Explanation of Test

I hereby consent to voluntarily engage in an exercise test to determine my exercise capacity and state of cardiovascular health. I also consent to the taking of samples of my exhaled air during exercise to properly measure my oxygen consumption. I also consent, if necessary, to have a small blood sample drawn by needle from my arm for blood chemistry analysis, to the performance of lung function, body fat (skin fold pinch), and standard psychological tests. It is my understanding that the information obtained will help me evaluate future physical activities in which I may safely engage and aid my doctor in his determination of an appropriate medical treatment for me.

Before I undergo the test, I certify to the program that I am in good health and have had a physical examination conducted by a licensed medical physician within the last _____ months, and that my physician has recommended the exercise test and referred me to this particular center for performance of the test. Further, I hereby represent and inform the program that I have completed the pretest history interview presented to me by the program staff and have provided correct responses to the questions as indicated on the history form or as supplied to the interviewer. It is my understanding that I will be interviewed by a physician and perhaps another person prior to my undergoing the test. In the course of these interviews, it will be determined if there are any reasons which would make it undesirable or unsafe for me to take the test. Consequently, I understand that it is important that I provide complete and accurate responses to the interviewer and recognize that my failure to do so could lead to possible unnecessary injury to myself during the test.

The test that I will undergo will be performed on a motor-driven treadmill or bicycle ergometer with the amount of effort gradually increasing. As I understand it, this increase in effort will continue until I feel and orally report to the operator any symptoms such as fatigue, shortness of breath, or chest discomfort that may appear. It is my understanding and I have been clearly advised that it is my right to request that a test be stopped at any point if I feel unusual discomfort or fatigue. I have been advised that I should immediately, upon experiencing any such symptoms or if I so choose, inform the operator that I wish to stop the test at that or any other point. My wishes in this regard shall be absolutely carried out.

It is further my understanding that prior to beginning the test, I will be connected by electrodes and cables to an electrocardiographic recorder that will enable the program personnel to monitor my cardiac (heart) activity. During the test itself, it is my understanding that a physician or (if the physician is in a room nearby) his or her trained observer will monitor my responses continuously and take frequent readings of blood pressure, the electrocardiogram, and my expressed feelings of discomfort or effort.

Once the test has been completed, but before I am released from the test area, I will be given special instructions about showering and recognition of certain symptoms that may appear within the first 24 hours after the test. I agree to follow these instructions and promptly contact the program personnel or medical providers if such symptoms develop.

2. Risks

It is my understanding, and I have been informed, that there exists the possibility of adverse changes during the actual test. I have been informed that these changes could include abnormal blood pressure, fainting, disorders of heart rhythm, stroke, and very rare instances of heart attack or even death. Every effort, I have been told, will be made to minimize these occurrences by preliminary examination and by precautions and observations taken during the test. I have also been informed that emergency equipment and personnel are readily available to deal with these unusual situations should they occur. I understand that there is a risk of injury, heart attack, or even death as a result of my performance of this test but knowing those risks, it is my desire to proceed to take the test as herein indicated.

3. Benefits to be Expected and Alternatives Available to the Exercise Testing Procedure

I understand that the possible beneficial results of this test depend upon my doctor's medical reasons for requesting it. It may be helpful in determining my chances of having heart disease that should be treated medically. If my doctor suspects or knows already that I have heart disease, this test may help to evaluate how this disease affects my ability to safely do certain types of physical work or exercises and how to best treat the disease. Other tests for determining the presence or severity of heart disease may be available as alternatives to this exercise test, as are alternative ways to assess my physical fitness. I have had an opportunity to ask about these and have been given answers regarding advantages/disadvantages as noted below:

_____

4. Confidentiality and Use of Information

I have been informed that the information that is obtained in this exercise test will be treated as privileged and confidential and will consequently not be released or revealed to any person without my express written consent. I do, however, agree to the use of any information for research or statistical purposes so long as same does not provide facts that could lead to the identification of my person. Any other information obtained, however, will be used only by the program staff to evaluate my exercise status or needs.

5. Inquiries and Freedom of Consent

I have been given an opportunity to ask questions as to the procedure. Generally, these requests, which have been noted by the testing staff, and their responses are as follows:

_____

_____

I further understand that there are also other remote risks that may be associated with this procedure. Despite the fact that a complete accounting of all remote risks is not entirely possible, I am satisfied with the review of these risks that was provided to me and it is still my desire to proceed with the test.

I acknowledge that I have read this document in its entirety or that it has been read to me if I have been unable to read same.

I consent to the rendition of all services and procedures as explained herein by all program personnel.

Date _____   _____
                                                              Patient's Signature

_____
Witness' Signature

_____
Test Supervisor's Signature

_____

Appendix B

Informed Consent for Exercise Rehabilitation of Patients With Known or Suspected Heart Disease

Name _____

1. Purpose and Explanation of Procedure

In order to improve my physical exercise capacity and generally aid in my medical treatment for heart disease, I hereby consent to being placed in a rehabilitation program that will include cardiovascular monitoring, physical exercises, dietary counseling, stress reduction, and health education activities. The levels of exercise that I will perform will be based upon the condition of my heart and circulation as determined through a laboratory graded exercise evaluation given at the beginning of the program. I will be given exact instructions regarding the amount and kind of exercise I should do. I agree to participate three times per week in the rehabilitation program. A physician will be present at each session and professionally trained clinical personnel will provide leadership to direct my activities and monitor my electrocardiogram and blood pressure to be certain that I am exercising at the prescribed level. I understand that I am expected to attend every session and to follow physician and staff instructions with regard to any medications that may have been prescribed, exercise, diet, stress management, and smoking cessation. If I am taking prescribed medications, I have already so informed the program staff and further agree to so inform them promptly of any changes that my doctor or I have made with regard to use of these. I will be given the opportunity for periodic reevaluation with laboratory evaluations at 3 and 6 months after the start of my rehabilitation program. Should I remain in the program beyond 6 months, less frequent evaluations will also be provided. The program physicians may change the foregoing schedule of evaluations for individuals if it is considered necessary for medical management.

I have been informed that in the course of my participation in exercise I will be asked to complete the activities unless such symptoms as fatigue, shortness of breath, chest discomfort, or similar occurrences appear. At that point, I have been advised it is my complete right to stop exercise and that it is my obligation to inform the program personnel of my symptoms. I recognize and hereby state that I have been advised that I should immediately, upon experiencing any such symptoms or if I so choose, reduce or stop exercise and inform the program personnel of my symptoms.

I understand that during the performance of exercise, a trained observer will periodically monitor my performance and perhaps take my electrocardiogram, pulse, or blood pressure or make other observations for the purposes of monitoring my progress and/or condition. I also understand that the observer may reduce or stop my exercise program when findings indicate that this should be done for my safety and benefit.

2. Risks

It is my understanding, and I have been informed, that there exists the possibility during exercise of adverse changes including abnormal blood pressure, fainting, disorders of heart rhythm, and very rare instances of heart attack, stroke, or even death. Every effort, I have been told, will be made to minimize these occurrences by proper staff assessment of my condition before each exercise session, staff supervision during exercise, and my own careful control of exercise effort. I have also been informed that emergency equipment and personnel

443

are readily available to deal with unusual situations should these occur. I understand that there is a risk of injury, heart attack, stroke, or even death as a result of my exercise, but knowing those risks, it is my desire to participate as herein indicated.

3. Benefits to be Expected and Alternatives Available to Exercise

I understand that this medical treatment may or may not benefit my health status or physical fitness. Generally, participation will help determine what recreational and occupational activities I can safely and comfortably perform. Many individuals in such programs also show improvements in their capacity for physical work. For those who are overweight and able to follow the physician's and dietitian's recommended dietary plan, this program may also aid in achieving appropriate weight reduction and control.

4. Confidentiality and Use of Information

I have been informed that the information that is obtained in this rehabilitation program will be treated as privileged and confidential and will consequently not be released or revealed to any person without my express written consent. I do, however, agree to the use of any information for research or statistical purposes as long as same does not identify my person or provide facts that could lead to my identification. Any other information obtained, however, will be used only by the program staff in the course of prescribing exercise for me, planning my rehabilitation program, or advising my personal physician of my progress.

5. Inquiries and Freedom of Consent

I have been given an opportunity to ask certain questions as to the procedures of this program. Generally, these requests, which have been noted by the interviewing staff member, and his/her responses are as follows:

_____

_____

I further understand that there are also other remote risks that may be associated with this program. Despite the fact that a complete accounting of all remote risks is not entirely possible, I am satisfied with the review of these risks that was provided to me and it is still my desire to participate.

I acknowledge that I have read this document in its entirety or that it has been read to me if I have been unable to read same.

I consent to the rendition of all services and procedures as explained herein by all program personnel.

Date _____   _____
                                        Participant's Signature

_____

Witness' Signature

_____

Program Supervisor's Signature

_____

PART VI

Cardiac Rehabilitation in Perspective

Chapter 30

Future Directions in Cardiac Rehabilitation

Nanette K. Wenger

Almost 30 years ago, a World Health Organization (WHO) seminar report described rehabilitation for cardiac patients as "the sum of activities required to ensure them the best possible physical, mental, and social conditions so that they may, by their own efforts, resume and maintain as normal a place as possible in the community" (1). These recommendations addressed predominantly patients recovered from myocardial infarction (MI), emphasized exercise training and return to work (2), and utilized the medical personnel and resources that were available in major medical centers in industrialized nations. A sharp contrast is offered by the recommendations of a WHO Expert Committee on Rehabilitation after Cardiovascular Diseases convened in October 1991; it was my privilege to chair this committee. Cardiac rehabilitation was delineated as an essential component of the comprehensive care that should be available for *all* cardiac patients, and guidelines for implementation were described for both industrialized and developing countries (3). The goals of rehabilitation include improvement in functional capacity, alleviation or amelioration of activity-related symptoms, decrease in unwarranted invalidism, and return of the patient to a useful and personally satisfying societal role. As previously, the categories of cardiac rehabilitation interventions that were addressed involved both physical training—involving varied intensities and modalities of exercise—and health education and counseling, but far greater emphasis is currently devoted to the importance of the latter for many categories of cardiac patients. Also emphasized was the importance of individualization of rehabilitative care based on clinical status, requirements for specific interventions, the patient's personal expectations and desires, and the medical setting in which the rehabilitative care is provided.

This chapter highlights advances in the care of cardiac patients, as well as the scientific data base developed during the past quarter century that enabled the transformations in rehabilitative care based on these guidelines; these advances chart the course for the future.

Increased Spectrum of Cardiac Patients Eligible for Exercise Rehabilitation: Role of Risk Stratification

The spectrum of the population considered eligible for exercise rehabilitation has widened substantially since the initial descriptions of the benefits of exercise training for patients with coronary artery disease (CAD) (4,5). Children with congenital and acquired cardiac disease, both with and without surgical correction, are considered candidates for exercise rehabilitation, and large populations of elderly cardiac patients, previously arbitrarily excluded because of age, have also been shown to benefit from individually prescribed exercise and now constitute a sizeable component of the population undertaking exercise rehabilitation. Since CAD among women predominantly affects those of older age, a greater proportion of women are likely to require cardiac rehabilitative care as the population ages. Although women who participate in exercise rehabilitation programs achieve functional improvement comparable to that of their male counterparts, adherence to an exercise program is far lower among women. Whether this reflects their increased severity of coronary illness, lack of social support, cultural factors, comorbid problems, or the relative unsuitability of an exercise program scheduled and tailored to meet the needs of the predominant population (working middle aged men) must be ascertained. An unmet need is the access to and maintenance of rehabilitative care for women with CAD and possibly other heart disease (6). Cardiac rehabilitation must also be comprehensively applied to children and young adults, in whom contemporary medical and surgical treatments of a variety of cardiovascular problems have dramatically improved their survival; however, many children fail to achieve optimal functional recovery even following successful surgery. Both physical activity regimens and education and guidance of the patient and family (including career counseling) can effect personal and societal gains.

Among coronary patients, the severity of their disease also shows greater diversity. The application of thrombolytic therapy and of myocardial revascularization procedures, either percutaneous transluminal coronary angioplasty (PTCA) or coronary artery bypass graft surgery (CABG), has lessened both the mortality from and the severity of an acute episode of MI. Patients incur limited damage to the myocardium, have few symptoms and little or no residual myocardial ischemia, and little functional impairment and thus have both a better prognosis and an improved ability to resume far earlier an active lifestyle, including return to work. At the other end of the spectrum are the often elderly, medically complex, coronary patients, many of whom survived prior episodes of MI and some of whom have undergone prior myocardial revascularization procedures. Their late presentation is typically that of ischemic cardiomyopathy, often with serious arrhythmia; cardiac transplantation is often the only option remaining for the younger of these patients. Even small improvements in physical work capacity may have a major impact on the quality of life of severely disabled cardiac patients, enabling them to maintain a reasonably independent lifestyle. For both populations, the development of a variety of risk stratification test procedures has enabled the delineation of those patients for whom early resumption of activity is safe and appropriate, those categorized as being at low risk because of their minimal likelihood of proximate coronary events and favorable long-term prognosis; and those considered as being at high risk for early recurrence of a coronary event, for whom intensive diagnostic intervention is often applied and in whom, at least initially, the recommendations are for supervision of exercise training. Risk stratification typically involves exercise-based assessments. Low-risk patients can perform reasonable levels of activity without adverse consequences, whereas high-risk patients are characterized by a low peak exercise capacity and the early onset of myocardial ischemia, serious arrhythmias, or ventricular dysfunction (7).

Only in recent decades have patients with angina pectoris or with symptomless ischemia (detected at exercise testing) been enrolled in exercise rehabilitation programs. Of value has been the information that exercise training can produce a beneficial effect in coronary patients receiving a variety of antianginal medications; these anti-ischemic drugs may improve the ability to exercise by reducing myocardial oxygen demand, lessening symptoms, and allowing training to proceed. The goals of exercise training for coronary patients have changed as well. Although, based on meta-analytic data (8,9), exercise rehabilitation was shown to effect an improvement in survival and lessening of reinfarction that was not evident in individual studies, this improvement in survival is less likely to be demonstrable in contemporary low-risk coronary patients and is far less often the goal either of patients in undertaking exercise or of their physicians in recommending exercise training. The desired outcome is an improvement in functional status and a limitation of activity-related symptoms—that is, improved life quality.

Recent studies have shown that patients with compensated congestive heart failure (CHF) or with severe left ventricular dysfunction of many etiologies can safely exercise and that modest improvement in their functional capacity (often paired with the teaching of techniques of work simplification) can enable prolongation of an independent lifestyle (10). Exercise regimens appropriate for these patients are characterized by lower intensity and longer duration of exercise sessions and, at times, alternating periods of rest and exercise (4). Maintenance of independence has assumed greater importance as contemporary therapies have improved the duration of survival of patients with heart failure. It is now recognized that exercise training exerts its benefits in the improvement of functional capacity and the lessening of exercise-induced symptoms predominantly owing to peripheral adaptations to exercise. These include changes in intact exercising skeletal muscle that permit improved extraction of oxygen from the perfusing blood and lessen the myocardial oxygen demand at submaximal levels of exercise, redistribution of the exercise cardiac output to provide blood flow to exercising muscles, and a decrease in systemic vascular resistance, and a variety of autonomic adaptations that enable a lower heart rate (HR) and systolic blood pressure (BP) for the same intensity of activity. Therefore, it should not be surprising that even patients with severe ventricular dysfunction can train their reasonably intact skeletal musculature. Further, in

Index

Page numbers in italics refer to figures and tables.

A

AACVPR. *See* American Association of Cardiovascular and Pulmonary Rehabilitation (AACVPR)
Abdominal body fat, 6, 15, 139-140. *See also* Obesity
Abramov, L., 369
Abrams, H.L., 95
Acclimatization, 311-312, 315, 330-332, *331*
Accreditation, of programs, 223, 241, 297-300, *300*
Accreditation Manual for Hospitals, 223, 299
ACE inhibitors (Angiotensin-converting enzyme inhibitors), 128, 344, 353, 379, 385, *385*
Acid aerosols, 336-337
ACLS (Advanced cardiac life support), 95, 189, 194, 220-221, 235, 430
ACP. *See* American College of Physicians (ACP)
ACSM. *See* American College of Sports Medicine (ACSM)
Activities, METs for, *260*
Activity schedules, 203, *204*
Actuarial models of exercise benefits, 173
Actuarial Mortality Follow-up Study, 137
Acute hypoxia, and high altitude, 310
Acute myocardial infarction (MI). *See* Myocardial infarction (MI)
Adams, K.F., 338
Adenosine, 86-88
Ad Hoc Task Force on Cardiac Rehabilitation (of ACC), 224
Adiposity. *See* Obesity
Administration. *See also* Staff
  and accreditation, 221-223, 241, 297-300, *300*
  budgets of, *192*, 192-195
  business plans for, 189
  and evaluation, 222-223
  leadership in, 187-189
  long-range plans for, 189-190
  and program certification, 294-295, 297, 299, *300*
  of programs, 187-200, *188*, *199*
Admission diagnosis, 232-233
Adoption stage, in behavior therapy, 165-166
Adrenergic activation, 312-313, 352
Adsett, C.A., 50
Adult learners, and education in rehabilitation, 277-280
Advanced cardiac life support (ACLS), 95, 189, 194, 220-221, 235, 430
Aerobic exercise capacity, 147-150
Aerobics Center Longitudinal Study, *172*, 173
Age. *See also* Biological risk factors; Elderly
  and air pollutants, 336, 339-340
  and cholesterol levels, 122
  and disease rates, 3-4
  and heat stress, 269, 327, *328*, 331-332
  and hypertension, 343, 347-349
  and rehabilitation needs, 448
  and return to work, 406

  as risk factor, 10, 41, 66, 117-118
  and sexual relations, 367-369, *368*
  and Type A behavior, 44, 46
Agency for Health Care Policy and Research (AHCPR), 224, 291, 295-296
Agreements, for exercise programs, 163, *164*
AHA. *See* American Heart Association (AHA)
Air Dyne cycle ergometers, 263
Air pollutants
  acid aerosols, 336-337
  carbon monoxide, 133, 135-137, *337*, 337-339
  effects of, 334, 339-340
  nitrogren oxide, 336
  ozone, 334-336, *335*, *336*
  and return to work, 409-410
  sulfur dioxide, 336-337, *337*
Ajzen, I., 162
Akin, Cary, 44
Alameda County, CA, study, 173-175, *174*
Alcohol consumption
  and cholesterol levels, 126
  effects on heart disease, 6, *9*, 15, 34
  and environmental conditions, 318, 331
  and sexual dysfunction, 367-368
Allegheny General Hospital, performance objectives of, 189-190
Allen, F.M., 357
Allison, T., 332
Almeida, D., 407
Alpha-blocking agents, 352
Altitude. *See* High altitude
AMA (American Medical Association), 223-224
Ambrose, J.A., 97
Ambulatory activities, 253-254, 413
American Association of Cardiovascular and Pulmonary Rehabilitation (AACVPR)
  on exercise therapy, 243, 248, 257-258, 265-266, 429
  formation of, 287
  guidelines of, 190, 194, 224, 277, 290-293, 423, 430-431
  on risk stratification, 244, 428
  standards of, 188, 223, 435-436
American Association of Respiratory Care, 194
American Cancer Society, 138
American College of Cardiology (ACC)
  on angiography, 95-97
  on exercise testing, 57
  guidelines of, 69, 224, 292, 423, 428-429, 435
American College of Physicians (ACP)
  on exercise testing, 71, 76, 429
  recommendations of, 224, 292, 296
  on risk stratification, 244, 423, 428
American College of Sports Medicine (ACSM)
  certification by, 189, 194, 234, 435
  on exercise therapy, 243, 248, 253, 257-259, 261, 265-266, 270
  group insurance of, 240
  guidelines of, 210, 223, 290-293, 333, 435-436
  on risk stratification, 244

455

Additional cardiac rehabilitation resources from Human Kinetics

Guidelines for Cardiac Rehabilitation Programs
(Second Edition)
American Association of Cardiovascular and Pulmonary Rehabilitation

Exercise Testing and Training in the Elderly Cardiac Rehab Patient
[Current Issues in Cardiac Rehabilitation Series, Monograph 1]
Mark A. Williams, PhD

Developing and Managing Cardiac Rehabilitation Programs
Linda K. Hall, PhD, Editor

Cardiac Rehabilitation
Exercise Testing and Prescription
[Volume II]
Linda K. Hall, PhD, and G. Curt Meyer, MS, Editors

Cardiac Rehabilitation
Exercise Testing and Prescription
Linda K. Hall, PhD, G. Curt Meyer, MS, and Herman K. Hellerstein, MD, Editors

Guidelines for Pulmonary Rehabilitation Programs
American Association of Cardiovascular and Pulmonary Rehabilitation
Gerilynn Connors, BS, RCP, RRT, and Lana Hilling, RCP, Editors